T0332741

FOURTH EDITION

Therapeutic Exercise
for Children With Developmental Disabilities

FOURTH EDITION

Therapeutic Exercise
for Children With Developmental Disabilities

Edited by

Barbara H. Connolly, PT, DPT, EdD, C/NDT, FAPTA

Professor Emeritus
University of Tennessee Health Science Center
Barbara Connolly Associates, LLC
Melbourne Beach, Florida

Patricia C. Montgomery, PT, PhD, FAPTA

Pediatric Private Practice
Fort Myers, Florida

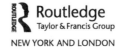

Routledge
Taylor & Francis Group

NEW YORK AND LONDON

Instructors: *Therapeutic Exercise for Children With Developmental Disabilities, Fourth Edition* includes ancillary materials specifically available for faculty use. Included are PowerPoint slides and the *Instructor's Manual*. Please visit http://www.routledge.com/9781630915766 to obtain access.

First published 2020 by SLACK Incorporated

Published 2024 by Routledge
605 Third Avenue, New York, NY 10158

and by Routledge
4 Park Square, Milton Park, Abingdon, Oxon OX14 4RN

Routledge is an imprint of the Taylor & Francis Group, an informa business

Cover Artist: Katherine Christie

Library of Congress Cataloging-in-Publication Data

Names: Connolly, Barbara H., editor. | Montgomery, Patricia C., editor.
Title: Therapeutic exercise for children with developmental disabilities /
    edited by Barbara H. Connolly, Patricia C. Montgomery.
Other titles: Therapeutic exercise in developmental disabilities
Description: Fourth edition. | Thorofare, NJ : SLACK Incorporated, [2020] |
    Preceded by Therapeutic exercise in developmental disabilities / [edited
    by] Barbara H. Connolly, Patricia C. Montgomery. 3rd ed. c2005. |
    Includes bibliographical references and index.
Identifiers: LCCN 2019040703 (print) | ISBN 9781630915766 (hardcover)
Subjects: MESH: Developmental Disabilities--rehabilitation | Disabled
    Children--rehabilitation | Child | Infant | Physical Therapy Modalities
Classification: LCC RJ506.D47 (print) | NLM WS 368 |
    DDC 618.92/8588--dc23
LC record available at https://lccn.loc.gov/2019040703

ISBN: 9781630915766 (hbk)
ISBN: 9781003526797 (ebk)

DOI: 10.4324/9781003526797

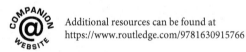

Additional resources can be found at
https://www.routledge.com/9781630915766

DEDICATION

This book is dedicated to children with developmental disabilities and the physical therapists and families who work together to manage their care and enrich their lives.

Contents

Instructors: *Therapeutic Exercise for Children With Developmental Disabilities, Fourth Edition* includes ancillary materials specifically available for faculty use. Included are PowerPoint slides and the *Instructor's Manual*. Please visit http://www.routledge.com/9781630915766 to obtain access.

Acknowledgments

We would like to acknowledge the artwork of Sandy Lowrance that was initially prepared for the *First Edition* of this text and has been reprinted in this edition. We also acknowledge Cayce Cloud, who provided artwork for this edition. Our appreciation goes out to the authors of the individual chapters for being so prompt and efficient in submitting their manuscripts. We wish to acknowledge our families for their support and patience during the many long hours we have spent away from them during the process of writing and editing this *Fourth Edition*.

About the Editors

Barbara H. Connolly, PT, DPT, EdD, C/NDT, FAPTA received her BS degree in Physical Therapy from the University of Florida, a DPT degree from the University of Tennessee, an MEd degree in Special Education with a minor in Speech Pathology, and an EdD in Curriculum and Instruction from the University of Memphis. She is a Professor Emeritus at the University of Tennessee Health Sciences Center, where she was a faculty member for 37 years, served as Chair of the Physical Therapy Department for 24 years, and as Interim Dean of the College of Allied Health Sciences for 2 years. Dr. Connolly has taught in physical therapy programs at numerous academic institutions, including the University of Mississippi, the University of Miami, and the University of Indianapolis. She served as a Trustee for the Foundation for Physical Therapy, a foundation dedicated to funding physical therapy research, for 9 years and was President from January 2015 to December 2016. She served as President of the International Organization of Physical Therapists in Pediatrics, a subgroup of the World Confederation of Physical Therapy, from its inception in 2007 until 2015. She also has served on the American Physical Therapy Association (APTA) Board of Directors, on the APTA Pediatric Specialty Council, and the American Board of Physical Therapy Specialists. She was President of the Section on Pediatrics of the APTA from 2002 to 2006. She received the Bud DeHaven Leadership Award, the Research Award, and the Jeanne Fischer Distinguished Mentorship Award from the Section on Pediatrics. She is a recipient of the Golden Pen Award from the APTA for her publications. In 2002, she received one of the highest honors from the APTA when she was named a Catherine Worthingham Fellow. In 2014 she received the Marilyn Moffat Leadership Award, and in 2015 she received a Lucy Blair Service Award. She is the first author of more than 32 publications in peer-reviewed journals, has written 21 book chapters, and has coauthored or edited 7 textbooks for physical therapists. She is certified in neurodevelopmental treatment and in sensory integration. She continues to provide professional development courses both nationally and internationally.

Patricia C. Montgomery, PT, PhD, FAPTA received her BS degree in Physical Therapy from the University of Oklahoma, Norman, and her MA in Educational Psychology and PhD in Child Psychology from the University of Minnesota, Minneapolis. Dr. Montgomery's clinical pediatric experience includes working in an outpatient hospital setting, a newborn intensive care unit, and for the St. Paul, Minnesota, Public School System. She also had a private practice and was the owner of a home health agency providing pediatric services in the Twin Cities area. Dr. Montgomery served on the APTA Board of Directors and as President of the Minnesota Chapter, APTA. Dr. Montgomery received the Pediatric Section, APTA, Research Award and the Bud DeHaven Award; the Minnesota Chapter, APTA, Outstanding Service Award; and the APTA Dorothy Briggs Memorial Scientific Inquiry Award and Lucy Blair Service Award. She also gave the inaugural Luise Lynch Lectureship at the University of Oklahoma, the Third Annual John H. P. Maley Lecture at the APTA Annual Conference, and the Fifth Annual Jack Allison Memorial Lectureship at the University of Minnesota. Dr. Montgomery is the first author of 17 publications in peer-reviewed journals and has coauthored several textbooks for physical therapists. Dr. Montgomery taught in physical therapy programs at several academic institutions, including the University of Minnesota, Minneapolis; Hahnemann University, Philadelphia, Pennsylvania; and the University of Tennessee Health Sciences Center. She continues to provide continuing education courses on the topic of children's brains and neuroplasticity.

Contributing Authors

Rona Alexander, PhD, CCC-SLP, BCS-S, C/NDT (Chapter 8)
Speech-Language Pathologist
Rona Alexander, PhD, CCC-SLP, Ltd.
Wauwatosa, Wisconsin

Joanell A. Bohmert, PT, DPT, MS (Chapters 6 and 15)
Anoka Public Schools and Fix It Physical Therapy
Anoka, Minnesota

David D. Chapman, PT, PhD (Chapter 9)
Associate Professor
St. Catherine University
St. Paul, Minnesota

Susan K. Effgen, PT, PhD, FAPTA (Chapter 10)
Professor
University of Kentucky
Lexington, Kentucky

Elizabeth Ennis, PT, EdD, PCS, ATP (Chapter 16)
Associate Professor
Belleramine University
Louisville, Kentucky

Roberta Gatlin, PT, DScPT, PCS (Chapter 7)
Assistant Professor
Emory and Henry University
Bristol, Tennessee

Dora J. Gosselin, PT, DPT, PCS, C/NDT (Chapter 12)
Assistant Professor and Director of Clinical Education
High Point University
High Point, North Carolina

Maria Jones, PT, PhD (Chapter 11)
Clinical Professor and Program Director
Oklahoma City University
Oklahoma City, Oklahoma

Lisa K. Kenyon, PT, DPT, PhD, PCS (Chapter 11)
Associate Professor
Grand Valley State University
Grand Rapids, Michigan

Helen L. Masin, PT, PhD (Chapter 4)
Clinical Associate Professor (Retired)
University of Miami
Miami, Florida

Anita Witt Mitchell, PhD, OTR, FAOTA (Chapter 13)
Associate Professor
University of Tennessee Health Science Center
Memphis, Tennessee

Anne H. Zachry, PhD, OTR/L (Chapter 13)
Assistant Professor
University of Tennessee Health Science Center
Memphis, Tennessee

PREFACE

The primary focus in the *First Edition* (1993) of *Therapeutic Exercise for Children With Developmental Disabilities* was on therapeutic techniques. The *Second* and *Third Editions* incorporated more empirical evidence to support intervention strategies. This *Fourth Edition* continues the process of updating empirical evidence relevant to clinical practice.

Five case studies of children with developmental disabilities continue to be used throughout the text to facilitate a practical problem-solving approach to the focus of individual chapters. A major change in the application of the case studies is a focus on the World Health Organization's *International Classification of Functioning, Disability and Health—Children and Youth* (ICF–CY) model. Although students may use a bottom-up process of identifying Impairments, then Activity Limitations and Participation Restrictions, we requested that authors use a top-down strategy by first identifying Participation Restrictions, then Activity Limitations and Impairments, before determining intervention objectives and goals.

The *Fourth Edition* emphasizes examples of treatment activities to achieve the Participation and Activity outcomes proposed for the children. Physical therapy students and clinicians with limited experience in pediatrics will benefit from having specific examples of treatment activities in addition to general intervention strategies. The primary goal of physical therapy intervention is to promote optimal functional independence for children with integration into home, school, and community life. We hope that this text is valuable to students and clinicians and, in turn, to the children they treat.

Foundational Sciences for Intervention

Patricia C. Montgomery, PT, PhD, FAPTA

When designing intervention for children with developmental disabilities, physical therapists apply principles derived from various fields of research, including motor control, motor learning, motor development, and neuroplasticity. Having studied these foundational sciences, therapists consciously or unconsciously subscribe to theories of how the central nervous system (CNS) is organized and how children develop and learn motor skills. Theories then are used clinically in the following ways:

1. To select tests and examinations that identify children's participation restrictions, impairments, and activity or functional limitations
2. To set objectives for intervention
3. To plan and sequence intervention activities

In the best of worlds, sufficient research would be available to guide decision making across the range of functional limitations and impairments demonstrated by children with developmental disabilities. As a profession, the American Physical Therapy Association continues to emphasize and support basic and clinical research to expand evidence-based practice. Yet, much of what we currently do has not been researched, and we often must rely on theoretical models for decision making. This chapter focuses on reviewing the foundational fields of science that guide physical therapy practice with children.

BASIC DEFINITIONS

Motor Control

The term *motor control* refers to processes of the brain and spinal cord that govern posture and movement. Neuroscientists initially focused their research on neural processes underlying animal movements. Investigations centered on the chemical or electrical activity of single nerve cells or nuclei to understand the organization of spinal motor mechanisms and mechanisms of higher control mediated by various brain structures. With the advent of noninvasive methods, such as

Connolly BH, Montgomery PC, eds. *Therapeutic Exercise for Children With Developmental Disabilities, Fourth Edition* (pp 1-23).
© 2020 Taylor & Francis Group.

functional magnetic resonance imaging (fMRI), to study the human brain, neuroscientists now are able to study more complex processes within the CNS. Many of these techniques have been safely employed with infants and young children, enhancing our understanding of neural functions and motor control.

Motor Learning

Schmidt and Lee[1] defined *motor learning* as a set of processes associated with practice or experience that lead to a relatively permanent change in skilled action. The specialized area of motor learning grew out of a subdiscipline within the field of psychology interested in high-level skills. Early research questions related to what elements of practice enhanced, what elements had a detrimental effect, or if there was no impact on learning of the variable being studied. Information on motor learning principles refocused physical therapists' attention solely from "treatment" as an intervention to "teaching" of motor skills.

Motor Development

Motor development is the study of life span change in motor behavior. Motor development, defined here as age-related change in motor behavior, results from internal and external influences and often has been attributed to processes such as maturation, growth, or learning. Developmental change in motor behavior also can be affected by external influences from the environment, such as the teaching of specific skills or from cultural expectations.[2] Early developmentalists studied body actions within specific tasks, such as rolling (eg, from supine to prone leading with hips or shoulders), as well as acquisition of motor milestones.[3]

Neuroplasticity

Doidge[4] described *neuroplasticity* as the (lifelong) property of the brain that enables it to change its own structure and functioning in response to activity and mental experience. Because plasticity of the brain underlies all cognitive, perceptual, and motor skill learning, principles of brain plasticity should serve as a framework for physical therapy intervention and will be discussed in more detail later in this chapter.

Differences and Similarities

Although neural processes underlie motor control, learning, and development, one difference is the time frame in which they occur. Motor control mechanisms typically are carried out in seconds and milliseconds. Learning motor skills often takes days and months or, in the case of world-class athletes, perhaps many years. Life span development is studied in relation not only to months and years, but also over several decades into adulthood and old age.

Separating underlying processes can be difficult. For example, movement can be categorized into 2 general classes.[1] One class of movements, such as control of our limbs and walking, appears to be determined primarily by genetic makeup or through growth and development. These movements are fairly stereotyped across members of the same species. What CNS structures are involved and how the CNS organizes individual and coordinated movements of the limbs and body are basic questions in the study of motor control.

A second class of movements, such as riding a bicycle, writing, or performing a somersault, can be considered "learned." These movements do not appear to be genetic and require varying (usually long) periods of practice and experience to master. How movements are produced as the result of practice or experience is the major question in the study of motor learning.

Attempting to classify the relative contributions of genetics and experience in human development, however, always results in a "nature vs nurture" debate. Issues of motor control and motor learning in relation to movement (genetic or practiced) may be somewhat differentiated in "normal" individuals; however, the distinction becomes blurred in the child with pathology of the CNS. Hadders-Algra[5] discussed Edelman's neuronal group selection theory of motor development, which consists of 2 phases of variability. An initial phase of "primary variability" in the newborn infant is characterized by abundant variation of movements brought about by explorative activity of the CNS. There is variation in motor behavior in the newborn, but limited ability to adapt to specifics of the situation. Over time, the CNS uses information related to behavior and experience, and selection of motor behavior that fits the situation best is possible (ie, "secondary variability"). (See Video 1-1.)

If there is CNS damage, the repertoire of motor strategies is reduced, resulting in less variability and more stereotypical motor behaviors. With limited primary variability, secondary variability is limited and strategies for movement are reduced. For example, if a child has damage to the CNS structures that produce a specific movement pattern, such as components of the gait cycle, he or she may have to practice or adapt the movements as able to produce or develop ambulation. In this case, ambulation could be considered a "skill" and is perhaps a better example of motor learning than motor control.

Motor Control Theories

Reflex Hierarchical Model

Sherrington,[6] a renowned neuroscientist, won a Nobel Prize in 1932 for his work describing the function of neurons and reciprocal inhibition. In terms of motor control, Sherrington believed all movements were the result of, or in response to, sensory input. This "reflexology model" of motor control came to dominate neuroscience. Sherrington's studies of animals undergoing deafferentation procedures (eliminating sensory input) appeared to support his theory. After loss of sensory input, animals in his studies did not produce active movement.

Sherrington's theory was combined with Hughlings Jackson's[7] view proposed in the late 1800s of the CNS as a strict hierarchy of functions with lower, middle, and higher levels. This reflex, hierarchical model (Figure 1-1) was the prevalent view of motor control used as a framework for intervention by physical therapy clinicians beginning in the 1940s and persisted for many years.[8-11]

Motor Programming Theory

In the 1970s, Taub conducted studies similar to those of Sherrington[12,13] and assessed movement potential in the impaired upper extremity of monkeys following deafferentation. When Taub allowed the monkeys to recover spontaneously, his results were similar to those of Sherrington— no active movement in the impaired limb. However, when Taub restricted use of the monkeys' uninvolved arm, the monkeys began to use the impaired extremity. This result presented a direct challenge to reflexology theory. Although initially resistant, neuroscientists gradually accepted the fact that the CNS could produce movement in the absence of sensory input.

Preprogrammed motor actions are considered to be "open loop" (feed-forward and absent sensory information). Other motor programs are "closed loop" (reliant on sensory information). In general, open-loop movements are too fast to rely on sensory feedback *during* the movement. Examples are snapping your fingers or throwing a ball. Sensory information would be used *after* the movement to provide feedback. Closed-loop movements are generally slow, and sensory information is used during the movement to continuously monitor and guide performance. Examples of closed-loop movements are steering a tricycle or tracing a circle.[1]

Figure 1-1. The reflex hierarchy represents a model of neural organization and development. A staircase of levels of neuroanatomical structures and reflexive behaviors is surmounted with volitional behavior controlled in the cerebral cortex. Neuromotor development in this model is hypothesized to proceed from Level 1 up to Level 4.

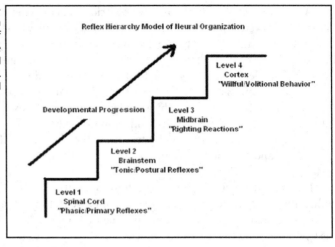

Systems Approach

Early theories of motor control emphasized functions of the CNS with little concern to the musculoskeletal system. Bernstein,[14] a Russian physiologist, introduced the concept that the *motor pattern* represents the CNS's solution to the problem of controlling a multitude of muscles and joints throughout the body. From a biomechanical perspective, the human body can be modeled as a series of rigid segments (such as an arm or a forearm) connected by joint structures that permit as well as restrict motion between the links. In determining possible movement combinations in the cardinal planes, beginning proximally at the shoulder girdle and moving distally to the terminal phalanx of a finger, it becomes obvious that the brain faces an enormous task to control so many possible combinations of movements at the joints. This is known as the *degrees of freedom* problem in motor control.[1] By establishing functional linkages or motor patterns to define relationships between groups of muscles, motor control becomes simplified. The terms *motor patterns, motor synergies,* and *coordinative structures* have been used to refer to the functional units of neuromotor organization that ensure the CNS need not control so many different combinations of action, but rather solves the degrees of freedom problem through an efficient system of muscle linkages.[15]

Physical therapists are aware of how biomechanical and anthropometric factors influence children's movements. Musculoskeletal impairments that interfere with children's ability to produce functional movements are addressed and included in the overall treatment plan.

Dynamic Systems Theory

Dynamical pattern theory, developed by Kelso and his colleagues,[16,17] includes general principles of motor coordination that can be used to explain the motor behavior of a variety of animal forms including man. The theory includes 2 main concepts: *order parameters* and *control parameters.*

Order parameters are variables that represent the action of many subsystems and can be used to characterize coordinated behavior of the system. For example, the timing of action between the 2 limbs during walking could be an order parameter. Variables that can initiate change in order parameters are termed control parameters.[18] In a study of individuals moving from the floor to standing, King demonstrated that constraints to ankle motion provided by ankle-foot orthoses triggered movement pattern changes.[19] The change in an order parameter (the movement pattern used to rise) resulted when a critical value of a control parameter (in this example, ankle motion) was reached. Thelen and Fisher, in an elegant series of studies, demonstrated that rather than cortical maturation, increasing weight of the lower limbs might be one reason why babies stop stepping.[20]

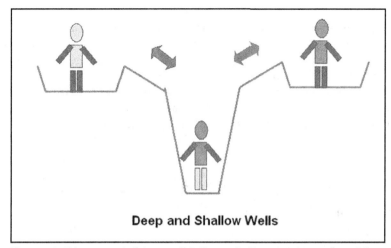

Deep and Shallow Wells

Figure 1-2. This portrayal of deep and shallow wells illustrates the number of times a child demonstrated specific sets of movement patterns during performance of the task of rising. The child was asked to rise from a supine position on a floor mat 10 consecutive times. The shallow well to the left represents performance of 2 of 10 trials of rising from the floor. The center deep well is reflective of 6 of 10 trials that were performed using a movement strategy that differed from the shallow well strategy both in head and trunk and lower limb patterns. The movement pattern strategy represented by the deep well could also be called an attractor pattern. The shallow well on the right illustrates another 2 of the 10 trials that were performed with upper limb and head and trunk patterns the same as the deep well strategy; only lower limb patterns differed. An interpretation of this mapping of one child's preferred patterns of rising illustrate a deep well strategy that is commonly performed and 2 shallow well strategies that are less commonly observed.

Some behavioral patterns are more common than others. In dynamic systems terms, these patterns are called *attractors*.[18] Attractors are preferred patterns of the system. Attractors are further described as having deep or shallow attractor wells. Deep attractor wells can be used to portray behavior that is quite stable and relatively difficult to change. Shallow attractor wells are characteristic of behaviors that are easily changed (Figure 1-2).

Developmental change is brought about by control parameters reaching critical values that bring the system to a period of instability. During developmental transitions from one stable attractor state to another, individuals are particularly sensitive to control variables. During phase transitions, very small influences can have a major impact on behavior. Therapists should be sensitive to phase transitions in their patients and try to discover the control parameter that is driving the system to new forms of behavior. Dynamic systems theory, as well as ecological theory, made therapists aware of the interaction of elements in a complex system that include the child, the child's environment, and the motor tasks the child is required to perform.

Ecological Theory

Gibson[21,22] proposed a perceptual-action theory of development in which perceptual systems are considered critical for any action system. Motor development is equally a function of perceptual system change as it is a function of change in motor systems. Perception plays a greater role in action than sensation and is a process of "detecting" information in the environment for possible actions by the child. The environment, therefore, is evaluated in terms of "affordances" for motor behavior.

Adolph and colleagues conducted a number of studies examining how typically developing (TD) children acquire perceptual-motor learning.[23-25] Two types of learning were described:

"learning sets," studied in rolling, crawling, cruising, and walking and "association" learning, which occurs typically when visual information is not helpful and physical interaction with a support surface is necessary. Visual information is crucial in learning sets, for example, in deciding whether or not to crawl up a 30-degree slope. Vision is not helpful in determining how "slippery" the surface is until the child tries to crawl up the slope ("association learning"). Surprisingly, there is no transfer of skills (decision making) from one learning set to another (eg, crawling to walking). Research by Adolph and colleagues makes therapists aware of how important it is for the child to move through the environment in as many positions as possible as perceptual-motor learning is "task specific."

Motor Learning Principles

Because most of the functional tasks we want children with disabilities to perform require a combination of motor control and motor learning, applying principles of motor learning to physical therapy intervention is essential. Many principles of motor learning are based on years of research with normal adult participants.[1] However, more recent studies of TD children and children with specific disabilities have questioned the application of all these principles to pediatric populations. Differences in motor learning principles with children may relate to their individual motor abilities, cognitive skills, sensory processing abilities, and ability to sustain attention.

Selected motor learning issues and their application to pediatrics are described briefly in the following sections.

Performance Versus Learning

Motor learning is not directly observable. Therapists must be able to distinguish between improved performance, which is observable during or at the end of a therapy session, and actual motor learning. When a physical therapist facilitates movement through manual guidance (ie, handling), such as assisting the child with shoulder protraction during reaching, the child's "performance" at that moment is affected and can be observed. It would be evident that the child had "learned" that skill only if he or she consistently and appropriately used protraction of the shoulder in daily activities over a period of time without intervention. Physical therapy that has as its end result only changes in performance is not cost effective and is of limited value to the child. The goal in physical therapy is for children to acquire motor skills that will increase their independence in a variety of natural environments ("participation") and decrease their dependence on the physical therapist or others.

A major issue for researchers in motor learning is to differentiate "performance" variables (effect while present) from "learning" variables (effect while present and when removed).[1] When comparing intervention variables in groups of individuals on a specific task, a "retention" period (rest period of a few hours, days, or longer) following training is used. Another method after skill acquisition is to transfer all individuals to a common condition ("transfer" design).

In some cases, a variable that improves performance may not be the most effective variable to promote learning. Herrin and Geil[26] compared 2 treatment strategies for children described as idiopathic toe-walkers. During intervention, one group wore an articulated ankle-foot orthosis, which provided better control of toe-walking than a rigid carbon footplate worn by a comparison group. However, when both groups walked later without orthotics ("transfer" design), it was the children who wore a rigid carbon footplate who sustained their improvements. In this case, a variable that enhanced performance was not the variable that best improved motor learning.

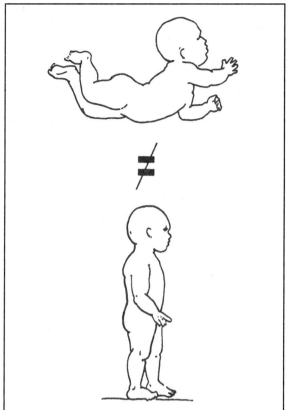

Figure 1-3. Trunk extension in upright position may have different requirements of motor control than extension in prone. (Reprinted with permission from Montgomery PC, Connolly BH. *Clinical Applications for Motor Control.* Thorofare, NJ: SLACK Incorporated; 2003.)

Transfer of Learning

Transfer of learning refers to a gain (or loss) in the capability for producing a movement or performing a task as the result of practice or experience of another movement or task. Transfer can be "near" (to a similar task) or "far" (to a dissimilar task). According to Schmidt and Lee,[1] in research on transfer of learning in adults, 2 major points emerge: (1) the amount of positive transfer between tasks appears to be quite small, and (2) the amount of transfer depends on the similarity of the tasks. The more similar the tasks, the more likely transfer will occur. Bonney et al[27] reviewed 2 theoretical constructs for transfer. One is the *identical elements theory*—the greater the number of common elements, the stronger the transfer effect. The second is the *transfer-appropriate processing theory*—transfer depends on the similarity of cognitive processing factors rather than motor elements.

One assumption made in some clinical approaches is that a motor skill learned in one position will provide positive transfer to a skill in another position. For example, it may be assumed that having a child practice trunk extension in prone will assist with trunk extension in sitting and standing. Another example is the hypothesis that facilitating balance reactions while the child sits on a therapy ball will improve his or her balance while sitting on the floor.

In the first example, prone extension is a different task for the CNS to organize from trunk extension in sitting and standing, where the biomechanical constraints and pull of gravity vary (Figure 1-3). In the second example, responses to externally produced perturbations present control issues for the CNS that are different from those for achieving and maintaining sitting balance through a feed-forward mechanism (see Chapter 10). The biomechanical aspects of the 2 sitting positions also vary.

In perceptual-motor studies of TD infants learning to crawl up and down slopes, then eventually to walk up and down slopes, Adolph et al demonstrated there was no transition of learning from crawling to walking.[25] Instead, infants who had become competent at crawling up and down slopes had to learn all over again how to cope with slopes when in an upright position. Additional studies demonstrated that deciding when to crawl or walk over a "step" or a "cliff" also was experience dependent.[28,29] There was no transfer in skill level or perceptual decision making from crawling to walking.

Until research studies offer a clearer understanding of the positive transfer of experience between specific movements and skills in children with various impairments, therapists can ensure a comprehensive approach to treatment by having children practice the specific target movements or tasks in addition to those prerequisite movements or tasks assumed to provide positive transfer. This means that, in addition to practicing trunk extension in prone, children will practice trunk extension in sitting and standing; and, in addition to facilitating balance reactions while sitting on a therapy ball, children are provided with ample opportunities to practice independent floor sitting.

Part-to-Whole Transfer

Another technique used by therapists is to have children practice components of a motor task before attempting to practice the entire task (ie, *part-to-whole transfer*). For example, children may work in a standing position on balance and lower extremity control, such as kicking a ball, before walking. According to Schmidt and Lee, the problem may be that "practice on a part in isolation may so change the motor programming of the part that for all practical purposes it is no longer the same as it is in the context of the total skill."[1(p382)] In walking, there are precise temporal and spatial relationships among and between the muscles of each leg that are difficult to separate and practice.

Part-to-whole transfer might also depend on the extent to which the movement is governed by a single motor program. Generally, if a movement is fast, it probably is governed by a single program and should be practiced as a whole. Throwing a ball is an example of a ballistic-type feed-forward movement that is better practiced as a whole (ie, open loop). Multilimb, simultaneous movements may be governed by a single program. There is, however, little research to guide physical therapists in determining which movements and tasks may benefit from part-to-whole transfer. In summary, the assumption that breaking down a task for practice always will improve performance on the whole task can be challenged. Therapists should include practice on the whole task as well as practice of component parts in treatment.

Variable Versus Repetitive and Random Versus Constant Practice

Research with adults has demonstrated that after skill acquisition performance on transfer and retention tasks is better when practice has been variable rather than repetitive.[1] One hypothesis is that each time a component of a task or the task itself is varied, the individual must concentrate anew and problem solve in relation to the required movements or task, thereby enhancing motor learning. In contrast, when practicing with numerous repetitions, movement becomes automatic and the individual may concentrate less and not be required to actively problem solve regarding the motor requirements.

Prado et al[30] used a maze task to compare performance in the transfer phase with random compared with constant practice in a group of children with cerebral palsy (CP) and a group of TD children. Similarly to adults, children in both groups performed better with random practice than those with constant practice. Kwon and Ahn[31] also demonstrated positive effects of task-oriented and high-variability practice in children with spastic diplegia CP on gross motor performance and functional independence.

In contrast, Bonney et al[27,32] compared the type of practice (variable or repetitive) on transfer tasks in children with developmental coordination disorder and TD children using an active video game (Nintendo Wii Fit). Results documented that children in both groups demonstrated positive transfer effects to real-life skills irrespective of the practice schedule. These authors suggested blocked or repetitive training might be more effective early in the learning process. A certain level of experience might be required for variable training to have a superior effect.

Repetition is an essential element in improving motor control. Undoubtedly there must be a sufficient number of repetitions to receive feedback about movements, or success in accomplishing a task, to engage in trial-and-error learning. The therapist must look for cues that the child is performing movement in a rote fashion with little attention to the task, and, at that point, vary the task requirements. Treatment sessions should be structured to accommodate differences in attention level, and activities should be motivating. A practical example would be to have the child change positions and practice various skills several times within a 45-minute treatment session, dictated by his or her attention span and the difficulty of the tasks. This would be preferable to predetermining the structure of a treatment session, for example, working 15 minutes on prone extension, 15 minutes on sitting balance, and 15 minutes on gait. Although research in adults suggests blocked (constant) practice and drills are highly ineffective ways to generate learning, the exception would be very early practice when a child is initially acquiring a movement or basic skill. Schmidt and Lee suggested that once a movement can be performed, practice should be randomized.[1] A related point is that practice needs to be somewhat difficult and require effort. The challenge for the therapist is to find activities that entice the child to attempt and repeat movements that require effort and concentration.

Guidance

Guidance refers to a number of procedures ranging from physically assisting movement (ie, facilitation/handling) to verbally talking the child through a task. In general, guidance tends to prevent the child from making errors. One hypothesis in support of guidance is that improved quality of movement will be produced and the child will be less apt to learn incorrect movements and, therefore, will not repeat or learn these less desirable movements. In an opposite view, motor learning appears to be most effective in trial-and-error situations. The child must learn which internal commands lead to effective or ineffective outcomes, and the only way to learn this is to make and try to correct errors.

Although research is limited, it appears that guidance is most effective in early practice of new, unfamiliar tasks.[1] Guidance also may be more effective for slow movements for which feedback may be used for control and monitoring (closed loop). Physical guidance may be beneficial in showing the child what to do and perhaps in reducing fear when having the child attempt new motor skills. The therapist initially assists the child in producing a response or movement; less guidance is used as the child takes more responsibility for producing the movement.

Too much guidance, however, may act as a "crutch," preventing the child from experiencing errors and learning from his or her own attempts at movement. In the presence of a damaged CNS, it may be idealistic to assume that we can facilitate "normal" movement. The goal of physical therapy should be for the child to produce the most efficient and effective movements to accomplish functional tasks. The therapist must decide when facilitation designed to improve "quality of movement" should be discarded and emphasis placed on alternative strategies for accomplishing a motor task. (See Video 1-2.)

MOTOR DEVELOPMENT

Critical Periods

Critical periods can be considered optimal "windows of opportunity" for development and achievement of specific functions. During these periods, the organism is especially susceptible to, and often may require, specific environmental influences to develop normally.[33] "Imprinting" studies in animals demonstrate the importance of early models and experiences to develop species-specific behaviors.[34] Although critical periods in some species may occur shortly after birth, critical periods in humans are much more protracted.

In TD human infants, the first 2 years of life is a critical period in gross motor skill development.[35-37] Fine motor skills become more refined in the following years. In children with CP, the greatest rate of progress in developing gross motor skills is between birth and ages 3 to 4 years.[38,39] The ability to achieve gross motor skills in this population appears to plateau around age 7 years. Gabbard[40] speculated that the critical period for most behavioral functions in TD children ends around age 10 years.

Hubel and Wiesel demonstrated, in a series of studies with cats, that different parts of the cortex processed lines, orientation, and movements of visually perceived objects. They also discovered that 3 to 8 weeks after birth was a critical period for the newborn kitten to develop normal vision. If one eye was prevented from processing visual information during that period, that area of the visual brain map failed to develop, which left the kitten blind in that eye for life.[41]

Critical periods have been studied in the visual system of children. Children born with dense cataracts can achieve vision when their cataracts are surgically removed.[12,42] Eye patching or use of atropine (forced usage) is most successful for children with amblyopia when initiated before age 3 years, with improvement up to age 7 years.[43] Critical periods for processing auditory inputs also have been studied in TD children and those with hearing impairments. Young infants of any culture can "hear" language sounds of any other culture.[12] Over time children become less responsive to non-native sounds in relation to native sounds to which they are exposed.[44,45] Sharma and colleagues[46] provided evidence that the sensitive period for central auditory development is about birth to age 3.5 years, with some variability in the data from age 3.5 to 7 years. In all likelihood, the sensitive period ends around age 7 years. Children receiving cochlear implants before age 3 to 4 years have significantly better speech and language skills than children receiving implants after age 6 to 7 years. Research suggests cortical plasticity in visual and auditory language systems of TD children lasts until around age 7 to 8 years.[12]

The "Normal Developmental Sequence"

Normal motor development has been considered the gold standard for movement and early neurophysiologic theorists and clinicians used the "normal developmental sequence" as a basic principle in their approaches. Unfortunately, the incorrect assumption that there is a single, best developmental sequence for achieving gross motor skills is widely accepted and has achieved "myth" status. In addition, age ranges for the development of a skill, such as sitting, are often specified. Empirical evidence, however, supports a wide range of ages for achieving a specific motor skill as well as a variety of sequences that can be employed when achieving developmental skills leading to ambulation.[47]

Cultural and environmental differences play an important role in motor skill development, and cross-cultural research has documented extraordinary diversity in motor skill acquisition.[2] Daily child-rearing practices, in particular, are related to accelerated or delayed onset of motor skills. For example, Karasik and colleagues[48] made a cross-cultural comparison of sitting in 5-month-old TD infants. Only 17% of American and South Korean children sat independently compared with 67% and 92% of Kenyan and Cameroonian infants, respectively. Proficiency in sitting varied considerably within and between cultural groups.

TD children also demonstrate varying strategies for early floor mobility, including crawling on hands and knees, hands and feet crawling, step-crawl mix, belly crawling, and scooting in a seated position.[49] Within these different movement strategies, children demonstrate organized, rhythmic interlimb coordination.

Bottos et al[50] completed a prospective study of 424 children: 270 infants cared for in a neonatal intensive care unit and 154 infants without perinatal complications who served as a control group. They documented a number of different locomotor strategies used by both the preterm and full-term children before the acquisition of independent walking. For example, 9% of the children never crawled on hands and knees, but moved by shuffling on their bottoms (ie, "hitching") and 12% just stood up and walked. Therefore, more or less typical sequences of motor development were documented. Follow-up data until the children were age 5 years demonstrated that the children who chose alternative patterns (such as bottom shuffling or "just walking") did not demonstrate intellectual or language delays any more frequently than infants who belly crawled or crawled on hands and knees before walking. Adolph et al[23-25] also demonstrated that motor development does not adhere to a strict progression of obligatory, discrete stages.

How did the myth of a single best developmental sequence occur? Ulrich pointed out that individual behavior was a hallmark of early descriptions of motor behavior by early developmentalists, but by collapsing observations into normative age means and categories, these differences were obscured. She stated that infants "who are typically and atypically developing skip common milestones, revert to earlier patterns after more complex ones emerge, and produce their own unique patterns under varied environmental contexts, and their own performance goals."[51(p1870)]

Karasik et al[48] stated that motor development—perhaps more than any other area of developmental science—falls victim to assumptions of universality. These authors also attributed these assumptions to standardization of motor skills in the 1930s and 1940s. Since then, observations of non–middle class infants of European descent often are typically described as "precocious" or "delayed" relative to norms established with Western infants.

Vereijken stated that "as soon as one is willing to move away from normative data and sample averages, the complexity of childhood development unveils itself in the many individual pathways children weave through development."[47(p1851)]

Descriptions of early motor skills provide physical therapists information regarding components of movements and patterns used by TD children. Developmental motor milestones are important functional goals. However, they do not have to be achieved in a specific sequence. Karel and Berta Bobath recognized this many years ago, stating in 1984: "However, we soon found that it was not enough—indeed it was wrong—to try to follow the normal developmental sequence too closely. We had made the child rigidly go through the stage of rolling over, before going on to sitting, side-sitting, kneeling, kneel-standing, half-kneeling, crawling and then finally standing; one stage after the other. But that sequence is not followed faithfully by normal children. Contrary to the impression that could be gained from charts of development … development often does not proceed in a definite sequence, in which 'milestones' follow each other."[52(p9)]

An alternative approach to using a predetermined developmental sequence is to have the child practice a variety of age-appropriate functional tasks that he or she might reasonably be expected to accomplish. A child age 2 years with spastic diplegia CP, for example, may have difficulty maintaining floor sitting because of increased muscle activity or tightness of the hamstrings, yet he or she may be able to control his or her balance in upright using a walker. This child may never master the task of independent floor sitting and, if the developmental sequence were followed prescriptively, he or she would not be allowed to practice ambulation skills. Children with spastic hemiplegia might never crawl on their hands and knees because their involved upper extremity will not support their weight. Research has shown that most, if not all, children with spastic hemiplegia become ambulatory.[52-55] To prevent the child with hemiplegia from ambulating until he or she could crawl on hands and knees would be illogical. The alternative approach is to work on a variety of skills simultaneously, allowing the child to progress with the acquisition of skills at varying rates as allowed by neurological, biomechanical, cognitive, and other factors.

MOTOR CONTROL, MOTOR LEARNING, AND MOTOR DEVELOPMENT—MAJOR CONCEPTS

Active Organism

At one time, the CNS was viewed as a system of reflexes arranged in a hierarchy of complexity with volitional processes dominating or controlling the reflexive base. The parallel model of motor development would portray the infant primarily as a reflexive being, acting solely in response to the environment. Only when the cerebral cortex became mature and exerted control over lower-level reflexes would complex volitional behavior become possible.

We now recognize the active role of the CNS in the creation and control of body actions.[56] From the "active organism" perspective, the CNS is viewed as capable of anticipating the demands of the environment and planning ahead. The process of planning, originating, and controlling motor acts requires an active CNS.

Research supporting the active organism concept required physical therapists to develop models of evaluation and treatment consistent with this perspective. In current practice, therapists do not rely on reflex tests to determine developmental levels of neural organization and control. Instead, emphasis is on documenting behaviors that are considered to be spontaneous or self-generated by the child.

Motor Pattern

Because postures and movements appear well organized and have characteristic forms, such as those observed in walking, running, or moving from sitting to standing, we know that processes of motor control are not random. In fact, postures and movements are composed of well-defined patterns of action, and it is these action patterns that behavioral scientists and physical therapists observe and study to better understand invisible internal control processes mediated by neural structures.

Despite the insufficiency of reflex theory in explaining spontaneous and volitional movement, the reflex was useful in explaining stereotyped patterns of posture and movement that could be evoked with specific types of sensory stimulation. This reflex, by definition, encompasses a well-organized, patterned motor response. Reflex responses involve consistent temporal and spatial relationships among muscle groups. For example, even in the simplest stretch reflex, muscles are controlled in relation to one another (agonists are activated, antagonists are inhibited) and produce observable behaviors. These stable relationships among muscle groups are termed *postural or movement patterns* (see Chapter 10).

The underlying neural representations of these observable response patterns dissociated or uncoupled from the stimuli that produce them are examples of motor patterns. The motor pattern specifies distinct temporal and spatial relationships between muscles. The concept of a motor pattern has a decided advantage over the concept of a reflex because the motor pattern is more versatile. The motor pattern need not be bound to a specific sensory stimulus. A motor pattern could be brought into action either by sensory stimuli or by internal processes within the CNS. If one considers the motor pattern, rather than the reflex, as the basic unit of neuromotor organization, it is possible to explain why, for example, there are so many different stimuli that can be used to evoke a specific movement pattern seen in an infant. This concept also explains why a child with hemiplegia demonstrates the same movement pattern both during volitional effort and in response to a variety of sensory stimuli.

Feedback/Knowledge of Results

One of the most important variables enhancing motor learning is feedback or information that is provided to children about their performance as they attempt to move or accomplish a task. *Intrinsic feedback* refers to information obtained through sensory systems (eg, visual, somatosensory, vestibular) as movement is attempted or produced. Feedback, as an integral element of motor control, provides the capacity to compare the intended with the actual result of an activity.

Only through a process of comparison can unsuccessful actions be identified and changed. Without feedback and comparison between intended and resultant actions, the CNS is destined to either repeat the same patterns without modification or to be totally dependent on someone in the external environment to affect change in motor behavior. When the CNS is afforded the capacity to compare intention with outcome, an element of control is removed from the environment and the individual need not wait for an external source to provide a correcting stimulus to change motor behavior. During intervention the child is capable of judging and correcting actions and can be encouraged to do so.

Extrinsic feedback refers primarily to verbal information (eg, from a therapist) related to performance. Extrinsic feedback also can be provided through nonverbal means, such as a switch device that activates a musical toy each time the child lifts his or her head to an upright position in sitting.

Knowledge of Performance Versus Knowledge of Results

Gentile[57] distinguished between knowledge of performance (KP—feedback about the movement itself) and knowledge of results (KR—feedback about the outcome of the movement). Providing the child information on how effectively the back muscles are contracting (KP) vs providing information on how effectively he or she is maintaining an upright sitting posture (KR) is a specific example. Most research to date has focused on information regarding movement outcome (KR), and the current assumption is that the mechanisms of KR and KP are similar.[1]

Thorpe and Valvano[58] compared the effects of presenting KP vs KP augmented by a cognitive strategy to 13 children with CP during practice of a novel skill (ie, moving a Pedalo/standing therapeutic exercise equipment). Results suggested that some of the children benefited greatly from KP and the use of cognitive strategies as they practiced the task.

Adult Versus Pediatric Populations

Studies of adult learners suggest reduced-feedback conditions are preferable to 100% feedback (ie, KR provided following every practice trial). Studies of KR frequency both with TD children and children with disabilities have produced inconsistent conclusions regarding frequency of feedback.

Sullivan and colleagues[59] compared frequency of feedback on a discrete arm movement task in a group of young adults and a group of TD children. As expected, adults with reduced feedback performed more consistently during the retention test than adults receiving 100% feedback. In contrast, the children in the reduced feedback group performed with less accuracy and consistency than children receiving 100% feedback. A discrete, coordinated arm movement task also was used by Burtner and colleagues[60] to compare the performance of TD children and children with CP. TD children performed with significantly less error during acquisition, retention, and reacquisition with 100% feedback vs 62% feedback. The children with CP mirrored this effect, although the difference between 100% and 62% feedback was not statistically significant. In both groups, 100% feedback was preferable to reduced feedback.

In another study, the opposite was found when reduced feedback was preferable to 100% KR.[61] The effect of frequency of feedback on learning dart throwing was studied in children (age 7 to 15 years) with CP. Different frequencies of feedback were compared. Acquisition was measured immediately following the last practice session and retention 3 days later. Because children receiving 50% KR performed better than children receiving 100% KR, the authors concluded that too much feedback in this task interfered with learning.

A mixed result regarding frequency of feedback was found by Sidaway et al.[62] In this study, TD fourth- and fifth-grade children threw beanbags at an unseen target (over a barrier) while walking or standing still. These 2 levels of task difficulty were crossed with 2 frequencies of feedback (33% and 100%). Retention tests (without feedback) were performed at 5 minutes and 1 week post–skill acquisition. Learning was improved on the easy version of the task with 33% KR frequency. In contrast, learning was improved on the difficult version of the task with 100% KR frequency.

An early view of feedback was that feedback that was more frequent, more immediate, more accurate, or produced more information had the most positive effect on learning.[1] However, in some instances, although frequent feedback may enhance motor performance, it may be detrimental to motor learning. One hypothesis is that feedback that is provided too frequently interferes with the child's ability to learn to detect and correct errors. Less frequent feedback or fading feedback in some instances may be more beneficial for motor learning.

More research needs to occur in pediatric populations to develop clinical guidelines regarding the appropriate frequency of feedback. The Challenge Point Framework[63] suggests motor learning is related to the interaction of the information-processing capacity of the learner, the task difficulty, and the conditions of practice. Therefore, physical therapists will need to use clinical decision-making skills to apply appropriate frequency of feedback. More frequent feedback may be appropriate for difficult tasks and for the child with intellectual and sensory-processing deficits. Less frequent feedback will be appropriate once a skill becomes easier and will allow more trial-and-error learning.

Schedules of Feedback

Various schedules of feedback have been examined experimentally and have been reviewed elsewhere.[1] An alternative to constant feedback would be to provide feedback in summary form after several trials. Another alternative is "bandwidth KR," in which feedback is given only if the movement or performance is outside a given error range. The absence of KR informs the child that his or her movement is acceptable. A practical example would be monitoring the child's tendency to "W-sit" during a treatment session. The child can be instructed that kneel-sitting on the feet is acceptable, but kneel-sitting while internally rotating the hips with the feet out to the side of the body with the buttocks on the floor is unacceptable (Figures 1-4 and 1-5).

The therapist decides to call the child's attention to his or her W-sitting position whenever the child sits in this position for more than 30 seconds. The absence of feedback at other times informs the child that his or her sitting posture is acceptable. Bandwidth KR can be used to allow more variability of movement, prevent too-frequent feedback (after every trial), and allow the child to concentrate on intrinsic feedback to monitor his or her movements.

Application to Pediatric Populations

Several principles of KR have special applicability in the treatment of children. When KR is provided, it is provided during or immediately after a movement or task is completed. The interval between completion of a movement and feedback from the therapist should be "empty." In other words, children should not be asked to perform other movements or be distracted by the therapist or the environment. It is hypothesized that children may be retaining in short-term memory kinesthetic information regarding the movement and that this process should proceed without distractions. Therapists should be cautious about distracting children unnecessarily by talking or calling attention to toys or other objects in the environment.

In research with children, performance often is disrupted when shortening the period of time following KR and when a subsequent attempt is made to repeat the movement or task.[1] The assumption is that new solutions to motor problems are being processed and a certain amount of time is necessary for this to occur. Children should be allowed to initiate repetitions of movements and tasks at self-determined speeds.

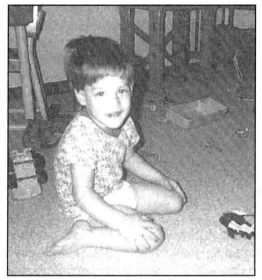

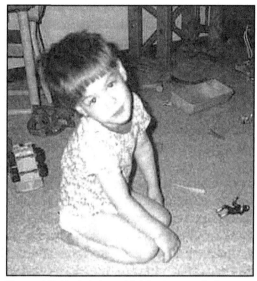

Figure 1-4. W-sitting with hips internally rotated and buttocks flat on floor.

Figure 1-5. Heel sitting with hips in neutral alignment and buttocks resting on feet.

Distributed Control

The model of the CNS as a strict hierarchy of function is no longer viable. A large body of science has demonstrated that human behaviors are a product of complex, multilevel, and recurrent networks within the CNS.[64] Although the idea of feedback is not new, the effects of feedback loops within the CNS is an important concept. Feedback loops, particularly those that link lower levels to the uppermost levels of the CNS, challenge the concept of hierarchical control. If information from lower levels is relayed to the top level (ie, cerebral cortex) and, as a result of feedback, actions are modified, then what level of the system is really in control? Could it not be argued that the lower level centers control the higher levels? Where does control reside in such a model? The concept of a "distributed" model of neuromotor control can help resolve this dilemma and explicit behaviors are recognized as a product of the system.

Memory

Another important concept related to motor control and learning is memory. Successful motor acts include elements of preplanning. For example, to be successful in a wheelchair transfer to a toilet, a child must position the chair in expectation of the activity that will follow, such as opening a door to a bathroom stall. The child must adjust the distance between his or her body and the door handle to successfully reach and pull the door open. The child needs to anticipate the arc of the door as it is opening. From where does this capacity to anticipate or predict the outcome of action arise? The ability to plan successful action is based on previous experiences. Whereas practice usually is considered to be the reason for success, practice is more than just repeating an act over and over. The key to the child's future motor success is the ability to use the result of one act to make the next motor act more successful. Key information related to the solution of the motor problem must be used to be successful in a situation not previously encountered. Commonly, the theoretical construct of memory is used to explain how an individual benefits from prior experience. The theory has been that practice permits the formation of memory structures that can be used in novel situations. Storing the exact solution for every problem encountered would not enable transfer of motor abilities to a novel situation. What has been proposed is that general rules, or *schema,* that specify the relationships among the conditions surrounding performance, the intended action, and the results of the action are stored in memory.[1] These schema enable the individual to solve novel motor problems.

NEUROPLASTICITY

Research Methods

Animal Models

In animal models, the rat has played a crucial role.[37] Although starkly different from the human brain in appearance and size, at a cellular level there are many similarities. The organization of the cerebral cortex is similar, and rat and human neurons both wire up in the same way and go through the same developmental stages. The rat can be trained to perform specific tasks and concurrent changes in neural activity can be assessed.

Brain mapping of the sensory cortex in animals can be conducted with microelectrodes that are so small that firing from a single neuron can be detected.[12] Using microelectrodes is a time-consuming surgical process because mapping 1 to 2 mm of a brain area might require hundreds of insertions over several days. Resulting "maps," however, can be very precise. Conversely, intra-cortical microstimulation can be performed to stimulate the motor cortex and resulting muscle activity recorded and mapped.

One sensory principle (in adult animal studies) is that simple exposure to sensory stimuli causes little or no long-latency changes in receptive field properties.[65] There must be context-dependent reinforcement. This would suggest active movement or responses concurrent with sensory processing would be important for neuroplastic change to occur. Following training of a specific task, related changes that occur in sensory and motor areas of the brain, such as synaptogenesis and map reorganization, are not general but are very specific in relation to the learned behavior.

Human Studies

Beginning in the 1930s, Penfield, a neurosurgeon, performed electrical stimulation of various areas of the human brain during surgery (with patients' permission).[12,66-67] The patients were conscious and could report sensations they felt in their body. Penfield correlated specific areas of the brain with thoughts, motor behaviors, and sensations. A major discovery was that sensory and motor brain maps are topographical. Areas adjacent to each other on the body surface are generally adjacent to each other on the brain maps. The size of representation of individual body parts in the brain, however, is proportional to how often and how precisely that body part is used, and not to actual size in the body. Penfield's work provided the first sensory and motor topographic maps of the human brain (cortical homunculus; Figure 1-6).

Since Penfield's early work, noninvasive neural imaging methods have been developed to identify areas of the brain active during performance of a variety of activities.[1] For example, sensory maps can be detected with fMRI. This type of MRI detects changes in blood supply, with areas where oxygen is being metabolized showing brighter than areas that are not active. In another type of imaging study, a small amount of radioactive glucose is injected into the bloodstream and positron emission tomography scans detect levels of activity in various brain areas.

Pascual-Leone and colleagues[68] were the first researchers to use transcranial magnetic stimulation to map motor areas of the human brain. An electric current is run through a "paddle" containing a copper wire, which generates a changing magnetic field inducing an electric current around it. When placed above the area of the motor cortex, neurons beneath the paddle are stimulated and resulting movements monitored and motor areas mapped.

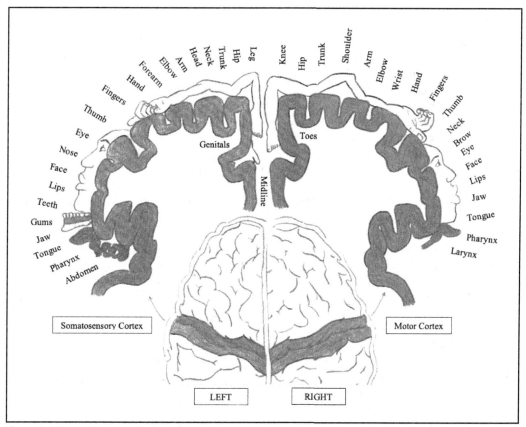

Figure 1-6. Sensory or motor homunculus.

Results of studies using transcranial magnetic stimulation demonstrate that motor maps vary among individuals and are constantly changing. Motor maps also are *fractionated*, which means they contain multiple overlapping representations of movements. Remodeling of the motor cortex occurs as a consequence of skill training. One hypothesis is that learning a skill requires creation or building of synergistic movements encompassing multiple joints and muscles and that a "functional cortical module" is formed.[65]

Task-Specific Versus General Activity

One principle of motor learning is that increases in motor activity in the absence of motor skill acquisition are insufficient to drive neurophysiologic changes in the motor cortex. Nudo[65] emphasized that plasticity in the motor cortex is skill or learning dependent, rather than strictly use dependent. Tasks that require acquisition of new motor skills induce neurophysiologic and neuroanatomic changes in the motor cortex, but simple repetitive motion or strength training tasks do not. In a comparison of 2 interventions in children with hemiparesis, only a structured motor skill training program with progressively more difficult and functional goals produced changes in size of the affected hand map and amplitudes of motor evoked potentials.[69] Children receiving the same amount of intervention, but unstructured bimanual activities, improved in bimanual hand use and dexterity but did not demonstrate the same CNS changes.

Aerobic Activity

Intervention designed to promote specific skills will result in specific changes in the brain. However, general or "unskilled" movements that are aerobic in nature also are important. Aerobic activity results in the release of several chemicals in the brain, including brain-derived neurotrophic factor, that assist in the processes of synaptogenesis and neurogenesis. Glial-derived neurotrophic factor promotes survival of many types of neurons. Both are growth factors that consolidate new neuronal connections so they will wire together and fire together.[4,12,64]

Aerobic exercise has been shown in mice[70,71] and humans[72-74] to promote neurogenesis in the hippocampus. Neurogenesis is the formation of new neurons and the hippocampus is vital for memory functions, which, in turn, are crucial in most aspects of human behavior and motor learning.

Chaddock-Heyman[75] demonstrated that aerobic fitness was associated with greater estimates of white-matter microstructure in the brains of 9- to 10-year-old TD children. The mapping of white-matter tracts was performed using diffusion tensor imaging, a type of MRI that characterizes 3-dimensional diffusion of water molecules along the axis of myelinated axons.[76] White-matter tracts provide the basis of the "internet" effect of connections within the CNS, which are necessary for complex behaviors. Studies of children with Down syndrome,[77] developmental coordination disorder,[78,79] autism,[80] attention-deficit hyperactivity disorder,[81] and CP[82-84] have demonstrated differences in amounts and distribution of white-matter tracts (eg, decreased volume, fewer distant connections) as compared with TD control individuals.

Kim and So[85] demonstrated a positive relationship between cognitive and memory functions in relation to the number of physical education (PE) classes attended per week. In a study of more than 75,000 Korean adolescents, 3 or more PE classes per week correlated with improved school performance. Fewer than 3 PE classes per week had a negative correlation with school performance. The supportive role of aerobic activity in neuroplasticity supports providing PE or "recess" in academic settings to enhance processes related to cognitive and motor learning.

Although aerobic activity appears to be beneficial to the CNS throughout the life span, it may be even more important during early brain development, when synaptogenesis is occurring rapidly.[86] Aerobic activity should be considered an important component of the overall physical therapy plan for children with disabilities.

Influence of Age

Remodeling of the brain occurs throughout the life span; however, plasticity processes vary with age.[64] In the perinatal period and during early childhood, almost all inputs continuously engage in competitive plasticity processes. In older children and adults, moment-by-moment control of change when specific contextual conditions are present is required to enable or trigger plasticity (ie, a function of behavioral outcomes).

Potential for Plasticity in Children With Disabilities

Staudt[87] reviewed mechanisms of reorganization following pre- and perinatally acquired unilateral brain lesions. Unilateral damage to the lateral corticospinal tract can lead to maintenance of normally transient ipsilateral corticospinal projections from the contralesional hemisphere. In some children this reorganization can enable active grasp of the paretic hand. Age is relevant, as by age 3 years the lateral corticospinal tract is much larger than the ipsilateral tract, so neuroplasticity of this type might be reduced with later-occurring brain injury. Periventricular lesions can be compensated for by thalamocortical projections, which form "bypasses" around defective white matter to reach the postcentral gyrus. All sensory processes except olfaction are received by the thalamus, and connections from the thalamus to the sensory cortex are essential as a precursor for efficient learning and motor behavior.

Moutard and colleagues completed a 10-year follow-up of children with isolated corpus callosum agenesis.[88] Of the 11 children completing the follow-up, 3 had borderline intelligence and 8 were within normal range, although half of these experienced some mild learning difficulties.

Children with intractable epilepsy may receive a hemispherectomy, which involves removing or disconnecting one cerebral hemisphere (half the brain). Although children have varying degrees of hemiparesis postsurgery, functional abilities may be greatly improved with half a brain as compared to presurgery with a dysfunctional brain.[89,90]

There appears to be great potential for various types of neuroplasticity to occur in the human CNS.[5,12,91-93] One consistent finding in brain research is *sensory and/or motor map expansion* in relation to specific types of learning or experience. *Sensory reassignment* can occur, for example, when the visual cortex in blind individuals processes tactile information. *Compensatory masquerade* (alternative strategy or unmasking of unused pathways) takes advantage of the fact that there is more than one way for the brain to approach a task. *Mirror region takeover* refers to the opposite hemisphere performing a function typically performed by the contralateral hemisphere. An example of mirror region takeover is evidenced by language functions being taken over by the right hemisphere in cases of left hemispheric damage.

Role of Attention and Reward/Motivation

In the animal model, attention must be paid to the task to be learned. Long-lasting plastic changes occur only when the animal pays *close attention*.[64] Brain maps can change when animals perform tasks automatically, but the neural changes do not last. In animal studies, the correct performance is met with a "reward" (eg, food pellet). Children also need "rewards." Rewards can be extrinsic, such as Cheerios or toys. A feeling of accomplishment (intrinsic reward) can be the most positive reward. An optimal approach to therapy intervention is to select tasks that are highly motivating and engage the child, because the more important the behavior/task is to the child, the more important it will be to the brain.[12,64]

Role of Therapists in Neuroplasticity

Because neural plasticity is the mechanism that accounts for learning and functional recovery, it is important to understand the elements necessary for neuroplastic changes to occur in the brain. The manipulation of tasks (ie, task-specific training) is the primary mode of intervention because children learn in a functional context. Physical therapists are responsible for selecting the task, structuring the task and environment, varying the task, progressively increasing task difficulty and complexity, and making the decision to switch to new tasks.

Although in its earliest stages, Merzenich et al[64] suggested the primary goal in therapeutic programs is shifting beyond behavioral improvement to the potential renormalization of dysfunctional brain systems. Based on animal and human studies, the critical elements to enhance brain plasticity appear to be attention, reward, sensory input, skilled exercise or experience (motor skills or tasks), and general aerobic exercise. Incorporation of these elements in conjunction with motor learning principles will maximize potential for acquisition of motor skills and recovery of function following CNS injury or dysfunction. A number of questions are relevant when designing intervention:

> Are the activities "task specific" (ie, do they reflect the proposed outcomes)?
> Is adequate sensory information available?
> Is the child receiving intrinsic and extrinsic feedback?
> Is there a component of aerobic activity to support neuroplastic changes?
> Is the child motivated and engaged in the activities (ie, paying close attention)?
> Does the child attempt activities independently for trial-and-error learning?

> Is the child "rewarded" for attempts at movement or to complete tasks?
> Can motor learning be differentiated from motor performance?
> Have affordances in the environment been optimized for motor behaviors?
> Is emphasis on long-term goals of "participation"?

SUMMARY

When applying foundational sciences in physical therapy, it is important to remember that models and theories are somewhat simplified abstract representations of complex processes. Their usefulness is in helping therapists design and evaluate effective intervention strategies. As research in foundational sciences expands, new findings will lead to changes in clinical practice. Physical therapists should heed the words of the Spanish philosopher José Ortega y Gasset: "Our strongest convictions are the most suspect; they mark our limitations and our bounds."[94] We must remain open to new information, and as a profession continue to embrace evidence-based practices for the benefit of the children in our care.

ACKNOWLEDGMENT

The editors wish to express appreciation to Ann VanSant, PT, PhD, FAPTA for contributions to this chapter in previous editions.

REFERENCES

1. Schmidt RA, Lee TD. *Motor Control and Learning. A Behavioral Emphasis.* 5th ed. Champaign, IL: Human Kinetics; 2011.
2. Karasik LB, Adolph KE, Tamis-LeMonda CS, Bornstein MH. WEIRD walking: cross-cultural research on motor development. *Behav Brain Sci.* 2010;33(2-3):95-96. doi:10.1017/S0140525X10000117.
3. McGraw MB. *The Neuromuscular Maturation of the Human Infant.* New York, NY: Hafner Publishing; 1966.
4. Doidge N. *The Brain's Way of Healing.* New York, NY: Penguin Books; 2015.
5. Hadders-Algra M. Variation and variability: key words in human motor development. *Phys Ther.* 2010;90(12):1823-1837. doi:10.2522/ptj.20100006.
6. Sherrington CS. *The Integrative Action of the Nervous System.* New Haven, CT: Yale University Press; 1906.
7. Hughlings Jackson J. The Croonian Lectures on evolution and dissolution of the nervous system. *Br Med J.* 1884;1(1214):660-663. doi:10.1136/bmj.1.1215.703
8. Bobath B. *Abnormal Postural Reflex Activity Caused by Brain Lesions.* 3rd ed. Rockville, MD: Aspen Systems; 1985.
9. Brunnström S. *Movement Therapy in Hemiplegia: A Neurophysiological Approach.* New York, NY: Harper & Row; 1970.
10. Knott M, Voss DE. *Proprioceptive Neuromuscular Facilitation: Patterns and Techniques.* 2nd ed. New York, NY: Harper & Row; 1968.
11. Stockmeyer SA. An interpretation of the approach of Rood to the treatment of neuromuscular dysfunction. *Am J Phys Med.* 1967;46(1):900-956.
12. Doidge N. *The Brain That Changes Itself.* New York, NY: Penguin Books; 2007.
13. Taub E, Perrella P, Barro G. Behavioral development after forelimb deafferentation on day of birth in monkeys with and without blinding. *Science.* 1973;181(4103):959-960. doi:10.1126/science.181.4103.959.
14. Bernstein N. *The Coordination and Regulation of Movement.* New York, NY: Pergamon Press; 1967.
15. Kelso JAS. On the self-organizing origins of agency. *Trends Cogn Sci.* 2016;20(7):490-499. doi:10.1016/j.tics.2016.04.004.
16. Kelso JAS, Tuller B. A dynamical basis for action systems. In: Gazzaniga MS, ed. *Handbook of Cognitive Neuroscience.* New York, NY: Plenum Press; 1984:321-356.
17. Perone S, Simmering VR. Applications of dynamic systems theory to cognition and development: new frontiers. *Adv Child Dev Behav.* 2017;52:143-180. doi:10.1016/bs.acdb.2016.10.002.
18. Kelso JA, Dumas G, Tognoli E. Outline of a general theory of behavior and brain coordination. *Neural Networks.* 2013;37:120-131. doi:10.1016/j.neunet.2012.09.003.

19. King LA, VanSant AF. The effect of solid ankle foot orthoses on movement patterns used to rise from supine to stand. *Phys Ther.* 1995;75(11):952-964.

20. Thelen E, Fisher DM. Newborn stepping: an explanation for a disappearing reflex. *Dev Psyc.* 1982;18(5):760-775. doi:10.1037/0012-1649.18.5.760.

21. Gibson JJ. *The Ecological Approach to Visual Perception.* Boston, MA: Houghton Mifflin Co; 1979.

22. Gibson JJ, Gibson EJ. Perceptual learning: differentiation or enrichment? *Psychol Rev.* 1955;62(1):32-41. doi:10.1037/h0048826.

23. Adolph KE. Learning in the development of infant locomotion. *Monogr Soc Res Child Dev.* 1997;62(3):I-VI, 1-158. doi:10.2307/1166199.

24. Adolph KE, Vereijken B, Denny MA. Learning to crawl. *Child Dev.* 1998;69(5):1299-1312. doi:10.1111/j.1467-8624.1998.tb06213.x.

25. Adolph KE, Berger SE, Leo AJ. Developmental continuity? Crawling, cruising, and walking. *Dev Sci.* 2011;14(2):306-318. doi:10.1111/j.1467-7687.2010.00981.x.

26. Herrin K, Geil M. A comparison of orthoses in the treatment of idiopathic toe walking: a randomized controlled trial. *Prosthet Orthot Int.* 2016;40(2):262-269. doi:10.1177/0309364614564023.

27. Bonney E, Jelsma LD, Ferguson Smits-Engelsman BCM. Learning better by repetition or variation? Is transfer at odds with task specific training? *PLoS One.* 2017;12(3):e0174214. doi:10.1371/journal.pone.0172/214.

28. Adolph KE, Specificity of learning: why infants fall over a veritable cliff. *Psychol Sci.* 2000;11(4):290-295. doi:10.1111/1467-9280.00258.

29. Kretch KS, Adolph KE. Cliff or step? Posture-specific learning at the edge of a drop-off. *Child Dev.* 2013;84(1):226-240. doi:10.1111/j.1467-8624.2012.01842.x.

30. Prado MTA, Fernani DCGL, da Silva TD, Smorenburg ARP, de Abreu LC, Monteiro CBdMM. Motor learning paradigm and contextual interference in manual computer tasks in individuals with cerebral palsy. *Res Dev Disabil.* 2017;64(5):56-63. doi:10.1016/j.ridd.2017.03.006.

31. Kwon HY, Ahn SY. Effect of task-oriented training and high-variability practice on gross motor performance and activities of daily living in children with spastic diplegia. *J Phys Ther Sci.* 2016;28(10):2843-2848. doi:10.1589/jpts.28.2843.

32. Bonney, E, Jelsma D, Ferguson G, Smits-Engelsman B. Variable training does not lead to better motor learning compared to repetitive training in children with and without DCD when exposed to active video games. *Res Dev Disabil.* 2017;62(3):124-136. doi:10.1016/j.ridd.2017.01.013.

33. London SE. Developmental song learning as a model to understand neural mechanisms that limit and promote the ability to learn [published online ahead of print November 20, 2017.] *Behav Processes.* doi:10.1016/j.beproc.2017.11.008.

34. Ohki-Hamazaki H. Neurobiology of imprinting [in Japanese]. *Brain Nerve.* 2012;64(6):657-664.

35. Basu AP. Early intervention after perinatal stroke: opportunities and challenges. *Dev Med Child Neurol.* 2014;56(6):516-521. doi:10.1111/dmcn.12407.

36. Reid LB, Rose SE, Boyd RN. Rehabilitation and neuroplasticity in children with unilateral cerebral palsy. *Nat Rev Neurol.* 2015;11(7):390-400. doi:10.1038/nrneurol.2015.97.

37. Eagleman D. *The Brain. The Story of You.* New York, NY: Pantheon Books; 2015.

38. Palisano RJ, Hanna SE, Rosenbaum PL, et al. Validation of a model of gross motor function for children with cerebral palsy. *Phys Ther.* 2000;80(10):974-985. doi:10.1093/ptj/80.10.974.

39. Rosenbaum PL, Walter SD, Hanna SE, et al. Prognosis for gross motor function in cerebral palsy. Creation of motor development cures. *JAMA.* 2002;288(11):1357-1363. doi:10.1001/jama.288.11.1357.

40. Gabbard C. Windows of opportunity for early brain and motor development. *J Phys Educ Recreat Dance.* 1998;69(8):54-55. doi:10.1080/07303084.1998.10605614.

41. Hubel DH, Wiesel TN. The period of susceptibility to the physiological effects of unilateral eye closure in kittens. *J Physiol.* 1970;206(2):419-436. doi:10.1113/jphysiol.1970.sp009022.

42. Vera L, Lambert N, Sommet J, Boulkedid R, Alberti C, Bui Quoc E. Visual outcomes and complications of cataract surgery with primary implantation in infants. *J Fr Ophthalmol.* 2017;40(5):386-393. doi:10.1016/j.jfo.2016.12.010.

43. Pediatric Eye Disease Investigator Group, Repka MX, Kraka RT, et al. A randomized trial of atropine vs patching for treatment of moderate amblyopia: follow-up at age 10 years. *Arch Ophthalmol.* 2008;126(8):1039-1044. doi:10.1001/archopht.126.8.1039.

44. Sebastián-Gallés N. Native language sensitivities: evolution in the first year of life. *Trends Cogn Sci.* 2006;10(6):239-241. doi:10.1016/j.tics.2006.04.009.

45. Tsao FM, Liu HM, Kuhl PK. Perception of native and non-native affricate-fricative contrasts: cross-language tests on adults and infants. *J Acoust Soc Am.* 2006;120(4):2285-2294. doi:10.1121/1.2338290.

46. Sharma A, Nash AA, Dorman M. Cortical development, plasticity and reorganization in children with cochlear implants. *J Commun Disord.* 2009;42(4):272-279. doi:10.1016/j.jcomdis.2009.03.003.

47. Vereijken B. The complexity of childhood development: variability in perspective. *Phys Ther.* 2010;90(12):1850-1859. doi:10.2522/ptj.20100019.

48. Karasik LB, Tamis-LeMonda CS, Adolph KE, Bornstein MH. Places and postures: a cross-cultural comparison of sitting in 5-month-olds. *J Cross Cult Psychol.* 2015;46(8):1023-1038. doi:10.1177/0022022115593803.

49. Patrick SK, Noah JA, Yang JF. Developmental constraints of quadrupedal coordination across crawling styles in human infants. *J Neurophysiol.* 2012;107(11):3050-3061. doi:10.1152/jn.00029.2012.

50. Bottos M, Dalla Barba B, Stefani D, Pettenà G, Tonin C, D'Este A. Locomotor strategies preceding independent walking: prospective study of neurological and language development in 424 cases. *Dev Med Child Neurol.* 1989;31(1):25-34. doi:10.1111/j.1469-8749.1989.tb08408.x.

51. Ulrich BD. Opportunities for early intervention based on theory, basic neuroscience and clinical science. *Phys Ther.* 2010;90(12):1868-1880. doi:10.2522/ptj.20100040.

52. Bobath B, Bobath K. The neuro-developmental treatment. In: Scrutton D, ed. *Management of the Motor Disorders in Cerebral Palsy.* Clinics in Developmental Medicine #90. London, England: Spastics International Medical Publications; 1984:6-18.

53. Bottos M, Puato ML, Viancello A, Facchin P. Locomotion patterns in cerebral palsy syndromes. *Dev Med Child Neurol.* 1995;37(10):883-899. doi:10.1111/j.1469-8749.1995.tb11941.x.

54. Bleck EE. Locomotor prognosis in cerebral palsy. *Dev Med Child Neurol.* 1975;17(1):18-25. doi:10.1111/j.1469-8749.1975.tb04952.x.

55. Molnar GE, Gordon SU. Cerebral palsy: predictive value of selected clinical signs for early prognostication of motor function. *Arch Phys Med Rehabil.* 1976;57(4):153-158.

56. Lobo MA, Harbourne RT, Dusing SC, McCoy SW. Grounding early intervention: physical therapy cannot just be about motor skills anymore. *Phys Ther.* 2013;93(1):94-103. doi:10.2522/ptj.20120158.

57. Gentile AM. A working model of skill acquisition with application to teaching. *Quest.*1972;17(1):3-23. doi:10.10 80/00336297.1972.10519717.

58. Thorpe DE, Valvano J. The effects of knowledge of performance and cognitive strategies on motor skill learning in children with cerebral palsy. *Pediatr Phys Ther.* 2002;14(1):2-15. doi:10.1097/00001577-200214010-00002.

59. Sullivan KJ, Kantak SS, Burtner PA. Motor learning in children: feedback effects on skill acquisition. *Phys Ther.* 2008;88(6):720-732. doi:10.2522/ptj.20070196.

60. Burtner PA, Leinwand R, Sullivan KJ, Goh HT, Kantak SS. Motor learning in children with hemiplegic cerebral palsy: feedback effects on skill acquisition. *Dev Med Child Neurol.* 2014;56(3):259-266. doi:10.1111/dmcn.12364.

61. Hemayattalab R, Rostami LR. Effects of frequency of feedback on the learning of motor skills in individuals with cerebral palsy. *Res Dev Disabil.* 2010;31(1):212-217. doi:10.1016/j.ridd.2009.09.002.

62. Sidaway B, Bates J, Occhiogrosso B, Schlagenhaufer J, Wilkes D. Interaction of feedback frequency and task difficulty in children's motor skill learning. *Phys Ther.* 2012;92(7):948-957. doi:10.2522/ptj.20110378.

63. Pollock CL, Boyd LA, Hunt MA, Garland SJ. Use of the Challenge Point Framework to guide motor learning of stepping control for improved balance central in people with stroke: a case series. *Phys Ther.* 2014;94(4):562-570. doi:10.2522/ptj.20130046.

64. Merzenich MM, Van Vleet TM, Nahum M. Brain plasticity-based therapeutics. *Front Hum Neurosci.* 2014;8:385. doi:10.3389/fnhum.2014.00385.

65. Nudo RJ. Recovery after brain injury: mechanisms and principles. *Front Hum Neurosci.* 2013;7:887. doi:10.3389/fnhum.2013.00887.

66. Kean S. *The Tale of the Dueling Neurosurgeons.* New York, NY: Little, Brown & Company; 2014.

67. Jasper H, Penfield W. *Epilepsy and the Functional Anatomy of the Human Brain.* New York, NY: Little Brown & Company, 1951 (2nd ed. 1954).

68. Pascual-Leone A, Valls-Solé J, Wassermann EM, Hallett M. Responses to rapid rate transcranial magnetic stimulation of the human motor cortex. *Brain.* 1994;117(Pt 4):847-858. doi:10.1093/brain/117.4.847.

69. Friel KM, Kuo HC, Fuller J, et al. Skilled bimanual training drives motor cortex plasticity in children with unilateral cerebral palsy. *Neurorehabil Neural Repair.* 2016;30(9):834-844. doi:10.1177/1545968315625838.

70. Pereira AC, Huddleston DE, Brickman AM, et al. An in vivo correlate of exercise-induced neurogenesis in the adult dentate gyrus. *Proc Natl Acad Sci U S A.* 2007;104(13):5638-5643. doi:10.1073/pnas.0611721104.

71. Van der Borght K, Kóbor-Nyakas DE, Klauke K, et al. Physical exercise leads to rapid adaptations in hippocampal vasculature: temporal dynamics and relationship to cell proliferation and neurogenesis. *Hippocampus,* 2009;19(10):928-936. doi:10.1002/hipo.20545.

72. Eriksson PS, Perfilieva E, Björk-Eriksson T, et al. Neurogenesis in the adult human hippocampus. *Nat Med.* 1998;4(11):1313-1317. doi:10.1038/3305.

73. Erickson KI, Voss MW, Prakash RS, et al. Exercise training increases size of hippocampus and improves memory. *Proc Natl Acad Sci U S A.* 2011;108(7):3017-3022. doi:10.1073/pnas.1015950108.

74. Spalding KL, Bergmann O, Alkass K, et al. Dynamics of hippocampal neurogenesis in adult humans. *Cell.* 2013;153(6):1219-1227. doi:10.1016/j.cell.2013.05.002.

75. Chaddock-Herman L, Erickson KI, Chappell MA, et al. Aerobic fitness is associated with greater white matter integrity in children. *Dev Cogn Neurosci.* 2016;20(8):52-58. doi:10.1016/j.dcn.2016.07.001.

76. Basser PJ, Mattiello J, LeBihan D. MR diffusion tensor spectroscopy and imaging. *Biophys J.* 1994;66(1):259-267. doi:10.1016/S0006-3495(94)80775-1.

77. Gunbey HP, Bilgici MC, Asian K, et al. Structural brain alterations of Down's syndrome in early childhood evaluation by DTI and volumetric analyses. *Eur Radiol.* 2017;27(7):3013-3021. doi:10.1007/s00330-016-4626-6.

78. Wilson PH, Smits-Engelsman B, Caeyenberghs K, et al. Cognitive and neuroimaging findings in developmental coordination disorder: new insights from a systematic review of recent research. *Dev Med Child Neurol.* 2017;59(11):1117-1129. doi:10.1111/dmcn.13530.

79. Williams J, Kashuk SR, Wilson PH, Thorpe G, Egan GF. White matter alterations in adults with probable developmental coordination disorder: a MRI diffusion tensor imaging study. *Neuroreport.* 2017;28(2):87-92. doi:10.1097/WNR.0000000000000711.

80. Vogan VM, Morgan BR, Leung RC, Anagnostou E, Doyle-Thomas K, Taylor MJ. Widespread white matter differences in children and adolescents with autism spectrum disorders. *J Autism Dev Disord.* 2016;46(6):2138-2147. doi:10.1007/s10803-016-2744-2.

81. Onnink AM, Zwiers MP, Hoogman M, et al. Deviant white matter structure in adults with attention-deficit hyperactivity/disorder points to aberrant myelination and affects neuropsychological performance. *Prog Neuropsychopharmacol Biol Psychiatry.* 2015;63:14-22. doi:10.1016/j.pnpbp.2015.04.008.

82. Englander ZA, Pizoli CE, Batrachenko A, et al. Diffuse reduction of white matter connectivity in cerebral palsy with specific vulnerability of long range fiber tracts. *Neuroimage Clin.* 2013;2:440-447. doi:10.1016/j.nicl.2013.03.006.

83. Papadelis C, Ahtam B, Nazarova M, et al. Cortical somatosensory reorganization in children with spastic cerebral palsy: a multimodal neuroimaging study. *Front Hum Neurosci.* 2014;8:725. doi:10.3389/fnhum.2014.00725.

84. Laporta-Hoyos O, Pannek K, Ballester-Plané J. White matter integrity in dyskinetic cerebral palsy: relationship with intelligence quotient and executive function. *Neuroimage Clin.* 2017;15:789-800. doi:10.1016/j.nicl.2017.05.005.

85. Kim SY, So WY. The relationship between school performance and the number of physical education classes attended by Korean adolescent students. *J Sports Sci Med.* 2012;11(2):226-230.

86. Chaddock-Heyman L, Hillman CH, Cohen NJ, Kramer AF. The importance of physical activity an aerobic fitness for cognitive control and memory in children. *Monogr Soc Res Child Dev.* 2014;79(4):25-50. doi:10.1111/mono.12129.

87. Staudt M. Brain plasticity following early life brain injury: insights from neuroimaging. *Semin Perinatol.* 2010;34(1):87-92. doi:10.1053/j.semperi.2009.10.009.

88. Moutard ML, Kieffer V, Feingold J, et al. Isolated corpus callosum agenesis: a ten-year follow-up after prenatal diagnosis (how are the children without corpus callosum at 10 years of age?). *Prenat Diagn.* 2012;32(3):277-283. doi:10.1002/pd.3824.

89. Lee YJ, Kim EH, Yum MS, Lee JK, Hong S, Ko TS. Long-term outcomes of hemispheric disconnection in pediatric patients with intractable epilepsy. *J Clin Neurol.* 2014;10(2):101-107. doi:10.3988/jcn.2014.10.2.101.

90. Pascoal T, Paglioli E, Palmini A, Menezes R, Staudt M. Immediate improvement of motor function after epilepsy surgery in congenital hemiparesis. *Epilepsia.* 2013;54(8):e109-e111. doi:10.1111/epi.12244.

91. Grafman J. Conceptualizing functional neuroplasticity. *J Commun Disord.* 2000;33(4):345-355; quiz 355-356. doi:10.1016/S0021-9924(00)00030-7.

92. Holmström L, Vollmer B, Tedroff K, et al. Hand-function in relation to brain lesions and corticomotor-projection pattern in children with unilateral cerebral palsy. *Dev Med Child Neurol.* 2010;52(2):145-152. doi:10.1111/j.1469-8749.2009.03496.x.

93. de Bode S, Chanturidze M, Mathern GW, Dubinsky S. Literacy after cerebral hemispherectomy. Can the isolated right hemisphere read? *Epilepsy Behav.* 2015;45:248-253. doi:10.1016/j.yebeh.2015.01.007.

94. Ortega y Gasset J. *Man and People.* New York, NY: WW Norton & Company; 1963.

Examination and Evaluation
Tests and Measures

Barbara H. Connolly, PT, DPT, EdD, C/NDT, FAPTA

The use of standardized norm-referenced and criterion-referenced tests and measures has become a mainstay in the day-to-day practice of the physical therapist and occupational therapist. These instruments may be used to determine a baseline level of performance to qualify a child for therapy services, measure the child's performance over time, or to predict future performance. The type of instrument used is based on the type of information needed at the time the child is examined and an assessment is performed. Additionally, using the *International Classification of Functioning, Disability and Health—Children and Youth* (ICF–CY) model,[1] the instrument selected is based on whether the assessment is at the level of body functions and structures, activities, or participation. *Body Functions and Structures* is defined as the physiological functions of body systems and anatomical elements such as organs, limbs, and their components. Impairments are problems in body function, such as a significant deviation or loss. Measures of Body Functions and Structures might include assessment of sensory functions and pain, neuromusculoskeletal and movement-related structures and functions, and function and structure of the cardiovascular system. *Activities and Abilities* are defined as the execution of specific tasks or actions by an individual. Activity Limitations are difficulties an individual may have in executing these tasks and actions. *Participation* is defined as involvement in a life situation. Participation Restrictions are problems an individual may experience in day-to-day life activities. Measures of Activities and Participation might include assessment of learning and applying knowledge, communication, mobility, self-care, interpersonal interaction and relationships, and community and social life. Another way to view the ICF model is that "body functions and structures" is functioning at the level of the body; "activities" is functioning at the level of the individual; and "participation" is the functioning of an individual as a member of society. ICF–CY terminology would be used in describing a child in the following example: A child who has dyspraxia may have low muscle tone (a body functions and structures problem), difficulty walking a narrow aisle at school (an activity limitation), and may be unable to play with classmates during recess (a participation restriction). Thus, tests and measures are used initially to identify impairments and activity limitations or participation restrictions in the child; then to help establish a diagnosis, prognosis, and plan of care; and, finally, to select appropriate interventions.

Connolly BH, Montgomery PC, eds. *Therapeutic Exercise for Children With Developmental Disabilities, Fourth Edition* (pp 25-93).
© 2020 Taylor & Francis Group.

Tests and measures that are used as a part of the initial examination allow the therapist to confirm or reject hypotheses about the factors that may contribute to the child's current level of functioning. Additionally, the tests and measures may be used to support the therapist's clinical judgments about necessary interventions, appropriate goals, and expected outcomes for the child. The information obtained through tests and measures is used in the dynamic process of evaluation in which the therapist makes clinical judgments based on data gathered during the examination. Additional data may be gathered during the examination process by obtaining a history, performing a systems review, and gathering information about the child's family and environment. Therefore, the use of standardized tests and measures is but a small part of the larger processes of examination and evaluation. Assessment of a child involves more than merely the administration of a test and is qualitative as well as quantitative.

Tests and measures also are used after the initial examination and evaluation to indicate achievement of outcomes that are indicated at specific points of care (eg, short- and long-term goal attainment) or at the end of an episode of care. *Reexamination* as defined in the *Guide to Physical Therapist Practice 3.0*[2] is:

> The process of performing selected tests and measures after the initial examination to evaluate progress and to modify or redirect intervention. Reexamination may be indicated more than once during a single episode of care. It also may be performed over the course of a disease, disorder, or condition, which for some individuals may be over the life span. Indications for reexamination include new clinical findings or failure to respond to physical therapist intervention.

With the pediatric population, reexamination may occur at the end of short periods of time (eg, 1 month) or at the end of an academic school year. Some standardized tests and measures perform the function of guiding interventions by stating functional goals that can be placed directly into the child's plan of care. For example, the School Function Assessment (SFA) identifies those functional skills needed in a school-based program for children between the ages of 5 to 12 years.[3] The Gross Motor Function Measure (GMFM)[4] also allows for the placement of test items directly into the child's Individualized Family Service Plan or the Individualized Education Program (IEP). The authors of the SFA stated that the use of specific skills from the test can appropriately be used in the child's IEP. For younger children, items from the Sensory Processing Measure—Preschool (SPM–P)[5] can be used to measure changes over time in areas such as body awareness, planning and ideas, and participation. However, other tests and measures, such as the Bruininks-Oseretsky Test of Motor Proficiency, Second Edition (BOT–2),[6] should not have items from the examination used in the child's IEP because these items represent novel and new tasks and not functional activities.

When a child is being assessed, the therapist must consider more than just the passing or failing of an item on a test or measurement. The therapist should consider the child's ability to perform a variety of tasks in a variety of settings or contexts, the meaning of his or her performance in terms of total functioning, and the likely explanation for those performances. Using this level of analysis, the therapist must consider other factors that might influence the child's performance at any given time. These factors include current life circumstances, health history, developmental history, cultural influences, and extrapersonal interactions. Current life circumstances relate to the child's current health, the day-to-day functioning of the family unit, as well as the family's living arrangements. For example, if the child is not feeling well during the examination, the therapist may not get an accurate picture of his or her abilities. If the family is in crisis because of illness of family members, transient living arrangements, or day-to-day life disruptions, the child may not have been able to adjust to these changes. This may affect how he or she performs during an examination, particularly if the child's sleep cycles or eating habits have been disrupted.

The child's health history is an important factor in the acquisition of certain motor skills. The child who has had poor health or nutrition is apt to be delayed in the acquisition of skills such as sitting, creeping, and walking. Delays in overall development may be seen if the child has a history of repeated hospitalizations. Additional musculoskeletal problems may be noted. For example, torticollis may be present if the child has been unable to lie on the stomach and remained in a supine position for extended periods of time. These musculoskeletal problems may interfere with the attainment of certain developmental skills, such as holding the head in midline or bringing the hands to midline.

Examination of the child's developmental history is important in determining the child's past rate of achievement of developmental milestones and in deciding what performance might be expected in the future. Even with the best intervention, the child who progressed only 2 months in gross motor skills during a 12-month period will probably not progress 12 additional months during the next 12-month period. The developmental history also allows the therapist to identify events that might have affected the child, either physically or psychologically.

Therapists, as well as other professionals, are becoming more aware of ethnicity influences on development in infancy and early childhood. Ethnicity encompasses the individual's cultural background, religion, language, and nationality. Ethnicity differs from race in that ethnicity refers to social characteristics, whereas race designates a group of individuals with specific physical characteristics. However, race is never independent of environmental and cultural contexts. Typically, Hispanic Americans, Asian Americans, Native Americans, and African Americans are considered both as racial and ethnic categories whereas Italian Americans, Irish Americans, and Polish Americans, for example, are referred to as ethnic groups. In examining ethnicity, the examiner must consider the environment in which the child is developing, including values, birth order, employment status of the parent or parents, and family unit in which the child (with or without siblings) is being raised. The family composition, a single mother or father, grandparents serving as parents, or foster parents, also must be taken into consideration. Handling practices may vary greatly among cultures. Certain activities may be practiced repeatedly, leading to differences in the age of sitting or standing.[7,8] For example, infants in Cameroon are expected to sit well by age 5 months, much earlier than children in other cultures.[7] Hopkins and Westra[8] found Jamaican, English, and Indian mothers differed in their expectations of motor skills development in their infants. The Jamaican mothers expected their infants to sit and to walk significantly earlier than did the Indian and English mothers.[7] Kolobe, in a study of Mexican American mothers in the United States, found evidence of differences among mothers' childrearing practices and parenting behaviors based on the level of acculturation.[9] Differences in childrearing and parenting behaviors also were related to the mother's level of education and socioeconomic status. In contrast to early accelerated motor development in children in some cultures, if the cultural expectations are to restrict movement in the infant (such as through swaddling), sitting and walking may be delayed if compared with Western norms.[10] Thus, if the examiner is unaware of the attitudes and values of the child's immediate family, an inaccurate picture may be obtained, especially during the early years. Of note, cultural practices may affect the pattern of early development but do not appear to have long-term consequences.

The effects of race and ethnicity have been studied for many years. Researchers using the Peabody Developmental Gross Motor Scales, Second Edition (PDMS–2)[11] found that the gross motor maturation of children of Hispanic descent was similar to that of children of Caucasian descent.[12] However, the authors concluded that children of African American descent consistently achieved gross motor skills at an earlier age than the normative sample of children from the PDMS–2. Thus, if these ethnicity differences were not taken into consideration when using the PDMS–2, the outcome of the tests might indicate that the child of African American descent was performing gross motor skills at an age-appropriate level when in fact the child actually had a delay when compared with peers. The use of culturally sensitive standardized tests and measures would most likely control for these variables when the therapist attempts to identify "typical" and "atypical" development.

The acculturation of the child also plays a major role in the assessment. Children who have limited exposure to toys may respond differently from the described "standard" response on a certain test. If the child has never seen a yellow tennis ball, but has seen yellow apples, he or she is apt to try to eat the ball rather than toss it.

Extrapersonal interactions to be considered during the assessment include the reaction of the child to the examiner and the conditions under which he or she is observed. Gender "mismatches" may affect the outcome of the testing. For example, if the only men that a child has been exposed to in the home environment were abusive, then his or her response to a male therapist might be affected. In other situations, a male therapist might be a great role model for a young boy in therapy, and the interaction would be strikingly different from the first scenario. Likewise, young boys who do not like girls because they have "cooties" might not respond appropriately to a female therapist. A child may not perform well because he or she refuses to cooperate with the examiner or refuses to separate from the parent. Some children may participate well under all circumstances and with any examiner, whereas other children might participate only in familiar surroundings. Communication problems with the parents also may interfere with obtaining adequate information about the child during the examination. Identification of ethnicity issues that might interfere with the establishment of rapport with the parent would be crucial prior to the examination if the test relies heavily on a parental questionnaire, such as the SPM–P.[5] The interpretation of the child's performance must be tentative, particularly if these extrapersonal interactions are affecting the assessment of the child. The child may actually be able to function at a higher level than what was formally assessed.

PURPOSES OF TESTS AND MEASURES

Tests and measures may be performed for the purposes of discrimination or placement, assessment of progress, or predicting outcomes. Tests and measures may be used to discriminate immature or atypical behaviors from "typical" behaviors. Very often these tests and measures are used for screening children to determine whether therapy services are necessary. Norm-referenced tests (those standardized on groups of individuals) must be used in this discrimination process to determine whether a child's performance is typical of a child of a similar age. Scores from norm-referenced tests usually are expressed as a percentile rank or a z-score. On some tests an age-equivalent score or a motor quotient may be given. Norm-referenced tests may allow the examiner to determine the developmental age of the child and to compare the child's performance with typically developing (TD) children. Tests such as the PDMS–2,[11] the BOT–2,[6] or the Test of Gross Motor Development, Second Edition (TGMD–2)[13] may be administered to determine which children need placement into intervention programs based on the developmental scores obtained. These norm-referenced tests also may be used for program placement, an important aspect of managing the child with special needs. The therapist must assess the level of the child's current functioning and then plan activities that will help the child progress in his or her abilities. A criterion-referenced test (one that measures a child's development of particular skills in terms of absolute levels of mastery) also may be appropriate for such program planning. Scores from criterion-referenced tests usually are expressed as a percentage of items passed or a scaled score. Items on the criterion-referenced tests may be linked directly to specific instructional objectives and therefore facilitate the writing of behavioral objectives for the child. Examples of criterion-referenced tests that serve this function are the GMFM–88 or GMFM–66[4] and the SFA.[3] The use of selective items from a norm-referenced test to develop behavioral objectives should be discouraged because this may lead to "teaching the test" and developing splinter skills. An example of this would be selecting items from the BOT–2 and then using the items and materials from the BOT–2 during the child's therapy sessions. Assessment of the child's progress using the same criterion-referenced test used for program planning is appropriate because the examiner wishes to determine whether he or she has achieved mastery of certain skills. Norm-referenced tests may be used, but the tests should be used only once or twice yearly so teaching the test does not occur. Overall program evaluation may be an important purpose of assessment. If one is comparing a new method of teaching gross or fine motor skills with a current method, assessment of the children in each group using a norm-referenced test would be imperative. The therapist would need to be able to compare the overall performance of each group of children with their peers as established by the norm-referenced tests.

Another classification of tests and measures may be described as "hybrids." These tests may allow for description of the child, such as "normal, at risk, or deficient." However, these terms represent a normal curve of functioning with a mean (normal), 1 standard deviation (SD) below the mean (at risk), and 2 SD below the mean (deficient).[14] Another example of terms used is from the Sensory Profile 2.[15] On the Sensory Profile 2, the child may be described as much less than other children, less than other children, like other children, more than other children, or much more than other children. These descriptive terms are based on a normal curve with like other children representing a mean score; less than or more than other children representing 1 ± SD from the mean; and much less and much more representing 2 ± SD from the mean.

Few tests used in physical therapy allow for prediction of outcomes based on a predictive index that classifies individuals based on what is believed or expected will be their future status. However, the Test of Infant Motor Performance (TIMP)[16] has been shown to predict the gross motor scores on the PDMS–2[11,17] when a child is preschool age and on the BOT–2[6] when a child is school age.[18] The motor growth curves that have been developed from the GMFM–66[4] for children with cerebral palsy (CP) also assist in estimating a child's future motor capabilities.[19]

Norm-Referenced Versus Criterion-Referenced Tests

The purposes of norm-referenced and criterion-referenced tests were described briefly in the preceding section. More delineation, however, needs to be made between the 2 types of tests. As previously stated, norm-referenced tests have standards or reference points that represent average performances derived from a representative group. *Criterion-referenced tests* have reference points that may not be dependent on a reference group. In other words, with criterion-referenced tests the child is competing against him- or herself, not a reference group. *Norm-referenced tests* may not overlap with actual objectives of instruction, whereas criterion-referenced tests are directly referenced to the objectives of instruction. Therefore, norm-referenced tests may not be as sensitive to the effects of instruction as criterion-referenced tests. Table 2-1 presents a comparison of norm-referenced and criterion-referenced tests in more detail.

Psychometric Characteristics of Tests

Norm-referenced tests must meet minimal standards of reliability and validity before being widely accepted. As with other tests, tests of motor abilities should be both reliable and valid. *Reliability* refers to the consistency between measures in a series. Types of test reliability include alternate forms, interrater, split–half (internal consistency), and test-retest. Alternate forms reliability assesses the relationship of scores by an individual on 2 parallel forms of the test. Interrater reliability examines the relationship between items passed and failed between 2 independent observers. Split–half reliability is the measure of internal consistency of a test. The test is split into 2 halves, and the scores obtained on the 2 halves by the individual are correlated. Test–retest reliability refers to the relationship of an individual's score on the first administration of the test to his or her score on the second administration. Test–retest reliability scores may be adversely affected by practice or memory. Scores for reliability often are expressed as percent agreement or correlational values obtained through statistical tests such as Spearman rho, Pearson product moment coefficient, intraclass correlation (ICC), or kappa.

Validity is the extent to which a test measures what it purports to measure. For example, the PDMS–2[11] is valid for measuring gross and fine motor skills, but not developmental reflexes or muscle tone. Three types of validity—construct, content, and criterion—are used to assess the viability of a test. Construct validity examines the theory or hypothetical constructs underlying

TABLE 2-1. COMPARISON OF NORM-REFERENCED AND CRITERION-REFERENCED MEASUREMENTS

NORM-REFERENCED	CRITERION-REFERENCED
Standard or reference points are average, relative points derived from the performance of a group	Reference points are fixed at specified cutoff points and do not depend on a reference group
Evaluates individual performance in comparison with a group of individuals; child competing against others	Evaluates individual performance in relation to a fixed standard; child competing against self
May or may not have a relationship to a specific instructional content	Is content specific
Tests may have a low degree of overlap with actual goals and objectives	Tests are directly referenced to the goals and objectives of instruction
Does not indicate when individuals have mastered a segment of the spectrum of goals and objectives	Identifies the goals and objectives that the individual has mastered
Designed to maximize variability and produce scores that are normally distributed	Variability of scores is not desired; a large number of perfect or near-perfect scores is desired
Designed to maximize differences among individuals	Designed to discriminate between successive performances of one individual
Requires good diagnostic skills	Geared to provide information for use in planning instruction
Tests are not sensitive to effects of the instruction	Tests are very sensitive to the effects of instruction
Is generally not concerned with task analysis	Depends on task analysis
Is more summative (used at the end of instruction) than formative, or is strictly diagnostic	Is more formative (used at various points during instruction) than summative, although it can be used both ways

the test. For example, the SFA[3] is based on the theory that children with functional limitations at school can be identified using the scales. Content validity refers to test appropriateness, or how well the content of the test samples the subject matter or behaviors about which conclusions are to be drawn. The specific items on the test must be representative of the behaviors to be assessed. Construct and content validity are determined not by using single measures of correlation but rather by examining the results of the tests. Criterion-related validity is measured by examining concurrent validity and predictive validity. Concurrent validity represents the relationship of the performance on the test with performance on another well-reputed test. Predictive validity examines the relationship of the test to some actual behavior of which the test is supposed to be predictive. For example, scores on the TIMP[16] for preterm infants have been shown to be predictive of later motor scores on the PDMS–2[11,17] at preschool age or on the BOT–2 at school age.[6,18]

Accuracy refers to the ability of a test to provide either positive predictive validity or negative predictive validity. *Sensitivity* indicates the ability of a measurement to detect dysfunction/

abnormality (ie, to identify those individuals with a positive finding who already have or will have a particular characteristic or outcome).[20] *Specificity* indicates the ability of a measurement to detect normality (ie, the proportion of people who have a negative finding on a test and who do not exhibit a certain particular characteristic). Newer tests often will provide this information for the clinician. For example, the sensitivity of the DeGangi-Berk Test of Sensory Integration[14] ranges from 0.66 for reflex integration to 0.84 for bilateral motor integration. The specificity of the DeGangi-Berk Test of Sensory Integration ranges from 0.64 for bilateral motor integration to 0.85 for the total test.

STANDARDIZED TESTS AND MEASUREMENTS USED IN PEDIATRIC PHYSICAL THERAPY

Standardized refers to tests commercially available to physical therapists that include directions for administration. These directions for administration allow the tests to be given in a "standard" format by a variety of individuals. Examples of standardized tests are the Timed Up and Go (TUG),[21-23] the Timed Up and Down Stairs (TUDS),[24] and the 6-Minute Walk Test (6MWT).[25,26] Standardized tests may be norm-referenced or criterion-referenced. Standardized tests may include just a test manual or a test manual as well as test materials. Other standardized tests may be found in a journal article that provides instructions for administration. The following section presents a description of selected tests and measurements used in pediatric physical therapy. The section is not all encompassing but rather presents tests and measurements frequently used for the purposes of examination and assessment in the evaluation process.

Newborn Developmental and Screening Assessments

NEUROLOGICAL ASSESSMENT OF THE PRETERM AND FULL-TERM INFANT[27]

1981

Dubowitz and Dubowitz

ICF Domains:	Body Functions and Structures; Activities
Purpose:	The purpose of the test is to provide information relative to neurologic maturation and changes in infants. The test documents deviations in neurologic signs and their eventual resolution.
Ages:	Full-term infants up to the third day of life; preterm infants up to term gestational age beginning when infant can tolerate handling and is medically stable.
Time:	10 to 15 minutes for testing and scoring
User Qualifications:	Medical professionals who have knowledge of neonatal neurology
Test Materials:	Consists of manual and score sheets
Test Areas:	Test items are drawn from the assessment tools of Saint-Anne Dargassies,[28] Prechtl,[29] Parmelee,[30] and Brazelton.[31] Areas assessed include habituation, movement and tone, reflexes, and neurobehavioral.
Administration:	The infant is assessed two-thirds of the time between feedings. Scoring is performed on a 5-point ordinal scale. All the items do not have to be administered with each infant, and no single total score is achieved. The pattern of responses, however, is examined and compared with case histories described in the test manual. Infants are categorized as normal, abnormal, or borderline depending on tone, head control, or a number of deviant signs noted during the examination.
Psychometric Properties:	**Criterion-referenced** No **reliability** information is reported on the scale by the authors. **Concurrent validity** was determined by comparing the results on the scale with ultrasound scans used to detect intraventricular bleeds. The results revealed that 24 of 31 infants born at less than 36 weeks' gestation with ultrasound evidence of a bleed had 3 or more abnormal clinical signs out of 6 items administered, as compared with only 2 of 37 infants of the same gestational age without evidence of intraventricular bleeds.[27] Of the 37 infants without evidence of intraventricular bleeds, 21 had no abnormal clinical signs as compared with only 1 of the 31 infants with documented bleeds. **Predictive validity** was determined by comparing scores for 66 very low birth-weight infants tested at term and then followed at 4 months post-term with a magnetic resonance imaging assessment. **Sensitivity** was found to be 88% and **specificity** was 46%.[32]

NEONATAL BEHAVIORAL ASSESSMENT SCALE (NBAS)[31,33]

1984

Brazelton

ICF Domains:	Body Functions and Structures; Activities
Purpose:	The purpose of the test is to provide a behavioral scale for infants from birth to the approximate post-term age of 2 months and to describe an infant's interaction with the caregiver. The NBAS is not considered a neurologic assessment, although it contains some neurologic items as outlined by Prechtl.[34]
Ages:	Full-term neonates, 37 to 48 weeks postconceptual age; additional items are given for infants born before 37 weeks
Time:	The test takes 30 to 35 minutes to administer. An additional 10 to 15 minutes are required for scoring.
User Qualifications:	A training program is recommended for examiners to become reliable in administration.
Test Materials:	Consists of manual and score sheets
Test Areas:	Includes assessment of the infant's state of consciousness and use of state to maintain control of his or her reactions to environmental and internal stimuli, which is thought to be an important mechanism reflecting the infant's potential for organization of sensory input. For each of the behavioral items, the appropriate state of consciousness for testing is indicated.
	Areas tested include the following: (1) ability to organize states of consciousness; (2) habituation of reactions to disturbing events; (3) attention to and processing of simple and complex environmental events; (4) control of motor activity and postural tone; and (5) performance of integrated motor acts.
	Nine supplementary items are used for the preterm or fragile infant and address the quality of alert responsiveness, cost of attention, examiner persistence, general irritability of the neonate, robustness and endurance, regulatory capacity, state regulation, balance of muscle tone, and reinforcement value of the infant's behavior.
Administration:	The initial test is conducted ideally on the third day after birth (because the infant may be disorganized during the first 48 hours) and between feedings. Each of the biobehavioral items is scored individually according to the criteria given in the test manual. The mean score for each item is based on the behavior exhibited by an average full-term (7 pounds [3.2 kg]), normal Caucasian infant with an Apgar scale score of no less than 7 at 1 minute and 8 at 5 minutes, and whose mother did not have more than 100 mg of barbiturates for pain or 50 mg of other sedative drugs as premedication in the 4 hours prior to delivery. The infant is scored on his or her best, not average, performance. Seven total cluster scores for the infant are obtained.

continued

NEONATAL BEHAVIORAL ASSESSMENT SCALE (NBAS)[31,33]

Psychometric Properties:

Criterion-referenced

Construct and **content validity** were demonstrated by Tronick and Brazelton,[35] who showed that NBAS was superior to a standard neurologic examination given during the neonatal period.

Predictive validity demonstrated through prediction of mental and motor scores on the Bayley Scales of Infant Behavior with correlation scores of 0.67 to 0.80.[33] Bakow et al reported good correlations between the test's items of alertness, motor maturity, tremulousness, habituation, and self-quieting with infant temperament at 4 months.[36] Ohgi and colleagues,[37] in a sample of 209 preterm infants (born 36 to 38 weeks, 40 to 42 weeks, or 44 to 46 postmenstrual age [PMA]) who were again tested at age 5 years, assessed the sensitivity and specificity of the NBAS. Of these infants the sensitivity was 50% to 78% for classification as mild disability and 71% to 85% for correct classification as severe disability. The specificity was found to be 94% to 97%.

Interrater reliability is stated to be at 0.90 if one completes training at 1 of the 6 training sites.

Test–retest reliability: Sameroff[38] found low test-retest relationships between days 2 and 3 in a group of full-term infants. Test-retest reliabilities, however, may be affected by changes in the infant's chronological age, behavioral state, and internal physiologic state.

TEST OF INFANT MOTOR PERFORMANCE (TIMP)[16]

2001

Campbell

ICF Domains:

Body Functions and Structures; Activities

Purpose:

Comprehensive assessment of developing head and trunk control as well as selective control of arms and legs. The test is currently in its fifth version.

Ages:

The test is given 34 weeks PMA to 4 months postterm in premature infants; 4 months chronologic age (CA) in term-born infants. Age-related standards based on performance of white (non-Hispanic), black (African and African American), and Latino (Mexican and Puerto Rican) infants from the Chicago metropolitan area.

Time:

The test takes 25 to 45 minutes to administer and score.

User Qualifications:

Physical therapists, occupational therapists, and other professionals in the neonatal intensive care unit

Test Materials:

Consists of test manual and score sheets; need rattle, squeaky toy, bright red ball, and soft cloth

continued

TEST OF INFANT MOTOR PERFORMANCE (TIMP)[16]

Test Areas: The TIMP has 2 sections: (1) observed scale of 13 dichotomously scored items used to examine spontaneous movements, such as head centering and individual finger, ankle, and wrist movements; and (2) elicited scale of 29 items scored on 5-, 6-, or 7-point scales, which assesses the infant's responses to placement in various positions and to sights and sounds.

Administration: All observations and test procedures should be conducted with infants in state 3, 4, or 5 as defined by Brazelton in the NBAS. Verbal and/or visual prompts may be used. No more than 3 trials are allowed for each item. If the infant fails to meet the full criterion, the behavior is scored at the next lower response level. Based on the infant's outcome on the test, he or she is described as average, low average, below average, or far below average. A shorter version, the Test of Infant Motor Performance Screening, is now available for screening purposes. This version takes about half the time to administer and is useful when assessing infants who are fragile or who need rapid screening.

Psychometric Properties:

Norm-referenced

Content validity: Expert review of items by experienced pediatric physical therapists, occupational therapists, and psychologists. Item analysis was funded by the Foundation for Physical Therapy.

Construct validity: The TIMP has been found to be sensitive to age changes with scores being highly correlated with age ($r = 0.83$).[39]

Discriminative validity is supported by cross-sectional studies using TIMP that demonstrated that children with many medical complications have significantly lower scores than healthier children.[40]

Concurrent validity: Correlation between raw scores on the TIMP and on the Alberta Infant Motor Scales (AIMS)[41] was $r = 0.64$.[42] The correlation between the TIMP raw scores and the AIMS percentile ranks was $r = 0.60$ ($P = .0001$). The TIMP score also identified 80% of infants at the same level as the AIMS.

Predictive validity was assessed by comparing scores on the TIMP in 96 infants who were assessed at 32 weeks PMA to 4 months CA and then assessed at age 6 months using the AIMS.[43]

Sensitivity was found to be 62.5% and **specificity** was 77.4%. However, for infants reassessed at 9 months, the sensitivity was 91.5% and specificity was 75.7%. Kolobe et al found that gross motor outcomes on the PDMS–2 for at-risk preterm infants could be predicted by the TIMP when these children were preschool age.[17] In another study of 35 preterm and term infants who were assessed at 32 weeks PMA to 4 months CA and then again at age 4 years 9 months using the BOT–2, sensitivity was found to be 50% and specificity was 100%.[18]

Test–retest reliability was assessed over a 3-day period on 106 infants (White, Black, and Latino). The participants ranged in age from 32 weeks post-CA to 16 weeks post-term. Reliability was found to be $r = 0.89$ ($P < .0001$), with 54% of the scores varying less than 8 points out of a possible 170 points.[44]

Interrater reliability of $r = 0.949$ was found if the therapists were trained. The test developers recommend that rate agreement of 90% on item ratings with experienced testers should be obtained when training new TIMP users.

GENERAL MOVEMENTS ASSESSMENT (GMA)[45]

2001

Prechtl

ICF Domains:	Body Functions and Structures; Activities
Purpose:	The purpose of the test is to identify infants at risk for impairments and to predict later adverse neurodevelopment outcomes.
Ages:	Birth to 20 weeks post-term (corrected for prematurity)
Time:	The test takes 10 to 30 minutes.
User Qualifications:	Formal training required; basic and advanced courses are available.
Test Materials:	Manual
Test Areas:	General movements involve the whole body with a variable sequence of arm, leg, neck, and trunk movements, which wax and wane in intensity and force. These general movements are present from 9 weeks to 48 weeks PMA. At term age, these general movements are described as writhing movements and involve small to moderate amplitude ellipsoid form movements with slow to moderate speed. Fidgety movements are present from 9 to 20 weeks post-term and are small movements of moderate speed and variable acceleration of neck, trunk, and limbs in all directions. Abnormal general movements include: poor repertoire (monotonous movements with complexity); cramped synchronous (rigid movements with lack of fluency and simultaneous contraction of limb and trunk muscles); chaotic (large amplitude movements with no fluency or smoothness); absent fidgety (a total absence of fidgety movements); and abnormal fidgety (exaggeration of amplitude, speed, and jerkiness of fidgety movements).
Administration:	The infant is observed lying supine while calm and alert. The infant should not have any toys or pacifiers. Parents may be watching but not interacting with their baby. The baby is observed or videotaped for 3 to 5 minutes and then scored on the type of movements seen.
Psychometric Properties:	**Criterion-referenced** **Construct validity:** General movements at one month and 3 months are strongly correlated with white-matter abnormalities on magnetic resonance imaging at term and general movements correlate with neurological examinations.[3,46-49] **Concurrent validity:** Low correlation between the GMA and the TIMP has been documented. **Predictive validity:** Summary estimates of **specificity** scores of 91% and **sensitivity** scores of 98% have been reported. The persistence of cramped synchronous movements and the absence of fidgety movements have been reported as predictors of cerebral palsy when the assessment is performed during the time frame of fidgety movements.[46,50,51] However, lower specificity (48%) and sensitivity (88%) were found in a group of very low birth-weight infants at 4 months postterm.[32] **Interrater reliability** of 90% has been shown when assessed with trained examiners using videos.

Screening Tests

QUICK NEUROLOGICAL SCREENING TEST, THIRD EDITION (QNST–3)[52]

2012

Mutti, Martin, Sterling, and Spalding

ICF Domains:	Body Functions and Structures; Activities
Purpose:	This test was developed to provide an empirically based assessment of the development of motor coordination and sensory integration tasks considered soft neurological signs. The original QNST was published in 1974, revised in 1978, and reprinted with minor revisions in 1998 as the QNST–II. The QNST–3 is intended to be used only as a screening instrument for soft neurological signs that may be associated with learning and everyday functions. However, the QNST–3 provides norms based on a nationally representative sample that extend from childhood through geriatrics.
Ages:	5 years through geriatrics (older than age 80 years)
Time:	This test takes approximately 20 minutes to administer and 10 minutes to score.
User Qualifications:	Psychologists, rehabilitation specialists, occupational therapists, and physical therapists
Test Materials:	The test manual has complete instructions for administration.
Test Areas:	Consists of 15 tasks that have been adapted from standard traditional neurological exams and developmental scales. Allows for observation of motor maturity and development, sensory processing, gross and fine muscle control, motor planning and sequencing, sense of rate and rhythm, spatial organization, visual and auditory perception, balance and vestibular function, and disorders of attention.
Administration:	The test is composed of 15 tasks:

- Hand skill
- Figure recognition and production
- Palm form recognition (graphesthesia)
- Eye tracking
- Sound patterns
- Finger to nose
- Thumb and finger circle
- Double simultaneous stimulation of hand and cheek
- Rapidly reversing repetitive hand movements (diadochokinesia)
- Arm and leg extension
- Tandem walk
- Stand on one leg
- Skipping

continued

QUICK NEUROLOGICAL SCREENING TEST, THIRD EDITION (QNST–3)[52]

- Left-right discrimination
- Behavioral irregularities

Each task is scored based on the types of errors observed. The error scores are given a weight of either 1 or 3; scores are tallied for each task, and then summed across all tasks for an overall score. The score sheet provides criteria for scores of 0, 1, or 3. The raw scores for each task and the overall raw score are interpreted according to cutoff scores, which allow for the child to be described as having no discrepancy (at or above the 25th percentile), a moderate discrepancy (between the 24th and 6th percentiles), or a severe discrepancy (at or below the 5th percentile) in function.

Psychometric Properties:

Criterion-referenced

Standardization for the Third Edition was performed on 1400 individuals between the ages of 4 years 0 months and 97 years. Testing was conducted at 43 sites in 21 states across the US. Institutions included public, private, and parochial schools; clinics; and private practice settings.

Content and **construct validity** of the test were developed through use of tasks commonly used in standard neurological exams. Additionally, developmental changes, motor skills, cognitive ability, and clinical group differences were considered in the selection of tasks. Factor analyses were used to further explore the relationships among the tasks.

Internal consistency was assessed by examining the item difficulty index. Because the motor tasks used in the QNST–3 are expected to have been developed by late childhood, high item difficulty indices were expected and found during the examination.

Test–retest reliability when the test was given on an average of 20 days apart was found to be at or above 0.70, demonstrating sufficient stability over time.

BRUININKS-OSERETSKY TEST OF MOTOR PROFICIENCY, SECOND EDITION (BOT–2)[6]

2005

Bruininks and Bruininks

The short form of the BOT–2 can be used for screening purposes, such as early identification of motor problems. Discussion on the use of the BOT–2 will be included in the section on comprehensive developmental testing.

Motor Development and Motor Control Tests

ALBERTA INFANT MOTOR SCALES (AIMS)[41]

1994

Piper and Darrah

ICF Domains:	Body Structures; Activities
Purpose:	The AIMS was developed to be used in the identification of motor delay (discrimination), the evaluation of change in motor performance over time resulting from maturation or intervention, and the provision of useful information for treatment planning.
Ages:	Birth to 18 months
Time:	This test takes 20 to 30 minutes to administer and score.
User Qualifications:	Physical therapists
Test Materials:	A test manual and score sheets are included. No specific toys, prompts, or conditions are used.
Test Areas:	The infant is tested in 4 positions (supine, prone, sitting, and standing). A total of 58 gross motor skill items are included. Three aspects of motor performance are observed: weight-bearing, posture, and anti-gravity movement.
Administration:	The test can be conducted in the clinic or the home. The infant should be unclothed and allowed to set the pace and momentum of the test. Minimal handling should be performed by the therapist. Each item on the test is scored as "observed" or "not observed." For each of the 4 positions, the sum of the observed items is a positional score. The sum of the positional scores is the total score that is then converted to a percentile rank.
Psychometric Properties:	**Norm-referenced**

A normative sample consisted of 2202 infants from Alberta, Canada, who were chosen based on age and sex. However, no information was provided regarding the race or ethnicity of children used in the norming. Questions regarding the use of the AIMS with children from different races or ethnicity have been raised.[53]

Construct validity was determined by comparing scores from infants who were identified as at risk or with known motor delays against the norms that had been established.[54] The authors stated that using the scores allowed the identification of infants as "abnormal," "at risk," or "normal."[55]

For **concurrent validity,** the total scores on the AIMS of 103 TD infants and 68 abnormal or at-risk infants were correlated with the PDMS gross motor raw scores and with the motor scales of the Bayley Scales of Infant Development. Correlation coefficients between 0.84 and 0.99 were determined for the TD infants and between 0.93 and 0.95 with the abnormal and at-risk infants.[53]

continued

ALBERTA INFANT MOTOR SCALES (AIMS)[41]

Interrater reliability was assessed using 2 therapists and 253 TD infants. Using the Pearson product moment coefficient, r values ranged from 0.96 to 0.99.

Test–retest reliability was assessed using the same 253 infants. Using the Pearson product moment coefficient, r values ranged from 0.86 to 0.99 when the same assessor scored the AIMS on both testing days. However, the r values ranged from 0.82 to 0.94 if a different assessor performed the test–retest. The lowest reliability scores were noted in the infants who were birth to age 3 months. (See Figure 2-1.)

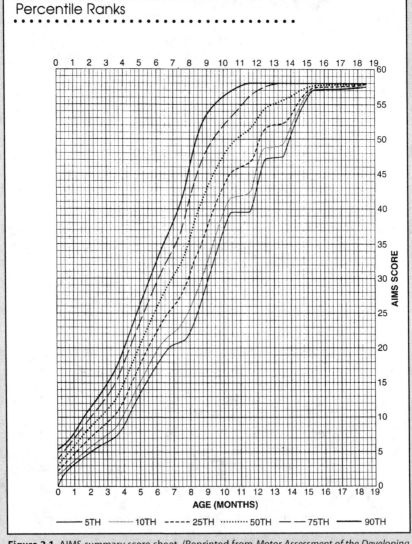

Figure 2-1. AIMS summary score sheet. (Reprinted from *Motor Assessment of the Developing Infant*, Piper MC, Darrah J. Copyright 1994, with permission from Elsevier.)

TODDLER AND INFANT MOTOR EVALUATION (TIME)[56]

1994

Miller and Roid

ICF Domains:	Body Structures; Activities
Purpose:	The TIME has 3 specific purposes: (1) to identify those children who are suspected to have motor delays or deviations, (2) to develop appropriate interventions, and (3) to conduct treatment efficacy research.
Ages:	4 months to 3 years 6 months
Time:	Administration time for entire assessment ranges from 10 to 20 minutes for young children and 20 to 40 minutes for older children. Scoring takes additional time and amount of time depends on examiner's familiarity with the test. The functional performance subtest interview requires an additional 15 minutes.
User Qualifications:	Occupational therapists and physical therapists
Test Materials:	The test manual and score sheets are very thorough. Written descriptions and line drawings are given for each item. The child is engaged in play in a familiar environment with a varying sequence of task presentation.
Test Areas:	Five primary subtests include mobility, motor organization, stability, functional performance, and social/emotional abilities. Three optional subtests are recommended to be used by advanced clinicians and researchers. These include component analysis, quality rating, and atypical positions.
Administration:	The test has a specific order of administration with the subtests given in the following order: social/emotional, mobility or motor organization, stability, and functional performance. The social/emotional abilities subtest is completed before and after the test session and addresses state/activity level, attention, and emotions/reactions. The mobility and motor organization subtests are scored during observations of the parent or parents playing with the child. The items are grouped into 4 developmental levels and are scored on a pass/fail scale. Stability is assessed and scored based on observations of the child during the mobility and motor organization subtests. The functional performance subtest is administered by the examiner through an interview with the parents. The subtest includes questions related to self-care, self-management/mastery, relationships/interactions, and function in the community. The 5 primary subtests yield scaled scores.

continued

TODDLER AND INFANT MOTOR EVALUATION (TIME)[56]

Psychometric
Properties:

Normed-referenced for the 5 primary subtests; the optional subtests are not norm-referenced.

Norming occurred on a sample of 731 children from across the United States who did not have motor delays or deviations. The sample was stratified by age, race/ethnicity, gender, and socioeconomic status. Children with biological or environmental risk for developmental delays were not included in the sample.

Construct validity was determined by analyzing children with and without motor delays using the test. A standardized mean difference between groups with and without delays averaged 1.5 SD. Age trend analysis also showed that with increasing age, children performed an increasing number of items and mastered increasingly more difficult items.[59]

Interrater reliability of the test has been found to range from 0.88 for motor organization to 0.99 for mobility when using the Pearson product moment correlation.[56]

Test–retest reliability using the same examiner is reported to range from $r = 0.96$ for mobility to $r = 0.99$ for motor organization and atypical positions.[56]

Specificity scores have been reported for mobility (92.6%), stability (96.9%), and atypical positions (98.6%).

Sensitivity scores have been reported for mobility (88.2%), stability (80.6%), and atypical positions (97.2%).

BAYLEY SCALES OF INFANT AND TODDLER DEVELOPMENT, THIRD EDITION (BAYLEY–III)[57]

2006

Bayley

ICF Domains:	Body Structures; Activities
Purpose:	The primary purpose is to identify developmental delay and to monitor a child's developmental progress.
Ages:	1 to 42 months
Time:	The test takes 25 minutes to 1 hour dependent on the child's age.
User Qualifications:	Psychologists, physical therapists, occupational therapists
Test Materials:	The test manual for the Bayley–III provides in-depth explanations of how the test is to be administered.
Test Areas:	The Bayley–III consists of 5 distinct scales: 3 scales administered to the infant or toddler by an evaluator (Cognitive scale, Language scale, and Motor scale), and 2 scales completed by the parent or main caregiver (the Social-Emotional scale and the Adaptive Behavior scale). The Motor scale includes a Fine Motor subtest and Gross Motor subtest.
Administration:	The test is individually administered with scoring according to the test manual. Types of scores that are available from the Bayley–III scales and subtests are scaled scores, percentile ranks, confidence intervals, and developmental age equivalents (AEs). The Bayley–III composite scores are derived from the sum of subtest scaled scores.
Psychometric Properties:	**Norm-referenced**

The Bayley–III represents a revision of the Bayley Scales of Infant Development, Second Edition. The Bayley–III was standardized using a random sample of 1700 American children aged 1 to 42 months. There were equal numbers of boys and girls selected to give the same proportions indicated in the US 2000 Census for parent education level, race/ethnicity, and geographic region. The goals of the revision were to: (1) update reference data, item administration, and stimulus materials; (2) develop 5 distinct scales (Cognitive, Language, Motor, Social-Emotional, and Adaptive Behavior); (3) strengthen the psychometric quality of the instrument; (4) improve the clinical utility of the instrument; and (5) simplify administration procedures.

Construct validity: The Bayley–III Motor Scale has demonstrated a very high level of internal consistency ($r=0.92$). Very high levels of internal consistency for special groups within subtests also were reported in the technical manual (fine motor, $r=0.94$, and gross motor, $r=0.98$). Special group studies included children with high incidence characteristics (eg, premature birth) and/or clinical diagnoses, such as pervasive developmental disorder, Down syndrome (DS), language impairments, small for gestational age, prenatal alcohol exposure, CP, and intrapartum asphyxia.

continued

BAYLEY SCALES OF INFANT AND TODDLER DEVELOPMENT, THIRD EDITION (BAYLEY–III)[57]

Concurrent validity: When scores on the Bayley–III Motor Scale were compared with scores of motor ability from several other motor development assessments, the correlations were found to range from low to moderate, with the majority being of moderate strength. Correlations between the Bayley–III and other tests that were lower included the PDMS–2 (total motor 0.57, fine motor 0.48, gross motor 0.51); Adaptive Behavior Assessment System, Second Edition (total motor 0.33, fine motor 0.14, gross motor 0.42); and the Vineland Adaptive Behavior Scale, Interview Edition (total motor 0.62).[57] Connolly et al studied 48 children representing 4 age groups (< 6 months, 6 to 12 months 15 days, 12 months 16 days to 18 months, > 18 months) using the Bayley–III and the PDMS–2. Moderate to very high correlation for all groups was found between the Bayley–III composite scores and the PDMS–2 Total Motor quotient scores (0.69 to 0.95). High correlations (0.90 to 0.94) were found between the Bayley–III composite scores and the PDMS–2 Gross and Fine Motor Quotients (age groups 12 to 26 months), high correlations (0.83) were found between the Bayley–III and the PDMS–2 Gross Motor quotient (6 to 12 months), and moderate correlations (0.59) were found for younger age groups. High concurrent validity (0.74 to 0.94) for AE scores was found only in the group above 18 months. Low to Moderate (−0.23 to −0.40) negative correlations were found in the group of children between ages 6 months to 12 months 15 days. Correlations between all AE scores for the younger than 6 months and the 12 months 16 days to 18 month age were low.[58] Milne and colleagues also reported that the use of composite scores for the Bayley–III underestimates the degree of developmental delay among children assessed for diagnosis of disability. They suggest the use of developmental quotients rather than composite scores may allow the full range of developmental disabilities to be identified.[59]

Test–retest reliability correlations are reported in the technical manual as being high (0.79 to 0.94).

Interrater reliability has been reported as high (0.76).[57]

PEABODY DEVELOPMENTAL MOTOR SCALES, SECOND EDITION (PDMS–2)[11]

2000

Folio and Fewell

ICF Domains:	Body Functions and Structures; Activities
Purpose:	The PDMS–2 was designed to (1) estimate a child's motor competence, (2) compare gross and fine motor disparity, (3) provide qualitative and quantitative aspects of individual skills, (4) evaluate a child's progress, and (5) provide a research tool.
Ages:	Birth to 6 years
Time:	Total test requires 45 to 60 minutes. Each section requires 20 to 30 minutes to administer.
User Qualifications:	Physical therapists, occupational therapists, early-intervention specialists, adapted physical educators, psychologists
Test Materials:	The PDMS–2 materials include the Examiner's Manual, Profile/Summary Form, Examiner Record Booklet, Guide to Item Administration, Motor Activities Program, Peabody Motor Development Chart, manipulatives, and optional computerized scoring program.
Test Areas:	The PDMS–2 comprises 6 subtests:

- Reflexes (Gross Motor, Birth to 11 months)
- Stationary (Gross Motor)
- Locomotion (Gross Motor)
- Object Manipulation (Gross Motor, 12 months to 6 years)
- Grasping (Fine Motor)
- Visual-Motor Integration (Fine Motor)

Administration:	The Guide to Item Administration provides detailed descriptions of each item. Each item description includes: (1) the age at which 50% of the children in a normative sample mastered the item, (2) the testing position, (3) the stimulus (if needed), (4) the procedure to be used to test the item, (5) the criteria for scoring the item, and (6) an illustration of a child performing the item. The testing environment may be in a room, hallway, or even outdoors. The child should wear nonslippery shoes or be barefoot. For seated items, the child's feet should touch the floor. If necessary, the parent or caregiver may remain during the testing. Items are scored on a 3-point scale. Raw scores are converted to AE, percentiles, and standard scores. Standard scores are converted to 3 indexes of motor performance: gross motor, fine motor, and total motor.

continued

PEABODY DEVELOPMENTAL MOTOR SCALES, SECOND EDITION (PDMS–2)[11]

Psychometric
Properties:

Norm-referenced

Norming took place on a sample of 2003 children residing in 46 states and one Canadian Province during winter 1997 and spring 1998. The demographics used for the norming mirrored the US Bureau of the Census data.

Construct validity has been addressed through **convergent validity** of the Movement Assessment Battery for Children (Movement–ABC) and the PDMS–2 with fair to good correlations (0.71 to 0.76).[60]

Content validity was used to determine whether the test content covered a representative sample of the behavior domain to be measured. The PDMS–2 items were based on a developmental framework and a taxonomy of psychomotor domain that incorporated hierarchical sequencing.[61] The gross motor quotient has good to high internal consistency (0.96).[11] Content validity also was assessed through item analysis and item response theory modeling.

Criterion-predictive validity studies compared the scores on the PDMS–2 with the original PDMS and with the Mullen Scales of Early Learning (MSEL:A). Correlation values between the PDMS–2 and the PDMS were 0.84 for the gross motor quotient and 0.91 for the fine motor quotient. Correlation values between the PDMS–2 and the MSEL:A were 0.86 for the gross motor scores and 0.80 for the fine motor scores.[11] The gross motor quotient for the PMDS–2 has variable concurrent validity with other gross motor tests (0.30 to 0.86).[11,58,62-64]

Interrater reliability was assessed using 2 examiners who reviewed 30 completed protocols for 3- to 11-month-old infants and 30 completed protocols for 15- to 36-month-old children.

Interscorer reliability values ranged from 0.96 (total motor scores) to 0.99 (locomotion).[11]

Test–retest reliability testing was performed on children in the 2 age groups of 2 to 11 months and 12 to 17 months. The Pearson product moment coefficients were found to range from 0.73 (fine motor quotient in 2- to 11-month-old infants) to 0.96 (total motor quotient for 12- to 17-month-old infants). Wang and colleagues found test–retest reliability to be high to very high (ICC = 0.88 to 1.00) in children with CP.[65] (See Figure 2-2.)

continued

PEABODY DEVELOPMENTAL MOTOR SCALES, SECOND EDITION (PDMS–2)[11]

PDMS-2

Profile/Summary Form

Peabody Developmental Motor Scales
Second Edition

Section I.   Identifying Information

Child's Name _ELIZABETH S._   Female ☒   Male ☐

	Year	Month	Day	
Date Tested	02	05	09	Examiner's Name
Date of Birth	00	07	08	Examiner's Title ___
Chronological Age	61	10	01	
Prematurity Adjustment	—	—		
Corrected Age	___	___	___	
Age in Months	___			

Section II.   Record of Scores

PDMS-2	Raw Score	Age Equivalent	%ile		Standard Scores	
Reflexes					___	___
Stationary	36	11 months	4	7		___
Locomotion	80	15 months	2	4		___
Object Manipulation	6	13 months	5	5		___
Grasping					___	___
Visual–Motor Integration	___	___	___		___	___

Sum of Standard Scores   [16]   [ ]   [ ]

	GMQ	FMQ	TMQ
Quotients	(70)	( )	( )
Percentiles	2%	___	___

Section III.   Profile of Scores

Standard Scores	Reflexes	Stationary	Locomotion	Object Manipulation	Grasping	Visual–Motor Integration	Standard Scores	Quotients	Gross Motor	Fine Motor	Total Motor	Quotients
20	.	.	.	.	.	.	20	150	.	.	.	150
19	.	.	.	.	.	.	19	145	.	.	.	145
18	.	.	.	.	.	.	18	140	.	.	.	140
17	.	.	.	.	.	.	17	135	.	.	.	135
16	.	.	.	.	.	.	16	130	.	.	.	130
15	.	.	.	.	.	.	15	125	.	.	.	125
14	.	.	.	.	.	.	14	120	.	.	.	120
13	.	.	.	.	.	.	13	115	.	.	.	115
12	.	.	.	.	.	.	12	110	.	.	.	110
11	.	.	.	.	.	.	11	105	.	.	.	105
10							10	100				100
9	.	.	.	.	.	.	9	95	.	.	.	95
8	.	.	.	.	.	.	8	90	.	.	.	90
7	.	.	.	.	.	.	7	85	.	.	.	85
6	.	.	.	.	.	.	6	80	.	.	.	80
5	.	.	.	.	.	.	5	75	.	.	.	75
4	.	.	.	.	.	.	4	70	.	.	.	70
3	.	.	.	.	.	.	3	65	.	.	.	65
2	.	.	.	.	.	.	2	60	.	.	.	60
1	.	.	.	.	.	.	1	55	.	.	.	55

Figure 2-2. Profile/summary form for PDMS–2. (Reprinted with permission from Folio MR, Fewell RR. *Peabody Developmental Motor Scales.* 2nd ed. Austin, TX: Pro-Ed; 2000.)

Test of Gross Motor Development, Second Edition (TGMD–2)[13]

2000

Ulrich

ICF Domains:	Body Functions and Structures; Activities
Purpose:	The test was developed to assess gross motor functioning in children. The author states that test can be used for identification and screening, instructional programming, assessment of individual progress, program evaluation, and as a research tool.
Ages:	3 to 10 years
Time:	The test takes 15 to 20 minutes to administer and score.
User Qualifications:	Physical therapists
Test Materials:	Test manual and score sheets included in test materials. Examiner must supply materials, which are described in the manual. Comes with software for quick scoring entry.
Test Areas:	(1) Locomotor and (2) object control
Administration:	Items are individually administered to the child. The test conditions should be arranged prior to testing to facilitate ease of administration. Children should wear rubber-soled shoes or be barefoot during the testing. Each item on the test contains 3 to 4 specific performance components that indicate mastery of the skill. Each of the performance components is scored as 1 if observed for 2 of 3 trials and 0 if not observed for 2 of 3 trials. Practice and 3 test trials are given for each component. Raw scores are converted to percentiles, standard scores, and AE scores for the 2 areas (locomotor and object control) in addition to a total gross motor quotient.
Psychometric Properties:	**Norm-referenced**

Ulrich used the 1997 US Census to ensure that the normative sample represented the nation as a whole using geographic area, sex, race, residence, educational attainment of parents, disability status, and age as the stratification criteria (1208 children from 10 states were used in the normative sampling).[13]

Content validity was based on discriminative powers of the test, which identified children who were significantly behind their peers.
Criterion-predictive validity study revealed that scores on the TGMD–2 compared positively to scores on the Comprehensive Scales of Student Abilities. When the tests were administered 2 weeks apart, a moderate correlation of 0.63 was found.[13]

Content sampling was performed to assess internal consistency. R values ranged from 0.76 to 0.94.[13]

Interrater reliability on the test was found to be very high, with correlational values of 0.98 found for locomotor, object control, and the gross motor quotient.[13]

Test–retest reliability scores for a sample of children between ages 3 and 10 years ranged from 0.88 to 0.96.[50] (See Figure 2-3.)

continued

TGMD-2

Test of Gross Motor Development–Second Edition

Profile/Examiner Record Form

TEST OF GROSS MOTOR DEVELOPMENT, SECOND EDITION (TGMD-2)[13]

Section I. Identifying Information

Name

Male ☐   Female ☐   Grade

Date of Testing

Date of Birth

Age

School

Referred by

Reason for Referral

Examiner

Examiner's Title

Section II. Record of Scores

First Testing

	Raw Score	Standard Score	Percentile	Age Equivalent
Locomotor				
Object Control				

Sum of Standard Scores

Gross Motor Quotient

Second Testing

	Raw Score	Standard Score	Percentile	Age Equivalent
Locomotor				
Object Control				

Sum of Standard Scores

Gross Motor Quotient

Section III. Testing Conditions

A. Place Tested

	Interfering				Not Interfering
B. Noise Level	1	2	3	4	5
C. Interruptions	1	2	3	4	5
D. Distractions	1	2	3	4	5
E. Light	1	2	3	4	5
F. Temperature	1	2	3	4	5
G. Notes and other considerations					

Section IV. Other Test Data

Name of Test	Date	Standard Score	TGMD-2 Equivalent

Section V. Profile of Standard Scores

Standard Scores	Locomotor	Object Control	Standard Scores	Quotients	Gross Motor Quotient	Quotients
20			20	150		150
19			19	145		145
18			18	140		140
17			17	135		135
16			16	130		130
15			15	125		125
14			14	120		120
13			13	115		115
12			12	110		110
11			11	105		105
10			10	100		100
9			9	95		95
8			8	90		90
7			7	85		85
6			6	80		80
5			5	75		75
4			4	70		70
3			3	65		65
2			2	60		60
1			1	55		55

Copyright © 2000, 1985 by PRO-ED, Inc.
3   4   5   04   03   02   01

1

Figure 2-3. Profile/examiner record form. (Reprinted with permission from Ulrich D. *Test of Gross Motor Development*. 2nd ed. Austin, TX: Pro-Ed; 2000.)

BRUININKS-OSERETSKY TEST OF MOTOR PROFICIENCY, SECOND EDITION (BOT–2)[6]

2005
Bruininks and Bruininks

ICF Domains:	Body Functions and Structures; Activities; Participation
Purpose:	The purpose of the test is to assess gross and fine motor skills in children and to assist in decision making about appropriate educational and therapeutic placement. The short form of the test can be used for screening for special purposes, such as early identification of developmental problems.
Ages:	4 to 21 years
Time:	The complete battery typically takes 45 to 60 minutes to administer whereas the short form can be administered in 15 to 20 minutes. Software for quick scoring entry is provided to save time.
User Qualifications:	Physical therapists, occupational therapists, psychologists, physical educators, special education teachers
Test Materials:	Easel-based instructions, largely image-based for universal utility and minimal verbal components. Certain items on the tests are identified for use as a short form and can be administered for screening. Most equipment for the test is included in the test materials.
Test Areas:	The test comprises 4 subscale areas: (1) Fine Manual Control, (2) Manual Coordination, (3) Body Coordination, and (4) Strength and Agility. The Fine Manual Control subtests address fine motor precision and fine motor integration, which represent control and coordination of distal musculature needed for grasping, writing, and drawing. The Manual Coordination subtests address manual dexterity and upper-limb coordination, which represent control and coordination needed for object manipulation. Subtests addressing bilateral coordination and balance are in the Body Coordination subscale. The Strength and Agility subscale addresses running speed and agility and strength, which are needed for locomotion and recreational/competitive sports.
Administration:	Items are individually administered to the child. All items on the test are to be administered, although some items may be difficult for younger children. Raw scores from each of the subtests can be converted into point scores and scale scores that may be further converted to standard scores for each of the 4 subscales. From the standard scores, a total motor composite score and a percentile rank for each of the subscales can be calculated. In addition, age-equivalent levels for each of the specific subtests in the subscales can be determined.
Psychometric Properties:	**Norm-referenced** The BOT–2 was standardized on a nationally representative sample of 1520 children ages 4 to 21 years. Twelve age groups were included in the sample with equal numbers of boys and girls included. The sample selection was random and stratified based on the most current US Census across sex, race/ethnicity, region of the US, socioeconomic status, and disability status in each age group.[6]

continued

BRUININKS-OSERETSKY TEST OF MOTOR PROFICIENCY, SECOND EDITION (BOT–2)[6]

Validity: The manual reports that validity of the BOT–2 is based on how well it assesses the constructs of motor development or proficiency.

Construct validity is stated to be present because of the statistical characteristics of the test.

Content validity has been established by experts, revealing anticipatory improvements with aging.[6] Validity also was assessed by comparing the scores of TD children with the scores of children with developmental coordination disorder (DCD), mild to moderate intellectual disabilities, and high-functioning autism/Asperger disorder. Wuang and Su, in a study of children with intellectual disability, found internal consistency of the total scale to be excellent (ICC = 0.99).[66]

Concurrent validity was supported by the relationship of the BOT–2 and the PDMS–2 in children ages 4 and 5 years. Correlation between the BOT–2 total motor composite and the PDMS–2 total motor quotient was found to be 0.73.[6] The relationship between the BOT–2 fine motor subtests and the Test of Visual Motor Skills–Revised has been examined and a high relationship found (0.74).

Split–half reliability has been reported as ranging from the high 0.70s to the mid-0.90s for the subscales, composites, and short form scores.[6]

Interrater reliability correlations have been reported to be very high (0.92 to 0.99) for all subtests except for Fine Motor Precision, which had a high (0.86) interrater reliability.[6]

Test–retest reliability has been reported to be between 0.69 to the low 0.80s for the subscale scores and from the mid to upper 0.80s for the total motor composite as well as for the short form.[6]

GROSS MOTOR FUNCTION MEASURE 88 (GMFM–88)[4]

2002

Russell, Rosenbaum, Avery, and Lane

ICF Domain:	Activities
Purpose:	The purpose of this observational instrument is to measure change in gross motor function over time. Therapists have indicated that the test is also useful for (1) describing the child's current level of motor function, (2) determining treatment goals, and (3) providing easy explanations to parents concerning their child's progress.
Ages:	The original validation sample included children ages 5 months to 16 years; GMFM–88 or GMFM–66 is appropriate for children whose motor skills are at or are below those of a 5-year-old child without any motor disability.

continued

GROSS MOTOR FUNCTION MEASURE 88 (GMFM–88)[4]

Time:	The test takes 45 to 60 minutes. An additional session can be scheduled for a child who tires before completing the entire test. However, the second session should be held within one week and any item completed during the first session should not be retested. The GMFM–66 takes less time to administer because there are fewer items.
User Qualifications:	Physical therapists
Test Materials:	Test materials required to administer the GMFM–88 generally are found in a physical therapy department. The test manual is essential for scoring of the test forms.
Test Areas:	Eighty-eight items are used to assess activities of motor function in 5 dimensions: (1) lying and rolling; (2) sitting; (3) crawling and kneeling; (4) standing; and (5) walking, running, and jumping. The GMFM–66 is composed of a subset of the 88 items identified as contributing to the measure of gross motor function in children with CP.
Administration:	The test should be administered in an environment that is comfortable for the child. The floor should be a smooth, firm surface and there should be adequate room for the child to move freely. The test items are individually administered with a demonstration and 3 trials for each item. A generic scoring system is present based on how much of each activity the child can complete. Each item is scored on a 4-point rating scale. In addition to a total score, a score may be obtained for each of the 5 dimensions. Each dimension score and the total score are converted to a percentage of the maximum score for that dimension. The GMFM–66 requires a computer program (the GMAE) for scoring.
Psychometric Properties:	**Criterion-referenced**

The GMFM–88 has been validated on children between ages 5 months and 16 years. The total validation sample included 111 children with CP, 25 with head injury, and 34 preschoolers with no known physical disabilities.[67] Of the 111 children with CP, 88 had spastic CP and 23 had nonspastic CP. Russell et al also have shown that the GMFM–88 is a valid measure of change in gross motor function in children with CP.[68] The total GMFM score was correlated with parents' judgments of change in motor function (0.54) and therapists' judgments (0.65). Additionally, Trahan and Malouin found the GMFM–88 was sensitive to changes over an 8-month period in gross motor performance in a group of children with different types of CP.[69] Russell and colleagues have shown that the GMFM–88 is a valid measure of change for children with DS and is responsive to differences in potential for change among children with DS.[70] The GMFM–66 is valid only for children with CP because the scaling was developed only from children with CP.[19] The GMFM–66 scaling allows for the (1) ordering of difficulty of all of the GMFM–66 items, (2) creation of an "item map" that displays the relative level of difficulty of each step of each item, and (3) provision of an "interval level measure."

continued

GROSS MOTOR FUNCTION MEASURE 88 (GMFM–88)[4]

Interrater reliability ICCs for children with CP range from 0.87 (lying and rolling) to 0.99 (standing, walking, running, and jumping; total).[67] Ruck-Gibis et al found ICCs for interrater reliability to be 0.98 for the lying and rolling dimension and 0.99 for the other dimensions and total score when testing children diagnosed with osteogenesis imperfecta (OI).[71] In children with DS, ICCs for interrater reliability have been reported as ranging from 0.73 (lying and rolling) to 0.98 (standing).[70]

Intrarater reliability ICCs computed for children with CP range from 0.92 for standing to 0.99 for all other dimensions as well as the total score.[67] The intrarater reliability ICCs for children with OI were calculated to be 0.99 for all 5 dimensions and the total score.[71]

Test–retest reliability has been assessed with children with DS and found to be very high. The ICCs were found to range from 0.87 (crawling and kneeling) to 0.99 (standing).[67] The high test–retest reliability indicates the GMFM is stable over a short period of time when no real change in the child's function is expected to occur. (See Figure 2-4.)

GMFM

SUMMARY SCORE

DIMENSION	CALCULATION OF DIMENSION % SCORES	GOAL AREA (indicated with ✓ check)
A. Lying & Rolling	$\dfrac{\text{Total Dimension A}}{51} = \dfrac{33}{51} \times 100 = \underline{65}\ \%$	A. ☐
B. Sitting	$\dfrac{\text{Total Dimension B}}{60} = \dfrac{33}{60} \times 100 = \underline{55}\ \%$	B. ☑
C. Crawling & Kneeling	$\dfrac{\text{Total Dimension C}}{42} = \dfrac{15}{42} \times 100 = \underline{36}\ \%$	C. ☑
D. Standing	$\dfrac{\text{Total Dimension D}}{39} = \dfrac{1}{39} \times 100 = \underline{3}\ \%$	D. ☑
E. Walking, Running & Jumping	$\dfrac{\text{Total Dimension E}}{72} = \dfrac{0}{72} \times 100 = \underline{0}\ \%$	E. ☐

TOTAL SCORE $= \dfrac{\%\,A + \%\,B + \%\,C + \%\,D + \%\,E}{\text{Total \# of Dimensions}}$

$= \dfrac{65 + 55 + 36 + 3 + 0}{5} = \dfrac{159}{5} = 32\ \%$

Figure 2-4. GMFM summary score sheet. (Reprinted with permission from Russell DJ, Rosenbaum PL, Avery LM, Lane M. *Gross Motor Function Measure [GMFM–66 and GMFM–88] User's Manual.* London, England: Mac Keith Press; 2002.)

PEDIATRIC BALANCE SCALE (PBS)[72]

2003

Franjoine, Gunther, and Taylor

ICF Domains: Body Functions and Structures; Activities; Participation

Purpose: The purpose of the test is to measure balance in school-age children with mild to moderate motor impairments.

Ages: 3 to 15 years; most appropriate for children ages 3 to 6 years[73]

Time: This test takes approximately 20 minutes.

User Qualifications: Physical therapists, occupational therapists

Test Materials: Instructions and score sheets from Franjoine et al.[72] The PBS requires a minimal use of specialized equipment, all of which must be supplied by the examiner.

Administration: The test is composed of 14 tasks. Each task is demonstrated and written instruction is given to the child. Each child receives a practice trial, and a second trial may be given if there is a question about the ability of the child to understand the directions. Each item is scored using a 0- to 4-point scale with a maximum total score of 56. A higher score indicates better balance performance. Multiple trials are allowed on many of the items. The child's performance is scored based on the lowest criteria, which describe the child's best performance.

Psychometric Properties: **Criterion-referenced**

Construct validity: An average range of scores for TD children has been determined and published.[73] The PBS was administered to 643 TD children ages 2 years 4 months to 13 years 7 months. However, although typical performance ranges and cut points based on 95% confidence intervals of the means were suggested, differentiation of performance was limited in children developing typically beyond the age of 6 years.

Reliability studies were performed using 20 children ranging in age from 5 to 15 years with mild to moderate motor impairments.

Test–retest reliability was assessed with the initial test and repeat testing being conducted within 14 days. Test–retest reliability was found to be 0.998. The test–retest reliability for individual items ranged from 0.89 to 1.0 when using the Spearman signed ranked correlation.

For **interrater reliability**, 10 pediatric physical therapists with varied clinical experience viewed and scored the videotaped performance of 10 children. High interrater reliability was demonstrated via an ICC $(3.1) = 0.997$.

PEDIATRIC REACH TEST (PRT)[74]

1994

Donahoe, Turner, and Worrell

ICF Domain:	Activities
Purpose:	The purpose of the test is to measure balance and postural control in sitting and standing through forward reaching and side reaching.
Ages:	5 to 15 years
Time:	The test takes approximately 15 minutes.
User Qualifications:	Physical therapists, occupational therapists
Test Materials:	Instructions and score sheets are available at Donahoe et al.[74] The PRT requires minimal use of equipment (measuring tape, benches of different heights), all of which must be supplied by the examiner.
Administration:	Testing is performed with the child sitting on a bench and then in standing. In sitting, the child is instructed to lift his or her preferred arm forward to 90 degrees, make a fist, and then reach forward as far as possible. The distance between the starting position and the ending position of the hand is determined. The reaching motion is repeated to the right side and then to the left side. The test is then repeated in standing. The difference between the start and the end positions are determined for each of the reaches. A total score is obtained by summing the interval data as measured in cm. Information about an average total reach in cm for ages 5 to 6 years, 7 to 8 years, 9 to 10 years, 11 to 12 years, and 13 to 15 years is available.[74] Additionally, an average total reach in cm is available based on height in 7- to 16-year-old children.[75]
Psychometric Properties:	**Criterion-referenced** **Construct validity** has been supported with the observation of high correlations between the standing section of the PRT and a laboratory test of steadiness in quiet stance (–0.79) and age (–0.83). Construct validity was also supported with a high correlation between the total PRT score and the Gross Motor Function Classification System (GMFCS) level (–0.88) among a sample of children with CP.[74] **Concurrent validity** has been supported with the observation of moderate to high correlations between the standing section of the PRT and laboratory tests of limits of stability (0.42 to 0.77).[76] **Reliability** studies were performed using 10 children with CP ages from 2.6 to 14.1 years.[74] **Test–retest reliability** was determined using 2 pediatric physical therapists who assessed each of these 10 children twice, 2 weeks apart. ICCS were found to be between 0. 54 to 0.88 for the total test scores and scores on the individual items on the test. For **interrater reliability,** the same 2 pediatric physical therapists assessed each of the 10 children. An interrater reliability of 0.50 was found for the first assessment of the children and 0.93 for the second assessment.

TIMED UP AND GO (TUG)[21,22]

1991: Podsiadlo and Richardson

2000: Shumway-Cook

ICF Domain:	Activities
Purpose:	Purposes of the test are to measure functional ambulation, mobility, and dynamic balance.
Ages:	3 years to adult; reference values for different ages have been reported.[23,77]
Time:	The test takes 5 minutes.
User Qualifications:	Physical therapists
Test Materials:	The TUG requires minimal equipment: a stopwatch, chair, and tape or other marker, all of which must be supplied by the examiner.
Administration:	The TUG was originally developed for use with adults. However, in children the protocol has been modified to allow for use of a chair with or without arms[78] or a backrest.[79] The protocol has also been modified to allow for a barefoot walk, a walk with footwear,[80,81] or a walk with orthotics.[80,81] Basic instructions are to measure, in seconds, the time taken by a child to stand up from an adjustable-height chair (with height of the seat adjusted so the child's knees and hips are flexed to 90 degrees when sitting with feet resting on the floor), walk a distance of 3 meters, turn, walk back to the chair, and sit down again.

Psychometric Properties:

Criterion-referenced

Construct validity has been supported with the observation that the TUG discriminates between GMFCS Levels I, II, and III in children with CP.[79,82]

Concurrent validity has been supported by studies that demonstrate the TUG correlates moderately to high with the GMFM–88 (–0.524, –0.89).[78,79] High inverse correlations have been found between the TUG and the Berg Balance Scale (–0.88) in children with CP.[78]

Test–retest reliability has been demonstrated to be high (ICC > 0.83) in children who are TD between the ages of 3 and 14 years,[83] in children with CP with GMFCS levels of I to III, and in children with DS. Test–retest reliability was found to be very high (ICC > 0.970).[82-85]

Interrater reliability and **intrarater reliability** have been shown to be excellent (ICC = 0.99) in TD children between the ages of 4 and 11 years[84] and 8 and 14 years.[79] In children with CP with GMFCS levels of I to III, interrater reliability was found to be high to very high (ICC = 0.834 to 0.996).[82-84]

6-Minute Walk Test (6MWT)[25]

2002
Guidelines from the American Thoracic Society

ICF Domain:	Activities
Purpose:	The purposes of the test are to measure functional exercise capacity in children, provide a screening tool and a method to monitor changes over time, and provide a method to evaluate the effects of interventions to improve functional mobility.
Ages:	4 to 11 years Reference values for different ages are available.[26,86] Reference values of children with spastic CP ages 4 to 17 years at GMFCS Levels I to III are available.[87]
Time:	The test takes 10 minutes.
User Qualifications:	Physical therapists
Test Materials:	Tape measure, tape or other marker
Administration:	A walking course is marked in a large open space (gym, large corridor) with tape. A cone or other marker is placed at the starting point of each lap. At "go," the child walks as fast as possible (without running) for 6 minutes. The therapist can provide verbal encouragement every 30 seconds. At the end of 6 minutes, laps completed are measured and converted to distance walked.
Psychometric Properties:	**Norm-referenced** **Construct validity** has been supported with the observation that the 6MWT discriminates between GMFCS Levels I and II in children with CP ages 10 to 16 years (0.948).[88] Significant differences ($P<.001$) between the 6MWT scores of children with CP across GMFCS Levels I to III and TD children also have been reported.[87] The 6MWT is viewed as a valid assessment of functional exercise capacity in children with juvenile idiopathic arthritis, end-stage renal disease, hemophilia, congenital heart disease, and cystic fibrosis.[89-92] **Concurrent validity** has been supported by a study of healthy children between the ages of 12 to 16 years that showed a moderate and significant correlation (0.44, $P<.0001$) between the 6MWT and peak oxygen uptake.[93] **Test–retest reliability** has been demonstrated to be very high in children with CP with GMFCS levels of I to III between ages 4 and 18 years (ICC=0.98)[94] and 11 and 17 years (ICC=0.98).[95]

Timed Up and Down Stairs (TUDS)[24]

2004

Zaino, Marchese, and Westcott

ICF Domains: Activities; Participation

Purpose: The purpose of the test is to measure functional mobility, which reflects the ability to be active in the community, home, and during recreational activities.

Ages: 8 to 14 years (can be used with younger children with caution)

Time: The test takes 5 minutes.

User
Qualifications: Physical therapists

Test Materials: One flight of stairs consisting of 14 steps (height 19.5 cm per step) and bilateral handrails.

Administration: The child is asked to stand 30 cm from the bottom of a 14-step flight of stairs. The instruction to "Quickly but safely go up the stairs, turn around on the top step (landing), and come all the way down until both feet land on the bottom step (landing)" is given. The child is allowed to choose any method of traversing the stairs. This includes using a step-to, a foot-over-foot pattern, running up the stairs, skipping stairs, or any other variation. However, the child is required to face in the direction of movement (up or down) during the stair climbing. The TUDS score is the time in seconds from the "go" cue until the second foot returns to the bottom landing. Shorter times indicate better functional ability.

Psychometric
Properties: **Criterion-referenced**

Construct validity has been examined by use of correlation and Kruskal-Wallis analysis of variance across ages and in 3 functional level groups according to the GMFCS in a sample of 47 children ages 8 to 14 years: 20 children with CP and 27 TD children. The correlation between the TUDS and age was moderate but significant, both for the CP (–0.61) and TD groups (–0.41). Significant differences in TUDS scores were found between all 3 functional level groups.[24]

Concurrent validity: Moderate to high Spearman rank correlations between the TUDS scores and performance on the TUG (0.78), the Functional Reach Test (–0.57), and a Timed One Legged Stance (–0.77) in a sample of 47 children ages 8 to 14 years (20 children with CP and 27 TD children) have been reported.[24]

Test–retest, interrater, and intrarater reliability were assessed in a sample of 47 children ages 8 to 14 years (20 children with CP and 27 TD children).[24] Interrater and intrarater reliabilities for the TUG and Timed One Legged Stance were very high with ICC (2,1) equal to 0.99.[83] The interrater and intrarater reliabilities for the Functional Reach Test also were very high with ICC (2,1) being 0.97 and 0.98, respectively. In a study of 12 children with DS between the ages of 3 and 17 years, test–retest reliability was found to be very high (ICC 2, 0.974).[85]

GOAL ATTAINMENT SCALE (GAS)[96]

1968

Kiresuk and Sherman

ICF Domains:	Body Functions and Structures; Activities; Participation Goals can be set for any of the ICF domains.
Purpose:	The purpose of the test is to measure change by defining an individualized set of goals; emphasis is placed on measurement of functioning that is not readily measured by traditional outcome measures.
Ages:	School-aged children
Time:	Varies
User Qualifications:	Physical therapists, occupational therapists
Test Materials:	None
Administration:	Goals are developed based on the student's specific areas of need based on the student, team, and family priorities. Goals are written to be relevant, understandable, measurable, attainable, and time limited.[97] A 5-point scale as developed by Kiresuk and Sherman is used to identify 5 possible outcomes for each goal. Table 2-2 represents the 5-point scale that is used for the GAS and how the goals might be charted.[96]
Psychometric Properties:	**Criterion-referenced**

Construct validity has been supported through studies with TD children and children with a variety of diagnoses.

Content validity and the responsiveness of the GAS was examined by Palisano in a study of 21 infants with motor delays. Ten physical therapists were asked to rate 10 randomly selected GAS-formatted goals on 3 dimensions. Palisano found 77% to 88% of the physical therapists' ratings for each of 3 different dimensions examined by the therapists met the criterion for content validity. Additionally, change that could not be measured with the behavioral objective format was measured with the GAS format for 61% of the goals.[98] Brown et al found the GAS to be responsive to change in a group of 24 children age 4 years who were born extremely preterm.[99]

Concurrent validity: Steenbeek et al assessed the responsiveness of the GAS compared with the Pediatric Evaluation of Disability Inventory (PEDI) and the GMFM–66 in a group of 23 children with CP ages 2 to 13 years. The contents of the 3 measures were compared using the ICF–CY codes. Spearman rho correlations between the GAS change scores and the change scores obtained with the PEDI functional skills scale and the GMFM–66 were calculated. Significant correlations were found between the GAS change scores and the PEDI mobility scale as measured by physical therapists (0.57, $P = .01$), between the GAS change scores and the PEDI Social Function scale as measured by speech pathologists (0.73, $P = .01$), and the GAS change scores and the

continued

Goal Attainment Scale (GAS)[96]

PEDI Self-Care scale as measured by occupational therapists (0.73, $P < .01$). However, 22% of the GAS items for the children in the study were not covered by items on the PEDI or the GMFM–66.[100]

Interrater reliability was determined by level of agreement among therapists trained on the GAS and the treating therapist on the amount of improvement 16 school-age children made in their goals. The level of agreement was found to be in the moderate range (0.60).[101] Steenbeek and colleagues examined interrater reliability of the GAS between scales constructed by the children's own therapists and by independent therapists for 23 children with CP. The scales constructed by the children's therapists had an interrater reliability of 0.82, whereas the reliability for the independent raters was 0.64. The disagreement was attributed to the professionals' interpretation of the children's capacities vs their actual performance during assessment.[102]

Table 2-2. The Five Levels of the Goal Attainment Scale

ATTAINMENT LEVEL	SCORE	ACTIVITY
Much less than expected	–2	
Somewhat less than expected	–1	
Expected performance or outcome	0	
Somewhat more than expected outcome	+1	
Much more than expected outcome	+2	

Adapted from Kiresuk TJ, Sherman RE. Goal attainment scaling: a general method for evaluating comprehensive community mental health programs. *Community Ment Health J.* 1968;4(6):443-453.

Sensorimotor Tests

SENSORY PROFILE 2[15]

2014

Dunn

ICF Domains:	Body Functions and Structures; Participation
Purpose:	The purpose of the test is to provide a set of standardized tools for evaluating a child's sensory processing patterns in the context of everyday life. The information from the test provides a way to determine how sensory processing may be contributing to or interfering with participation. When combined with other information about the child in context, professionals can plan effective interventions to support the child, family, and educators as they interact with each other throughout the day.
Ages:	Birth to 14 years 11 months
Time:	Varies based on the age of the child. Should take no more than 30 minutes to administer and 15 to 20 minutes to score.
User Qualifications:	Occupational therapists, physical therapists, psychologists, speech-language pathologists, teachers
Test Materials:	User manual and 5 rater questionnaires: • Infant Sensory Profile 2 (English and Spanish versions) • Toddler Sensory Profile 2 (English and Spanish versions) • Child Sensory Profile 2 (English and Spanish versions) • Short Sensory Profile 2 (English and Spanish versions) • School Companion Sensory Profile 2 (English version only)
Test Areas:	Each of the profiles contains questions related to general processing as well as auditory, visual, touch, vestibular, proprioceptive, and oral sensory processing. The Short Sensory Profile gives quick information on sensory processing for screening and research purposes. For the Toddler Sensory Profile 2, the Short Sensory Profile 2 ,and the School Companion Sensory Profile 2, a score is given for Behavioral Responses Associated with Sensory Processing. For the Child Sensory Profile 2, 3 scores are provided for Behavioral Responses: Conduct Associated with Sensory Processing, Social Emotional Responses Associated with Sensory Processing, and Attentional Responses Associated with Sensory Processing. Sensory Pattern scores also are obtained from the questionnaires. The child's pattern may be described as seeking/seeker, avoiding/avoider, sensitivity/sensor, or registration/bystander based on Dunn's Sensory Processing Framework. The School Companion Profile 2 contains 4 additional scores that reflect the teacher's point of view about the student. The School Factor scores reflect the student's need for external supports to participate in learning, the student's awareness and attention within the learning environment, the student's tolerance within the learning environment, and the student's availability for learning.

continued

SENSORY PROFILE 2[15]

Administration: Caregivers and teachers who have regular contact with the child complete a questionnaire that describes the child's responses to daily sensory experiences. The questionnaires are available for paper-based or web-based administration.

Each questionnaire includes a number of items:

- Infant Sensory Profile 2 to 25 items
- Toddler Sensory Profile 2 to 54 items
- Child Sensory Profile 2 to 86 items
- Short Sensory Profile 2 to 34 items
- School Companion Sensory Profile 2 to 44 items

Each item is scored on a scale that corresponds to the frequency the caregiver(s) observes the behavior:

- Almost always=5 points
- Frequently=4 points
- Half the time=3 points
- Occasionally=2 points
- Almost never=1 point
- Does not apply=0

Raw scores obtained in each of the areas then are compared with cut scores determined for each area. Based on the scores obtained, the child's performance in each of the areas may be described as much less than others (score more than –2 SD from the mean), less than others (score between –1 SD and –2 SD from the mean), just like the majority of others (score between –1 SD and +1 SD from the mean), more than others (score between +1 SD to +2 SD from the mean), or much more than others (score more than +2 SD from the mean).

Psychometric Properties:

Criterion-referenced

The national standardization sample study took place from 2012 to 2013 and included evaluations of 1791 children between the ages of birth and 14 years. A further 774 children with disabilities participated in the clinical validity studies (matched with 774 children without disabilities). This resulted in the overall inclusion of 75 infants (ages birth to 6 months), 404 toddlers (ages 7 months to 35 months), 1056 children for the Child Sensory Profile 2 (3 years to 14 years 11 months), and 1030 children for the School Companion Sensory Profile 2 (3 years to 14 years 11 months) with and without disabilities. Children were selected from 4 regions of the US (West, Midwest, South, and Northeast). The children included in the study were Caucasian, African American, Hispanic, Asian, and Other. Percentages of children in each of these groups were similar to the percentages found in the most recent US Census.

Construct and **content validity** were addressed through the use of literature review, expert review, and preliminary pilot studies.

continued

SENSORY PROFILE 2[15]

Convergence (concurrent) validity was assessed by comparing scores from the Sensory Profile 2 with scores from the original Sensory Profile Questionnaires, the Behavioral Assessment System for Children, Second Edition, Social Skills Improvement System Rating Scales (SSIS), Vineland–2, and the SFA. Detailed correlational values for each of the various questionnaires that comprise the Sensory Profile 2 are included in the user manual.

Discriminant validity was assessed by collecting data from parents and children in several vulnerable groups. These vulnerable groups included children with developmental delays, children with autism spectrum disorders, children with attention-deficit/hyperactivity disorder, children with learning disabilities, and gifted and talented children. In each case, a child was identified in the typical sample matched for age and sex to a child in a vulnerable group. A multivariable analysis of variance was conducted with each paired group to determine whether the appropriate form discriminated between the groups.

Internal consistency (reliability) was assessed using Cronbach alpha. The values for alpha for the various sections ranged from 0.57 to 0.93.

SENSORY PROCESSING MEASURE—PRESCHOOL (SPM–P)[5]

2010

Home Form: Ecker and Parham

School Form: Miller Kuhaneck, Henry, and Glennon

ICF Domains:	Body Functions and Structures; Participation
Purpose:	The purposes of the test are to provide norm-referenced indices of function in the visual, auditory, tactile, proprioceptive, and vestibular sensory systems, as well as the integrative functions of praxis and social participation; to provide descriptive clinical information on processing vulnerabilities within each sensory system; and to allow for comparisons of the child's functioning in home, preschool, and community environments.
Ages:	2 to 5 years
Time:	The test takes 15 to 20 minutes to administer and 5 to 10 minutes to score.
User Qualifications:	Occupational therapists, physical therapists, psychologists, speech-language pathologists, teachers
Test Materials:	User manual, SPM–P Home AutoScore Form, SPM–P School AutoScore Form

continued

SENSORY PROCESSING MEASURE—PRESCHOOL (SPM–P)[5]

Test Areas:

The SPM-P School Form and the SPM-P Home Form each has 75 items. Each form yields 8 norm-referenced standard scores: Social Participation; Vision; Hearing; Touch; Body Awareness; Balance and Motion; Planning and Ideas; and Total Sensory Systems.

Administration:

The SPM–P Home Form is completed by the child's parent or home-based care provider. The SPM–P School Form is completed by the child's primary preschool teacher or child care provider. Each item on the form is scored using a descriptor that corresponds to the frequency with which the caregiver(s) or teacher observes the behavior in the child:

- Never: The behavior never or almost never happens
- Occasionally: The behavior happens some of the time
- Frequently: The behavior happens much of the time
- Always: The behavior always or almost always happens

The standard score for each of the areas assessed allows for classification of the child's function into 1 of 3 interpretative ranges: Typical, Some Problems, or Definite Dysfunction. Table 2-3 provides examples of Body Awareness (proprioception) questions that would be asked on the Home Form and the School Form. In each of the areas assessed on the SPM–P, questions specific to the home or the school environment are asked. Additionally, an Environment Difference score allows comparison of the child's sensory functioning between home and preschool/child care environments.

Psychometric Properties:

Norm-referenced

The Home Form and School Form were standardized on a demographically representative sample of 651 TD children. The 2007 US Census data were used to select a sample that was a close approximation to Census figures. Separate norms were developed for 2-year-old and 3- to 5-year-old children because of the developmental differences between the 2 groups.

Content validity was addressed through the use of literature review and expert review.

Construct or **structural validity** was assessed through factor analysis, interscale correlations, item-scale correlations, and rating scale validity.

Convergence (concurrent) validity was assessed by comparing scores from the SPM-P with scores from the Short Sensory Profile,[103] the Infant/Toddler Sensory Profile,[104] and the Sensory Profile School Companion.[105] Detailed correlational values for these comparisons are included in the user manual.

Discriminant validity was assessed by using a separate sample of 242 children receiving occupational therapy intervention to verify that the scales could differentiate TD children from those with clinical disorders. The Home Form Total Sensory Systems cut score of 60 was found to have a sensitivity of 0.64 and specificity of 0.84. The School Form Total Sensory Systems cut score of 60 had a sensitivity of 0.52 and specificity of 0.82.

Internal consistency (reliability) for the Home Form ranged from 0.75 to 0.93 and for the School Form from 0.72 to 0.94.

Test–retest reliability for the Home Form ranged from 0.90 to 0.98 and for the School Form from 0.90 to 0.96.

TABLE 2-3. EXAMPLES OF BODY AWARENESS (PROPRIOCEPTION) QUESTIONS ON THE SENSORY PROCESSING MEASURE—PRESCHOOL

HOME FORM	SCHOOL FORM
Grasps objects so tightly that difficult to use objects	Moves chairs roughly
Grasps objects so loosely that difficult to use objects	Accidently breaks glue sticks, crayons, or pencils; tears paper from too much force
Lots of pushing, pulling, jumping	Jumps excessively; crash landings from heights
Exerts too much pressure during tasks	Bumps into peers excessively
Chews on toys, clothes, or other objects more than other children	Closes scissors forcefully with tight squeeze for each snip

Adapted from Miller Kuhaneck H, Ecker C, Parham LD, Henry DA, Glennon TJ. *Sensory Processing Measure—Preschool (SPM–P): Manual.* Los Angeles, CA: Western Psychological Services; 2010.

SENSORY PROCESSING MEASURE (SPM)[106]

2007

Home Form: Parham and Ecker

School Form: Miller Kuhaneck, Henry, and Glennon

ICF Domains:	Body Functions and Structures; Participation
Purpose:	The purpose of the test is to provide an integrated system of rating scales that enables assessment of sensory processing issues, praxis, and social participation in elementary school-aged children.
Ages:	5 to 12 years
Time:	The test takes 15 to 20 minutes to administer and 5 to 10 minutes to score.
User Qualifications:	Occupational therapists, physical therapists, psychologists, speech-language pathologists, teachers
Test Materials:	User manual, SPM Home Form, SPM Main Classroom Form, School Environments Form (on unlimited-use compact disc)
Test Areas:	The SPM Home Form consists of 75 items. The SPM Main Classroom Form has 62 items. Each form yields 8 norm-referenced standard scores: Social Participation; Vision; Hearing; Touch; Body Awareness (Proprioception); Balance and Motion (Vestibular); Planning and Ideas (Praxis); and Total Sensory Systems. The SPM School Environments Form is designed to be completed by teachers and other school staff members who work with and observe the child in the following 6 settings: Art Class, Music Class, Physical Education, Recess/Playground, Cafeteria, and School Bus. Each rating sheet has 15 items except for the School Bus sheet (10 items).

continued

Sensory Processing Measure (SPM)[106]

Administration: The SPM Home Form is completed by the child's parent or home-based care provider. The SPM Main Classroom Form is completed by the child's primary classroom teacher. Each item on the form is scored using a descriptor that corresponds to the frequency with which the caregiver(s) or teacher observes the behavior in the child:

- Never: The behavior never or almost never happens
- Occasionally: The behavior happens some of the time
- Frequently: The behavior happens much of the time
- Always: The behavior always or almost always happens

The standard score for each of the areas assessed allows for classification of the child's function into one of 3 interpretative ranges: typical, some problems, or definite dysfunction. Additionally, an environment difference score allows comparison of the child's sensory functioning between home and school environments.

Psychometric Properties: **Norm-referenced**
The Home Form and School Form were standardized on a demographically representative sample of 1051 typical children based on the 2007 US Census. Census data were used to select a sample that was a close approximation to the US population of children. A subsample of 360 children from the standardization study was used to develop scores and establish cutoff criteria for the School Environments Form.

Content validity was addressed through the use of literature review and expert review.

Construct or **structural validity** was assessed through factor analysis, interscale correlations, item-scale correlations, and rating scale validity.

Convergence (concurrent) validity was assessed by comparing scores from the SPM with scores from the Short Sensory Profile,[103] the Sensory Profile,[104] and the Sensory Profile School Companion.[105] Detailed correlational values for these comparisons are included in the user manual.

Discriminant validity was assessed by testing a separate sample of 345 children receiving occupational therapy intervention to verify that the scales could differentiate TD children from those with clinical disorders. The Home Form Total Sensory Systems cut score of 60 was found to have a sensitivity of 0.85 and specificity of 0.85. This means that 85% of children with sensory processing disorders have scores of 60 or greater and 85% of TD children had scores of 59 or less. The Main Classroom Form Total Sensory Systems cut score of 60 was found to have a sensitivity of 0.53 and specificity of 0.85.

Internal consistency (reliability) for the Home Form ranged from 0.77 to 0.93 and for the Main Classroom Form from 0.75 to 0.95.

Test–retest reliability for the Home Form ranged from 0.94 to 0.98 and for the Main Classroom Form from 0.95 to 0.98.

SENSORY PROFILE FOR ADOLESCENTS/ADULTS[107]

2002

Brown and Dunn

ICF Domains:	Body Functions and Structures; Participation
Purpose:	The purposes of the test are to capture information about an individual's sensory processing, link sensory processing with everyday experiences, provide information for theory-based decision making, and include the individual in the assessment and intervention process.
Ages:	11 to 65+ years
Time:	The test takes 10 to 15 minutes to complete and 20 minutes to score.
User Qualifications:	Occupational therapists, physical therapists, adult education teachers, psychologists, social workers, vocational counselors
Test Materials:	The profile consists of a user manual, a self-questionnaire, and a summary score sheet.
Test Areas:	Areas of assessment include taste/smell processing, movement processing, visual processing, touch processing, activity level, and auditory processing.
Administration:	The test is administered in 4 general ways: (1) the self-questionnaire can be sent to the individual with a cover letter explaining the purpose of the instrument; (2) the individual can complete the form while the therapist is present; (3) the therapist can administer the instrument by reading and recording the individual's responses to each item; or (4) the questionnaire can be completed in a group setting with the therapist present and available to answer questions.

Each item is scored on a scale that corresponds to the frequency with which the individual responds in the manner described:

- Almost always (100%)=5 points
- Frequently (75%)=4 points
- Occasionally (50%)=3 points
- Seldom (25%)=2 points
- Almost never (5%)=1 point

Raw scores obtained in each of the areas are then compared with cut scores that were determined for each area. Based on the scores obtained, the individual's performance in each of the areas may be described as much less than most people, less than most people, similar to most people, more than most people, or much more than most people.

continued

SENSORY PROFILE FOR ADOLESCENTS/ADULTS[107]

Psychometric Properties:

Criterion-referenced

Norming included a sample of 950 adolescents and adults without disabilities. The majority of the sample was Caucasian and from the Midwestern region of the US (92%).The sample was divided into 3 age groups: adolescent, adult, and older adult.

Construct and **content validity** were addressed through the use of literature review, expert review, and examination of the relationship of test scores to external variables.

Convergence (concurrent) and **discriminant validity** were assessed by comparing scores from the Adolescent/Adult Sensory Profile with scores obtained on the New York Longitudinal Scales Adult Temperament Questionnaire.[108] This study revealed moderate correlations between the profile and the following areas on the New York Longitudinal Scales: approach/withdrawal, adaptability, mood, and sensory threshold.

Internal consistency (reliability) was assessed using the coefficient alpha. The values for alpha for the various sections ranged from 0.639 to 0.775.

The standard error of measurement (SEM), an index of the degree to which obtained scores differ from true scores, is provided for each possible quadrant raw score total for each cut-score group. The more reliable the test, the smaller the SEM. SEM values for the profile ranged from 3.58 to 4.51.[107]

TEST OF SENSORY FUNCTIONS IN INFANTS (TSFI)[109]

1989

DeGangi and Greenspan

ICF Domain: Body Functions and Structures

Purpose: The TSFI was designed to measure sensory processing and reactivity in infants. The TSFI is intended as both a research and a clinical tool for infants with regulatory disorders (ie, difficult temperament, irritability), infants with developmental delays, and infants at risk for later learning and sensory processing disorders. The TSFI may be used in combination with other standardized developmental motor, neuromotor, and cognitive tests to determine the infant's developmental functioning.

Ages: 4 to 18 months

Time: The test takes 25 minutes to administer and score.

User Qualifications: Occupational therapists, physical therapists, pediatricians, psychologists, and infant educators

Test Materials: All materials needed for the test are included in the test materials. The test manual is comprehensive and scoring is easy to follow. Illustrations also are provided in the test manual.

continued

TEST OF SENSORY FUNCTIONS IN INFANTS (TSFI)[109]

Test Areas:
The TSFI is a 24-item test consisting of 5 subtests that assess 5 areas of sensory function: (1) Reactivity to Tactile Deep Pressure; (2) Visual-Tactile Integration; (3) Adaptive Motor Responses; (4) Ocular-Motor Control; and (5) Reactivity to Vestibular Stimulation.

Administration:
Individually administered to an infant who may sit on the caregiver's lap for all except the vestibular subtest. Test results classify an infant as normal, at risk, or deficient for the total test and in each of the 5 subtests. Cut scores are provided for 4 age groups: 4 to 6 months, 7 to 9 months, 10 to 12 months, and 13 to 18 months.

Psychometric Properties:
Criterion-referenced

Content validity was assessed by using a 2-stage judgmental review with a panel of 8 infant-assessment experts examining item-behavior congruence and representativeness. The judges used ratings of high, moderate, or poor for each item. Seventy-five percent to 85% of the ratings of item-behavior congruence were high for all items on the TSFI. Eighty-seven percent of the ratings of representativeness were high for all the subtests except Reactivity to Vestibular Stimulation, which was rated high 75% of the time. The panel concluded that (1) the test items measured the behaviors they were intended to measure and (2) the groups of items that constituted the individual subtests were representative of their respective domains. The content validity was stated to be moderate to high for the total test.

Construct validity was assessed through use of an analysis of item-discrimination indexes, the estimation of classification decision accuracy, and the interrelationships of different subtests. The TSFI was found to be most accurate for diagnostic purposes in identifying normal infants ages 4 to 18 months and infants with sensory dysfunction ages 10 to 18 months.[60] A false normal rate for the total test score was found to be 14% to 45%; a false delayed rate for the total test score was 11% to 19%.

Criterion validity was found to be low when compared with the Bayley–III,[110] the Bates Infant Characteristics Questionnaire,[111] and the Fagan Test of Infant Intelligence.[112] However, the authors stated that this signifies the specific nature of the areas of behavior stimulated by the TSFI.

Interrater reliability was determined by using an occupational therapist and a physical therapist who scored the same test behaviors on the same children at the same time. Using ICCs, coefficients from 0.88 to 0.99 were found for each of the 5 subtests and the total test scores. Interrater reliability of the TSFI has been evaluated with babies exposed to cocaine in utero.[113] Results showed the total test score to be highly reliable (0.92). However, the Ocular-Motor Control and Reactivity to Tactile Deep Pressure subtests were found to have lower interrater reliabilities (0.25 and 0.67, respectively).

continued

Test of Sensory Functions in Infants (TSFI)[109]

Decision-consistency reliability as well as **test–retest reliability** were examined. High levels of classification consistency were found throughout the test (81% to 96%). Pearson product moment coefficients between test–retest scores were measured to assess stability of separate scores. Stability of the total test was good (0.81). There was good stability determined for the Visual-Tactile Integration subtest (0.84) and the Ocular-Motor Control subtest (0.96). Stability was fair for the Reactivity to Tactile Deep Pressure subtest (0.77). Although test–retest reliability coefficients for vestibular and adaptive motor functioning domains were low (0.26 and 0.64, respectively), DeGangi and Greenspan stated that subtest results may still be incorporated into the total test score because of its reliability. Similar results were found on a test–retest reliability study conducted by Jirikowic and colleagues for infants with developmental delays.[114] (See Figure 2-5 and Videos 2-1 and 2-2.)

Test of Sensory Functions in Infants (TSFI)

Administration and Scoring Form

Georgia A. DeGangi, Ph.D., O.T.R., and Stanley I. Greenspan, M.D.

Published by
WPS WESTERN PSYCHOLOGICAL SERVICES
12031 Wilshire Blvd., Los Angeles, CA 90025-1251
Publishers and Distributors

Name of Infant: AA

Birth Date: 12-27-0 Date of Testing: 9-24-03

Age (in months): 9 mos Sex: ☐ M ☒ F

Reason for Referral: ? Hyper responsive to movement

Directions

Administer the test according to the instructions presented in the Manual (WPS Catalog No. W-262C). During administration, score the items and record the item scores on the other side of this form. Each item is scored using a numerical rating scale. The criteria for scoring are summarized on the back of this form and detailed in the Manual. Determine the infant's score on each item according to these criteria and enter the number on the right.

After administration, add the item scores for each subtest and enter the total next to the subtest name. Add the five subtest scores to obtain the Total Test Score and enter that number on the bottom right of the page. Then transfer the subtest scores and the Total Test Score to the profile form below by entering the scores in the appropriate boxes under the column heading "Score."

To use the profile form, place an "X" in the box that includes the infant's score on each subtest and the Total Test. Complete the profile by connecting the X's.

Profile Form

Subtest	Score	4-6 months			7-9 months			10-12 months			13-18 months		
		Normal	At Risk	Deficient	Normal	At Risk	Deficient	Normal	At Risk	Deficient	Normal	At Risk	Deficient
Reactivity to Tactile Deep Pressure	10	9–10	8	0–7	9–10	8	0–7	9–10	8	0–7	9–10	8	0–7
Adaptive Motor Functions	13	7–15	6	0–5	11–15	10	0–9	14–15	13	0–12	15	14	0–13
Visual-Tactile Integration	8	4–10	3	0–2	9–10	7–8	0–6	9–10	7–8	0–6	9–10	7–8	0–6
Ocular-Motor Control	2	1–2		0	2	1	0	2	1	0	2	1	0
Reactivity to Vestibular Stimulation	7	10–12	9	0–8	10–12	9	0–8	10–12	9	0–8	11–12	10	0–9
Total Test	40	33–49	30–32	0–29	41–49	38–40	0–37	44–49	41–43	0–40	44–49	41–43	0–40

W 262B

Figure 2-5. Sample of completed score sheet. (Material from the TSFI copyright © 1989 by Western Psychological Services. Reprinted by permission of the publisher, Western Psychological Services, 12031 Wilshire Blvd, Los Angeles, CA 90025, www.wpspublish.com. Not to be reprinted in whole or in part for any additional purpose without the expressed, written permission of the publisher. All rights reserved.)

DeGangi-Berk Test of Sensory Integration[14]

1983
DeGangi and Berk

ICF Domain:	Body Functions and Structures
Purpose:	The purpose of the test is to capture information about sensory processing for those children for whom Sensory Integration and Praxis Tests clinical observations are not appropriate. The tool is designed for early identification of sensory integrative dysfunction in preschool-age children.
Ages:	3 to 5 years
Time:	The test takes 30 minutes to administer and 20 minutes to score.
User Qualifications:	Occupational therapists, physical therapists
Test Materials:	All materials needed for the test are included in the test materials except for a rolling pin, a scooter board, and a hula hoop. The test manual is comprehensive with illustrations and scoring instructions.
Test Areas:	The test consists of 36 scores on 13 separate items in 3 areas:

Postural Control: Assesses antigravity postures necessary for stabilization of the neck, trunk, and upper extremities, as well as muscle co-contraction of the neck and upper extremities.

Bilateral Motor Integration: Emphasizes bilateral motor coordination. Components of laterality include trunk rotation; crossing midline; rapid unilateral and bilateral hand movements; stability of upper/lower extremities in bilateral symmetrical postures; and dissociation of trunk and arm movements.

Reflex Integration: Assesses asymmetrical tonic neck reflex (ATNR), symmetrical tonic neck reflex (STNR), and associated reactions.

Administration:	Each of the individual test items are weighted with point values ranging from 0 to 1 and 0 to 4. Criteria for the assigning of a point value are described in the test manual. Scores for Postural Control, Bilateral Motor Integration, and the Total Test are obtained from administration of the entire battery. These scores are then compared against "normed" scores for children between ages 3 to 4 years or age 5 years. Based on these "normed" scores, an individual child's score may be interpreted as normal, at risk, or deficient. The authors stated that these results can be used for either screening or diagnosis, depending on the needs of the child and examiner.

continued

DeGangi-Berk Test of Sensory Integration[14]

Psychometric
Properties:

Criterion-referenced

Construct validity of the test was assessed by using 2 criterion groups of normal and delayed children. A total of 139 children, 101 normal and 38 delayed, representing ages 3 to 5 years, and 3 ethnic groups (Black, Hispanic, and White), were used. Results from administration of the original 73 items to these groups of children aided in determining item validity, decision validity, and test structure. The authors found the total test scores could be used for screening decisions with better than 80% accuracy and a 9% false-normal error rate. The subtests of Postural Control and Bilateral Motor Integration were very accurate with false-normal error rates less than 7%. Based on the cutoff score used in the decision validity study, the test was found to be more effective in excluding TD children from a delayed population than excluding delayed children in a typical population.

Interrater reliability was assessed by using 3 different therapists and 2 independent samples of children, which included a total of 33 children (26 normal and 7 delayed). Interrater reliabilities of 0.80 to 0.88 were found for the Postural Control and Bilateral Motor Integration subtests. The reliability scores for the Reflex Integration subtest varied from 0.24 to 0.66. Therefore, the authors cautioned against using the Reflex Integration subtest alone in making diagnoses.

Decision consistency reliability was determined by using a sample of 29 children (23 normal and 6 delayed), who were tested twice during a 1-week retest interval. Three observers conducted the testing. High levels of classification consistency were found for all 3 subtests and for the total test, with reliability scores ranging from 0.79 to 0.93.

Test–retest reliability information was obtained from the decision consistency study cited above. The test–retest reliability coefficients ranged from 0.85 to 0.96 when each subtest, as well as the total test, were considered.

Sensitivity: 0.66 (reflex integration) to 0.84 (bilateral motor integration).

Specificity: 0.64 (bilateral motor integration) to 0.85 (total test).
(See Figure 2-6.)

continued

DeGangi-Berk Test of Sensory Integration[14]

Item Number	Description	Scoring Criterion	Postural Control	Bilateral Motor Integration	Reflex Integration
				Item Score	
1	**MONKEY TASK** Ability to hold position	Unable to hold .... 0 / Loses grip .... 1 / Head 6" below .... 2 / Head 2-6" below 3			
2	Number of seconds held	0 seconds .... 0 / 1-5 seconds .... 1 / 6-10 seconds .... 2 / 11-15 seconds .... 3 / 16 or more seconds 4			
3	**SIDE-SIT COCONTRACTION** Amount of resistance	None .... 0 / Slight .... 1 / Moderate to maximum 2			
4	Number of seconds held	0 seconds .... 0 / 1-5 seconds .... 1 / 6-10 seconds .... 2 / 11 or more seconds 3			
5	**ROLLING PIN ACTIVITY** Ability to maintain grasp / Left Side / Right Side	Loses grasp .... 0 / Maintains grasp .... 1 / Loses grasp .... 0 / Maintains grasp 1		0 / 1 / 0 / 1	
6	Crosses midline, left / Point A / Point B / Point C	Does not cross .... 0 / Crosses .... 1 / Does not cross .... 0 / Crosses .... 1 / Does not cross .... 0 / Crosses 1		0 / 1 / 0 / 1 / 0 / 1	
7	Crosses midline, right / Point D / Point E / Point F	Does not cross .... 0 / Crosses .... 1 / Does not cross .... 0 / Crosses .... 1 / Does not cross .... 0 / Crosses 1		0 / 1 / 0 / 1 / 0 / 1	
8	**PRONE ON ELBOWS** Amount of resistance	None .... 0 / 1-2" head movement .... 1 / No head movement 2			
9	**WHEELBARROW WALK** Elbow position	Slight to moderate flexion .... 0 / Extends arm 1			
10	Distance	0-1 foot .... 0 / 2-4 feet .... 1 / 5-8 feet .... 2 / 9-10 feet 3			
11	**AIRPLANE** Placement of support	Shoulder .... 0 / Mid-chest .... 1 / Waist .... 2 / Hips 3			

DeGangi-Berk Test of Sensory Integration
Protocol Booklet

Georgia A. DeGangi, Ph.D., OTR and Ronald A. Berk, Ph.D.

Published by:
WPS WESTERN PSYCHOLOGICAL SERVICES
12031 Wilshire Blvd, Los Angeles, CA 90025-1251
Publishers and Distributors

Name: BJ   Sex: (M) F   Test Date: ___ year ___ month ___ day

Address: ___   Birthdate: ___ year ___ month ___ day

School: ___   Grade: 3   Age: 3 1 29

Referred by: Teacher - Preschool   Examiner: BC

Reason for Referral: Poor coordination; gravitational insecurity

DIRECTIONS: Administer the test according to the instructions presented in the Manual. During administration, score the items and record the item scores in this booklet. Each item is scored using a numerical rating scale. The criteria for scoring are summarized in this booklet and detailed in the Manual. Determine the child's score on each item according to these criteria, and circle the corresponding number on the right.

After administration, add the item scores in each column across all pages. Enter the subtest scores in the boxes at the bottom of the columns on page 4. Then transfer the subtest scores to the boxes below, and add them to obtain the Total Test Score.

To use the profile for Postural Control, Bilateral Motor Integration, and the total test, place an "X" in the box which includes the child's score on each. Complete the profile by connecting the X's.

$$10 + 13 + 4 = 27$$

Postural Control Score + Bilateral Motor Integration Score + Reflex Integration Score = Total Test Score

PROFILE

Functioning Level	Postural Control		Bilateral Motor Integration		Total Test Score	
	Ages 3-4	Age 5	Ages 3-4	Age 5	Ages 3-4	Age 5
Normal	20-30	20-30	30-42	30-42	52-88	52-88
At Risk	17-19	26-29		26-29	47-51	
Deficient	0-16	0-19	0-25	0-29	0-46	0-51

Note: The Reflex Integration score should be used only to determine the Total Test Score.

W-190C

Figure 2-6. Sample of completed score sheet. (Material from the TSI copyright © 1983 by Western Psychological Services. Reprinted by permission of the publisher, Western Psychological Services, 12031 Wilshire Blvd, Los Angeles, CA 90025, www.wspublish.com. Not to be reprinted in whole or in part for any additional purpose without the expressed, written permission of the publisher. All rights reserved.)

Sensory Integration and Praxis Tests (SIPT)[115]

1989

Ayres

ICF Domain:	Body Functions and Structures
Purpose:	The tests were developed to measure the sensory integration processes that underlie learning and behavior.
Ages:	4 to 8 years 11 months
Time:	The entire test battery takes approximately 2 hours to administer. An additional 45 minutes to 1 hour is needed for scoring, and 1 additional hour for interpretation after the profile is developed.
User Qualifications:	Physical therapists, occupational therapists; certification in administration and interpretation of these tests is recommended for use of the test as a diagnostic tool.
Test Materials:	The SIPT test materials and score sheets are included in the test materials.
Test Areas:	The 17 subtests of the SIPT are categorized into 4 overlapping groups: Tactile, Vestibular, and Proprioceptive Sensory Processing Tests; Form and Space Perception and Visuomotor Coordination Tests; Praxis Tests; and Bilateral Integration and Sequencing Tests.
Administration:	The SIPT is individually administered. The tests then are computer-scored based on completed computer score sheets, which are sent to Western Psychological Services for weighting of scores and determination of standard scores based on available norms. Scoring also can be performed by the examiner if a computer scoring disc is purchased.
Psychometric Properties:	**Norm-referenced** The SIPT represents an evolution of the Southern California Sensory Integration Test (SCSIT)[116] and the Southern California Postrotary Nystagmus Test.[117] Ayres, during the 1960s and 1970s, performed numerous factor analyses on the subtests of the SCSIT.[118-121] Based on these factor analyses, several of the subtests from the SCSIT were not included on the new SIPT either because of their lack of clinical usefulness, the difficulty in administrating the subtest, or poor reliability in measurement of the function. In the development of the new subtests for the SIPT and in the revision of the SCSIT, field and pilot studies were conducted during the early 1980s. In these pilot studies, 3 criteria were used in the selection of the final tests and individual test items: (1)the capability of each item to distinguish between dysfunctional and normal children; (2) evidence of a logical association between items and functions under assessment; and (3) interrater/test–retest reliability. Based on these pilot studies, the final version of the SIPT was composed of tests designed to assess sensory perception and the processing of tactile, proprioceptive, vestibular, and visual input as well as several aspects of praxis. The SIPT was normed using the

continued

Sensory Integration and Praxis Tests (SIPT)[115]

1980 US Census to determine the appropriate representation of the US population in the normative sample. The variables considered in selecting the sample were age, sex, ethnicity, type of community, and geographic location. The final normative sample comprised approximately 2,000 children between the ages of 4 years 0 months to 8 years 11 months, with an almost equal number of boys and girls. Children in the sample were evaluated by selected examiners who were trained in the administration and scoring of the SIPT and who were tested on their administration skills at workshops held around the United States. Preliminary analyses of the normative sample revealed significant age and sex differences on the SIPT tests. Therefore, separate norms were established for boys and girls in 12 age groups. Additionally, means and SDs were computed for each of the normative subgroups. Most of the individual tests of the SIPT also yielded subscores for time and accuracy.

Content validity was established (according to Ayres) through the work that led to the development of the SCSIT, the refinement of the SCSIT, and through consultation with experts in the area of sensory integration.

Construct validity was examined through the use of numerous factor analyses conducted by Ayres and reported in the SIPT manual. Additionally, Ayres used multiple discriminant analyses with a matched sample of 352 children without dysfunction and children with sensory integrative problems. The weights for time and accuracy scores that adequately discriminated between the 2 groups of children were used in the final version of the test. In preliminary studies using the SIPT in various populations, each of the subtests of the SIPT discriminated between children without dysfunction and those with dysfunction at a statistically significant level ($P < .1$).[115] Construct validity has been further supported by Murray and colleagues, who studied 21 children with learning disabilities and 18 children without learning disabilities, ages 5 to 8 years, to determine the relationship between form and space perception, constructional abilities, and clumsiness.[122] The children with learning disabilities in the study were further divided into 2 groups, clumsy and nonclumsy, based on their scores on a test of motor behaviors. All children in the study were assessed using 6 of the SIPT subtests that measure form and space perception and visual construction. Results indicated both groups of learning disabled children scored lower than the nonlearning disabled children on 4 of the 6 SIPT subtests (space visualization, motor accuracy, design copying, and constructional praxis) at a significant level. Within the 2 learning disabled groups, the clumsy and nonclumsy children differed significantly from each other only on the Motor Accuracy and Design Copying subtests. The degree of clumsiness in the 12 children who were identified as clumsy was correlated significantly with 3 of the 6 subtests (Space Visualization, Motor Accuracy, and Design Copying).

continued

Sensory Integration and Praxis Tests (SIPT)[115]

Test–retest reliability coefficients for the 17 subtests of the SIPT were reported by Ayres as ranging from 0.48 to 0.93.[115] The praxis tests had the highest test–retest reliability, but reliabilities for most of the other tests were acceptable. Four of the tests had reliability coefficients below 0.70: Postrotary Nystagmus, Kinesthesia, Localization of Tactile Stimuli, and Figure Ground Perception. Ayres reported that the small sample size and the predominance of children with dysfunction in the test–retest reliability study, as well as the nature of the assessed neural functions in the SIPT, may have affected the test–retest reliability of these subtests.[115]

Interrater reliability studies for the SIPT revealed correlation coefficients for all of the major SIPT scores to be between 0.94 and 0.99 when trained examiners were used.[115]

Clinical Observations of Motor and Postural Skills (COMPS)[123]

2000

Wilson, Pollock, Kaplan, and Law

ICF Domain:	Body Functions and Structures
Purpose:	The purpose of the test is to screen children for the presence or absence of motor problems with a postural component.
Ages:	5 to 16 years
Time:	The test takes 15 to 20 minutes to administer.
User Qualifications:	Occupational therapists, physical therapists
Test Materials:	The test materials comprise a test manual, 2 ATNR measurement tools, and a score sheet.
Test Areas:	The COMPS consists of 6 items: (1) Slow Movements, (2) Rapid Forearm Rotation, (3) Finger-Nose Touching, (4) Prone Extension Posture, (5) Asymmetrical Tonic Neck Reflex, and (6) Supine Flexion Posture.
Administration:	The test should be administered in the sequence of the 6 items as outlined in the test manual. It is most important that the last 3 items be given in the order listed. Stretch to the flexor muscles is stated to have a facilitation effect on these muscles and thus the administration of the Supine Flexion item immediately following the Prone Extension could result in an exaggerated performance. The tool is not designed nor recommended to be used for children with known neurological or neuromotor problems.

continued

CLINICAL OBSERVATIONS OF MOTOR AND POSTURAL SKILLS (COMPS)[123]

Psychometric Properties:

Criterion-referenced

The test was originally developed for children between ages 5 and 9 years. The authors later tested 261 children between ages 10 and 16 years to develop standards for older children.

Interrater reliability ICCs were found to be 0.57 between occupational therapists with pediatric experience and those without when testing children with DCD. The ICC for occupational therapists with pediatric experience with this group of children was 0.76. When evaluating children without, the ICC between occupational therapists with experience and those without was found to be 0.81. The ICCs between occupational therapists with pediatric experience in the group of children without DCD was higher at 0.90.

Test–retest reliability using the ICC was found to be 0.87 for children with DCD and 0.76 for the non-DCD group.

The Cronbach coefficient alpha was used to assess **internal consistency**. The alpha coefficient for the total test with younger children was 0.77. The internal consistency for the older children was at 0.69. Both of these values were at an acceptable level of internal consistency.

Construct validity was assessed by the examination of the discriminant values of the test. The analysis showed that the COMPS discriminated between those children who had DCD and those who did not.

Concurrent validity was assessed by comparing scores on the COMPS with test performance of the younger DCD group and the non-DCD group on 6 measures other than the COMPS (Balance subtest from the Bruininks-Oseretsky Test of Motor Proficiency, the Motor Accuracy tests from the SIPT-dominant and nondominant hand, the Developmental Test of Visual Motor-Integration, and tests of Standing Balance eyes open and eyes closed). Scores ranged from 0.40 on the motor accuracy test to 0.48 on the Developmental Test of Visual Motor-Integration when using the Pearson *r*.

Sensitivity was found to be 82% to 100% for the younger children (ages 5 to 9 years) and 23% to 59% for the older children (ages 10 to 12 years and older).

Specificity was found to be 63% to 90% for the younger children and 88% to 98% for the older children.

SENSORY INTEGRATION INVENTORY—REVISED (SII–R)[124] FOR INDIVIDUALS WITH DEVELOPMENTAL DISABILITIES

1992

Reisman and Hanschu

ICF Domain:	Body Functions and Structures
Purpose:	The purpose of the test is to screen for clients who might benefit from a sensory integration treatment approach.
Ages:	Any age child or adult with developmental disabilities
Time:	The test takes 20 to 30 minutes to administer and score.
User Qualifications:	Occupational therapists, physical therapists
Test Materials:	The test comprises a test manual and a score sheet.
Test Areas:	The SII–R addresses the areas of tactile, vestibular, and proprioceptive processing, as well as general reactions to sensory input. The individual's responses to these sensory inputs are linked to the following areas:
	Tactile: Dressing, activities of daily living, personal space, social, self-stimulatory behaviors, and self-injurious behaviors
	Vestibular: Muscle tone; equilibrium responses; posture and movement; bilateral coordination; spatial perception; emotional expression; and self-stimulatory behaviors
	Proprioception: Muscle tone, motor skills (planning and body image), self-stimulatory behaviors, and self-injurious behaviors
Administration:	The inventory can be used in 2 ways. The first is by therapy staff who are familiar with the individual and who can complete the questionnaire. The second is as a semistructured interview of those who are most familiar with the individual. The individual questions on the inventory are scored as "yes" or "no." The item is scored as "yes" if the behavior is typical and has been observed, reported, or can be elicited through testing. The item is scored as "no" if the behavior is not typical or characteristic of the individual. A question mark can be used if the tester is unsure whether the behavior is typical even though it has been observed. There are no set numbers of questions that must be marked "yes" before an individual is considered to have sensory integrative dysfunction. The inventory is best used as a means of explaining an individual's behavior in his or her day-to-day environment.
Psychometric Properties:	**Criterion-referenced**
	The test was originally developed at the Cambridge Regional Human Service Center, which provided services for approximately 300 adults with intellectual deficits. The pilot for the tools was used to screen clients at the center. After the publication of the First Edition

continued

SENSORY INTEGRATION INVENTORY—REVISED (SII–R)[124] FOR INDIVIDUALS WITH DEVELOPMENTAL DISABILITIES

of the inventory, therapists reported that it was useful in assessing individuals who could not cooperate fully in a testing situation. These included children with autism and pervasive developmental disorders, and adults with schizophrenia, Alzheimer disease, and other psychogeriatric conditions.[77] No psychometric characteristics are reported in the test manual. (See Figure 2-7.)

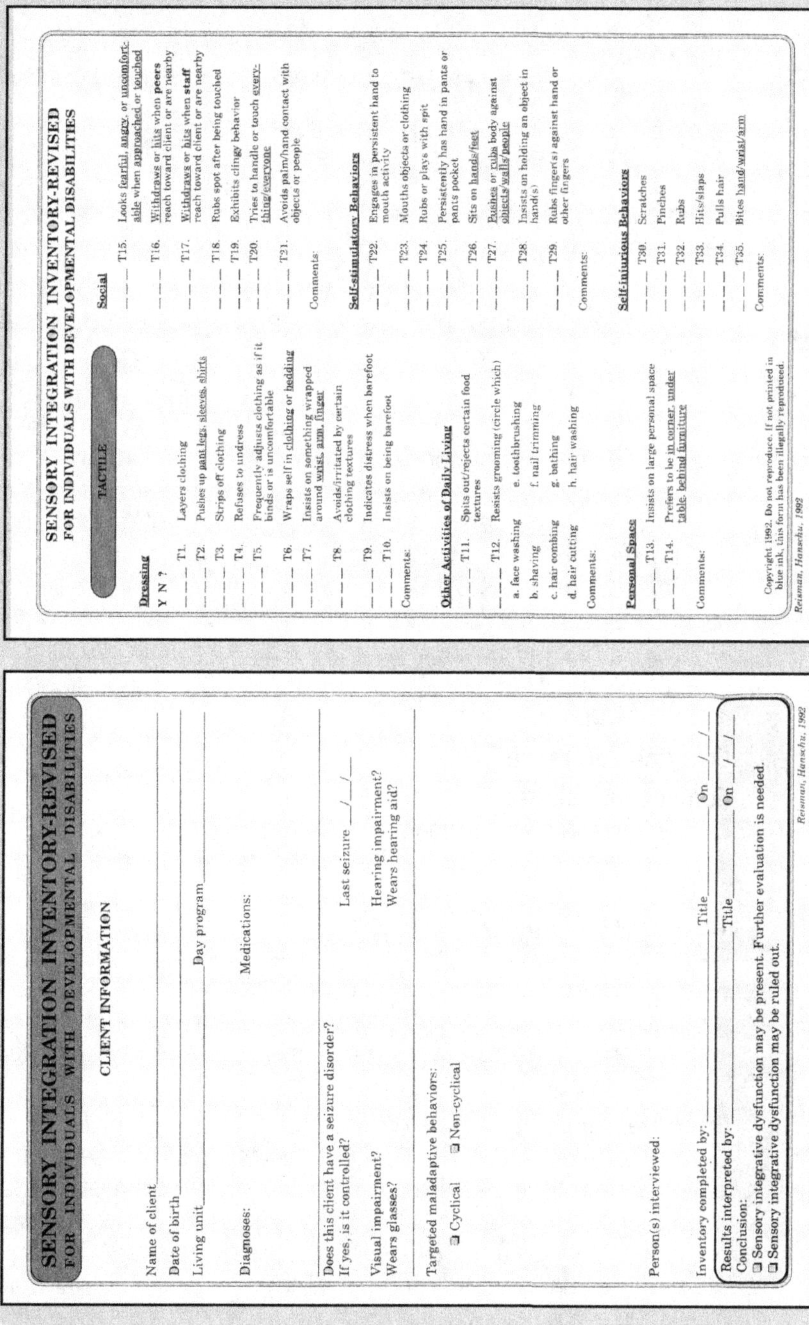

Figure 2-7. Sample score sheet (tactile). (Reprinted with permission from Reisman JE, Hanschu B. *Sensory Integration Inventory—Revised for Individuals With Developmental Disabilities.* Stillwater, MN: PDP Press, Inc; 1992.)

SENSORIMOTOR PERFORMANCE ANALYSIS (SPA)[125]

1989

Richter and Montgomery

ICF Domain:	Body Functions and Structures
Purpose:	The purpose of the test is to provide a qualitative record of an individual's performance on selected motor tasks.
Ages:	5 to 21 years
Time:	The test takes 30 to 45 minutes to administer and score.
User Qualifications:	Both physical therapists and occupational therapists with experience in pediatrics
Test Materials:	The test comprises a test manual and a score sheet. Minimal equipment is necessary for the administration: tape; tilt board; suspended tether ball; pencils; large paper; table and chairs; scissors; pellets; small bottle; and a drawing of a "+" and "o."
Test Areas:	The SPA tasks include: (1) rolling; (2) belly crawling; (3) bat the ball from 3 points; (4) kneeling balance; (5) pellets in a bottle; (6) paper and pencil task; and (7) scissor task.
Administration:	The SPA is individually administered to the child, and the criterion for each task is on the test form. The criterion is scored on a continuum from 1 to 5. Poor performance is represented by 1, inadequate by 3, and optimal by 5. Operational definitions for the scores for each item are presented in the test manual. Sixteen sensorimotor components are analyzed during each task on the test. These sensorimotor components include ATNR, STNR, antigravity extension, antigravity flexion, body righting, head righting, equilibrium/righting reactions, vestibular function, tactile processing, visual processing, bilateral integration, motor planning, tone/strength, stability/mobility, neurological status, and developmental level.
Psychometric Properties:	**Criterion-referenced** **Concurrent validity:** The test was originally developed for use with children with intellectual challenges. No specific sensorimotor tests were appropriate at the time of development of the SPA for examining concurrent validity. **Test–retest reliability** was assessed in a study with 10 children who were intellectually challenged (intelligence quotient between 50 and 80) who did not have accompanying physical disabilities, such as neuromotor disorders. The participants' performance on the SPA was compared with their performance 1 week later. Test–retest reliability coefficients ranged from 0.89 to 0.97. **Interrater reliability** was determined using the same children as those used for test–retest reliability. Using the first test session, a second observer simultaneously assessed and scored the children. Correlation coefficients ranged from 0.15 to 0.91. There was poor agreement between raters for the ATNR (0.21), STNR (0.15), and tactile processing (0.31). If these 3 scores were eliminated, an interrater reliability score of 0.76 was obtained. (See Figure 2-8.)

continued

Figure 2-8. Sample score sheet. (Reprinted with permission from Richter EW, Montgomery PC. *The Sensorimotor Performance Analysis.* Stillwater, MN; PDP Press; 1989.)

Functional Assessments

Standardized Assessments of Instrumental Daily Living Skills

PEDIATRIC EVALUATION OF DISABILITY INVENTORY—COMPUTER ADAPTIVE TEST (PEDI–CAT)[126]

2012

Haley, Coster, Dumas, Fragala-Pinkham, and Moed

ICF Domains:	Activities; Participation
Purpose:	The purposes of the test are to identify functional delay, examine improvement for an individual child after intervention, and to evaluate and monitor group progress in program evaluation and research.
Ages:	1 to 21 years
Time:	The PEDI–CAT has 2 versions. The Speedy version has less than 15 items and takes 10 to 15 minutes for all 4 domains. The Content Balanced version has up to 30 items and takes 20 to 30 minutes for all 4 domains.
User Qualifications:	Physical therapists, occupational therapists, speech-language pathologists, nurses, and educators
Test Materials:	No special environment, materials, or activities are necessary. The test focuses on typical performance at the present time. The PEDI–CAT is available for iPads and computers. Each download includes English and Spanish versions. A PEDI–CAT for autism spectrum disorders also is available.
Test Areas:	The PEDI–CAT captures functioning in 4 domains: (1) daily activities, (2) mobility, (3) social/cognitive, and (4) responsibility. Each domain is self-contained and can be used separately or with other domains. The daily activities domain is composed of 68 items in 4 content areas: (1) getting dressed, (2) keeping clean, (3) home tasks, and (4) eating and mealtime. The mobility domain is composed of 75 items in 5 content areas: basic movement and transfers; standing and walking; steps and inclines; running; and playing. The social cognitive domain is composed of 60 items in 4 content areas: (1) interaction, (2) communication, (3) everyday cognition, and (4) self-management. The responsibility domain (for ages 3 to 21 years) is composed of 51 items that assess the extent to which a young person is managing life tasks that enable independent living, such as organization and planning; taking care of daily needs; health management; and staying safe.
Administration:	An examiner should review the PEDI–CAT manual prior to administration to become familiar with administration procedures, instrument content, item intent, response scales, and score interpretation. Illustrations of daily activities and mobility items are included to facilitate understanding of the item intent. The PEDI–CAT is administered only on the computer. The PEDI–CAT uses an artificial intelligence to select only the most relevant items from a pool of validated items.

continued

PEDIATRIC EVALUATION OF DISABILITY INVENTORY— COMPUTER ADAPTIVE TEST (PEDI–CAT)[126]

Each item in the pool represents a different amount of difficulty. On the 3 functional skill domains of Daily Activities, Mobility, and Social/Cognitive, the child's ability is rated on a 4-point difficulty scale with responses of Unable, A Little Hard, Hard, and Easy. A response of "I don't know" is also available. The Responsibility domain is a 5-point scale with responses ranging from "adult/caregiver has full responsibility" to "child takes full responsibility without any direction, supervision, or guidance from an adult/caregiver." For each domain, all respondents begin with the same question in the middle of the scoring range. The initial response will dictate whether a harder or an easier item will be administered next. Not every item needs to be answered to get a score. The respondent can be the clinician, caregiver, or a combination of clinician and caregiver. The PEDI–CAT produces both normed standard scores (percentile and T-scores) and criterion-referenced scores (scaled scores) for analysis.[127]

Psychometric Properties:

Norm-referenced

The PEDI–CAT's normative standardization sample was recruited through an online panel and resulted in a nationally representative sample of 2205 parents of children younger than age 21 years in the contiguous United States.

Content validity was assessed through literature review, expert opinion, and item analysis. An expanded item set and response options were reviewed by clinician experts and examined at parent and clinician focus groups.

Concurrent validity: Dumas and Fragala-Pinkham, in a study of 35 children with neurodevelopmental disabilities, reported the strength of association between the PEDI–CAT Mobility domain and the PEDI full-scale and Mobility scale was good to excellent (0.82).[128] ICCs ranged from 0.339 to 1.00, and percent agreement results ranged from 60% to 100%. These findings indicate strong agreement between the original PEDI and the PEDI–CAT on identification of limitations. Concurrent validity also has been demonstrated between the AIMS and the PEDI–CAT.[129]

Discriminant validity has been documented by examining the accuracy and precision of the PEDI–CAT in TD children (n = 2205) and children with disabilities (n = 703). The clinical validation sample of 703 children with disabilities (behavioral, intellectual, and physical) was recruited through the online panel, as well as through 2 clinical sites in the Northwest Central and Northeastern United States. Factor analyses revealed excellent accuracy (ICC > 0.95) with the full item banks.[130] Additionally, discriminative validity was assessed in a prospective study of 102 children with and without disabilities[131] and in a study of children who used a walking aid or a wheelchair.[132]

Test–retest reliability was examined in a group of parents (n = 25) who completed the PEDI–CAT twice within 1 month.[131] Test–retest reliability estimates were high (ICC = 0.96 to 0.99) for all 4 domains of the PEDI–CAT.

School Function Assessment (SFA)[3]

1998

Coster, Deeney, Haltiwanger, and Haley

ICF Domains:	Activities; Participation
Purpose:	The purpose of the test is to measure a student's performance of functional tasks that support participation in the academic and social aspects of the educational environment between grades kindergarten through 6. An additional purpose is to facilitate collaborative program planning for students with varying disabling conditions.
Ages:	Children in kindergarten through sixth grade
Time:	New users of the SFA should allow a minimum of 1 and one-half to 2 hours to complete the assessment. Once familiar with the test, the time to administer individual parts or the entire scale should decrease. Typically, the assessment is not completed within a single day. However, the assessment period should not extend longer than 2 to 3 weeks.
User Qualifications:	Physical therapists, occupational therapists, speech-language pathologists, psychologists, and educators
Test Materials:	The test is composed of a user manual, a ratings scale guide, and a record form. The test manual is detailed and has operational definitions for scores for each part of the SFA.
Test Areas:	The SFA is divided into 3 parts. Each part has one or more scales. Part I, Participation, allows for assessment of the student's participation in 6 major school-related activity settings. Part II, Task Supports, is composed of 4 scales. Two types of support, assistance and adaptations, are rated for physical and cognitive/behavioral tasks. Part III, Activity Performance, is composed of 21 separate scales: Travel; Maintaining and Changing Positions; Recreational Movement; Manipulation with Movement; Using Materials; Setup and Cleanup; Eating and Drinking; Hygiene; Clothing Management; Up/Down Stairs; Written Work; Computer and Equipment Use; Functional Communication; Memory and Understanding; Following Social Conventions; Compliance with Adult Directives and School Rules; Task Behavior/Completion; Positive Interaction; Behavior Regulation; Personal Care Awareness; and Safety.

continued

SCHOOL FUNCTION ASSESSMENT (SFA)[3]

Administration: The SFA is a judgment-based questionnaire that is completed by one or more school professionals who know the student well. The ratings from Part I are summed to yield a Participation total raw score. In Part II, Task Supports, a total raw score for each of the following scales is generated: Physical Tasks Assistance, Physical Tasks Adaptation, Cognitive/Behavioral Tasks Assistance, and Cognitive/Behavioral Tasks Adaptations. A total raw score is generated for each of the 21 separate scales in Part III, Activity Performance. The raw scores obtained are converted to a criterion score using tables in the test manual. An SEM also is obtained for each criterion score. Two criterion cutoff scores are provided for each scale, one for children in grades kindergarten through 3 and one for children in grades 4 through 6. By using the criterion scores, the examiner can create a functional profile for the student by plotting the student's score for each scale on the profile graph.

Psychometric Properties:

Criterion-referenced

A sample of 363 students with disabilities participated in the standardization of the SFA. The children were drawn from 112 different sites in 40 states. Fifty-seven percent of the students were in regular classrooms and 43% were in special education, but with some degree of mainstreaming. More boys (66%) than girls (34%) were represented in the standardization. A total of 315 children who were in regular education comprised the remainder of the sample. Forty-seven percent of the students in regular education were male and 53% were female. The sample of special needs and regular-education students mirrored the race/ethnicity percentages of children in the 1990 Census of Population.

Two **content validity** studies were conducted during the development of the SFA using panels of experts.

Concurrent validity and **internal consistency** of the SFA were examined using the Cronbach coefficient alpha. These correlations were found to range between 0.92 to 0.98. A second method used was the consideration of fit statistics of each item within a scale. Analyses of the scales confirmed the coherence of the items within each scale.

Test–retest reliability was assessed on a convenience sample of 23 students who were examined twice over a 2- to 3-week period.

The **reliability coefficient** scores between the test and retest were between 0.82 and 0.98. Approximately 40% of the sample had been identified as having a motor impairment. In a second test–retest study on another sample of children with a variety of disabilities using the ICC 2, 1 revealed correlation coefficients ranging from 0.80 to 0.97 on Part II of the SFA. The correlation coefficients were higher for Part III, Activity Performance, with scores ranging from 0.90 to 0.98.

Child-Reported Instruments

CHILDREN'S ASSESSMENT OF PARTICIPATION AND ENJOYMENT (CAPE) AND PREFERENCE FOR ACTIVITIES OF CHILDREN (PAC)[133]

2004

King, Law, King, Hurley, Rosenbaum, Hanna, Kertoy, and Young

ICF Domains:	Activities; Participation
Purpose:	The purposes of the test are to provide an understanding of the social well-being and activity or performance of a child with disabilities. Activity types addressed in both measures include: recreational, physical, social, skill-based, and self-improvement.
Ages:	6 to 21 years
Time:	Test times are 30 to 45 minutes for the CAPE and 15 to 20 minutes for the PAC.
User Qualifications:	Physical therapists, occupational therapists
Test Materials:	Manual, record forms, and summary score sheets. CAPE and PAC may be used independently or together. CAPE/PAC activity cards are available.
Administration:	The CAPE is a 55-item questionnaire designed to examine how a child participates in everyday activities outside school. The questions on the CAPE address 5 types of activities: recreational, physical, social, skill-based, and self-improvement. Information is provided about the diversity (number of activities performed), intensity (frequency of participation measured as a function of the number of possible activities within a category), and enjoyment of the activities. The CAPE also gives information about the context in which the child participates in these activities (where and with whom). The PAC taps into the child's preference for involvement in each activity. There is a self-administered and an interviewer-assisted version of the CAPE and the PAC. Three levels of scoring are used for the CAPE and PAC: overall participation scores, scores for the 2 domains of formal and informal activities, and scale scores for the 5 types of activities. Scores can be computed for these 3 levels for each of the 5 dimensions of participation obtained from the CAPE and for the preference domain from the PAC.
Psychometric Properties:	**Criterion-referenced** **Construct** and **content validity** were obtained from a longitudinal study involving 427 children with physical disabilities from across Canada. Correlations that have been reported as evidence of construct validity are low.[134] **Internal consistency reliability** was assessed by using the Cronbach alpha to compare each item with the overall score and the other individual items. The overall CAPE scores were 0.42 (formal) and 0.76 (informal). The overall PAC scores were 0.76 (formal) and 0.84 (informal). **Test–retest reliability** was determined by assessing 3 CAPE subscales (diversity, intensity, and enjoyment). The *r* values ranged from 0.64 to 0.86, indicating moderate to high reliability.

PEDIATRIC QUALITY OF LIFE INVENTORY (PEDSQL 4.0)[135]

1999

Varni

ICF Domains:	Activities; Participation
Purpose:	The purpose of the test is to systematically assess physical, emotional, social, school functioning, and global health.
Ages:	2 to 18 years
Time:	The test takes 4 minutes.
User Qualifications:	Physical therapists, occupational therapists
Test Materials:	Scaling and scoring for the PedsQL are available online at www.pedsql.org, and include child self-report forms for children age 5 years and older, and parent proxy forms for children ages 2 to 18 years. Specific modules are available for children with CP (PedsQL 3.0), muscular dystrophy, asthma, rheumatology, diabetes, cancer, and cardiac conditions.
Administration:	The core scale consists of 23 items measuring the core dimensions of health from the World Health Organization: physical, emotional, and social functioning, as well as school functioning. A 5-point Likert scale from 0 (never) to 4 (almost always) is used to score each item on the Parent Report for Toddlers. For the Child and Parents Reports for Children and Teens, the 5-point Likert scale is used. However, for the Child and Parents Reports for Young Children, a 3-point scale of 0 (not at all), 2 (sometimes), and 4 (a lot) is used. Raw scores that trend toward smaller scores indicate an improvement since the scores are reverse scored and linearly transformed to a 0 to 100 scale. Higher scores on all the inventories indicate a better health-related quality of life. Table 2-4 presents examples of questions on the Physical Domain of the PedsQL and Scoring.
Psychometric Properties:	**Criterion-referenced** **Construct** and **content validity** have been demonstrated using the known-groups methods, correlations with indicators of morbidity and illness burden, and factor analyses, which have been shown to not only distinguish between healthy children and children with acute and chronic health conditions, but also to distinguish disease severity within a chronic health condition.[136] The PedsQL also has been shown to be reliable and valid for use with children with cancer.[135] **Internal consistency reliability** for the total scale score (Cronbach alpha=0.88 child, 0.90 parent report), Physical Health Summary Score (Cronbach alpha=0.80 child, 0.88 parent), and Psychosocial Health Summary Score (Cronbach alpha=0.83 child, 0.86 parent) were acceptable for group comparisons.[136]

TABLE 2-4. EXAMPLE OF QUESTIONS ON THE PHYSICAL DOMAIN SECTION OF THE PEDIATRIC QUALITY OF LIFE INVENTORY

- It is hard for me to walk more than one block.
- It is hard for me to run.
- It is hard for me to do sports activity.
- It is hard for me to lift something heavy.
- It is hard for me to take a bath or shower by myself.
- It is hard for me to do chores around the house.
- I hurt or ache.
- I have low energy.

Adapted from Varni JW, Seid M, Rode CA. The PedsQL: measurement model for the pediatric quality of life inventory. *Med Care.* 1999;37(2):126-139.

SUMMARY

This overview of selected standardized criterion-referenced and norm-referenced tests should supply the therapist performing examinations of children an understanding of the components of an acceptable test. The information provided for each of the tests also should assist the therapist in the selection of the appropriate test for a given child in a given situation. The pediatric therapist should be aware of other components of an examination in addition to the administration of a test and should use information gathered from other parts of the assessment in the total evaluation of the child.

REFERENCES

1. World Health Organization. *International Classification of Functioning, Disability and Health: Children and Youth Version.* Geneva, Switzerland: World Health Organization; 2007.
2. American Physical Therapy Association. Guide to physical therapist practice 3.0. http://guidetoptpractice.apta.org/. 2014.
3. Coster W, Deeney T, Haltiwanger J, Haley S. *School Function Assessment.* San Antonio, TX: Psychological Corporation; 1998.
4. Russell D, Rosenbaum P, Wright M. *Gross Motor Function Measure (GMFM-66 and GMFM-88) User's Manual.* London, England: Mac Keith Press; 2013.
5. Miller Kuhaneck H, Ecker C, Parham LD, Henry DA, Glennon TJ. *Sensory Processing Measure-Preschool (SPM-P): Manual.* Los Angeles, CA: Western Psychological Services; 2010.
6. Bruininks RH, Bruininks B. *BOT-2: Bruininks Oseretsky Test of Motor Proficiency.* 2nd ed. Bloomington, MN: PsychCorp; 2005.
7. Karasik LB, Tamis-LeMonda CS, Adolph KE, Bornstein MH. Places and posture: a cross-cultural comparison of siting in 5-month-olds. *J Cross Cult Psychol.* 2015;46(8):1023-1038. doi:10.1177/0022022115593803.
8. Hopkins B, Westra T. Maternal Expectations of Their Infants' Development: An Intracultural Study. *Genet Soc Gen Psychol Monogr.* 1988;114(3):377-408.
9. Kolobe THA. Childrearing practices and developmental expectations for Mexican-American mothers and the developmental status of their infants. *Phys Ther.* 2004;84(5):439-453. doi:10.1093/ptj/84.5.439.
10. Karasik LB, Robinson S, Abraham E, Mladenovic, Tamis-LeMonda CS, Adolph K. Baby in a bind: traditional cradling practices and infant motor development. *Dev Psychobiol.* 2015;57(S1):S19.
11. Folio MR, Fewell RR. *Peabody Developmental Motor Scales. Examiner's Manual.* 2nd ed. Austin, TX: Pro-Ed; 2000.
12. Cohen E, Boettcher K, Maker T, et al. Evaluation of the Peabody Developmental Gross Motor Scales for young children of African American and Hispanic ethnic backgrounds. *Pediatr Phys Ther.* 1999;11(4):191-197.

13. Ulrich D. *Test of Gross Motor Development–2.* Austin, TX: Pro-Ed; 2000.

14. DeGangi GA, Berk RA. *DeGangi-Berk Test of Sensory Integration.* Los Angeles, CA: Western Psychological Services; 1983.

15. Dunn W. *Sensory Profile 2. User's Manual.* Bloomington, MN: PsychCorp; 2014.

16. Campbell S. *The Test of Infant Motor Performance. Test User's Manual Version 3.0 for the TIMP Version 5.* Chicago, IL: Infant Motor Performance Scales, LLC; 2012.

17. Kolobe THA, Bulanda M, Susman L. Predicting motor outcome at preschool age for infants tested at 7, 30, 60 and 90 days after term age using the Test of Infant Motor Performance. *Phys Ther.* 2004;84(12):1144-1156. doi:10.1093/ptj/84.12.1144.

18. Flegel J, Kolobe THA. Predictive validity of the Test of Infant Motor Performance as measured by the Bruininks–Oseretsky Test of Motor Proficiency at school age. *Phys Ther.* 2002;82(8):762-771. doi:10.1093/ptj/82.8.762.

19. Rosenbaum P, Walter SD, Hanna S, et al. Prognosis for gross motor function in cerebral palsy: creation of motor development curves. *JAMA.* 2002;288(11):1357-1363. doi:10.1001/jama.288.11.1357.

20. Sackett DL, Strauss SE, Richardson WS, Rosenberg W, Haynes RB. *Evidence-Based Medicine: How to Practice and Teach EBM.* 2nd ed. New York, NY: Churchill Livingstone Inc; 2000.

21. Podsiadlo D, Richardson S. The Timed "Up & Go": a test of basic functional mobility for frail elderly persons. *J Am Geriatr Soc.* 1991;39(2):142-148. doi:10.1111/j.1532-5415.1991.tb01616.x.

22. Shumway-Cook A, Brauer S, Woollacott M. Predicting the probability for falls in community-dwelling older adults using the Timed Up & Go test. *Phys Ther.* 2000;80(9):896-903. doi:10.1093/ptj/80.9.896.

23. Itzkowitz A, Kaplan S, Doyle M, et al. Timed Up and Go: reference data for children who are school age. *Pediatr Phys Ther.* 2016;28(2):239-246. doi:10.1097/PEP.0000000000000239.

24. Zaino CA, Marchese VG, Westcott SL. Timed Up and Down Stairs Test: preliminary reliability and validity of a new measure of functional mobility. *Pediatr Phys Ther.* 2004;16(2):90-98. doi:10.1097/01. PEP.0000127564.08922.6A.

25. ATS Committee on Proficiency Standards for Clinical Pulmonary Function Laboratories. ATS statement: guidelines for the Six-Minute Walk Test. *Am J Respir Crit Care Med.* 2002;166(1):111-117. doi:10.1164/ajrccm.166.1.at1102.

26. Klepper SE, Muir N. Reference values on the 6-Minute Walk Test for children living in the United States. *Pediatr Phys Ther.* 2011;23(1):32-40. doi:10.1097/PEP.0b013e3182095e44.

27. Dubowitz L, Dubowitz V. *The Neurological Examination of the Full Term Newborn Infant.* Clinics in Developmental Medicine No. 79. Philadelphia, PA: JB Lippincott; 1981.

28. Saint-Anne Dargassies S. *Neurological Development in the Full-Term and Premature Neonate.* London, England: Excerta Medica; 1977.

29. Prechtl HFR. *The Neurological Examination of the Full-Term Newborn Infant.* Clinics in Developmental Medicine, No. 63. Philadelphia, PA: JB Lippincott; 1977.

30. Parmelee AH, Michaelis R. Neurological examination of the newborn. In: Hellmuth J, ed. *Exceptional Infant.* Vol. 2: Studies in Abnormalities. London, England: Butterworths; 1971.

31. Brazelton TB. *Neonatal Behavioral Assessment Scale.* Philadelphia, PA: JB Lippincott; 1973.

32. Woodward LJ, Mogridge N, Wells SW, Inder TE. Can neurobehavioral examination predict the presence of cerebral injury in the very low weight infant? *J Dev Behav Pediatr.* 2004;25(5):326-334. doi:10.1097/00004703-200410000-00004.

33. Brazelton TB. *Neonatal Behavioral Assessment Scale.* 2nd ed. Philadelphia, PA: JB Lippincott; 1984.

34. Prechtl HFR. Assessment methods for the newborn infant, a critical evaluation. In: Stratton P, Chichest J, eds. *Psychobiology of the Human Newborn.* New York, NY: Wiley; 1982.

35. Tronick E, Brazelton TB. Clinical uses of the Brazelton Neonatal Behavior Assessment. In: Friedlander BZ, Sterritt BM, Kirk GE, eds. *Exceptional Infant: Assessment and Intervention.* Vol. 3. New York, NY: Brunner/Mazel; 1975.

36. Bakow H, Samaroff A, Kelly P. Relation between newborn and motherchild interactions at four months. Paper presented at: biennial meeting of the Society for Research in Child Development; 1973; Philadelphia, PA.

37. Ohgi S, Arisawa K, Takahashi T, et al. Neonatal behavioral assessment scale as a predictor of later developmental disabilities of low birth-weight and/or premature infants. *Brain Dev.* 2003;25(50):313-321. doi:10.1016/S0387-7604(02)00233-4.

38. Sameroff AJ. Organization and stability of newborn behavior: a commentary on the Brazelton Neonatal Behavioral Assessment Scale. *Monographs of the Society of Research in Child Development.* 1978;43(5/6):46-59.

39. Campbell SK, Kolobe TH, Osten ET, Lenke M, Girolami GL. Construct validity of the Test of Infant Motor Performance. *Phys Ther.* 1995;75(7):585-596. doi:10.1093/ptj/75.7.585.

40. Barbosa VM, Campbell SK, Berbaum M. Discriminating infants from different developmental outcome groups using the test of Infant Motor Performance (TIMP) item responses. *Pediatr Phys Ther.* 2007;19(1):28-39. doi:10.1097/PEP.0b013e31802f65f9.

41. Piper MC, Darrah J. *Motor Assessment of the Developing Infant.* Philadelphia, PA: WB Saunders; 1994.

42. Campbell SK, Kolobe THA. Concurrent validity of the Test of Infant Motor Performance with the Alberta Infant Motor Scale. *Pediatr Phys Ther.* 2000;12(1):2-9. doi:10.1097/00001577-200012010-00002.

43. Campbell SK, Kolobe THA, Wright B, Linacre JM. Validity of the Test of Infant Motor Performance for prediction of 6-,9-, and 12 month scores on the Alberta Infant Motor Scale. *Dev Med Child Neurol.* 2002;44(4):263-272. doi:10.1111/j.1469-8749.2002.tb00802.x.

44. Campbell SK. Test-retest reliability of the Test of Infant Motor Performance. *Pediatr Phys Ther.* 1999;11(2):60-66. doi:10.1097/00001577-199901120-00002.

45. Prechtl HF. General movement assessment as a method of developmental neurology: new paradigms and their consequences. The 1999 Ronnie MacKeith Lecture. *Dev Med Child Neurol.* 2001;43(12):836-842. doi:10.1111/j.1469-8749.2001.tb00173.x.

46. Noble Y, Boyd R. Neonatal assessments for the preterm infant up to 4 months corrected age: a systematic review. *Dev Med Child Neurol.* 2012;54(1):129-139. doi:10.1111/j.1469-8749.2010.03903.x.

47. Einspieler C, Prechtl HF. Prechtl's assessment of general movements: a diagnostic tool for the functional assessment of the young nervous system. *Ment Retard Dev Disabil Res Rev.* 2005;11(1):61-67. doi:10.1002/mrdd.20051.

48. Hadders-Algra M. General movements: a window for early identification of children at high risk for developmental disorders. *J Pediatr.* 2004;145(suppl 2):S12-S18. doi:10.1016/j.jpeds.2004.05.017.

49. Romeo DM, Guzzetta A, Scoto M, et al. Early neurological assessment in preterm-infants: integration of traditional neurological examination and observation of general movements. *Eur J Paediatr Neurol.* 2008;12(3):183-189. doi:10.1016/j.ejpn.2007.07.008.

50. Einspieler C, Prechtl HF, Bos A, Ferrari F, Cioni G. *Prechtl's Method on the Qualitative Assessment of General Movement in Preterm, Term, and Young Infants.* London, England: Mac Keith Press; 2004.

51. Xie K, Zheng H, Li H, et al. The study of effect for general movements assessment in the diagnosis of neurological development disorders: a meta-analysis. *Clin Pediatr (Phila).* 2016;55(1):36-43. doi:10.1177/0009922815592878.

52. Mutti M, Martin NA, Sterling HM, Spalding NV. *Quick Neurological Screening Test.* 3rd ed. Novato, CA: ATP Assessments; 2012.

53. Coster W. Critiques of the Alberta Infant Motor Scale (AIMS). *Phys Occup Ther Pediatr.*1995;15(3):53-64. doi:10.1080/J006v15n03_04.

54. Piper MC, Pinnell LE, Darrah J, Maguire T, Byrne PJ. Construction and validation of the Alberta Infant Motor Scale. *Can J Public Health.* 1992;83(suppl 2):S46-S50.

55. Darrah J, Piper M, Watt MJ. Assessment of gross motor skills of at-risk infants: predictive validity of the Alberta Infant Motor Scale. *Dev Med Child Neurol.* 1998;40(7):485-491. doi:10.1111/j.1469-8749.1998.tb15399.x.

56. Miller LJ, Roid GH. *Toddler and Infant Motor Evaluation: A Standardized Assessment.* Tucson, AZ: Therapy Skill Builders; 1994.

57. Bayley N. *Bayley Scales of Infant and Toddler Development Technical Manual.* 3rd ed. San Antonio, TX: Psychological Corporation; 2006.

58. Connolly BH, McClune NO, Gatlin R. Concurrent validity of the Bayley III and the Peabody Developmental Motor Scale-2. *Pediatr Phys Ther.* 2012;24(4):345-352. doi:10.1097/PEP.0b013e318267c5cf.

59. Milne S, McDonald J, Comino EJ. The use of the Bayley Scales of Infant and Toddler Development III with clinical populations: a preliminary exploration. *Phys Occup Ther Pediatr.* 2012;32(1):24-33. doi:10.3109/01942638.2011.592572.

60. Van Waelvelde H, Peersman W, Lenoir M, Engelsman BC. Convergent validity between two motor tests: Movement-ABC and PDMS-2. *Adapt Phys Activ Q.* 2007;24(1):59-69. doi:10.1123/apaq.24.1.59.

61. Harrow AJ. *A Taxonomy of the Psychomotor Domain: A Guide for Developing Behavioral Objectives.* New York, NY: David McKay; 1972.

62. Provost B, Heimerl S, McClain C, Kim N, Lopez B, Kodituwakku P. Concurrent validity of the Bayley Scales of Infant Development II Motor Scale and the Peabody Developmental Motor Scales-2 in children with developmental delays. *Pediatr Phys Ther.* 2004;16(3):149-156. doi:10.1097/01.PEP.0000136005.41585.FE.

63. Connolly BH, Dalton L, Smith JB, Lamberth NG, McCay B, Murphy W. Concurrent validity of the Bayley Scales of Infant Development II (BSID-II) Motor Scale and the Peabody Development Motor Scale II (PDMS-2) in 12-month-old infants. *Pediatr Phys Ther.* 2006;18(3):190-196. doi:10.1097/01.pep.0000226746.57895.57.

64. Maring JR, Elbaum L. Concurrent validity of the early intervention developmental profile and the Peabody Developmental Motor Scale-2. *Pediatr Phys Ther.* 2007;19(2):116-120. doi:10.1097/PEP.0b013e31804a5786.

65. Wang HH, Liao HF, Hsieh CL. Reliability, sensitivity to change and responsiveness of the Peabody Developmental Motor Scales-second edition for children with cerebral palsy. *Phys Ther.* 2006;86(10):1351-1359. doi:10.2522/ptj.20050259.

66. Wuang YP, Su CY. Reliability and responsiveness of the Bruininks-Oseretsky Test of Motor Proficiency-Second Edition in children with intellectual disability. *Res Dev Disability.* 2009;30(5):847-855. doi:10.1016/j.ridd.2008.12.002.

67. Russell DJ, Rosenbaum PL, Avery LM, Lane M. *Gross Motor Function Measure (GMFM-66 and GMFM-88) User's Manual.* London, England: Mac Keith Press; 2002.

68. Russell D, Rosenbaum PL, Cadman DT, Gowland C, Hardy S, Jarvis S. The Gross Motor Function Measure: a means to evaluate the effects of physical therapy. *Dev Med Child Neurol.* 1989;31(3):341-352. doi:10.1111/j.1469-8749.1989.tb04003.x.

69. Trahan J, Malouin F. Changes in the Gross Motor Function Measure in children with different types of cerebral palsy: an eight- month follow-up study. *Pediatr Phys Ther.* 1999;11(1):12-17.

70. Russell D, Palisano R, Walter S, et al. Evaluating motor function in children with Down syndrome: validity of the GMFM. *Dev Med Child Neurol.* 1998;40(10):693-701. doi:10.1111/j.1469-8749.1998.tb12330.x.

71. Ruck-Gibis J, Plotkin H, Hanley J, Wood-Dauphinee S. Reliability of the Gross Motor Function Measure for children with osteogenesis imperfecta. *Pediatr Phys Ther.* 2001;13(1):10-17. doi:10.1097/00001577-200104000-00003.

72. Franjoine MR, Gunther JS, Taylor MJ. Pediatric Balance Scale: A modified version of the Berg Balance Scale for the school-age child with mild to moderate motor impairment. *Pediatr Phys Ther.* 2003;15(2):114-128. doi:10.1097/01.PEP.0000068117.48023.18.

73. Franjoine MR, Darr N, Held SL, Kott K, Young BL. The performance of children developing typically on the Pediatric Balance Scale. *Pediatr Phys Ther.* 2010;22(4):350-359. doi:10.1097/PEP.0b013e3181f9d5eb.

74. Donahoe B, Turner D, Worrell T. The use of functional reach as a measurement of balance in boys and girls without disabilities ages 5 to 15 years. *Pediatr Phys Ther.* 1994;6(4):189-193. doi:10.1097/00001577-199406040-00004.

75. Volkman KG, Stergiou N, Stuberg W, Blanke D, Stoner J. Factors affecting functional reach scores in youth with typical development. *Pediatr Phys Ther.* 2009;21(1):38-44. doi:10.1097/PEP.0b013e318196f68a.

76. Bartlett D, Birmingham T. Validity and reliability of a pediatric reach test. *Pediatr Phys Ther.* 2003;15(2):84-92. doi:10.1097/01.PEP.0000067885.63909.5C.

77. Nicolini-Panisson RD, Donadio MV. Normative values for the Timed 'Up and Go' test in children and adolescents and validation for individuals with Down syndrome. *Dev Med Child Neurol.* 2014;56(5):490-497. doi:10.1111/dmcn.12290.

78. Gan SM, Tung LC, Tang YH, Wang CH. Psychometric properties of functional balance assessment in children with cerebral palsy. *Neurorehabil Neural Repair.* 2008;22(6):745-753. doi:10.1177/1545968308316474.

79. Williams EN, Carroll SG, Reddihough DS, Phillips BA, Galea MP. Investigation of the Timed 'Up & Go' test in children. *Dev Med Child Neurol.* 2005;47(8):518-524. doi:10.1111/j.1469-8749.2005.tb01185.x.

80. Katz-Leurer M, Rotem H, Lewitus H, Keren O, Meyer S. Relationship between balance abilities and gait characteristics in children with post-traumatic brain injury. *Brain Inj.* 2008;22(2):153-159. doi:10.1080/02699050801895399.

81. Katz-Leurer M, Rotem H, Lewitus H, Keren O, Meyer S. Functional balance tests for children with traumatic brain injury within-session reliability. *Pediatr Phys Ther.* 2008;20(3):254-258. doi:10.1097/PEP.0b013e3181820dd8.

82. Carey H, Martin K, Combs-Miller S, Heathcock JC. Reliability and responsiveness of the Timed Up and Go Test in children with cerebral palsy. *Pediatr Phys Ther.* 2014;28(4):401-408. doi:10.1097/PEP.0000000000000301.

83. Held SL, Kott KM, Young BL. Standardized Walking Obstacle Course (SWOC): reliability and validity of a new functional measurement tool for children. *Pediatr Phys Ther.* 2006;18(1):23-30. doi:10.1097/01.pep.0000202251.79000.1d.

84. Dhote SN, Kharti PA, Ganvir SS. Reliability of "Modified Timed Up and Go" test in children with cerebral palsy. *J Pediatr Neurosci.* 2012;7(2):96-100. doi:10.4103/1817-1745.102564.

85. Martin K, Natarus M, Martin J, Henderson S. Minimal detectable change for TUG and TUDS tests for children with Down syndrome. *Pediatr Phys Ther.* 2017;29(1):77-82. doi:10.1097/PEP.0000000000000333.

86. Lammers AR, Hislop AA, Flynn Y, Haworth SG. The 6-Minute Walk Test: normal values for children of 4–11 years of age. *Arch Dis Child.* 2008;93(6):464-468. doi:10.1136/adc.2007.123653.

87. Fitzgerald D, Hickey C, Delahunt E, Walsh M, O'Brien T. Six-Minute Walk Test in children with spastic cerebral palsy and children developing typically. *Pediatr Phys Ther.* 2016;28(2):192-199. doi:10.1097/PEP.0000000000000224.

88. Nsenga Leunkeu A, Shephard RJ, Ahmaidi S. Six-Minute Walk Test in children with cerebral palsy gross motor function classification system levels I and II: reproducibility, validity, and training effects. *Arch Phys Med Rehabil.* 2012;93(12):2333-2339. doi:10.1016/j.apmr.2012.06.005.

89. Lelieveld OT, Takken T, van der Net J, van Weert E. Validity of the 6-Minute Walk Test in juvenile idiopathic arthritis. *Arthritis Rheum.* 2005;53(2):304-307. doi:10.1002/art.21086.

90. Takken T, Engelbert R, van Bergen M, et al. Six-Minute Walking Test in children with ESRD: discrimination validity and construct validity. *Pediatr Nephrol.* 2009;24(11):2217-2223. doi:10.1007/s00467-009-1259-x.

91. Cunha MT, Rozov T, de Oliveira RC, Jardim JR. Six-Minute Walk Test in children and adolescents with cystic fibrosis. *Pediatr Pulmonol.* 2006;41(7):618-622. doi:10.1002/ppul.20308.

92. Moalla W, Gauthier R, Maingourd Y, Ahmaidi S. Six-minute walking test to assess exercise tolerance and cardiorespiratory responses during training program in children with congenital heart disease. *Int J Sports Med.* 2005;26(9):756-762. doi:10.1055/s-2004-830558.

93. Li A, Yin Y, Yu CCW, et al. The Six-Minute Walk Test in healthy children: reliability and validity. *Eur Respir J.* 2005;25(6):1057-1060. doi:10.1183/09031936.05.00134904.

94. Thompson P, Beath T, Bell J, et al. Test-retest reliability of the 10-Metre Fast Walk Test and 6-Minute Walk Test in ambulatory school-aged children with cerebral palsy. *Dev Med Child Neurol.* 2008;50(5):370-376. doi:10.1111/j.1469-8749.2008.02048.x.

95. Maher CA, Williams MT, Olds TS. The Six-Minute Walk Test for children with cerebral palsy. *Int J Rehabil Res.* 2008;31(2):185-188. doi:10.1097/MRR.0b013e32830150f9.

96. Kiresuk TJ, Sherman RE. Goal attainment scaling: a general method for evaluating comprehensive community mental health programs. *Community Ment Health J.* 1968;4(6):443-453. doi:10.1007/BF01530764.

97. King GA, McDougall J, Palisano RJ, Gritzan J, Tucker MA. Goal Attainment Scale: its use in evaluating pediatric therapy programs. *Phys Occup Ther Pediatr.* 1999;19(2):31-52. doi:10.1080/J006v19n02_03.

98. Palisano RJ. Validity of Goal Attainment Scaling in infants with motor delays. *Phys Ther.* 1993;73(10):651-658; discussion 658-660. doi:10.1093/ptj/73.10.651.

99. Brown L, Burns YR, Watter P, Gray PH. Goal Attainment Scaling to evaluate intervention on individual gains for children born extremely preterm. *Pediatr Phys Ther.* 2017;29(3):215-221. doi:10.1097/PEP.0000000000000388.

100. Steenbeek D, Gorter JW, Ketelaar M, Galama K, Lindeman E. Responsiveness of Goal Attainment Scaling in comparison to two standardized measures in outcome evaluation of children with cerebral palsy. *Clin Rehabil.* 2011;25(12):1128-1139. doi:10.1177/0269215511407220.

101. King G, Tucker MA, Alambets P, et al. The evaluation of functional school-based therapy services for children with special needs. A feasibility study. *Phys Occup Ther Pediatr.* 1998;18(2):1-27. doi:/10.1080/J006v18n02_01.

102. Steenbeek D, Ketelaar M, Lindeman E, Galama K, Gorter JW. Interrater reliability of goal attainment scaling in rehabilitation of children with cerebral palsy. *Arch Phys Med Rehabil.* 2010;91(3):429-435. doi:10.1016/j.apmr.2009.10.013.

103. Parham LD, Ecker C, Miller Kuhaneck H, Henry DA, Glennon TJ. *Sensory Processing Measure (SPM): Manual.* Los Angeles: Western Psychological Services; 2007.

104. Dunn W. *Short Sensory Profile.* San Antonio, TX: Psychological Corporation; 1999.

105. Dunn W. *Infant Toddler Sensory Profile User's Manual.* San Antonio, TX: Psychological Corporation; 2002.

106. Dunn W. *Sensory Profile School Companion User's Manual.* San Antonio, TX: Harcourt Assessment; 2006.

107. Brown CE, Dunn W. *Sensory Profile for Adolescents/Adults User's Manual.* San Antonio, TX: Psychological Corporation; 2002.

108. Chess S, Thomas A. *The New York Longitudinal Scales Adult Temperament Questionnaire Test Manual.* Scottsdale, AZ: Behavioral Developmental Initiatives; 1998.

109. DeGangi GA, Greenspan SI. *Test of Sensory Functions in Infants (TSFI).* Los Angeles, CA: Western Psychological Services; 1989.

110. Bayley N. *Bayley Scales of Infant Development.* New York, NY: Psychological Corporation; 1969.

111. Bates JE. *Infant Characteristics Questionnaire, Revised.* Unpublished questionnaire. Bloomington, IN: Indiana University; 1984.

112. Fagan JF III. New evidence of the prediction of intelligence from infancy. *Infant Ment Health J.* 1982;3(4):219-228. doi:10.1002/1097-0355(198224)3:4<219::AID-IMHJ2280030404>3.0.CO;2-L.

113. Benson AM, Lane SJ. Interrater reliability of the Test of Sensory Functions in Infants as used with infants exposed to cocaine in utero. *OTJR.* 1994;14(2):170-177. doi:10.1177/153944929401400304.

114. Jirikowic TL, Engel JM, Deitz JC. The Test of Sensory Functions in Infants: test–retest reliability for infants with developmental delays. *Am J Occup Ther.* 1997;51(9):733-738. doi:10.5014/ajot.51.9.733.

115. Ayres AJ. *Sensory Integration and Praxis Tests.* Los Angeles, CA: Western Psychological Services; 1989.

116. Ayres AJ. *Southern California Sensory Integration Tests (rev. ed.).* Los Angeles, CA: Western Psychological Services; 1980.

117. Ayres AJ. *Southern California Postrotary Nystagmus Test Manual.* Los Angeles, CA: Western Psychological Services; 1975.

118. Ayres AJ. Patterns of perceptual-motor dysfunction in children: a factor analytic study. *Percept Mot Skills.* 1965;20(4):335-368. doi:10.2466/pms.1965.20.2.335.

119. Ayres AJ. Deficits in sensory integration in educationally handicapped children. *JOLD.* 1969;2(3):160-168. doi:10.1177/002221946900200307.

120. Ayres AJ. Types of sensory integrative dysfunction among disabled learners. *Am J Occup Ther.* 1972;26(1):13-18.

121. Ayres AJ. Cluster analyses of measures of sensory integration. *Am J Occup Ther.* 1977;31(6):362-366.

122. Murray EA, Cermak SA, O'Brien A. The relationship between form and space perception, constructional abilities, and clumsiness in children. *Am J Occup Ther.* 1990;44(7):623-628. doi:10.5014/ajot.44.7.623.

123. Wilson BN, Pollock N, Kaplan BJ, Law M. *Clinical Observations of Motor and Postural Skills.* 2nd ed. Framingham, MA: Therapro, Inc; 2000.

124. Reisman JE, Hanschu B. *Sensory Integration Inventory–Revised for Individuals With Developmental Disorders.* Stillwater, MN: PDP Press; 1992.

125. Richter EW, Montgomery PC. *The Sensorimotor Performance Analysis.* Stillwater, MN: PDP Press; 1989.

126. Haley S, Coster W, Dumas H, Fragala-Pinkham M, Moed R. *Evaluation of Disability Inventory Computer Adaptive Test: Development, Standardization and Administration Manual.* Boston, MA: Health and Disability Research Institute; 2012.

127. Dumas HM, Fragala-Pinkham MA, Haley SM, et al. Item bank development for a revised Pediatric Evaluation of Disability Inventory (PEDI). *Phys Occup Ther Pediatr.* 2010;30(3):168-184. doi:10.3109/01942631003640493.

128. Dumas HM, Fragala-Pinkham MA. Concurrent validity and reliability of the Pediatric Evaluation of Disability Inventory—Computer Adaptive Test Mobility Domain. *Pediatr Phys Ther.* 2012;24(2):171-176; discussion 176. doi:10.1097/PEP.0b013e31824c94ca.

129. Dumas HM, Fragala-Pinkham MA, Rosen EL, Lombard KA, Farrell C. Pediatric Evaluation and Disability Inventory Computer Adaptive Test (PEDI–CAT) and Alberta Infant Motor Scale (AIMS): validity and responsiveness. *Phys Ther.* 2015;95(11):1559-1568. doi:10.2522/ptj.20140339.

130. Haley SM, Coster WJ, Dumas HM, et al. Accuracy and precision of the Pediatric Evaluation of Disability Inventory—Computer Adaptive Tests (PEDI–CAT). *Dev Med Child Neurol.* 2011;53(12):1100-1106. doi:10.1111/j.1469-8749.2011.04107.x.

131. Dumas HM, Fragala-Pinkham MA, Haley SM, et al. Computer adaptive test performance in children with and without disabilities: prospective field study of the PEDI–CAT. *Disabil Rehabil.* 2012;34(5):393-401. doi:10.3109/09638288.2011.607217.

132. Dumas HM, Fragala-Pinkham MA, Feng T, Haley SM. A preliminary evaluation of the PEDI–CAT mobility item bank for children using walking aids and wheelchairs. *J Ped Rehabil Med.* 2012;5(1):29-35. doi:10.3233/PRM-2011-0184.

133. King G, Law M, King S. *Children's Assessment of Participation and Enjoyment (CAPE) and Preferences for Activities of Children (PAC).* San Antonio, TX: Pearson; 2004.

134. King G, Law M, King S, et al. Measuring children's participation in recreation and leisure activities: construct validation of the CAPE and PAC. *Child Care Health Dev.* 2007;33(1):28-39. doi:10.1111/j.1365-2214.2006.00613.x.

135. Varni JW, Seid M, Rode CA. The PedQL: measurement model for the Pediatric Quality of Life Inventory. *Med Care.* 1999;37(2):126-139. doi:10.1097/00005650-199902000-00003.

136. Varni JW, Seid M, Kurtin PS. PedsQL 4.0: reliability and validity of the Pediatric Quality of Life Inventory version 4.0 generic core scales in healthy and patient populations. *Med Care.* 2001;39(8):800-812. doi:10.1097/00005650-200108000-00006.

Establishing Functional Goals and Organizing Intervention

3

Patricia C. Montgomery, PT, PhD, FAPTA

When providing services to the pediatric population, the physical therapist is responsible for determining the treatment techniques to be used, when to use them, and how long intervention should continue. Making the transition between didactic information and theoretical frameworks to actual "hands-on" intervention can be a long, frustrating, and anxiety-producing experience both for the therapist and the child. If the primary focus in the academic program was on techniques, the physical therapist new to pediatrics may not have experience in development of strategies for planning and sequencing treatment. The purpose of this chapter is to identify some of the variables that influence treatment planning. A method for selecting appropriate treatment techniques and sequence of application is suggested by using the World Health Organization's *International Classification of Functioning, Disability and Health* (ICF) model.[1] In this framework outcome goals are established by determining the child's Participation Restrictions, which reflect the child's inability to function in typical life situations.

The information presented in this chapter is intended to serve as one possible process for developing a strategy for organizing treatment and involves a number of therapist and patient variables that will alter its applicability in different situations. Many experienced clinicians have no difficulty determining the content of individual treatment sessions in relation to therapeutic goals. These clinicians, however, may not be able to describe the cognitive processes they use to make such determinations. Therefore, a specific strategy for treatment planning and sequencing may be useful to many physical therapists, particularly students, new graduates, and clinicians with limited clinical experience in pediatrics.

In addition, documentation of patient progress in relation to intervention is essential in clinical as well as research settings. The approach of goal setting and use of measurable behavioral objectives in relation to treatment outcome will be emphasized.

Connolly BH, Montgomery PC, eds. *Therapeutic Exercise for Children With Developmental Disabilities, Fourth Edition* (pp 95-111).
© 2020 Taylor & Francis Group.

Variables Influencing Treatment Planning

The theoretical framework a physical therapist uses to plan intervention will be affected by the understanding of and degree of agreement with specific theories of motor control, motor learning, and motor development. Although physical therapy curricula contain similar content in therapeutic exercise, there will be differences between which theories are emphasized and which therapeutic techniques are taught depending on physical therapy faculty, and, in turn, their training and clinical experiences. This is not a negative but a positive phenomenon because it provides the physical therapist several approaches to treatment that eventually can be validated or invalidated by clinical research. The current emphasis in physical therapy is on evidence-based practice.[2] Whenever possible the physical therapist uses empirical evidence to support intervention strategies with pediatric patients. An attempt has been made throughout this text to present the most recent empirical evidence in areas relevant to making clinical decisions.

Another variable affecting treatment planning is the physical therapist's ability to integrate general evaluation and intervention strategies taught in the basic curriculum with specific techniques used in the treatment of the pediatric population. For example, techniques for improving strength, endurance, and flexibility are essential in the treatment of many children. Orthopedic and cardiovascular considerations in relation to exercise, weight-bearing positions, various activities, and the use of adaptive devices also are important.

The selection of examination tools will be determined by the therapist's knowledge of tests and measures appropriate for the pediatric population. Norm-referenced tests are designed primarily to detect whether a child has a motor delay in relation to a same-age, nondisabled peer group.[3] Criterion-referenced tests measure a child's performance against set criteria or his or her own previous performance, therefore providing information on the most appropriate focus of treatment. Generally, the more physically and intellectually challenged the child is, the more difficult it is to determine current abilities and potential for change, and fewer standardized examination tools are available. An in-depth discussion of tests and measures currently used in pediatrics was provided in the preceding chapter.

Physical therapists rely on clinical observations or qualitative assessments of sensory and motor abilities to supplement the results of formal examinations. These clinical observations also may be used as a substitute for unavailable or inappropriate examination tools. The applicability of qualitative clinical information in relation to choosing specific treatment techniques is documented in subsequent chapters.

Another variable affecting the process of treatment planning is clinical experience in determining participation restrictions and functional goals, as well as observing change resulting in attainment or failure to accomplish specific objectives. For example, motor milestones, such as rolling, sitting, and crawling, may be used as functional outcomes. The physical therapist working with the child with severe disabilities, however, may discover that these outcomes must be broken down into smaller goals to effectively measure progress over specified periods of time.

Developing a Strategy for Planning Treatment

The first step in developing a strategy for planning treatment is for the physical therapist to assess his or her own level of knowledge. Has the physical therapist's academic and clinical training provided a foundation for working with pediatric patients? A basic prerequisite is a thorough understanding of normal motor development that is necessary for optimal examination, evaluation, and intervention. The physical therapist needs to determine what areas of knowledge need to be supplemented with additional information or training. If the therapist's caseload consists of children with learning disabilities who demonstrate subtle motor problems, for example, additional study of pertinent resource material may be necessary. The physical therapist must assume the responsibility of being adequately prepared to plan intervention for specific children.

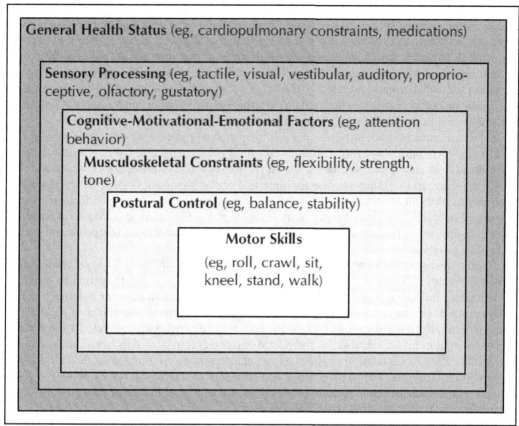

Figure 3-1. Intrinsic variables that interact in the development of motor skills. Extrinsic variables include cultural and environmental factors.

Although various intervention approaches can be employed, a systems perspective suggests numerous variables will interact to affect outcome. Some of these variables are intrinsic (eg, degree of pathology to the central nervous system, cognitive status) while others are extrinsic (eg, cultural influences, environmental factors). Figure 3-1 illustrates some of the intrinsic factors that should be considered in pediatric examination, evaluation, and intervention. Each physical therapist will address the mental organization of these variables differently, but should create a framework useful in evaluating and treating children in a holistic manner.

The physical therapist also must choose appropriate examination tools. Most normative tests provide information as to whether the child is performing below, at, or above expectations as compared with a typically developing child of the same age. Few tests will provide information regarding what to do to improve the child's performance. Normative and criterion-referenced tests, however, may reveal areas of deficits and test results that can be used for monitoring developmental change. Clinical measurements, such as the 6-Minute Walk Test and Goal Attainment Scale, also can be used to document progress (see Chapter 2).

During the examination process, the physical therapist summarizes what the child can and cannot do. Identifying sensory tasks or motor activities the child should be accomplishing is helpful. Emphasis should be on the functional movements and tasks the child needs to perform optimally in natural environments, such as home, child care, preschool, school, and community ("Participation"). The most difficult aspect of the assessment process is to determine why the child cannot perform the tasks or movements. The examination and evaluation procedures throughout this text are intended to assist the physical therapist in delineating specific problem areas. Different phases in the lifespan require different skills. Early childhood is characterized by the expansion of basic motor abilities, such as independent sitting, crawling, and walking. With increasing age various forms of locomotion develop (eg, running, hopping, skipping, jumping, riding a tricycle). When the child begins school, an increasing emphasis is on fine motor skills required for drawing, cutting, pasting, and printing or using a keyboard. With maturation the child may participate in team or individual sports and select hobbies that satisfy individual interests. Focusing on age-appropriate tasks that match varying needs within the lifespan is important to the child's motivation and success in participating in natural environments.

A decision must be made as to whether it is reasonable to project long-term outcomes for the child in relation to normal or typical skills. For the high-risk preterm infant who is mildly delayed in motor skills at an adjusted age of 6 months, the use of typical developmental skills, such as rolling, crawling, and walking, may be appropriate. For the 5-year-old child with severe spastic quadriplegia, who will not attain typical motor skills, goals that reflect improved independence or obtainment of specific functional skills are more appropriate. For example, a long-term outcome may be "to improve voluntary use of one upper extremity so the child can independently punch the keys on a keyboard."

Finally, treatment planning is performed within a general framework of appropriate intervention for children. In an old paradigm, "optimizing development" meant getting to the next developmental milestone, and individual treatment plans in rehabilitation for children usually were organized with motor milestones as goals.[4] Using the ICF model, the ability of children to function optimally in life situations ("Participation") is the desired outcome. Activity limitations refer to restrictions in individual skills, and related impairments in Body Functions and Structures then are identified. Goals relate to intended impact of intervention on functioning (body functions and structures, activities, and participation), and outcomes are the actual results of intervention. A distinction is made between capacity (what can be accomplished in a controlled environment) and performance (what children typically accomplish).

DETERMINING ACTIVITY AND PARTICIPATION GOALS

One of the most important responsibilities of the physical therapist is to determine intervention strategies and functional goals for the child. Although the therapist may know what "improving ambulation skills" refers to, various therapists may use different observational data to support the conclusion that this therapeutic goal has been met. Our responsibility, then, is to describe the behavior or set of behaviors that allows other observers (eg, therapists, physicians, parents, teachers) to arrive at the same conclusion regarding the child's level of function. Precise, unambiguous specifications regarding a behavior also decrease the amount of subjectivity in the assessment process. For example, the objective "the child will ambulate independently with a walker" does not specify if there are any constraints on the child's abilities. If we state "the child will ambulate independently with a reverse walker in the home and school environment during daily activities," the behavioral objective and the desired participation outcome are clarified.

Behavioral objectives consist of a behavior that can be observed and measured. Specific criteria describing the behavior may include the conditions under which the behavior will occur. Using successful completion of a minimum number of trials or performance of a behavior during a percentage of a set time period would be examples of specified conditions.

Activity or functional limitations identified in a child are related to theoretical perspectives. If a child cannot maintain an upright head position and sitting balance, for example, one can hypothesize that there are deficits in postural control, deficient strength in the neck and trunk muscles, deficits in cognitive and motivational functions, or a combination of factors. The physical therapist can be accurate in describing the child's posture and movement, but can only hypothesize about underlying causes or impairments.

Physical therapy interventions and goals for the child also depend on the theoretical framework of the physical therapist. In hierarchical models, goals often relate to altering muscle tone, decreasing reflex patterns of movement, achieving developmental motor milestones, and improving sensory processing. In more contemporary models, goals relate to the development of functional skills, which are "essential activities required in natural environments—such as communication, personal care, ambulation, transfers, and manipulation."[5] Traditional goals of physical therapy intervention, such as those addressing strength, endurance, and flexibility, also are used in pediatrics. Goals in various frameworks overlap. The essential element that ties them together is the use of measurable objectives.

If a goal of improving postural control in a child with spastic quadriplegia is selected, how is success following intervention determined? The ICF model suggests the first step is to identify participation restrictions that, in this case, would relate to postural control. Then the activity limitations and impairments that contribute to these participation restrictions can be hypothesized and intervention strategies determined. Finally, specific, measurable functional goals within a specific time frame are used to measure progress.

In the following section, examples of participation restrictions related to gross motor and mobility skills, upper extremity skills, sensorimotor processing, and cognitive functions are provided. The participation restriction is identified first, followed by activity/functional limitation(s), and hypothesized contributing impairments. Examples of physical therapy interventions and related functional and participation goals to be achieved with intervention are provided.

Gross Motor and Mobility Skills

Example 1

> *Participation Restrictions:* In prone, infant cannot maintain neutral head position to view objects in his or her environment.
> *Activity Limitations:* In prone, infant does not lift his or her head off the floor, but can only slide it from side to side to clear the airway.
> *Impairments:* Deficits in motor control that limit ability to control head position; weakness in trunk and neck muscles; limited tolerance for prone position.
> *Interventions:* Improve head control in prone position, increase strength in trunk and neck extensors, facilitate prone-on-elbows position.
> *Functional/Participation Goals:* In prone, infant will lift his or her head 45 to 90 degrees, 2 out of 3 trials, and maintain this position for 10 seconds to view an object/toy.

Example 2

> *Participation Restrictions:* While sitting on the floor, the child is unable to make transitions of movement to play effectively with peers and/or toys.
> *Activity Limitations:* Child is able to transition from prone to sitting only by pushing up on extended arms, pulling legs underneath trunk, and W-sitting. He or she then is unable to alter this position.
> *Impairments:* Deficits in motor control, poor motor planning, limited trunk rotation.
> *Interventions:* Increase variety of movement transitions from prone to sitting and from sitting to hands and knees, increase trunk and hip flexibility, encourage ring- and side-sitting positions.
> *Functional/Participation Goals:* When placed on the floor in prone, the child will use more than one movement pattern to transition into sitting at least once during 5 trials. The child will assume 2 different sitting positions over a 5-minute observation period of free play with a peer.

Example 3

> *Participation Restrictions:* Child often falls when sitting and play interactions with peers are disrupted. He or she occasionally hits head when falling, and injury is a concern to the parents, so play dates with friends are limited.

> *Activity Limitations:* When child loses balance in sitting, he or she does not always attempt to catch him- or herself with arms.

> *Impairments:* Deficits in motor control, poor sitting balance, slow or inadequate processing of sensory information regarding position in space.

> *Interventions:* Improve motor control and sitting balance, improve reaction time to sensory input, improve protective responses to loss of balance.

> *Functional/Participation Goals:* When placed in ring-sitting, the child will prop on extended arms for 1 minute without collapsing. In ring-sitting, child will successfully catch him- or herself in 2 of 3 trials when slowly pushed off balance in a lateral direction. In a 5-minute play period, the child will successfully catch him- or herself when losing balance while in a ring-sitting position.

Example 4

> *Participation Restrictions:* Child is not allowed to walk down the halls in his or her school alone. A classroom aide accompanies him or her, limiting independence and interactions with peers.

> *Activity Limitations:* The child is ambulatory, but must wear a helmet and be supervised because he or she does not protect him- or herself adequately when falling.

> *Impairments:* Deficits in motor control, slow or inadequate processing of sensory information regarding position in space, weakness of upper extremities.

> *Interventions:* Improve motor control, increase response time to sensory input, increase strength of upper extremities, teach protective strategies.

> *Functional/Participation Goals:* The child will be able to deliberately fall forward and sideways from a standing position and catch him- or herself with his or her arms. The child will be able to deliberately fall backward from a standing position and "sit down" with protective reactions of the arms. In walking during the school day, the child will not hit his or her head on the floor if falling and will be allowed to walk down the halls without assistance from the classroom aide.

Example 5

> *Participation Restrictions:* The child needs the assistance of an adult to dress lower extremities (eg, socks, shoes, pants), an activity easily accomplished by younger siblings. He or she also has difficulty riding a tricycle and keeping up with peers, limiting independent mobility and social interactions.

> *Activity Limitations:* The child tends to use both legs together. For example, in sitting he or she cannot shift weight onto one hip and flex opposite hip and knee to put on a sock.

> *Impairments:* Deficits in motor control with poor lower extremity dissociation and poor postural control; lower extremity and trunk weakness; deficits in motor planning.

> *Interventions:* Improve lower extremity control of isolated movements, increase general lower extremity and trunk strength, improve balance, improve motor planning.

> *Functional/Participation Goals:* In sitting on the floor, the child will shift his or her weight and leave one leg extended while flexing the opposite leg to put on socks or pants. Child will crawl on hands and knees with a reciprocal lower extremity pattern with verbal reminders. The child will independently ride a tricycle for a distance of 6 feet.

Example 6

> *Participation Restrictions:* The child is unable to participate in classroom activities performed in a standing position and is not at the same level as peers to maintain good eye contact and socialize.

> *Activity Limitations:* In ambulation using a reverse walker, the child walks too slowly to keep up with his or her peers in the classroom or hallways at school, so he or she uses a manual wheelchair.

> *Impairments:* Deficits in motor control, poor motor planning, decreased strength and endurance, poor balance.

> *Interventions:* Increase speed of ambulation with walker, increase endurance for standing with walker, improve motor planning.

> *Functional/Participation Goals:* The child will march in place (20 steps per minute or faster) to fast music while standing with his or her walker. The child will ambulate independently with the walker 20 feet (6 m) in 10 seconds in the classroom. The child will keep up with his or her peers while walking with the walker for a distance of 50 feet (15 m).

Upper Extremity Skills

Example 1

> *Participation Restrictions:* In supine, the infant cannot transfer a toy from one hand to the other or bring toy to mouth efficiently for sensory exploration and play.

> *Activity Limitations:* In supine, the infant cannot bring hands to mouth or hands together at midline of body.

> *Impairments:* Deficits in motor control, decreased strength in upper extremities, limited shoulder range of motion (ROM).

> *Interventions:* Improve ability to volitionally control upper extremity movements in supine position, increase active ROM in shoulders.

> *Functional/Participation Goals:* In supine, infant will be able to bring either hand to his or her mouth. In supine, the infant will be able to bring his or her hands together at midline for hand-to-hand contact and to manipulate toys.

Example 2

> *Participation Restrictions:* The child is unable to eat finger food independently during snack time at preschool and must rely on adult for assistance, limiting independence and social interactions with peers.

> *Activity Limitations:* The child uses gross grasp and release and cannot move objects to the radial side of the hand or orient the hand to get objects or food to the mouth.

> *Impairments:* Deficits in upper extremity control, limited control over individual fingers.

> *Interventions:* Improve hand skills and isolated use of fingers.

> *Functional/Participation Goals:* The child will be able to grasp a bread stick and bring it to the mouth independently. In 5 out of 10 attempts, the child will grasp small objects with the radial portion of the hand. In 1 of 5 trials, the child will use a 3-finger pinch to pick up a Cheerio.

Example 3

> *Participation Restrictions:* The toddler is limited in activities that require both hands to be used simultaneously (bilateral activities) and cannot manipulate some toys when playing with peers.

> *Activity Limitations:* The toddler does not use right upper extremity during play or when large toys requiring bilateral upper extremity control are presented for him or her to hold.

> *Impairments:* Deficits in motor control, impaired somatosensory processing from right upper extremity.

> *Interventions:* Increase frequency of attempts at independent movement with right upper extremity, increase sensory input/awareness to right upper extremity, promote bilateral upper extremity activities.

> *Functional/Participation Goals:* In ring-sitting, the toddler will use his or her right arm, with verbal reminders, to pick up 3 of 5 puzzle pieces placed to the right. The toddler will use his or her right hand spontaneously to clap in a game of patty-cake, imitating the therapist on 5 of 10 attempts. Toddler will use both hands to hold a 12-inch (30-cm) diameter ball and roll it to parent in 3 of 5 trials.

Example 4

> *Participation Restrictions:* At school, the child uses a manual wheelchair, rather than his or her power wheelchair, which requires assistance and limits independence and social interactions.

> *Activity Limitations:* The child can independently control his or her power wheelchair, but runs into objects, walls, and people.

> *Impairments:* Deficits in fine motor control, intellectual deficits, poor motor planning.

> *Interventions:* Improve fine motor control, improve general motor planning.

> *Functional/Participation Goals:* In his or her power wheelchair, child will successfully complete a 20-foot obstacle course 2 of 3 trials without hitting walls or 2 of 3 obstacles. When using a rear-view mirror mounted on the wheelchair, the child will successfully back up 3 feet (1 m). The child will be able to turn the wheelchair around in a 4-foot (1.2 m) square space in the classroom. The child will be able to use his or her power wheelchair without accidents in the school environment.

Sensory/Perceptual Processing

Example 1

> *Participation Restrictions:* The child does not interact with peers during many gross motor activities, especially on the playground, where he or she avoids moveable equipment.

> *Activity Limitations:* The child does not enjoy or tolerate movement activities. He or she will not attempt to play on moveable equipment or toys.

> *Impairments:* Hypersensitivity to vestibular stimulation, "postural insecurity" (ie, deficient postural control), poor motor planning.

> *Interventions:* Decrease sensitivity to vestibular stimulation, improve balance, increase confidence in participating in gross motor activities, improve motor planning skills.

> *Functional/Participation Goals:* The child will tolerate swinging slowly on a playground swing for 3 minutes. The child will participate in scooter board games with his or her peers.

Example 2

- › *Participation Restrictions:* The child fusses during activities of daily living and during play and school activities that involve tactile input. His or her behavior affects personal hygiene, as well as social and learning opportunities.
- › *Activity Limitations:* The child is sensitive to tactile input. He or she does not like to be touched, wear new clothes, or have face or hair washed. He or she does not use hands to explore or play in various textured mediums.
- › *Impairments:* Hypersensitivity to tactile stimulation.
- › *Interventions:* Decrease tactile hypersensitivity, develop strategies to increase tolerance to various textures of clothing.
- › *Functional/Participation Goals:* The child will seek out hugs from adults. Child will not cry or scream when his or her hair is washed. The child will participate with classmates for 5 minutes to complete a finger-painting project.

Example 3

- › *Participation Restrictions:* The child does not visually interact socially with peers or adults.
- › *Activity Limitations:* The child does not consistently look at objects placed in his or her visual field and does not maintain eye contact with adults or peers for more than 1 to 2 seconds.
- › *Impairments:* Deficits in visual focus and tracking, possible cognitive/emotional deficits (eg, autism), poor head control, poor eye-head coordination.
- › *Interventions:* Improve visual focus and tracking, improve eye-head coordination, increase interest in environmental objects and people.
- › *Functional/Participation Goals:* The child will orient 2 of 3 trials to an object lit by a flashlight. The child will maintain visual focus on a specific toy for 10 seconds. He or she will turn eyes and head in 2 of 3 trials to follow a moving object. The child will maintain eye contact with an adult 50% of the time during a 1-minute social interaction.

Example 4

- › *Participation Restrictions:* The child often ignores people to his or her left side and occasionally bumps into objects on the left while moving through his or her environment, limiting social interactions and independence.
- › *Activity Limitations:* The child tends to neglect the left side of his or her body and space during motor activities, usually orienting to his or her right and demonstrating difficulty with bilateral activities.
- › *Impairments:* Deficits in somatosensory processing from the left side of the body, deficits in visual perception, deficits in motor control.
- › *Interventions:* Improve somatosensory and visual awareness of left side of the body and left side of space, increase spontaneous use of left side of body, increase frequency of orientation to the left side.
- › *Functional/Participation Goals:* The child will actively remove sticky tape or stickers placed on his or her left arm. The child will "twirl" to the left and right when "dancing" to music. The child will walk through a crowded classroom without bumping into objects.

Intellectual Functions

Example 1

▸ *Participation Restrictions:* Siblings and parents consistently assist the child, decreasing opportunities for the child to practice motor skills and increase his or her independence.

▸ *Activity Limitations:* The child is slow to initiate movement in response to verbal requests and relies on family for activities of daily living.

▸ *Impairments:* Deficits in motor control, sensory processing deficits, intellectual/motivational deficits.

▸ *Interventions:* Improve speed in initiation of movement, teach the family behavioral strategies to encourage the child's independence.

▸ *Functional/Participation Goals:* In sitting, the child will initiate reaching for a toy less than 5 seconds after a verbal request to "get the toy." In prone, the child will begin to belly crawl toward a toy within 5 seconds after the toy is placed near him or her on floor. The child will assist in dressing and undressing tasks.

Example 2

▸ *Participation Restrictions:* In the school lunchroom, the child often eats the majority of meals seated by him- or herself, limiting social interaction.

▸ *Activity Limitations:* The child moves very slowly when feeding him- or herself and takes more than 60 minutes to finish a meal.

▸ *Impairments:* Poor oral-motor skills, attention deficit (ie, increased distractibility).

▸ *Interventions:* Improve oral-motor skills and attention during mealtime, develop behavior modification strategies for school staff to implement during lunch.

▸ *Functional/Participation Goals:* The child will feed him- or herself and complete a meal within 30 minutes with occasional verbal encouragement from an adult.

Example 3

▸ *Participation Restrictions:* The child cannot walk without classroom aide from the classroom to the gym at school, which limits his or her social interaction and development of independence.

▸ *Activity Limitations:* When walking without a classroom aide in the school hallways, the child lags behind classmates or stops walking, becoming distracted by other children.

▸ *Impairments:* Intellectual and motivational deficits, attention deficits.

▸ *Interventions:* Improve selective attention for gross motor tasks, use behavioral cues and rewards in hallway to facilitate progress.

▸ *Functional/Participation Goals:* The child will walk independently from classroom to gym within 3 minutes, 100% of the time when no other children are present in the hallway. The child will walk independently from classroom to gym within 5 minutes, 100% of the time when other children are present in the hallway.

Short-Term Goals

In the previous examples, goals are the intended impact on functioning, including body functions and structures, activities, and participation.[1] Outcomes are the actual results of intervention. Outcomes can be determined only at the conclusion of intervention either by achieving a specific long-term outcome or as a result of post-testing on a specific variable.

One example of a long-term outcome is that "the child will ambulate independently with a walker in the home during all daily activities." The therapist analyzes this task in relation to the child's abilities and develops short-term goals that are appropriate for eventually reaching the long-term outcome. Examples of short-term goals for this functional skill might include:

> The child will pull to stand at furniture 2 of 3 trials when a toy is placed out of reach on the furniture.
> The child will cruise to the left or right a distance of 3 feet (1 m) at furniture to obtain toys.
> When placed, the child will maintain balance in upright with the walker for 5 minutes.
> The child will make forward progress with the walker on a smooth surface for a distance of 10 feet (3 m).
> The child will make forward progress with the walker on a carpeted surface for a distance of 10 feet (3 m).
> The child will demonstrate the ability to motor plan a distance of 15 feet (4.5 m) and turn the walker to avoid 2 obstacles in his or her path.
> The child will demonstrate protective reactions each time he or she falls or attempts to lower him- or herself from the walker.
> The child will be able to lower him- or herself independently from the walker to the floor or transfer to a chair in 2 of 3 attempts.
> The child will be able to get into his or her walker from the floor or a chair independently in 2 of 3 attempts.

After determining the long-term outcome and short-term goals, the therapist then selects appropriate treatment techniques to enable the child to achieve the desired outcome (refer to subsequent chapters). During treatment, the therapist continually evaluates the effectiveness of treatment techniques, adding, omitting, or revising intervention as necessary for the child's success. As the child makes progress, long-term outcomes may be altered or added and short-term goals reestablished. In the current example, once the child has achieved the outcome of using the walker in all daily activities at home, a new long-term outcome may be initiated. For example, it may be appropriate to initiate short-term goals to achieve a new long-term outcome of using the walker independently in the school classroom.

Organizing Treatment

Environmental Considerations

In Gibson's theoretical model for understanding human behavior, the child and the environment are linked.[6] Objects in the environment are described in terms of "affordances" or what possibilities they offer the child for action in relation to his or her action capabilities. For example, while observing a 7-month-old child belly crawling on the floor, a toy is placed on an 18-inch (45 cm) high sofa (Figure 3-2). The child sees the toy and appears interested in it, but does not attempt to reach the toy. If the sofa cushion (6 inches [15 cm] in height) is placed on the floor and the toy is placed on top of the cushion, the child reaches up to the sofa cushion, pulls him- or herself up on his or her knees, and reaches for the toy (Figure 3-3). The top of the sofa was too high for the child to reach from a prone position and, therefore, did not "afford" the child a surface to pull up on. The sofa cushion on the floor, however, was of an appropriate height and "afforded" the child the opportunity to pull to a kneeling position to obtain the toy.

The physical therapist working with children constructs "affordances" in the environment to elicit functional movements. A parental self-report to assess quantity and quality of affordances in home and child care environments that are conducive for infants between 3 and 18 months has been developed.[7-9] Affordances in natural environments can be very successful in allowing

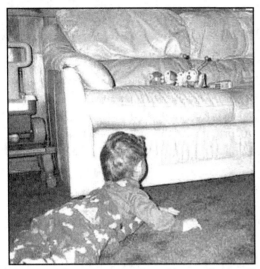

Figure 3-2. From prone, child is unable to pull to kneeling at a sofa.

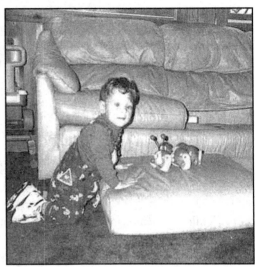

Figure 3-3. From prone, child is able to pull to kneeling at a sofa cushion.

children to explore movement options. For example, stairs can be used for sliding and climbing up and down, sitting, jumping, or kneeling. A variety of movements such as climbing on hands and knees, climbing on hands and feet, standing on 2 feet, sitting with feet on the step below, kneeling and playing with toys, or sitting sideways on a step with legs extended are possible. Most children will explore options for movement if given the opportunity and encouragement. Practicing skills in relevant environments, such as school and community, which relate to long-term functional outcomes also is important. The child needs to be able to perform specific skills, such as ambulation, in a variety of environments (ie, different contexts). Being able to walk safely in a therapy room with a tile floor and few obstacles or distractions does not ensure that the child will be able to walk safely on carpet; in a cluttered, noisy, and visually distracting classroom; or in a variety of community settings.

To ensure use of the same skill in varied contexts, the physical therapist has the child practice the skill in each environment and makes modifications or alters training as necessary. This often is a difficult concept for some third-party payers, which prefer to reimburse physical therapy services that are delivered on an inpatient or outpatient basis in a hospital or medically related facility. Medicare guidelines for home-based services frequently are inappropriately applied to children, and some payers will allow only home-based services for children who are medically fragile and unable to leave the home environment. This is an inefficient protocol that should be discarded. Environments in which it is important for children to function include the home, school, neighborhood, and community settings including church, shopping mall, and playground. Several physical therapy sessions spent on the neighborhood playground may appear frivolous to a third-party payer. This is the best context, however, in which children can learn skills that will enable them to effectively and safely move and interact with peers in a playground setting. (See Video 3-1.)

Physical therapists in inpatient and outpatient settings have to make a concentrated effort to provide caregivers appropriate suggestions for carryover in home, school, or community environments. There are instances, however, when outpatient physical therapy may be the most efficient setting for providing pediatric services, such as when specific equipment is needed (eg, whirlpool, treadmill) or when children do not perform well in the home environment and are more cooperative in an outpatient setting. It is hoped that third-party payers will be flexible in allowing physical therapy services to be provided in the settings in which therapy will be most effective in achieving improved functional independence.

Quality of Movement

The issue of "quality" of movement is controversial. One opinion is that the best strategy is to strive for normal quality of movement. There are many children, however, who do not have the ability to produce typical movements, and valuable time may be lost working toward unattainable goals when the major objective of the physical therapist should be to improve children's functional abilities to optimize participation in real-life environments.

How basic motor skills are accomplished does not need to mirror "normal." Consider the child with arthrogryposis who is limited in how he or she moves because of lack of specific muscles and certain joint limitations. This child will not be able to produce "typical" movement patterns using the same muscles and joint ROM of nondisabled peers. Yet, by using the muscles and joint ROM available, the child with arthrogryposis may be able to accomplish the motor skills necessary to function independently. Is the "quality" of this child's movements poor because they do not "look like" the movements produced by a typically developing peer? It is important for the physical therapist not to judge the child against a standard of "normal" or typical. If the child's performance does not meet a specific standard, the child may infer failure from the therapist's negative feedback and may become dependent on external standards for judging the motor performance. This may result in the child losing the desire to practice or acquire skills independently.

Latash and Anson[10] suggested that under certain conditions, as in the child with motor impairments, the central nervous system might reconsider its priorities. Perhaps the changed motor patterns that result should not be considered pathological, but rather adaptive to a primary disorder and may even be viewed as optimal for a given state. For each particular motor task, these authors suggested that the main criterion is functional success and that movements should be judged primarily by their effectiveness in accomplishing a task.

If children with developmental disabilities are able to accomplish the functional components of ambulation, perhaps the "quality" of their movements should be considered good, regardless of how closely they approximate typical movement patterns. Moore and colleagues[11] found, for example, that oxygen cost was higher for reciprocal walking than for a swing-through gait in adolescents with low lumbar myelomeningocele. The authors suggested a swing-through gait was the more efficient walking pattern for this group of individuals. Energy consumption is a critical variable to consider during motor tasks. Franks et al[12] demonstrated that the high energy cost of walking (compared with using a wheelchair) may have adversely affected certain aspects of school performance in 3 students (ages 9, 10, and 15 years) with myelomeningocele.

Another important issue in evaluating the quality of movement is to determine the potential for the development of secondary problems.[13] For example, W-sitting when used excessively may contribute to decreased ROM in hip external rotation, increased knee instability, and excessive ankle eversion, resulting in a poor base of support in standing. Reaching only with the forearm in a pronated position will limit active forearm supination and muscle tightness may result, adversely affecting the development of upper extremity control. Braendvik and colleagues[14] suggested that in high-functioning children and adolescents with cerebral palsy, limited active supination range and difficulties in generating and modulating force were strongly related to limitations in hand activity. Prolonged wearing of ankle-foot orthoses may result in decreased ankle plantar flexion ROM that will make floor mobility (eg, crawling on all fours, tall kneeling) and dressing and undressing the lower extremities more difficult. Children and their families must be informed about the risk of secondary problems and, together with the therapist, make decisions about which patterns of movements and positions should be promoted.

Sequencing Treatment

Usually several impairments occur simultaneously in children with developmental disabilities. For example, children may demonstrate deficits in sensory processing, motor control, strength, and attention. In organizing treatment and attempting to address various problem areas simultaneously, there are 2 general treatment sequences to consider. The first is the overall sequence of treatment over an extended period of time, for example, a 2- or 3-month period or a school year. Careful formulation of short-term goals and long-term outcomes will aid the therapist in obtaining a mental overview of the necessary emphasis in treatment. The second consideration is sequencing treatment within an individual treatment session, which may vary from one-half hour to 1 hour or longer.

Variables to be considered when determining the content of an individual treatment session are the intellectual abilities of the child, motivation, age, and endurance. A "play" vs a "work" approach can be varied depending on the age, personality, and interests of the child. Toys can be used quite effectively to motivate the young child and infant and to maintain interest during therapy. If a child resists or fatigues during certain activities, such as abdominal strengthening, 3 or 4 treatment techniques designed to strengthen the abdominal muscles can be interspersed during an individual session.

Techniques for behavior management can be employed to assist in specific sensory or motor tasks and also as a way to modify negative behavior during therapy. Checklists of exercises, which when completed yield a reward, often are helpful to motivate the child and to help the child be more organized during therapy. A small kitchen timer can be used to designate specific "work" (15 minutes) vs "play" (3 minutes) sessions, or specific rewards can be given for each 15 minutes of "crying-free" period of time.

A final, but perhaps the most important, consideration is the availability of caregivers for carryover of treatment. Whenever possible, the physical therapist should involve the family, school personnel, and other caregivers in the child's therapy program. Clearly defined behavioral objectives will assist in this process, and the therapist can facilitate the child's progress by training others in the child's environment(s) in related therapeutic activities and, when necessary, the use of adaptive equipment (see Chapter 14).

DOCUMENTING PROGRESS

The physical therapist is responsible not only for determining functional outcomes for the child, but also for determining whether the objectives have been met. Various methods for charting progress can be employed. An important component is to differentiate motor performance from motor learning (see Chapter 1). One method used to determine whether functional objectives have been achieved is to observe the child at the beginning of the treatment session to document his or her performance before treatment begins. Another method is to have the parent or teacher chart specific movements or tasks (eg, number of times the child assumes all fours independently per day) between treatment sessions. Post-testing performance on specific tests or measures can be compared with preintervention performance and also used to document progress.

EPISODE OF CARE

According to the *Guide to Physical Therapist Practice,*[2] intervention occurs in set time periods (short or continuous, or a series of intervals marked by brief separations of care) and are described as *episodes of care.* An episode of care can be concluded when anticipated goals and expected outcomes have been achieved. An episode of care also can conclude when the patient or caregiver declines further intervention, the patient is unable to continue progress toward outcomes because of medical or other complications, because financial/insurance resources have been expended, or the physical therapist determines that the patient will no longer benefit from intervention. The child with a lifelong disability may require multiple episodes of care following changes in physical status (eg, growth or surgical interventions), caregivers, environments, or task demands.

As part of the physical therapy diagnosis and prognosis, the plan of care should include criteria for decreasing frequency of physical therapy intervention and concluding the episode of care (discharge). Beginning with the initial evaluation, the plan of care should be a component of documentation. Early discussion of criteria for decreasing frequency of intervention and eventual discharge from physical therapy will educate the child's caregivers about the focus of physical therapy (ie, improving function and independence) and possible strategies for motor interventions for the child with lifelong disabilities (eg, transitioning from private clinic or home-based services to school physical therapy services, transitioning from direct to indirect physical therapy services, transitioning from physical therapy to adapted physical education or community-based motor activities, transitioning to activities with emphasis on lifelong fitness).

The concept of "episodic care" can be introduced through the plan of care so caregivers can be reassured that concluding an episode of care may not be final, but that reassessment and intervention can occur if new problems are identified. The plan of care also is helpful to payers to provide an idea of the anticipated frequency and duration of therapy services. Several examples of appropriate Plans of Care are listed next.

Sample Plans of Care

Example 1

> *Child:* Angela, age 2 months, birth asphyxia (not yet demonstrating a significant delay, prognosis is poor and therapist anticipates increasing frequency)
> *Initial Plan of Care:* Owing to Angela's young age, it is difficult to anticipate the duration of physical therapy services. She is at risk for developmental delay because of her birth history. Her progress will be reassessed every 2 to 3 months and, based on achievement of developmental motor skills and rate of progress, recommendations for frequency of services will be made. Bimonthly visits are recommended at this time with a possible increase to weekly when Angela begins to work on gross motor skills, such as rolling, crawling, and sitting.

Example 2

> *Child:* Devin, age 12 months, Down syndrome (mild impairments, currently pulling to stand and cruising, prognosis is good for independent ambulation)
> *Plan of Care:* Frequency of home-based physical therapy services was decreased when Devin began to pull to stand and cruise around furniture. This episode of weekly direct physical therapy services will end when he begins to walk independently. However, he will be monitored every 3 months for continued progress in his gross motor skills.

Example 3

> *Child:* Brittany, age 3 years 2 months, gross motor delay and intellectual impairments (child is demonstrating poor motivation and very slow progress toward independent ambulation, has been cruising at furniture for 12 months; therapist is trying to decrease frequency of intervention and the family is resisting any decrease in services)
> *Plan of Care:* It is anticipated that Brittany will need physical therapy services until she reaches her full potential for independent ambulation. Her motor skills and progress toward goals are reassessed every 3 months with recommendations made for frequency of physical therapy services. Now that Brittany is able to work on her upright mobility skills (ie, cruising and walking with assistance), frequency of physical therapy can be decreased from weekly to 2 times a month. If Brittany's motor skills plateau over the next 3- to 6-month period, frequency of physical therapy can be decreased further to periodic monitoring of her program.

Example 4

> *Child:* Billy, age 4 years 3 months cerebral palsy/visual impairment/Gross Motor Function Classification System Level II (child recently began walking independently, although balance is poor. Private clinic-based therapist anticipates his needs can be met by the school physical therapist who currently sees him 2 times/month)

> *Plan of Care:* Billy is currently being followed every other week for private clinic-based physical therapy. His program has been coordinated with his school physical therapist. Billy has met the long-term outcome of walking independently. Additional therapy goals can be met by the school physical therapist and vision specialist. He will be discharged from private physical therapy services at the end of this month.

Example 5

> *Child:* Hannah, age 6 years 6 months, L2, 3 myelomeningocele (child appears to be functioning at the highest level possible within the constraints of her impairments; therapist would like to discharge her from services and resume therapy at some future point if her needs change, that is, "episodic care")

> *Plan of Care:* At this time, it appears that Hannah is performing to the best of her capability within the limits of her disability. It is recommended that physical therapy sessions be decreased to twice per month for the next month, then once per month for 3 months, at which time she will be discontinued from services. A follow-up visit will be made in 6 months to determine whether she is able to maintain her level of function. If any problems develop or medical interventions occur, Hannah's physical therapy needs will be reassessed.

Example 6

> *Child:* John, age 8 years, developmental coordination disorder (child has significant motor planning problems and generally poor physical fitness; he is receiving private physical therapy services during the summer months when school therapy services are not provided)

> *Plan of Care:* John will participate in 8 physical therapy sessions over the summer to work on specific goals related to his coordination and physical fitness. One session will be made to consult with his new karate instructor. In September John will be discharged from private clinic-based therapy services, and staff in his school program will be updated on his progress and motor status. Motor-related services in his educational program will then be coordinated between his school physical therapist and adapted physical education teacher.

SUMMARY

Developing a strategy for planning and sequencing treatment requires physical therapists to impose organization on the many variables affecting this process. Although individual therapists will have differing theoretical frameworks, the use of well-defined, long-term outcomes, short-term goals, and behavioral objectives, as well as a clearly proposed plan of care, will improve communication among professionals, parents, other caregivers, and third-party payers about the child's current functioning, physical therapy intervention, and progress.

References

1. International Classification of Functioning, Disability and Health: ICF. Geneva, Switzerland: World Health Organization; 2001. http://www.int/classifications/icf/en/.
2. American Physical Therapy Association. Guide to physical therapist practice 3.0. http://guidetoptpractice.apta.org/, 2014.
3. Montgomery PC, Connolly BH. Norm-referenced and criterion-referenced tests: use in pediatrics and application to task analysis of motor skill. *Phys Ther.* 1987;67(12):1873-1876. doi:10.1093/ptj/67.12.1873.
4. Pellegrino L. Cerebral palsy: a paradigm for developmental disabilities. *Dev Med Child Neurol.* 1995;37(9):834-838. doi:10.1111/j.1469-8749.1995.tb12068.x.
5. Haley SM, Andrellos PJ, Coster WJ, Haltiwanger JT, Ludlow LH. *Pediatric Evaluation of Disability Inventory (PEDI).* Boston, MA: New England Medical Center Hospitals; 1992.
6. Osiurak F, Rossetti Y, Badets A. What is an affordance? 40 years later. *Neurosci Biobehav Rev.* 2017;77(16):403-417. doi:10.1016/j.neubiorev.2017.04.014.
7. Caçola P, Gabbard C, Santos DC, Batistela AC. Development of the Affordances in the Home Environment for Motor Development–Infant Scale. *Pediatr Int.* 2011;53(6):820-825. doi:10.1111/j.1442-200X.2011.03386.x.
8. Caçola PM, Gabbard C, Montebelo MI, Santos DC. The new Affordances in the Home Environment for Motor Development–Infant Scale (AHEMD-IS): versions in English and Portuguese languages. *Braz J Phys Ther.* 2015;19(6):507-525. doi:10.1590/bjpt-rbf.2014.0112.
9. Müller AB, Valentini NC, Bandeira PFR. Affordances in the Home Environment for Motor Development: validity and reliability for the use in daycare setting. *Infant Behav Dev.* 2017;47(5):138-145. doi:10.1016/j.infbeh.2017.03.008.
10. Latash ML, Anson JG. What are "normal movements" in atypical populations? *Behav Brain Sci.* 1996;19(2):55-106. doi:10.1017/S0140525X00041467.
11. Moore CA, Nejad B, Novak RA, Dias LS. Energy cost of walking in low lumbar myelomeningocele. *J Pediatr Orthop.* 2001;21(3):388-391. doi:10.1097/01241398-200105000-00024.
12. Franks CA, Palisano RJ, Darbee JC. The effect of walking with an assistive device and using a wheelchair on school performance in students with myelomeningocele. *Phys Ther.* 1991;71(8):570-577. doi:10.1097/01241398-199205000-00057.
13. Gudjonsdóttir B, Mercer VS. Hip and spine in children with cerebral palsy: musculoskeletal development and clinical implications. *Pediatr Phys Ther.* 1997;9(4):179-185. doi:10.1097/00001577-199700940-00005.
14. Braendvik SM, Elvrum AK, Vereijken B, Roeleveld K. Relationship between neuromuscular body functions and upper extremity activity in children with cerebral palsy. *Dev Med Child Neurol.* 2010;52(2):29-34. doi:10.1111/j.1469-8749.2009.03490.x.

Communications to Establish Rapport With Children and Their Families

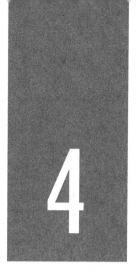

Helen L. Masin, PT, PhD

Physical therapists, occupational therapists, and speech-language pathologists are in a unique clinical situation when working with children. They must relate successfully to children and family/caregivers alike to provide patient-centered therapy. One strategy for enhancing communication is called *patient-centered care* (PCC). PCC was described in an Institute of Medicine report as "care that is respectful of and responsive to individual patient preferences, needs, and values" and that ensures "that patient values guide all clinical decisions."[1(p780)] PCC has patients and caregivers working together to produce optimal outcomes[1] and is recognized as a core value in family medicine. It has been associated with reduction of malpractice complaints and improved physician satisfaction, consultation time, patients' emotional state, and medication adherence. PCC also may increase patient satisfaction and empowerment, as well as reduce severity of symptoms, use of health care resources, and health care costs.[2]

In pediatric therapy, the child's age may range from birth through 21 years. The clinician must recognize the child's developmental age, at every age, and adjust the examination, evaluation, and treatment plan so it is age appropriate and patient centered. The settings in which pediatric physical therapists work include hospitals, outpatient clinics, schools, and the patient's home.

To work with children and caregivers in diverse settings, pediatric therapists must be not only excellent clinicians, but also excellent communicators. Information in this chapter provides strategies and tools for enhancing communication interactions with pediatric clients and their families/caregivers. In addition, an overview of the role of communication in pediatric patient care and strategies for developing effective communication skills in pediatric settings are provided. Evidence-based literature related to effective communication in health care is included along with interview data from experienced pediatric physical therapists working in a variety of pediatric settings. The interview data provide clinical insights into the complex interactions that the clinicians have experienced with their pediatric patients and families. Throughout this chapter, the term "family" is used to refer to children's families/caregivers.

The critical role of communication has been described in evidence-based articles regarding the importance of communication for the pediatric physician. Mărginean et al[3] cited the American Academy of Pediatrics statement in which effective communication is identified as the cornerstone

Connolly BH, Montgomery PC, eds. *Therapeutic Exercise for Children With Developmental Disabilities, Fourth Edition* (pp 113-130).
© 2020 Taylor & Francis Group.

of care. They stated that communication in pediatrics can be more challenging than in the care of adult patients because there are a minimum of 3 individuals involved in the interaction—the child, the parent, and the physician. Four critical aspects of the pediatricians' interactions were identified: (1) informativeness, (2) interpersonal sensitivity, (3) interest in the caregivers and pediatric patient's feelings and concerns, and (4) partnership building. Additional studies were cited that found the greatest factors for effective communication among patients/families and physicians were caring, interest, warmth, and responsiveness.

Although communication was cited as probably the most common "procedure" in medicine, these authors found that communication training often was neglected in medical universities. They recommended that communication skills be provided to all medical students from the beginning of medical school training to develop practical abilities in developing an effective doctor-patient relationship. Medical education needs to encourage physician responsiveness to the patient's unique experience and encourage the perception of reaching common ground.[4]

Although the studies cited above refer to medical education, there also are multiple physical therapy resources that encourage the teaching of communication skills for physical therapists. In physical therapy education, there are guiding documents that promote the development of effective communication skills for all physical therapy students.

The importance of communication in physical therapy also has been described in resources related to the development of professional behaviors[5] and in chapters and journal articles describing professional communication in physical therapy.[6-10] The professional behaviors in physical therapy that are directly related to pediatrics are communication, interpersonal skills, and professionalism. The items for communication include the ability to communicate effectively (ie, verbal, nonverbal, reading, writing, and listening) for varied audiences and purposes. The interpersonal objectives include the ability to interact effectively with patients, families, colleagues, other health care professionals, and the community in a culturally aware manner. In addition, the professionalism objectives include the ability to exhibit appropriate professional conduct and to represent the profession effectively while promoting the growth/development of the physical therapy profession.[11]

A Delphi study by Lopopolo and colleagues[12] found that the top-ranked skill for physical therapy managers was communication. Communication had the highest median score among management skills and, therefore, was cited as the most important category. The findings of this study found novice physical therapists need "extensive knowledge" of communication techniques and should be "skilled" in using these techniques in a clinical setting.

SKILLS NECESSARY FOR PATIENT-CENTERED CARE

There are many skills that promote PCC with children, their families, and other health professionals. These include tools for conveying rapport, respect, empathy, and compassion. Research indicates that PCC uses language and nonverbal cues that lead to increased patient satisfaction. Evidence also indicates that better communication promotes better patient adherence to treatment and better clinical outcomes. In addition, evidence suggests effective and compassionate communication promotes decreased costs and fewer malpractice cases.[13]

Throughout this chapter, self-reflective questions are printed in italics to promote thoughts about your personal communication style and preferences. To understand one's communication with patients, one must first understand one's own communication style and preferences. For example, I have worked with several students who are perceived as "soft spoken" by their clinical instructors, but the students perceived themselves as "loud." The feedback from their clinical instructors indicated a need to increase their volume as a way of reflecting confidence in what they were recommending for the children and their families. Once these students recognized how they were being perceived by others, they were able to increase their volume as a way of establishing better rapport and building confidence with the patients and their families. In another clinical setting, one student was talking too much and patients became confused. Once the student recognized how he was being perceived, he talked less and looked for signs of understanding in his patients' verbal and nonverbal behaviors.

What does communication mean to you?

Merriam-Webster describes communication as "a process by which information is exchanged between individuals through a common system of symbols, signs, or behavior."[14]

Think about a recent visit to a health care professional in your own experience. What did you notice about him or her? Did you feel comfortable with that professional? Why or why not? What are the characteristics that you expected when interacting with that health professional? What did you feel during the interaction? What went well? What could be improved? How did the communication with the professional affect you?

Multiple types of communication systems exist. These include verbal, nonverbal, listening, reading, writing, and electronic communication and social media.

Verbal and Nonverbal Communication

When individuals interact, there are verbal as well as nonverbal cues that convey the meaning of their message. You can hear their speech and observe their posture, gestures, and movements.

Mehrabian and Wiener[15] found that 60% to 90% of communication is transmitted nonverbally. Nonverbal cues include pitch, tonality, silence, pacing, touch, gesture, eye contact, and gaze aversion. If the verbal and nonverbal cues match each other, the communication is considered congruent. If the verbal and nonverbal cues do not match, there may be confusion as to the meaning of the communication. Therefore, verbal and nonverbal cues both have an important role in PCC.

Communication that occurs silently within an individual is called internal dialogue.[16] Internal dialogue is heard only by the individual as an inner voice and may or may not affect the nonverbal communication with others involved in the communication.

Think of a time when you were explaining a home program to the parent of a child in your clinical practice. You explain the home program but you notice that the parent seems distracted and is averting your gaze. You continue with the explanation but you wonder whether the parent has understood anything you have said. How do you know the parent is distracted? What can you do to facilitate more patient-centered communication?

As a clinician, you can observe verbal and nonverbal cues to determine whether a home program is being understood. You might ask the parent to tell you what was heard regarding the home program and request a demonstration. If the parent is able to tell you what was understood, then you know that you were heard. If the parent can demonstrate for you, you know the information can be applied. In this way, you will have a better understanding of the parental perception of what you are asking. If the parent is unable to tell you or demonstrate, then you know you need to modify your communication to facilitate understanding.

Communication also occurs in groups. Verbal and nonverbal cues alike are sent by the group members to each other. We cannot NOT communicate. Communication occurs every time we interact with each other—even if nothing is said verbally. By being present, we are communicating nonverbally by our affect, posture, and body language.

Think of a time when you were leading a parent support group for Parent to Parent in your community. Some parents were enthusiastically sharing their experiences with the group, but others appeared to be sleepy and uninterested in the discussion. What assumptions did you make about the parents who appeared sleepy and lacked interest? What behaviors led you to make those assumptions? What could you have done to facilitate more PCC in the group?

As the facilitator of the Parent to Parent group, you may want to ask the group members who are sleepy or quiet whether they have anything to add. By asking for their input, you give them permission to participate because you have acknowledged their presence and requested their participation.

Active Listening

Active listening is another important skill when promoting PCC. Many people have difficulty actively listening because they are preparing a response to the speaker rather than truly listening to what the speaker is saying. By restating, reflecting, and clarifying what you heard the speaker say before you respond, you are letting the speaker know that you were actively listening. Active listening requires practice and is not easy. When working with children and families, active listening builds rapport.

Think of parents who tell you they are frustrated that their child is not walking after 6 months of therapy with you. You can restate that you understand they are feeling frustrated. You then reflect the content and the implied feelings that this is a difficult situation for these parents. You then clarify by summarizing the content and feelings by stating that you appreciate the parents' frustration and you are open to discussing the parents' concerns about their child's development.

Another powerful strategy that builds PCC is using acknowledgment, validation, and empathy when communicating with families. You verbally can acknowledge the parents' concerns, validate their feelings about their concerns, and provide empathy. In this way, parents recognize that you are actively listening to them with empathy and respect. This builds the parents' trust in you and demonstrates your genuine interest in their child's well-being.

Reading

Reading is another communication skill that is critical for clinicians. Professionals must be able to read and evaluate evidence-based literature and be able to determine which findings are useful in clinical practice. Each clinician must be able to analyze and interpret evidence-based literature to provide the most current approaches in PCC.

Writing

Writing skills are essential for communicating with children and families, as well as peers and other professionals. The home exercise program you provide gives important information to the family. One of the mothers with whom I worked told me to recommend only 3 exercises to work on each week. She said that 3 was a magic number of exercises to be practiced each week. She would proudly bring the paper with the home exercise program back each week, would demonstrate her child's progress, and then ask me to "grade" her performance. She felt that the home exercise program with the 3 items enabled her to focus on the most important skills to practice with her child each week. She saved the home programs and valued the "grades" that I gave her.

The accuracy of your writing skills also can affect your ability to obtain reimbursement for your services. If your documentation is unclear, third-party payers may reject your requests. In addition, if you are involved in research projects, your writing skills are essential for dissemination of your findings. Your ability to describe your research question, methodology, analysis, findings, and discussion will be critical to getting your research recognized and published.

Generational Issues in Communication

When practicing PCC, the clinician needs to be aware of the perceptions of different generations of caregivers relating to therapy.

When I first arrived in Miami, I was surprised that extended family members attended my physical therapy sessions. The family members often included mothers, grandmothers, and great-grandmothers. As a physical therapist in the northeastern United States, I usually had only the nuclear family in attendance at my sessions. However, in Miami, the family members who attended were primarily female. This may not be true in other areas of the country. To communicate effectively with the different generations, I modified my communication style to match that of the family members in attendance.

Through understanding the expectations of different generations, I was able to modify my communication to meet the needs of the different generations of children and family members. In the United States, there are 4 primary generations of caregivers that may be involved in caring for children. Each generation has characteristics unique to their generation. The generations include Traditionalists, Baby Boomers, Generation Xers, and Millennials.

Traditionalists are those individuals born before 1946. These might be the great-great-grandparents and great-great-aunts or uncles in the family. They may be hard of hearing or have visual losses. They may be taking a variety of medications for age-related disorders. Their opinions are important to younger family members.

Baby Boomers are those individuals born between 1946 and 1964. These might be the great-grandparents and great-aunts or uncles in the family. They may be helping the Traditionalists in the family with health issues and may have age-related disorders themselves. They are sometimes called "digital immigrants" because they learned to use electronic communication as adults. Their opinions are important to younger family members.

The Gen Xers are those individuals born between 1965 and 1981. They may be called "digital natives" because they have used electronic communication since childhood and are comfortable with it. These might be the grandparents, great-aunts or uncles, or parents in the family, and their opinions are valued. They have searched the web regarding the child's diagnosis and suggested treatment. They may ask you about what they found online.

The Millennials are individuals born between 1982 and 2000. They are the parents and aunts or uncles in the family. They are multitaskers and also are called "digital natives." They are comfortable with computers as well as social media and prefer electronic communication. They may have researched the diagnoses and treatment of the child's condition online and ask you questions related to what they have read.

When working with families, pediatric clinicians can adapt their teaching to meet the needs of each generation as a way of building trust in the relationship with the different family members. However, recognizing that each member of each generation is unique is important. That person *may* or *may not* reflect the generational characteristics described previously. The realization that within-group variation can be as great as between-group variation is important. By viewing each family member as unique, the pediatric clinician can provide the optimal PCC.[17]

Electronic Communication and Social Media

Electronic communication includes email, texting, tweets, social media, web surfing, and blogging. Social media includes tools that are used to produce, publish, and share online content with others. These may include blogs, podcasts, videos, microblogs, and wikis. The American Physical Therapy Association (APTA) suggests 7 steps related to social networking[18]:

1. Avoid becoming online "friends" with patients/clients.
2. Avoid including information gained from online social networking regarding your patients as part of the patient/client management process.
3. Avoid including information gained from online social networking regarding students' performance in clinical education.
4. Use caution when posting and disclosing personal information on social networking sites.
5. Check the social networking site's privacy settings and control who can access your online profile.
6. Avoid "venting" on blogs or social networks.
7. Have a strategy regarding social networking and commit to it.

Electronic communication can be considered a blessing and/or a challenge to PCC. It can be a blessing when used to transmit appropriate information quickly and efficiently. However, it can be a challenge when messages are sent that are misinterpreted, misunderstood, or inaccurate.

Think of a time when you sent a home program to a family via email because your treatment session started late. When the family returned for an appointment with you the following week, you realized that the family had misinterpreted your email and had been doing the home exercise program incorrectly.

Thinking back to the research by Mehrabian and Wiener,[15] you realize that 60% to 90% of your communication was lost because the home exercise program was sent in an email rather than discussed and demonstrated in a face-to-face interaction.

The difficulty with electronic communication occurs because it is essentially a one-way communication. The sender is unaware of how the receiver reacts to the communication. This increases the chances for misinterpretation and misunderstanding. In addition, emails can be inadvertently sent to individuals for whom they are not intended. This can result in legal challenges if the email contains inflammatory comments about the unintended receiver.

Optimal communication involves both the sender and the receiver interacting with each other in an empathetic dialogue. Since much of electronic communication occurs as a monologue from the sender to the receiver, it does not facilitate empathetic interaction. As a result, miscommunication and misunderstanding may occur.

As a result of these challenges, APTA developed standards of conduct for the use of social media by physical therapists, physical therapist assistants, and physical therapy students. Social media is here to stay. Guidelines for use are important for therapists, children, and their families to understand. The APTA Standards of Conduct for the use of social media were adapted by the APTA House of Delegates in 2016.[19] These standards provide guidelines regarding communication in a public forum such as electronic media.

The APTA also developed updated guidelines for succeeding and protecting yourself in social media in 2017.[20] Eight steps were suggested related to social media: (1) have a goal, (2) start small, (3) act professionally, (4) improve your brand, (5) think before you "friend" or "follow," (6) consider legal counsel, (7) learn your platform, and (8) engage with the APTA.

Establishing Rapport Using Neurolinguistic Programming

Rapport lays the foundation for effective communication. It is a critical component of communication described in neurolinguistic programming (also known as neurolinguistic psychology or NLP). NLP is a communication system that provides psychological skills for understanding and influencing people. NLP is based on the art and science of excellence, as well as being derived from studying how successful people in different fields obtained their outstanding results. NLP has been used in the fields of business, education, communication, and therapy through teaching communication skills that can be used to enhance effectiveness personally and professionally.[16]

Types of Rapport

In NLP, *rapport* is defined as an interaction marked by mutual collaboration and respect, but does not necessarily indicate agreement. Rapport can be present even when 2 parties disagree. There are 3 main types of rapport described in NLP—cultural, verbal, and behavioral.

Cultural Rapport

Cultural rapport is when the therapist wears the form of dress or greeting that is considered appropriate for the cultural group receiving therapy. In pediatric therapy, the therapist might wear casual clothing rather than a white lab coat. By dressing in casual clothes, the therapist avoids wearing a white lab coat that may frighten a child who has interacted with medical professionals who may be associated with injections or unpleasant interactions.

Another example of cultural rapport occurred in my first year as a pediatric physical therapist in Miami. When I first met families when they arrived for the child's physical therapy, they would kiss me on the cheek. Initially, I felt uncomfortable with the greeting because it was so different from what I was used to in the northeastern United States. This greeting is considered polite in many Latin cultural groups in Miami. Once I got used to this greeting, I felt very comfortable using it to build cultural rapport with the children and their families.

Verbal Rapport

Verbal rapport is when the therapist uses the same or similar descriptive phrases and conversational content as the families with whom he is speaking. For example, when working with a child or family member who asks to "see the home exercise program," the therapist might show the home exercise program and then ask the child or family member, "How does this look to you?" In this way, the therapist is matching the child or family's visual descriptors to build verbal rapport.

Behavioral Rapport

Behavioral rapport is when the therapist mirrors the posture and body language of the child or family member with whom he or she is speaking. The therapist also may match the child or family member's speed, tonality, and tempo of speech. For example, when working in early intervention, I positioned myself on the floor mat to work at the eye level of the child I was treating to build behavioral rapport with the child.

Behavioral rapport also can be used to establish rapport with a family member when a medical interpreter is present. The therapist can match the body language of the child's caregiver while actively listening to the medical interpreter. In this way, the therapist is developing behavioral rapport by matching the family member's posture even if the therapist does not speak the same language.

Another example of developing behavioral rapport occurred when I was working with a 3-year-old child with moderate hearing impairment, autistic-like behaviors, and minimal vocalization. His classroom teacher asked for my help because she said he "bounced off the walls in class." She could not get him to vocalize "AAH" or "BAA" as primary vocalizations. I moved the child and myself to a small room with minimal distractions. I put a medium-sized therapy ball between us and knelt opposite him on the floor at his eye level. Initially, he covered his eyes and looked away from me. So I matched his posture and covered my eyes too. After a few seconds, he began to peek out at me between his fingers and had a small smile. I matched his peeking and smiled back at him. We repeated this interaction several times and then he took his hands away from his face and looked at me directly. I took my hands away and looked at him directly too. He was smiling now so I tapped the therapy ball several times with a flat open hand creating a tap, tap, tap rhythm on the ball. For a few seconds nothing happened, but then he tap, tap, tapped the ball too. Since he was still smiling, I decided to see if he would tolerate bouncing on top of the ball while in sitting. I demonstrated sitting and bouncing on the ball and then offered the ball to him. He got onto the ball and let me bounce him in sitting on the ball. After a short time, he got off the ball and assumed a prone posture over the ball with his arms outstretched forward. He was enjoying being in prone so I started to roll him back and forth over the ball. He was quite happy in this position so I decided to introduce sounds into our activities. As he rolled forward I said "AAH" and "BAA," which were the vocalizations his teacher wanted him to develop. After several repetitions, he vocalized "BAA" loud and clear! We were both delighted! Matching had established rapport with a preverbal child with hearing impairments and autistic-like behaviors. This convinced me of the power of matching to create behavioral rapport. This interaction was the beginning of many successful interactions with him, his teacher, and his other classmates.

By matching and pacing his posture and movement, we were able to establish a functional communication system with him for the first time. Because he had a long latency of response to

TABLE 4-1. COMMUNICATION STYLE DIFFERENCES (OVERT ACTIVITY DIMENSION—NONVERBAL/VERBAL)			
AMERICAN INDIANS	**ASIAN AMERICANS, HISPANICS**	**EURO AMERICANS**	**AFRICAN AMERICANS**
Speak softly/slower	Speak softly	Speak loud/fast to control listener	Speak with affect
Indirect gaze when listening or speaking	Avoidance of eye contact when listening or speaking to high-status person	Greater eye contact when listening	Direct eye contact (prolonged) when speaking, but less when listening
Interject less/seldom offer encouraging communication	Similar rules	Head nods, nonverbal markers	Interrupt (turn taking) when can
Delayed auditory (silence)	Mild delay	Quick responding	Quicker responding
Manner of expression, low-key, indirect	Low-key, indirect	Objective, task oriented	Affective, emotional, interpersonal
Adapted from Sue DW, Sue D. *Counseling the Culturally Different: Theory and Practice.* New York, NY: John Wiley & Sons, Inc; 1990:67.			

stimuli, the pace of his classroom may have been too fast for him to adapt. As a result, he became overstimulated and "bounced off the walls." By matching his postures in our interactions, it became clear that he could interact effectively when given enough time to respond.

Match, Pace, Lead

When building rapport, the therapist must be aware both of verbal and nonverbal components of communication. Verbal components include language, pacing, tonality, and speed of communication. Nonverbal components include gesture, posture, haptics, proxemics, and oculesics (Table 4-1).

Learning Preferences

The therapist also can build rapport verbally by noticing the language patterns of the speaker to identify the learning preferences of the child or family member when teaching a home program of exercises. Preferences can be visual, auditory, or kinesthetic. By listening to the patterns of the speaker, the therapist can learn whether the speaker has visual, auditory, or kinesthetic preferences. For example, if the speaker asks, "Can I see how you do that?" the therapist can respond using a visual response, such as "How does that look to you?" If the speaker says, "Tell me how you do that," the therapist can respond by saying, "How does that sound to you?" If the speaker asks, "Can I feel how you do that?" the therapist can respond by saying, "Can you grasp that now?" In this way, the therapist matches the speaker's verbal preference as a way of building rapport.

Verbal Matching

Other verbal matching can include pacing, tonality, and speed of communication. The therapist can match the learner's pace of speaking by matching the learner's pauses or stops between words and thoughts. The therapist can match the tonality of the speaker depending on whether the speaker has low-, medium-, or high-pitched tones. The speed of the communication can be matched as slow, medium, or fast speed.

Nonverbal Matching

Nonverbal matching can include gesture, posture, haptics, proxemics, and oculesics. Gestural matching may include matching any movement of the hands and arms to mirror the gestures of the child or family member. Postural matching may include positioning of the whole body so it mirrors the body posture of the child or family member. Haptics is using touch in the same way as the child or family member.

Proxemics

Proxemics is the formal distance between 2 speakers, which varies based on cultural norms. For example, my first Spanish teachers suggested I watch novellas (soap operas in Spanish) to improve my Spanish language skills. I watched several novellas but discovered that I felt anxious while watching them. I realized that I was uncomfortable because the distance between the camera and the actor was too close for my comfort level. My preferred distance was an arm's length and the actors were at less than an arm's length. I realized that my proxemics were different from that of the actors and had caused my anxious response.

Oculesics

Oculesics is the process of observing the eye movements of the speaker and the listener. This often is determined culturally and may be direct eye contact, gaze aversion, or a combination of gaze aversion and eye contact. For example, in certain Native American groups, gaze aversion is a sign of respect when interacting with a medical professional.

Postural Matching

Studies have shown that people who assume similar postures have better rapport with each other than those who do not.[22] By developing rapport, the clinician builds trust and mutual respectful collaboration, which is the foundation of PCC. When therapists match the nonverbal behaviors of the child or family member, they indicate that they are paying attention and the interaction is harmonious. It is said to be "in sync." In contrast, poor rapport is described as awkward or "out of sync."[22]

Students in my class have mentioned they worry that the child or family member will notice that the therapist is matching them. In my 20 years of experience using matching to build rapport, this has not been a problem. Because body language is perceived at the subconscious level, the child or family member usually is not conscious of the matching.

Practice matching posture and gesture with someone at a low stress social event before using it with children or family members in your physical therapy practice. What did you discover? How did you feel? Did matching enhance your rapport with that person?

Pediatric therapists also must learn how to break rapport. This might be necessary in challenging situations in which inappropriate comments are being made or sexual harassment is occurring. In these cases, the therapist can mismatch the body language and verbal language of the challenging child or family member. For example, if the therapist is seated and is hearing offensive comments from the other person, the physical therapist can stand and verbally inform the other person that the comments are unacceptable in the clinical setting. By posturally and verbally mismatching the other person, the therapist breaks rapport and establishes boundaries before the situation escalates.

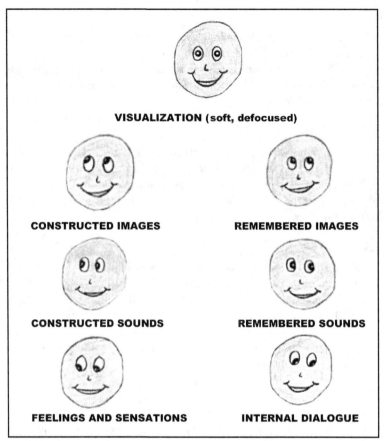

Figure 4-1. Eye accessing. (Adapted from Matthews P. What the eyes can tell you. People Alchemy. https://www.alchemyformanagers.co.uk/topics/smYYdfbXNeVJqfme.html.)

Eye Accessing

The NLP skill of observing eye accessing enables us to understand whether a person is think-ing in pictures (visual), sounds (auditory), or feelings (kinesthetic) during communications. Neurological studies have shown that eye movements are associated with activation of different parts of the brain. The eye accessing chart (Figure 4-1) demonstrates the eye movements that are associated with visual, auditory, or kinesthetic systems. When the eyes are defocused and looking straight ahead, the person is visualizing something. When the eyes move up and to the left, the person is remembering something (visually remembered). When the eyes move up and to the right, the person is constructing a visual image (visual construction). When the eyes move to the left in the middle, the person is remembering a sound (auditorily remembered). When the eyes move to the right in the middle, the person is constructing a sound (auditory construction). When the eyes move down and to the left, the person is having an internal dialogue. When the eyes move down and to the right, the person is experiencing feelings or body sensations. This eye accessing infor-mation can be helpful in understanding learning preferences and how the child or family member is processing directions.

For example, when children or family members are being asked a question, if they have visual preferences, they may look up and to the left to remember the answer. If they have auditory pref-erences, the may look to the middle left to hear the answer. If they have kinesthetic preferences, they may look down and to the left to access their internal dialogue. Once they have accessed the information, they will look back at the therapist, thus indicating that they have the answer. If the therapist knows about eye accessing, he or she will watch the eye movements and wait for the learner to look back at him or her before asking the next question.

In some cases, the person's eye accessing chart may be reversed. The therapist will need to ask multiple questions to determine whether the eye accessing for a child or family member may be reversed.

In the case of English as a second language, the learner may access the auditory remembered first to translate the question before being able to answer. In this way, the physical therapist recognizes when the person has processed the answer before posing another question or giving more instructions.

CROSS-CULTURAL ASPECTS OF COMMUNICATION

Pediatric therapists interact with a wide variety of children and families from diverse cultural backgrounds. Families may come from different ethnicities, religious backgrounds, socioeconomic levels, generations, sexual orientations, and/or health care orientations. To communicate effectively in diverse communities, the therapist must be culturally competent. This is defined as having behaviors, attitudes, and policies that come together in a health care system, agency, or individual practice to function effectively in cross-cultural interactions.[23] Cultural competency is described on a continuum. This theoretical model describes 6 behaviors, including cultural destructiveness, incapacity, blindness, precompetence, competence, and proficiency.[24] Agar, an anthropologist and linguist, writes that "communication in today's world requires culture. Problems in communication are rooted in who you are in encounters with a different mentality, different meanings, and a different time between language and consciousness. Solving the problems inspired by such encounters inspires culture."[25p23]

To appreciate cultures, one must first appreciate one's culture of origin. This involves reflection on your personal beliefs, attitudes, and behaviors as well as the beliefs, attitudes, and behaviors of the profession of physical therapy. For example, biomedical Western medicine places a strong emphasis on direct and linear verbal communication. However, other cultures may use indirect and abstract communication.

A tool that has helped me to decipher cultural constructs in my pediatric practice is the concept of high- and low-context cultural assumptions.[26] *Context* in communication refers to what gives "meaning" to a communication interaction. It is important for the therapist to be able to recognize and interpret both the verbal and nonverbal signals that patients demonstrate.

High-context assumptions also are called *collectivistic assumptions.*[26] In high-context cultures, the group is more important than the individual. The communication style is indirect, and spiral and circular logic are used. Meaning is determined based on implicit cues, such as where the interaction occurs, instead of what is said. Nonverbal nuances such as eye gaze, posture, and gesture are considered important. The communication is based on what the listener knows rather than what the speaker is saying. For example, the film *Crouching Dragon, Hidden Tiger* (Asia Union Film and Entertainment, Ltd, 2001) displays high-context cultural assumptions.[27] In the film, the protagonists have minimal dialogue but meaning is conveyed by eye movements, clothing, setting, posture, and gesture.

Is your communication style high context?

Low-context assumptions are based on individualistic assumptions that assume that the individual is more important than the group. The communication is direct, linear, and logical. The meaning is determined by explicit cues. In other words, "what you say is what you get." Communication is less dependent on nuances or contextual cues. The meaning is conveyed by what the speaker is saying rather than what the listener knows.[26]

Is your communication style low context?

Is the cultural context of your patients more high context or more low context?

The culture of biomedical Western medicine operates primarily from low-context assumptions. However, the culture of many of the families we serve may or may not be low context. If the family is high context and the therapist is low context, miscommunication can occur. Arthur Kleinman, a medical anthropologist and psychiatrist, stated that it is the responsibility of the practitioner to learn the explanatory model of the family as it relates to the condition of the child.[28] Kleinman's explanatory model addresses the family's beliefs about the child's condition based on the culture of the family. It explains the cause, onset of symptoms, pathophysiology, course of sickness, and treatment for the problem being addressed.

The Spirit Catches You and You Fall Down: A Hmong Child, Her American Doctors, and the Collision of Two Cultures by Fadiman is an ethnographic book that demonstrates how misunderstandings and miscommunication occurred with the care of Lia Lee and her family.[29] Lia was the daughter of a large Hmong family. Her family emigrated from the highlands of Cambodia to California. The Hmong culture is considered high context. The medical doctors caring for Lia came from a low-context biomedical Western culture. Lia was diagnosed with seizure disorder and the family was advised to give Lia antiseizure medicine to control her seizures. The family was not familiar with regular administration of medicine because of a variety of reasons related to their cultural background. The Lee family and Lia's doctors were operating from very different explanatory models.

The doctors evaluated Lia's condition and determined that her seizures were caused by abnormal electrical discharges in her brain that could be controlled by regular administration of antiseizure medications. In contrast, the Lee family believed that her seizures were caused by spiritual issues that were related to a condition known as "soul loss." To address the soul loss, the family invited a shaman from the community to perform a soul-retrieval ritual for Lia in their home. The family continued to administer the antiseizure medicine but did so on an irregular basis. Unfortunately, the irregular administration did not adequately control the seizures and Lia went back to the hospital. At one point, Lia was removed from her home by the state of California and placed in foster care. This was a huge blow to Lia's family and the local Hmong community. In high-context cultures such as the Hmong community, decisions are made by the extended family and the community regarding its members. The removal of Lia from the family was considered a tragedy for the family as well as the local Hmong community because children are deeply cherished in Hmong culture. As a result of Lia's going to foster care, her mother became very depressed and other family members experienced emotional problems. A social worker familiar with Hmong culture was able to interpret the situation for the medical community and Lia eventually was returned to her family. There had been a misunderstanding between the high-context assumptions of the Hmong community and the low-context assumptions of the hospital community, which resulted in multiple complications related to Lia's care.

At the conclusion of her book, Fadiman contacted Kleinman. She asked him if he thought the miscommunications with Lia and her family might have been avoided. He suggested that the medical team should have asked the following questions:

1. What do you call your problem? What name does it have?
2. What do you think caused your problem?
3. Why do you think it started when it did?
4. What does your sickness do to you: How does it work?
5. How severe is your sickness: How long do you expect it to last?
6. What do you fear most about your illness?
7. What are the biggest problems that your illness has caused for you?
8. What kind of treatment do you think you should receive? What are the most important results you hope to receive from treatment?

Kleinman suggested that Lia's situation may not have become so critical if the medical team had asked the family the 8 questions during the initial encounter and learned about the family's explanatory model. Their answers to the questions would have indicated that the family viewed Lia's seizures as a spiritual issue related to soul loss. By understanding the differences between the explanatory model of the family and the explanatory model of the medical team, a compromise may have been worked out.

After Fadiman's book was published, several educational institutions made her book required reading for professionals to increase their awareness of the critical nature of effective cross-cultural communication in health care.[30]

I personally experienced a life-threatening miscommunication that occurred with a 2-year-old boy who was a student in our early intervention program in Miami. He also was diagnosed with a seizure disorder. He was being followed in the pediatric neurology clinic and had been given liquid phenobarbital to control his seizures. His mother was very dedicated to him and to his care. However, he was still having breakthrough seizures during the early intervention program on a fairly regular basis.

The staff and I were very concerned about his well-being. We invited a medical interpreter to speak with his mother to determine what might be going wrong. His mother stated that she had the medicine and that she was giving it to him. From the interview, we did not discover any reason why he should still be having breakthrough seizures. We were at a loss as to what might be causing the seizures. We decided to have his mother return to our program and show us how she was administering the medicine. We were surprised when she asked us to give her a basin of water. We did so and she proceeded to put the liquid phenobarbital in the water. She stated that she had been bathing him in the phenobarbital-infused water. We were stunned! We explained that the medicine had to be administered by mouth to control the seizures. Once she understood this, his breakthrough seizures stopped. This was another example of how misunderstanding and miscommunication created a dangerous situation for this little boy and his mother. His mother's explanatory model for the treatment of the seizure disorder was to bathe him in the phenobarbital. Our explanatory model for the treatment of the seizure disorder was to take the medicine by mouth.

When I teach cross-cultural communication to students, I always ask them if they know why his mother administered the medicine by bathing her son in it. One of my students stated that the child's mother may have bathed her son in the medicine because medicine was typically administered topically in her country of origin rather than orally as in the United States. I remind students to consider possible cultural misunderstandings when problems being addressed do not respond in the way you expect. The differences may be related to cultural beliefs different from biomedical Western beliefs.

Another resource for solving cultural miscommunication is contacting cultural informants who can explain cultural issues with which you may not be familiar. In the early intervention program in Miami, I relied heavily on staff who came from different countries of origin to assist me in communicating effectively with our students and their families.

LANGUAGE CHALLENGES

Another issue in cross-cultural communication is the challenge of communicating with a child or family member who does not speak English or has limited English. If your client does not speak English, a medical interpreter should be involved in the communication.[31] You can build rapport with the family member who is the decision maker by matching his or her posture while actively listening to the medical interpreter. In some families, the decision maker may be an elder or a member of the extended family. Children who are family members should not be involved in translation because the topics being discussed may not be appropriate for the child to hear. Tips for communicating with individuals with limited proficiency in English are listed in Table 4-2.[32]

TABLE 4-2. TEN TIPS FOR COMMUNICATING DIRECTLY WITH LIMITED-ENGLISH–SPEAKING PATIENTS

1. Speak slowly, not loudly.
2. Face the patient and make extensive use of gestures, pictures, and facial expressions. Watch the patient's face, eyes, and body language carefully.
3. Avoid difficult and uncommon words and idiomatic expressions.
4. Don't "muddy the waters" with unnecessary words or information.
5. Organize what you say for easy access.
6. Rephrase and summarize often.
7. Don't ask questions that can be answered by "yes" or "no."
8. Check your understanding of the patient by paraphrasing what he or she has said.
9. Check the concept behind the word.
10. Don't burden the patient with decisions he or she is not prepared to make.

Adapted from Salimbene S. *What Language Does Your Patient Hurt In?* St. Paul, MN: EMC Paradigm; 2000.

You may want to work collaboratively with a culturally acceptable caregiver, such as the shaman in the Hmong community. By showing your respect for the indigenous caregiver, you build rapport by acknowledging this person's importance in the traditional culture of the family. This may indicate to the family that you respect their culture and you hope that they will respect yours.

I had an experience at the Children's Hospital in Montevideo, Uruguay, that dramatically taught me that language does not equal culture. I studied Spanish in Miami with teachers from Cuba and Puerto Rico. They informed me that there are some words in Caribbean Spanish that are considered rude in South American Spanish. At the Children's Hospital, I demonstrated a facilitation technique with an infant in the main auditorium with about 300 participants in the audience. I said a phrase that means "take the toy" in Caribbean Spanish. As soon as I said it, there was a shocked silence in the room. A medical interpreter ran over to me and told me another phrase to say. After the presentation, the interpreter told me that what I had said was considered very rude in Uruguay. It was an understandable error given my background in Caribbean Spanish. However, it made me realize how important it is to utilize a medical interpreter who is both multilingual and multicultural!

COMMUNICATING WITH SPECIAL POPULATIONS

Children and Families With Vision Loss

According to the 2015 American Community Survey, there are approximately 455,462 children with vision difficulties. The children in this survey ranged from ages 0 to 18 years.[33] In addition, according to the 2015 National Health Interview Survey, there are 16.4 million American adults between ages 18 and 64 years and 7.3 million adults ages 65 years and older who report significant vision loss.[34]

As pediatric therapists, it is important to know the prevalence of vision loss so we are prepared to work with children and their families who may experience vision loss. For example, when working in our early intervention program, our staff introduced ourselves to each child using both tactile and verbal cues before beginning a therapy session. We often made a tactile cue that included the first letter of our first name in sign language. We would touch the person with vision loss on the shoulder using this letter. In this way, the child or family member had a unique verbal and tactile prompt that they could associate with each of us.

Children and Families With Hearing Loss

According to the Hearing Loss Association of America, 2 to 3 children out of 1000 are born with a detectable hearing loss in one or both ears. Almost 15% of school-age children from ages 6 to 19 years have some loss of hearing. In adults, about 20% of adults experience some degree of hearing loss. At age 65 years, 1 out of every 3 adults has a hearing loss.[35]

As pediatric therapists, we frequently are involved with children with hearing loss, which may or may not be associated with other developmental delays. For example, our early intervention program served children with mild, moderate, and severe hearing losses. Many of the children in our program had cochlear implants and received physical therapy and speech therapy. Staff members were aware of the challenges faced by the children with hearing loss and its impact on the development of their speech and language skills.

QUALITATIVE FINDINGS FROM
FOUR EXPERIENCED PHYSICAL THERAPISTS

Interviews were audiotaped individually with 4 experienced pediatric clinicians in a variety of pediatric physical therapy settings in South Florida. The findings from the interviews were congruent with the findings in the evidence-based research on effective communication and PCC described in this chapter. The settings included a pediatric acute care hospital, a pediatric outpatient private practice, a pediatric home-based physical therapy program, and a pediatric early intervention program for children ages 0 to 3 years.

The same 5 interview questions were used with each of the clinicians. All of them mentioned the importance of communication using language that the child and the family can understand; waiting for the family to be ready to be involved in physical therapy; being respectful, compassionate, and sensitive to different cultural expectations; developing rapport with the family and working together; and empowering the family to make a difference in their child's development. For each of the 5 questions, I summarized the responses of the physical therapists and provide representative quotes.

Question 1: What role does effective communication play when working with children and their families in pediatric physical therapy? How do you know?

All the clinicians stated that communication is an essential component of their pediatric physical therapy practice. One practitioner said communication is the building block of "you being able to relate to a patient." The second practitioner said communication is the foundation for "establishing rapport with the family." The third practitioner said, "Communication is one of the most important and basic things that lets me proceed with my treatment ... the way that you transmit and communicate with the families will impact the life of that family and the child." The fourth practitioner stated, "We show the family ... what we're trying to explain."

Question 2: What are the communication issues that have affected your interactions with children and their families in pediatric physical therapy? How do you know?

All the therapists mentioned that cultural issues and personal challenges facing the families affected their interactions with the child and the families. One respondent stated, "There's challenges (culturally) because I'm WASPy and my upbringing is different than ... a Latino person or a Haitian ... and I have to communicate in a way that ... they can be receptive to what I am saying."

A second respondent said, "Like any families ... they have personal issues going on ... like a couple getting divorced (or) going through a lot of stress and sometimes that impact(s) your relationship with them." A third respondent stated, "Cultural (issues are) a big thing. I always try to find a way to enter those family's lives, to see how they live, where they live, what are their customs." A fourth respondent stated, "It's so important to try to engage ... the family ... first ... really make them a part of this."

Question 3: How have cultural issues affected your interactions with children and their families in pediatric physical therapy? How do you know?

All the clinicians reported a wide variety of cultural issues that affected their interactions with the children and families. These included discrimination toward Hispanic physical therapists, awareness of cultural forms of dress, confusion regarding their child's diagnoses, the presence of significant cultural artifacts in the home, and recognizing the beliefs of the family. Cultural respect and cultural humility on the part of the clinicians enhanced the cross-cultural interactions with families. One clinician stated that "families would bring their little girls in ... puffy skirts and ... they didn't want them to play on the floor and get dirty ... that was a challenge because culturally that was not their way." A second clinician stated, "I did encounter discrimination in a couple of occasions because of me being Hispanic." The Hispanic therapist working in rural North Carolina encountered "a family that was in the Ku Klux Klan ... had a dog named Wizard, and had a grand wizard's robe framed in the middle ... of their living room." A third clinician stated, "They don't even know what the doctor is talking about ... so I explain in the best way for her to understand ... why she's walking like that." A fourth clinician stated, "We have to respect the different beliefs [of the family]."

Question 4: What have been the most surprising elements related to communication issues when working with children and their families in pediatric physical therapy? How do you know?

The clinicians all cited surprising elements that occurred with the children and the families receiving their care. These included establishing a long-term relationship with children and families, becoming aware of how to balance playing with calming activities, that every day is a surprise related to communication with teachers and parents, and that clinicians can empower families to make a difference in their children's lives. One clinician stated, "The family left my practice because they didn't think I was listening to what they were saying ... and then years later they came back to me again and I saw them for quite some time because the parents trusted what I was saying." A second clinician stated the importance of gauging your responses: "When the child would withdraw from you because you were just being too much and you were overwhelming them." A third clinician stated, "I am always available for them ... they feel that you're there any time that they need ... and this approach helps me to accomplish the goals that I want for the kids in terms of function, gross motor movement." A fourth clinician stated, "We are going to guide them [the family], but they are the ones who control."

Question 5: What should I have asked you that I did not ask you about your experiences in pediatric physical therapy? Is there anything else you would like to share?

All the clinicians shared additional experiences related to communication. They shared that personal communication is important along with establishing rapport. One clinician mentioned a variety of ways to establish rapport including, "just talking to them ... asking them what they like and including them in the goals writing." He also mentioned singing, asking permission, and interpreting body language when the child does not want to be handled and respecting that choice. The second clinician stated, "Rapport is not only with the family and the children. It's also with coworkers ... and the physician or the orthotist." She also mentioned smiling as a way to establish rapport—"not an exaggerated smile, not overdoing it." The third clinician stated, "Communication ... with compassion and love ... is the way that you transmit the information you want to give to those parents and that probably will impact their lives forever." A fourth clinician stated, "Empower the family to be the ones who are going to lead ... really involve them [the family from] the beginning."

SUMMARY

Effective communication is a critical component of PCC and family-centered care in pediatric practice. The most effective therapist is both an excellent clinician and an excellent communicator. If you demonstrate rapport-building skills and interpret verbal and nonverbal cues, you can create an alliance with children and families. If you understand generations, socioeconomic levels, learning preferences, electronic media, belief systems, and cultural and language systems, then you have the ability to relate to patients from backgrounds different from your own. The reflective activities, evidence-based literature, suggested strategies, interviews, and tools described in this chapter should enhance your ability to build rapport, respect, empathy, and compassion with the children and families in your care.

REFERENCES

1. Barry MJ, Edgman-Levitan S. Shared decision making—the pinnacle of patient-centered care. *New Engl J Med.* 2012;366 (9):780-781. doi:10.1056/NEJMp1109283.
2. Hudon C, Fortin M, Haggerty JL, Lambert M, Poitras ME. Measuring patient perception of patient centered care: a systematic review of tools for family medicine. *Ann Fam Med.* 2011;9(2):155-164. doi:10.1370/afm.1226.
3. Mărginean CO, Meliţ LE, Chinceşan M, et al. Communication skills in pediatrics—the relationship between pediatrician and child. *Medicine (Baltimore).* 2017;96(43):e8399. doi:10.1097/MD.0000000000008399.
4. Levetown M; American Academy of Pediatrics Committee on Bioethics. Communicating with children and families: from everyday interactions to skill in conveying distressing information. *Pediatrics.* 2008;121(5):e1441-e1460. doi:10.1542/peds.2008-0565.
5. May WW, Morgan BJ, Lemke JC, Karst GM, Stone HL. Model for ability-based assessment in physical therapy education. *J Phys Ther Educ.* 1995;9(1):3-6.
6. Masin HL. Communicating with cultural sensitivity. In: Davis CM, Musolino GM. *Patient Practitioner Interaction: An Experiential Manual for Developing the Art of Health Care.* 6th ed. Thorofare NJ: SLACK Incorporated; 2016:199-222.
7. Masin HL. Communicating to establish rapport and reduce negativity. In: Davis CM, Musolino GM. *Patient Practitioner Interaction: An Experiential Manual for Developing the Art of Health Care.* 6th ed. Thorofare NJ: SLACK Incorporated; 2016:181-198.
8. Masin HL. Communication in physical therapy in the twenty-first century. In: Pagliarulo MA. *Introduction to Physical Therapy.* 5th ed. St Louis, MO: Elsevier; 2016:150-179.
9. Masin HL. Education in the affective domain: a method/model for teaching professional behaviors in the classroom and during advisory sessions. *J Phys Ther Educ.* 2002;16(1):37-45. doi:10.1097/00001416-200201000-00006.
10. Masin HL. Integrating the use of the generic abilities, clinical performance instrument, and neurolinguistic psychology processes for clinical education intervention. *Phys Ther Case Rep.* 2000;3(6):258-266.
11. May WW, Kontney L, Iglarsh A. Professional behaviors for the 21st century, 2009-2010. Unpublished research.
12. Lopopolo RB, Schafer DS, Nosse LJ. Leadership, administration, management and professionalism (LAMP) in physical therapy: a Delphi study. *Phys Ther.* 2004;84:137-150. doi:10.1093/ptj/84.2.137.
13. Palazzi DL, Lorin MI, Turner TL, Ward MA, Cabrera AG. Communicating with pediatric patients and their families: *The Texas Children's Hospital Guide for Physicians, Nurses and Other Healthcare Professionals.* 2015. www.bcm.edu/pediatrics/patient-communication-guide. Accessed January 9, 2018.
14. Merriam Webster online. www.merriam-webster.com/dictionary/communication. Accessed January 9, 2018.
15. Mehrabian A, Wiener M. Decoding of inconsistent communications. *J Pers Soc Psychol.* 1967;6(1):109-114. doi:10.1037/h0024532.
16. O'Connor J, Seymour J. *Introducing NLP Psychological Skills for Understanding and Influencing People.* 2nd ed. San Francisco, CA: Conari Press; 2011.
17. Lancaster L, Stillman D. *When Generations Collide: Who They Are, Why They Clash, How to Solve the Generational Puzzle at Work.* New York, NY: Harper Collins; 2002.
18. Bemis-Dougherty A. Professionalism and social networking. www.apta.org/PTinMotion/2010/6/Feature/Professionalissandsocialnetworking. Accessed February 6, 2018.
19. American Physical Therapy Association. Standards of conduct in the use of social media HOD PO6-12-17. nationalgovernance@apta.org. Accessed February 1, 2018.
20. American Physical Therapy Association. www.apta.org/SocialMedia/Tips/Succeeding. Accessed February 1, 2018.
21. Sue W, Sue D. *Counseling the Culturally Different: Theory and Practice.* New York, NY: John Wiley & Sons, Inc; 1990:67.

22. Bernieri B, Rosenthal R. *Interpersonal Coordination: Behavior Matching and Interactional Synchrony, Fundamentals of Nonverbal Behavior.* Cambridge, England: Cambridge University Press; 1991.

23. Cross TL, Bazron BJ, Dennis KW, Isaacs MR. *Toward a Culturally Competent System of Care.* Washington DC: CAASP Technical Assistance Center, Georgetown University Child Development Center; 1989.

24. Leavitt RL. *Cross-Cultural Rehabilitation: An International Perspective.* London UK: Saunders; 1994.

25. Agar M. *Language Shock—Understanding the Culture of Conversation.* New York, NY: Perennial; 1994.

26. Würtz E. Intercultural communication on web sites: a cross-cultural analysis of web sites from high-context cultures and low-context cultures. *J Comput Mediat Communi.* 2005;11(1):274-299. doi:10.1111/j.1083-6101.2006.tb00313.x.

27. Crouching Tiger, Hidden Dragon. http://www.imdb.com/title/tt0190332/?ref_=nv_sr_1. Released 2000. Accessed February 6, 2018.

28. Kleinman A. Concepts and a model for the comparison of medical systems as cultural systems. *Soc Sci Med.* 1978;12(2B):85-93. doi:10.1016/0160-7987(78)90014-5.

29. Fadiman A. *The Spirit Catches You and You Fall Down: A Hmong Child, Her American Doctors and the Collision of Two Cultures.* New York, NY: Farrar, Strauss, Giroux; 1997.

30. Taylor JS. Confronting "culture" in medicine's "culture of no culture." *Acad Med.* 2003;78(6):555-559. doi:10.1097/00001888-200306000-00003.

31. Lattanzi JB, Masin HL, Phillips A. Translation and interpretation services for the physical therapist. *HPA Resour.* 2006;6(4):1-5.

32. Salimbene S. *What Language Does Your Patient Hurt In?* St. Paul, MN: EMC Paradigm; 2000.

33. United States Census Bureau. 2015 American Community Survey. http://www.census.gov/acs. Accessed February 6, 2018.

34. Centers for Disease Control and Prevention. 2015 National Health Interview Survey. www.cdc.gov/nchs/nhis.htm. Accessed February 6, 2018.

35. US Department of Health & Human Services. National Institutes of Health. National Institute on Deafness and Other Communication Disorders (NIDCD). http://www.nidcd.nih.gov/health/statistics/quick.htm. Accessed February 6, 2018.

The Children
History and Tests/Measures

Barbara H. Connolly, PT, DPT, EdD, C/NDT, FAPTA
Patricia C. Montgomery, PT, PhD, FAPTA

One of the major problems experienced by the student, new graduate, or clinician inexperienced in pediatric developmental therapy is integrating theory with practice. A problem-solving approach can be helpful for developing skill in the practical application of examination, evaluation, and intervention strategies. To facilitate a problem-solving approach, we have selected 5 case studies of children with varying developmental problems representing typical issues encountered by the clinician. Contributing authors were asked to address these 5 children using the *International Classification of Functioning, Disability and Health—Children and Youth* (ICF–CY) model[1] (ie, Body Functions and Structures, Activities, and Participation) and to suggest appropriate intervention strategies from a variety of perspectives. Composite histories and a review of tests and measures categories are presented in this chapter for each of the children and should be reviewed briefly before proceeding to the subsequent chapters.

CASE STUDY #1: JASON

> *Medical Diagnosis:* Cerebral palsy, right hemiparesis
> *Gross Motor Function Classification System:* Level I
> *Age:* 24 months

Examination

History

Jason was the first born of preterm, nonidentical twins with a birth weight of 1660 grams. His Apgar scores were 7 at 1 minute and 9 at 5 minutes. He did not require mechanical ventilation and was discharged from the neonatal intensive care unit (NICU) after 40 days on caffeine-citrate due to bradycardia with feedings. Initial follow-up at age 2 months' gestational age was nonremarkable.

Connolly BH, Montgomery PC, eds. *Therapeutic Exercise for Children With Developmental Disabilities, Fourth Edition* (pp 131-139).
© 2020 Taylor & Francis Group.

At his follow-up visit at age 6 months definite asymmetries in stretch reflexes and voluntary use of his extremities were noted. Jason was referred for early intervention services. Jason is not on any medication and has not had any surgical procedures.

Tests and Measures Categories

> *Anthropometric Characteristics:* Jason is noted to have a slightly smaller right upper extremity (noticeable only in the upper arm) as compared with the left. He is of average height and weight for his age.

> *Mental Functions:* Testing indicates that Jason's intelligence quotient (IQ) falls within the average range. He has delayed expressive language and relies more on gestures for communication than other children his age.

> *Assistive Technology:* None.

> *Gait:* Jason began walking at age 15 months. His gait is characterized by a short swing phase on the right, short stride length with retraction of the pelvis on the right, minimal right knee and ankle flexion at mid-swing, short stance phase on the right with genu recurvatum, and a valgus position of the right foot at mid-stance. He initiates walking with the left side and turns and changes direction from the left side only.

> *Balance:* He falls frequently during the day.

> *Integumentary Integrity:* Normal.

> *Joint Integrity and Mobility:* Within normal range to passive movement.

> *Motor Function:* Jason is able to follow directions and attempts to imitate motor skills, although he has generally poor coordination of his right extremities. Isolated control of right forearm and finger movements is difficult.

> *Muscle Performance (Including Strength, Power, Endurance, and Length):* Weakness is evident in the right upper extremity, particularly in the triceps and supinators of the forearm. He also has generalized weakness in the right lower extremity.

> *Neuromotor Development and Sensory Processing:* Jason has good head control in all positions. He can assume an all fours position and bear partial weight on his right upper extremity. He can crawl, but occasionally collapses on the right arm. He can get into standing independently from the middle of the floor by assuming a bear stance and rising. He uses a gross grasp with the right hand for most fine motor tasks. He attempts to run, but is clumsy and usually falls. Gross motor skills range between 12 to 15 months. He has slow and often ineffective protective reactions on the right side. Tactile defensive behaviors occasionally are observed and tactile input generally results in an increased activity level.

> *Posture:* In standing, Jason demonstrates an asymmetrical posture with a slight anterior tilt of the pelvis and pelvic retraction on the right. He has an observable asymmetry in the rib cage. The right upper extremity usually is held in a position of shoulder retraction with elbow, wrist, and finger flexion.

> *Range of Motion:* Active reach of the right arm is limited to 90 degrees of humeral abduction. Jason also demonstrates tightness to passive stretch in the hip muscles and lateral trunk flexors on the right with limitation in trunk rotation.

> *Reflex Integrity:* Hyperactive stretch reflexes are present to tendon tap at the ankle (plantar flexors), knee (quadriceps), and elbow (biceps) on the right. Normal stretch reflexes are evident on the left side of the body.

> *Education Life:* He currently receives home-based services consisting of weekly visits from his local school district (alternating between teacher and occupational therapist) and once-per-week visits from a private speech-language pathologist and a private physical therapist.

- *Community, Social, and Civic Life:* Jason enjoys age-appropriate play activities and demonstrates typical behaviors for a 24-month-old child when his sibling or other children are present.
- *Self-Care and Domestic Life:* Jason drools occasionally, especially when concentrating on an activity. He is a "messy" eater, often losing food out of his mouth. He does not seem to notice when food escapes from his mouth. He is just beginning to assist with dressing and undressing activities. He also is beginning to show some interest in toilet training.
- *Sensory Integrity:* General neglect of the right side of the body, especially the right upper extremity, is noted.
- *Ventilation and Respiration:* Breathiness is noted during speech and consonants are limited in quantity and quality. He often gasps for breath after drinking.

Case Study #2: Jill

- *Medical Diagnosis:* Cerebral palsy, spastic quadriparesis, microcephaly, intellectual deficits, seizure disorder
- *Gross Motor Function Classification System:* Level V
- *Age:* 7 years

Examination

History

Jill was born full term following a normal pregnancy. Her Apgar scores were 5 at 1 minute and 8 at 5 minutes. Jill had seizures during the neonatal period and had an abnormal electroencephalogram. She was on mechanical ventilation for several days and initially had feeding difficulties. She was discharged from the NICU on antiseizure medication. At the time of discharge, she was drinking well from a bottle. At a 4-month follow-up visit with her pediatrician, decreased head growth was noted. She had a normal eye exam and brainstem auditory evoked response. Jill has continued to have occasional seizures. She had orthopedic surgery (heel cord and adductor releases) at age 5 years. Jill received weekly intervention services (occupational, speech, and physical therapy) through a private agency from the time of her discharge from the NICU until she entered a public school program full days at age 6 years.

Tests and Measures Categories

- *Anthropometric Characteristics:* Jill has microcephaly and is below the 10th percentile in height and weight for her age.
- *Mental Functions:* Testing indicates that Jill's IQ is below 50 (severe intellectual impairment). She often is lethargic, which appears to be related to her seizure medication. When she is alert, she is easily distracted and has poor selective attention. She is a sociable child, however, and is easily motivated. Jill has few words and communicates through variations in vocalization patterns.
- *Assistive Technology:* Jill has an adapted manual wheelchair. She has a prone stander at school and at home. Jill has static ankle-foot orthoses that she uses when in her stander.
- *Mobility (Including Locomotion):* Jill is nonambulatory and has poor potential for assisted ambulation.
- *Balance:* She is unable to maintain her balance in any position (eg, sitting, kneeling, all fours, standing).

- *Integumentary Integrity:* Skin integrity is normal, but Jill is at risk for skin irritation because of lack of active movement and prolonged positioning in sitting.
- *Joint Integrity and Mobility:* Rib cage and shoulder girdle immobility are noted.
- *Motor Function:* Motor control is very limited. Jill has poor head control in all positions. She attempts to grasp, but her hand often closes involuntarily prior to obtaining an object. Voluntary release is difficult, and she is unable to manipulate objects with her fingers. She has limited voluntary movement of her extremities.
- *Muscle Performance (Including Strength, Power, Endurance, and Length):* Jill has generalized weakness because of her limited motor control and paucity of active movement. Poor muscle development/bulk is noted throughout her extremities.
- *Neuromotor Development and Sensory Processing:* Gross motor skills are at approximately a 3-month level. Jill can lift her head momentarily in prone, but not in supine. She maintains her head in neutral when held vertically, but generally has poor head control. She is not able to sit without support. She can roll to side-lying from supine, but does not roll over. She has no independent floor mobility. Protective and equilibrium responses to movement are absent. Movement through space results in autonomic distress. She demonstrates hypersensitivity in the oral area with increased lip retraction and head extension. She also has poor ocular control and lacks downward gaze.
- *Posture:* A kyphotic posture is noted in the upper back with her head and neck often in hyper-extension. She has a mild scoliosis and an indented sternum.
- *Range of Motion:* Tightness is noted in capital extensors, pectorals, shoulder girdle muscles, hip flexors, and lumbar extensors. Active reach is 60 degrees of humeral abduction and passive range is limited to 90 degrees.
- *Reflex Integrity:* Hyperactive tendon reflexes are noted in upper and lower extremities (+3 to +4). Jill demonstrates increased resistance (stiffness) to passive movements of her extremities and trunk.
- *Education Life:* Jill is in an educational setting in a special education classroom. She is main-streamed with other children for part of each day. Jill needs adult assistance to participate in play and classroom activities. She receives occupational, speech, and physical therapy services (30 minutes per week each) on an indirect basis. Programming is carried out in the classroom with the help of a classroom aide.
- *Community, Social, and Civic Life:* Jill needs adult assistance to participate in play and leisure activities. She enjoys watching videos and children's television programs, but needs assistance or positioning for head control. She is participating in a community-sponsored adaptive aquatics class and therapeutic horseback riding (hippotherapy).
- *Self-Care and Domestic Life:* Jill's oral-motor skills are poor and she has difficulty eating and drinking. She demonstrates severe cheek/lip retraction and jaw thrusting. Her tongue is thick in contour and often retracted. Jill occasionally will assist in dressing by pushing her arms through sleeves and can assist in standing-pivot transfers, otherwise she is totally dependent on caregivers for self-cares. She is not toilet trained.
- *Sensory Integrity:* Vision is normal, although she has poor ocular-motor control. Hearing also is within the normal range. Jill demonstrates hypersensitivity to movement (vestibular stimulation) and to tactile stimulation in and around the mouth.
- *Ventilation and Respiration:* Jill's rib cage generally is immobile and she demonstrates an asynchronous respiratory pattern. Coordination with respiration during feeding is poor with much coughing and choking, therefore she is susceptible to upper respiratory infections.

CASE STUDY #3: TAYLOR

> *Medical Diagnosis:* Myelomeningocele, repaired L1-2
> *Age:* 4 years

Examination

History

Taylor was a full-term infant born by cesarean section because of fetal distress and breech presentation. At birth a large myelomeningocele was noted and was closed surgically. A ventricular-peritoneal shunt was surgically inserted on day 5. Taylor had increased apnea and was on a respirator. He had questionable seizures, but his electroencephalogram was normal. He had a suspected Arnold-Chiari malformation that was treated by surgical release of the posterior fossa. He had equinovarus deformities and underwent serial casting beginning at age 2 weeks. Following a 4-month hospital stay, Taylor was discharged home on a cardiorespiratory monitor for continued apnea. He was referred for physical therapy services at discharge. He subsequently had surgery to correct bilaterally dislocated hips.

Tests and Measures Categories

> *Anthropometric Characteristics:* Taylor's lower extremities are small in proportion to his upper extremities and trunk. His head is slightly larger (95th percentile) in proportion to his body because of hydrocephalus.
> *Mental Functions:* Taylor has visual perceptual problems, which has made cognitive testing difficult. His performance suggests his intellectual skills are in the low normal range. He has good attention skills and usually is cooperative and motivated in the classroom. He has a mean sentence length of 3 to 4 words, and sounds produced are within normal limits. He is being evaluated for speech and language services.
> *Assistive Technology:* Taylor currently uses an anterior walker and a reciprocating gait orthosis. He also has long leg braces and forearm crutches. He self-propels in a manual wheelchair.
> *Mobility (Including Locomotion):* External support is necessary for standing. Taylor ambulates with a reciprocating gait orthosis and a walker, but is working with crutches and long leg braces.
> *Balance:* Balance reactions are slow in sitting and standing. He has good protective reactions in sitting, but not in standing.
> *Integumentary Integrity:* Taylor has had frequent skin breakdowns in the sacral area and in his feet/ankles.
> *Joint Integrity and Mobility:* Mobility is limited in his feet, but his ankles can be positioned at 90 degrees of dorsiflexion for standing activities.
> *Motor Function:* Taylor has loss of motor function in his lower extremities. He has poor active trunk extension. He has good head control in all positions and normal upper extremity coordination.
> *Muscle Performance (Including Strength, Power, Endurance, and Length):* Generalized weakness is noted in upper extremities and trunk, especially in abdominal muscles. Overall endurance for physical activity is decreased compared with peers.
> *Neuromotor Development and Sensory Processing:* Taylor rolls with poor leg dissociation. He can get in and out of sitting and onto all fours independently. He attempts to pull to kneeling. He has normal grasp, manipulation, and release. He has visual acuity problems and wears glasses. He has particular difficulty with figure-ground discrimination and, when standing, bending his head to look at the floor disturbs his balance.

- *Posture:* On all fours, Taylor demonstrates a lordotic posture. In sitting, he slumps rather than using muscle activity to sit upright.
- *Range of Motion:* Taylor's range of motion is within functional limits. He has slightly tight hip flexors and hip adductors.
- *Reflex Integrity:* Tendon reflexes are absent in the lower extremities, normal in upper extremities.
- *Education Life:* Taylor attends a preschool program 3 mornings per week. He receives occupational therapy once each week and physical therapy twice each week in his preschool program. The school district is considering placement for Taylor in a regular kindergarten classroom next year.
- *Community, Social, and Civic Life:* Taylor is a sociable child who is interested in age-appropriate play and leisure activities. He is most interested in peer interaction in his home and classroom as he cannot keep up with peers outside or on the playground. He is enrolled in a Saturday karate class in the community that includes children who are nondisabled and disabled.
- *Self-Care and Domestic Life:* Taylor can put on and take off his T-shirts. He needs assistance for lower body dressing. Oral-motor skills are normal and there are no feeding problems. He needs assistance with other self-cares, such as toileting.
- *Sensory Integrity:* Taylor demonstrates loss of cutaneous and proprioceptive sensation below L1-2.
- *Ventilation and Respiration:* Taylor tends to hold his breath when using his upper extremities for weight-bearing or strenuous tasks. He has inadequate abdominal strength to support sustained exhalation.

Case Study #4: Ashley

- *Medical Diagnosis:* Down syndrome
- *Age:* 15 months

Examination

History

Ashley was a full-term infant born to a 26-year-old primipara mother who had experienced an uncomplicated pregnancy. Ashley was diagnosed with Down syndrome (DS) shortly after birth. She had esophageal atresia and primary repair was not possible. A gastrostomy was present for the first 6 months of age. She had a ventricular-septal defect that was surgically repaired at 8 months. Ashley has a history of chronic otitis media with mild conductive hearing loss. Pressure equalizing tubes were placed at 12 months.

Tests and Measures Categories

- *Anthropometric Characteristics:* Ashley's height and weight are within the normal range for children her age with DS. Facial features are characteristic of children with DS.
- *Mental Functions:* Formal IQ testing has not been completed on Ashley, although she has mild intellectual deficits associated with her medical diagnosis. She is a passive child, needing encouragement and stimulation to attend to motor and cognitive tasks. She has several words that she uses singly rather than in combination (eg, "more," "mama," "dada").
- *Assistive Technology:* None.

- *Mobility (Including Locomotion):* Ashley pulls to stand but is not yet attempting to cruise at furniture. She will walk with maximal assistance with 2 hands held.
- *Integumentary Integrity:* Normal.
- *Joint Integrity and Mobility:* Hypermobility is noted in all upper and lower extremity proximal and distal joints.
- *Motor Function:* Ashley appears to have a typical variety of movement patterns, but her movements are very slow. Postural reactions are delayed. Ashley needs multiple repetitions of cognitive and motor tasks for skill achievement and retention.
- *Muscle Performance (Including Strength, Power, Endurance, and Length):* Ashley has poor muscle definition throughout her body, particularly noticeable in the shoulders and hips. She tends to lock her elbows into extension and externally rotates her arms when making movement transitions. She has poor stability in weight-bearing positions (eg, all fours, kneeling).
- *Neuromotor Development and Sensory Processing:* Ashley has good head control in all positions. She rolls independently, and transitions in and out of sitting and in and out of a hands and knees position. She also pulls to kneeling and to stand at furniture. She tends to use straight plane movements without using trunk rotation. She has slow and usually ineffective protective and equilibrium reactions in sitting, all fours, and standing. She does not appear hypersensitive to tactile input. She generally is apprehensive about movement activities. She grasps objects but cannot release them with control. She cannot pick up pellet-sized objects.
- *Posture:* In standing, Ashley has a wide base of support with lumbar lordosis, knee hyperextension, and foot pronation. Her trunk posture is kyphotic in sitting, but lordotic in quadruped.
- *Range of Motion:* Hypermobility is noted in both proximal and distal joints of the extremities. She tends to keep her shoulders elevated with shortened capital extensor muscles.
- *Reflex Integrity:* Decreased tendon reflexes are present throughout her upper and lower extremities. Low muscle tone is noted throughout the face and trunk.
- *Education Life:* Although her parents were encouraged to contact local early intervention programs when Ashley was discharged from the hospital, they did not seek services until she was age 10 months. Ashley and her mother attend a parent/caregiver-infant early intervention program twice weekly with consultative physical therapy, occupational therapy, and speech therapy services available at each session. The family has declined home-based services.
- *Community, Social, and Civic Life:* Ashley observes other children but does not interact with them. She tends to fling objects or toys to dispose of them. Play is seldom goal directed.
- *Self-Care and Domestic Life:* Ashley has poor oral-motor skills. She uses a suckle pattern in feeding. Her tongue is thick in contour and protrudes from her mouth. She drinks from a cup only at snack time. Solids are inconsistently presented. She tends to lose food from her mouth. She does not assist in any other self-cares.
- *Sensory Integrity:* Vision is normal. Mild conductive hearing loss has been noted. Ashley tends to avoid movement-based activities.
- *Ventilation and Respiration:* Ashley has decreased respiratory-phonatory functioning. She is a mouth breather and occasionally drools.

CASE STUDY #5: JOHN

- *Medical Diagnosis:* Developmental coordination disorder/attention-deficit hyperactivity disorder
- *Age:* 5 years

Examination

History

John was a premature infant who spent a short time in the NICU before being discharged to home. He was noted to have slightly delayed motor milestones (sat at age 9 months, walked at 18 months). He always has been considered to be a very active child. He is easily frustrated with motor tasks and temper tantrums are frequent. He is noted to be "clumsy" and is unable to perform gross and fine motor tasks as well as his peers (eg, cannot ride a bike without training wheels, has poor tracing and coloring skills). He recently was evaluated by a developmental pediatrician and a neuropsychologist and received dual diagnoses of developmental coordination disorder/attention-deficit hyperactivity disorder. He has been placed on Ritalin (methylphenidate).

Tests and Measures Categories

- *Anthropometric Characteristics:* Average height and weight for his age.
- *Mental Functions:* John's attention span has improved since he began taking medication. He still has difficulty with selective attention and often has to be redirected to task. Formal IQ testing on the Stanford-Binet suggests above-average intelligence. John has an expressive language delay, often omitting consonants in words and words in sentences.
- *Assistive Technology:* None.
- *Gait:* John walks independently, but occasionally walks on his toes. He can walk with a heel-toe gait when reminded.
- *Balance:* He tends to walk too quickly with poor balance, often bumping into environmental objects or other people. He cannot walk a 4-inch (10 cm) balance beam without falling off and can maintain his balance on one foot for only 1 to 2 seconds.
- *Integumentary Integrity:* Normal.
- *Joint Integrity and Mobility:* Normal.
- *Motor Function:* John does not have an abnormal neurological examination that would indicate impaired motor control, although he is consistently characterized as being "clumsy." He has difficulty varying the speed of movement and coordinating his upper and lower extremities, such as required when performing jumping jacks. He has motor planning problems and has difficulty learning new motor skills. He requires more practice than his peers to master each motor skill, and skills do not generalize easily.
- *Muscle Performance (Including Strength, Power, Endurance, and Length):* Upper extremity strength is decreased for his age. For example, he has difficulty supporting his weight on his arms to "wheelbarrow." Endurance for age-appropriate activities, such as soccer, is decreased compared with peers.
- *Neuromotor Development and Sensory Processing:* John ambulates independently. He can run, although he does so in a poorly coordinated pattern. He cannot skip, but gallops instead. He has difficulty with ball skills (eg, catching, throwing, dribbling) and eye-hand coordination. He uses a modified lateral pinch for coloring and printing. He occasionally demonstrates signs of tactile defensiveness.
- *Posture:* John tends to walk with stiff legs and a decreased arm swing. He often leans forward as he walks.
- *Range of Motion:* Within normal limits.
- *Reflex Integrity:* Normal.
- *Education Life:* John is in a half-day kindergarten program, but does not qualify for special education services. He is receiving occupational and physical therapy (each 2 times per month) through a private agency.

➤ *Community, Social, and Civic Life:* John prefers video games to gross motor play. He avoids physical activity and group sports. His parents have been encouraged to explore community resources for John (eg, swimming, karate classes, T-ball, soccer) and to encourage his participation.

➤ *Self-Care and Domestic Life:* John has difficulty using utensils during meals and prefers finger foods. He is independent in dressing, but has difficulty with buttons, snaps, and zippers. He prefers Velcro closures, T-shirts, and sweatpants. He is independent in toileting, but needs to be monitored to do an adequate job bathing and tooth brushing.

➤ *Sensory Integrity:* Vision and hearing are normal. Testing indicates problems with tactile discrimination, kinesthesia, and stereognosis.

➤ *Ventilation and Respiration:* Normal.

Summary

The preceding 5 case descriptions can be used as references for information in this text. The authors of each chapter present a specific perspective for evaluation of and intervention for children with developmental disabilities. In some chapters the ages of the children have been modified to reflect age-appropriate interventions (eg, NICU, Early Mobility). Chapter 17 presents a comprehensive review of various proposed strategies in relation to each child in the 5 case studies. In addition, considerations relevant to case management for each child are discussed.

Reference

1.   World Health Organization. *International Classification of Functioning, Disability and Health: Children and Youth Version.* Geneva, Switzerland: World Health Organization; 2007.

Applying the
Guide to Physical Therapist Practice 3.0

Joanell A. Bohmert, PT, DPT, MS

The purpose of this chapter is to apply the *Guide to Physical Therapist Practice 3.0* (the *Guide 3.0*) to clinical practice.[1] The *Guide* is the primary resource document that describes the practice of the physical therapist. The *Guide* provides the concepts and framework with which physical therapists organize practice. Although the previous *Guide* was available in print and compact disc (CD), the *Guide 3.0* is available only online.[1] The *Guide 3.0* is free to American Physical Therapy Association (APTA) members and by subscription for institutions and individuals.

DEVELOPMENT OF THE *GUIDE*

The *Guide* was developed by the APTA based on the needs of members to justify physical therapy practice to state legislators. This process began in 1992 with a board-appointed task force and culminated in the publication of *A Guide to Physical Therapist Practice, Volume I: A Description of Patient Management* in 1995.[2]

Volume II described the preferred patterns of practice for patient/client groupings commonly referred for physical therapy and reflected current APTA standards, policies, and guidelines. The process for completion of Volume II was by expert consensus and included a project advisory group, a board oversight committee, and 4 panels. Membership review was provided throughout the development with more than 600 individual field reviewers and general input at various APTA-sponsored forums.[3] Volume I and Volume II became Part One and Part Two of the *Guide,* with Part Two reflecting information obtained in the development of Part Two. In late 1997, the *First Edition* of the *Guide* was published after having been approved by the APTA House of Delegates earlier that year.[4]

The *Guide* was developed as a "living" document that will need updating to reflect changes in the base of knowledge for physical therapists.[4] In addition, the *Guide* will need to reflect membership input, changes in APTA policies[5,6] and incorporate further description of practice. In 1998, APTA initiated Part Three and Part Four of the *Guide* to catalog the specific tests and measures used by physical therapists and to develop standardized documentation forms that incorporated

Connolly BH, Montgomery PC, eds. *Therapeutic Exercise for Children With Developmental Disabilities, Fourth Edition* (pp 141-176).
© 2020 Taylor & Francis Group.

the patient/client management process. This further development of the *Guide* also involved expert task force members, field reviews, and membership input at APTA forums. Documentation templates for inpatient and outpatient settings were developed, as was a patient/client satisfaction instrument, all of which were available in the *Guide*.[3]

During 1999 through 2001, work continued on reviewing tests and measures. Part Four was incorporated into Part Three, with the result being a listing of tests and measures that were used in Chapter 2 of the *Guide*. Part Three contained reference literature describing the tests and provided available data regarding each test's reliability and validity. Part Three, available only on CD, was searchable and linked to Chapter 2 as well as to specific patterns. The CD included the entire *Guide* (Parts One through Three). In 2001, the *Guide to Physical Therapist Practice, Second Edition*, which reflected input from membership, leadership, Part Three revisions, and changes in House policies, was published. After 2001, revisions were made to update the tests and measures and to expand content of the CD to include all aspects of the *Guide*. In 2010, the *Guide* went online with its own website: http://guidetoptpractice.apta.org.

The *Guide 3.0* was released in 2014 as an online-only resource (no print edition) on the *Guide*'s website. The *Guide 3.0* was the result of work that began in 2009 that included seeking input for revisions from all APTA components, a focus group, an expert panel, and a field review.[7] Significant changes that occurred with the *Guide 3.0* included the following[8]:

> ‣ Changing the focus of use of the *Guide* from a resource for those within the physical therapy community as well as for those outside physical therapy to being just a description of physical therapist practice for physical therapists and physical therapist assistants.

> ‣ Updating the Patient/Client Management Model to reflect current practice and updating language to reflect the *International Classification of Functioning, Disability and Health* (ICF).

> ‣ Removing the Preferred Practice Patterns. The Preferred Practice Patterns are still available in an edited form, Adapted Practice Patterns, for educational purposes through links in the *Guide 3.0*[9] and on APTA's website.[10]

As a dynamic, evolving document, the *Guide* will continue to be updated with posts on the APTA *Guide* home page. Readers are encouraged to access the *Guide 3.0* online for the most current version.

ORGANIZATION OF THE *GUIDE*

The *Guide 3.0* website is interactive, with links embedded throughout the document. The *Guide 3.0* is accessed from the home page with links to the Table of Contents, Updates and Summary of Revisions, and *Guide 3.0*: What You Need to Know.[1] To access the *Guide 3.0*, you must first log in. APTA members may access the site for free, and other individuals and institutions must purchase a subscription. Once you are logged in, you may access all areas of the *Guide 3.0*.

The *Guide 3.0* is composed of the following sections that are accessed from the Table of Contents:

> ‣ Chapter 1—Introduction to the *Guide to Physical Therapist Practice*
> ‣ Chapter 2—Principles of Physical Therapist Patient and Client Management
> ‣ Chapter 3—Measurement and Outcomes
> ‣ Chapter 4—Physical Therapist Examination and Evaluation: Focus on Tests and Measures
> ‣ Chapter 5—Interventions
> ‣ Appendix—History of Guide Development
> ‣ Glossary

Introduction to the Guide to Physical Therapist Practice

The Introduction includes the Purpose; Description of Physical Therapist Practice; Physical Therapist Direction and Supervision of Personnel; Constructs and Concepts That Inform Physical Therapist Practice; and Education, Specialization, and Licensure. The Purpose of the *Guide 3.0* is to describe physical therapist practice for the physical therapist, physical therapist assistant, and physical therapy community. This is accomplished by describing physical therapist practice; identifying roles, settings, and practice opportunities; standardizing terminology; reviewing educational preparation; and describing the patient/client management process that includes clinical decision making, the examination and evaluation process, the intervention process, and use of outcome measures.[11]

The Description of Physical Therapy Practice includes a general description of the physical therapy profession and the roles physical therapists play not only in patient/client care but also in the health care environment and health. These roles include but are not limited to primary, secondary, and tertiary care; prevention and promotion of health, wellness, and fitness; consultation; education; critical inquiry; and administration.[11]

Physical Therapist Direction and Supervision of Personnel addresses who may provide physical therapy. Physical therapy is not a generic term but a service provided by a licensed physical therapist or assisted by a physical therapist assistant under the direction and supervision of the physical therapist.

CONCEPTS OF THE *GUIDE*

The *Guide 3.0* has 4 key concepts on which it is based: (1) ICF and the biopsychosocial model, (2) evidence-based practice, (3) professional values and guiding documents, and (4) quality assessment.[11]

International Classification of Functioning, Disability and Health *and Biopsychosocial Model*

The first key concept that serves as the basis for physical therapist practice is a disablement-enablement model. Several models of disablement (Nagi, World Health Organization, National Center for Medical Rehabilitation and Research) have been developed and continue to be updated and revised.[12-17] These models use different terminology to describe the components of disablement with APTA using Nagi's terminology of pathology, impairment, functional limitation, and disability as the terminology for early versions of the *Guide*.[3]

In 1991, the Institute of Medicine introduced the concept of prevention being a factor that could affect the disablement model.[18] In this model of disablement, prevention is the act of providing intervention, before or within the disablement process, at the level of the components (ie, pathology, impairment, functional limitation, disability), or at the level of risk factors to positively affect the individual. This concept of affecting the process of disablement was expanded further by the Institute of Medicine in 1997 to include rehabilitation as a method of preventing disability, thereby resulting in "enabling" the individual and removing disability from the process.[19]

In 1997, Engle proposed a model for medicine that moved the traditionally used biomedical model (impact of illness and disease on the individual's biological system)[20,21] to a model that added the psychological and social components of the individual to the biological components, the "biopsychosocial" model. This model examines the impact of the disease or condition on an individual's biological system as well as on personal and social functions, in other words, how the disease or condition affects the individual's life. The World Health Organization incorporated the

TABLE 6-1. DISABLEMENT-ENABLEMENT DEFINITIONS USED IN THE *GUIDE 3.0*

HEALTH

A state of being associated with freedom from disease, injury, and illness that also includes a positive component (wellness) that is associated with a quality of life and positive well-being.

DISABILITY

An umbrella term for impairments, activity limitations, and participation restrictions. It denotes the negative aspects of the interaction between an individual with a health condition and that individual's contextual factors (environmental and personal factors).

ENVIRONMENTAL FACTORS

The physical, social, and attitudinal environment in which people live and conduct their lives. These are either barriers to or facilitators of the individual's functioning.

PERSONAL FACTORS

Contextual factors that relate to the individual, such as age, gender, social status, and life experiences.

Adapted from the American Physical Therapy Association. *Guide to Physical Therapist Practice 3.0.* Alexandria, VA: American Physical Therapy Association; 2014. http://guidetoptpractice.apta.org/.

biopsychosocial model into the framework of the ICF, recognizing that disease does not present the same in every individual and that it is important to consider individual and environmental factors in addition to biological factors as a measure of health and disability.[22]

The ICF provides the framework and classification system for measuring health and disability from the perspective of health domains using contextual factors of the individual and environment.[22] The *Guide 3.0* uses terminology based on ICF model, and the concepts of the disablement-enablement process serve as the basis for physical therapist practice. Table 6-1 provides the definitions of the disablement-enablement model used in the *Guide 3.0*.[23]

The disablement process incorporates 4 components: (1) health condition or pathology, (2) impairment of body functions and structures, (3) activity limitations, and (4) participation restrictions. Table 6-2 provides the definitions for these components. Disablement is not linear or unidirectional.

Health condition or pathology cannot be assumed to lead to impairments, that impairments lead to activity limitations, or that activity limitations lead to participation restrictions. There are many factors that can affect the process and change the relationship of the 4 components. These factors include those of the individual and those of the environment.

The following are individual factors:
› Those inherent to the individual (eg, biological and demographic)
› Those in which the individual makes choices (eg, health habits, personal behaviors, lifestyles)
› The psychological attributes of the individual (eg, motivation, coping)
› The individual's social support (social interactions and relationships)

The following are environmental factors:
› Available health care
› Physical therapy services

TABLE 6-2. COMPONENTS OF DISABLEMENT DEFINITIONS USED IN THE *GUIDE 3.0*

HEALTH CONDITION

An umbrella term for acute or chronic disease, disorder, injury, or trauma. It also may include other circumstances such as aging, stress, pregnancy, congenital abnormality, or genetic predisposition.

IMPAIRMENT

Problems in body functions and/or structures as a significant deviation or loss.

ACTIVITY LIMITATIONS

The difficulties an individual may have in executing activities.

PARTICIPATION RESTRICTIONS

Problems an individual may experience in involvement in life situations. The presence of a participation restriction is determined by comparing an individual's participation with that which is expected of an individual without a disability in a particular culture or society.

Adapted from the American Physical Therapy Association. *Guide to Physical Therapist Practice 3.0*. Alexandria, VA: American Physical Therapy Association; 2014. http://guidetoptpractice.apta.org/.

> Medications
> Other therapies
> The physical and social environment[3]

The disablement-enablement model is the model physical therapists use to view how an individual interacts with the environment and how that affects the individual's sense of well-being or health-related quality of life. The physical therapist observes how the patient/client is functioning then determines which factors are affecting the areas of difficulty. As a primary resource for physical therapist practice, the *Guide 3.0* incorporates the concepts of disablement-enablement through a number of ways:

> The 4 main components of the disablement process (health condition or pathology, impairments of body functions and structures, activity limitations, participation restrictions)
> Individual factors (risk reduction and prevention; health, wellness, and fitness; patient/client satisfaction)
> Environmental factors (risk reduction and prevention, societal resources)

These concepts are addressed throughout the continuum of service within the patient/client management model, concluding in outcomes.

Evidence-Based Practice

The second key concept is evidence-based practice (EBP). EBP incorporates 3 components: (1) the best available research, (2) the patient's/client's needs and values, and (3) the physical therapist's expertise and clinical judgment.

Physical therapists need to have an understanding of research design, measurement, and outcomes to evaluate the best available research. Physical therapists also need to learn and understand the needs and values of their patient/client, as the individual's perspective drives what evidence will be sought and how it may apply. Physical therapists also use their expertise in determining the best patient/client management process for a specific patient/client.

Access to literature, clinical practice guidelines, and systematic reviews are available to APTA members at PTNow.[24] PT Now: Tools to Advance Physical Therapist Practice has a website (https://www.ptnow.org) and serves as the home base and launch site for resources for physical therapist EBP. Resources include article search, rehabilitation reference center, clinical summaries, tests, clinical practice guidelines, and Cochrane Reviews.[24]

Professional Values and Guiding Documents

A third key concept is the incorporation of professional values and adherence to guiding documents that provide the foundation for physical therapist practice. Core values of accountability, altruism, compassion/caring, excellence, integrity, professional duty, and social responsibility result in patient-/client-focused practice.[25] These values also direct physical therapists to place the needs of the patient/client above those of institutions or organizations, to practice within the physical therapist's personal scope of practice, and to address the needs of society. Guiding documents for the physical therapist include the *Code of Ethics for the Physical Therapist*[26] and the accompanying *Guide for Professional Conduct,*[27] *Standards of Practice for Physical Therapy,*[28] and *Criteria for Standards of Practice for Physical Therapy.*[29] Guiding documents for the physical therapist assistant include the *Standards of Ethical Conduct for the Physical Therapist Assistant*[30] and the *Guide for Conduct of the Physical Therapist Assistant.*[31]

Quality Assessment

Quality of assessment is the fourth key concept of physical therapist practice. To provide quality services and programs, physical therapists perform ongoing quality assessments. These assessments address how service is structured, the processes of care, and measurement of outcomes of care.[11]

PATIENT/CLIENT MANAGEMENT MODEL

The patient/client management model is the clinical decision-making model for the provision of physical therapist service. The patient/client model includes the 5 essential elements of (1) examination, (2) evaluation, (3) diagnosis, (4) prognosis, and (5) intervention that result in optimal outcomes. Figure 6-1 illustrates the patient/client management process with a brief explanation of the 5 elements.[3] The patient/client management process is dynamic and allows the physical therapist to monitor the patient's/client's progress in the process, return to an earlier element for further analysis, refer the patient/client for further evaluation, or exit the patient/client from the process when the needs of the patient/client cannot be addressed by the physical therapist.

The patient/client management process incorporates the disablement-enablement model of the ICF throughout the 5 elements and outcomes and is to be used throughout the continuum of service in all settings. Descriptions of the elements of patient/client management is provided in the *Guide 3.0*: Chapter 2—Principles of Physical Therapist Patient and Client Management, Chapter 4—Physical Therapist Examination and Evaluation: Focus on Tests and Measures, and Chapter 5—Interventions. The Preferred Practice Patterns, which were examples of the patient/client management process in the 4 main body systems, are no longer a part of the *Guide 3.0* but have been adapted and are available as a teaching resource under Education Tools.[10]

DIAGNOSIS
Both the process and the end result of evaluating examination data, which the physical therapist organizes into defined clusters, syndromes, or categories to help determine the prognosis (including the plan of care) and the most appropriate intervention strategies.

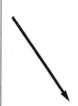

EVALUATION
A dynamic process in which the physical therapist makes clinical judgments based on data gathered during the examination. This process also may identify possible problems that require consultation with or referral to another provider.

PROGNOSIS
Determination of the level of optimal improvement that may be attained through intervention and the amount of time required to reach that level. The plan of care specifies the interventions to be used and their timing and frequency.

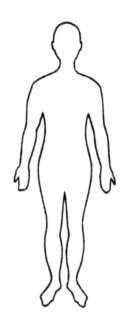

EXAMINATION
The process of obtaining a history, performing a systems review, and selecting and administering tests and measures to gather data about the patient/client. The initial examination is a comprehensive screening and specific testing process that leads to a diagnosis classification. The examination process also may identify possible problems that require consultation with or referral to another provider.

INTERVENTION
Purposeful and skilled interaction of the physical therapist with the patient and, if appropriate, with other individuals involved in care of the patient, using various physical therapy methods and techniques to produce changes in the condition that are consistent with the diagnosis and prognosis. The physical therapist conducts a reexamination to determine changes in patient status and to modify or redirect intervention. The decision to reexamine may be based on new clinical findings or on lack of patient progress. The process of reexamination also may identify the need for consultation with or referral to another provider.

OUTCOMES
Results of patient management, which include the impact of physical therapy interventions in the following domains: pathology/pathophysiology (disease, disorder, or condition); impairments, functional limitations, and disabilities; risk reduction/prevention; health, wellness, and fitness; societal resources; and patient satisfaction.

Figure 6-1. The elements of patient/client management leading to optimal outcomes. (Reprinted from http://guidetoptpractice.apta.org/, with permission of the American Physical Therapy Association. © 2019 American Physical Therapy Association. All rights reserved.)

Application of the *Guide 3.0* to Clinical Practice

The *Guide 3.0* can be applied in a number of ways. I will explain an application of the *Guide 3.0* by looking at the clinical decision-making process of the patient/client management process. The Adapted Practice Patterns provide an outline of the patient/client management process with examples of how to use the process within a specific body system and possible health condition.

You will need the *Guide 3.0* and the Adapted Practice Patterns to follow the examples. I will show you how the patient/client management process and the disablement-enablement model are integrated. I will then show you specific applications of the *Guide 3.0* for the case studies described in Chapter 5 of this text.

Adapted Practice Patterns

The Adapted Practice Patterns are the Preferred Practice Patterns that were deleted from the *Guide*. The patterns have been revised and adapted and continue to be organized in 4 body systems: Musculoskeletal (4A to J), Neuromuscular (5A to I), Cardiovascular/Pulmonary (6A to J), and Integumentary (7A to E).[9] The patterns are helpful as examples in using the patient/client management decision-making process in the 4 body systems for individuals with and without health conditions.

Whereas the patterns are grouped by 4 body systems, the physical therapist will need to address the "whole" patient/client to determine the system in which the primary impairment(s) that drive the intervention are located. The physical therapist should not assume that the patient/client automatically will be classified in the system of the associated pathology or condition. For example, in an individual with a pathology diagnosis of cardiovascular accident, the system of origin of the pathology is the cardiovascular system. The system of primary impact of the pathology is the neuromuscular system. The system of secondary or tertiary impact may be the musculoskeletal, cardiovascular/pulmonary, or integumentary system.

Likewise, the physical therapist should not assume that the patient/client will be automatically classified in the system of the most frequently seen impairments associated with the identified pathology or condition. Using the above example, the system of the primary impairment(s) that drives the intervention for this individual may be cardiovascular/pulmonary (aerobic capacity), neuromuscular (motor control), musculoskeletal (muscle performance), or integumentary (primary prevention/risk reduction for integumentary). Only through examination, evaluation, and diagnosis is the physical therapist able to identify the primary impairment(s) for a specific patient/client that will drive the interventions for this episode of care. Once the physical therapist has identified the primary impairments that are affecting the patient's/client's functional abilities, the physical therapist then can classify the patient/client in the appropriate pattern.

Pattern Title

The title of the pattern is the diagnostic classification or the diagnosis by the physical therapist for patients/clients grouped in this pattern. The titles are based on the impairment or group of impairments that drive the intervention for that patient/client grouping. Patterns may or may not have a condition or pathology associated with them. When there is only an impairment(s) listed in the title, the patient/client can be included with or without an associated condition or pathology. The physical therapist must decide whether the condition or pathology significantly alters the patient/client management from that described in the pattern and whether to make the decision to include the patient/client. Using the *Guide 3.0,* physical therapists need to classify/diagnose the patient/client by the impairment(s) that is(are) driving the intervention, not the associated condition or pathology. This concept is important to remember when classifying pediatric patients/

clients as many of them have pathologies/conditions that are lifelong, but the pathology/condition, in and of itself, is not the reason for the need for physical therapy.

The title also may specify an age range. If an age is not specified, the pattern applies to all ages. In the Adapted Practice Patterns there are 2 patterns that apply only to pediatric patients/clients: Pattern 5C: Impaired Motor Function and Sensory Processing Associated With Nonprogressive Disorders of the Central Nervous System—Congenital Origin or Acquired in Infancy or Childhood and Pattern 6G: Impaired Ventilation, Respiration/Gas Exchange, and Aerobic Capacity/Endurance Associated With Respiratory Failure in the Neonate. There is one pattern that begins in adolescence: Pattern 5D: Impaired Motor Function and Sensory Processing Associated With Nonprogressive Disorders of the Central Nervous System—Acquired in Adolescence or Adulthood. The remaining 31 patterns of the Adapted Practice Patterns are not age specific but are available for consideration when classifying pediatric patients/clients.

Inclusion

This section provides examples of examination findings that may support the inclusion in this pattern. The inclusion findings are organized in 2 categories and are specific to this pattern:

> Risk Factors or Consequences of Pathology/Pathophysiology (Disease, Disorder, or Condition)
> Impairments of Body Functions and Structures, Activity Limitations, or Participation Restrictions

Exclusion or Multiple-Pattern Classification

This section provides examples of examination findings that may support exclusion for this pattern or classification into additional patterns. The exclusion findings are organized in 2 different categories and are specific to this pattern:

> Findings That May Require Classification in a Different Pattern
> Findings That May Require Classification in Additional Patterns

Examination

Examination is required for all patients/clients and is performed prior to the initial intervention. The examination includes 3 components: patient/client history, systems review, and tests and measures. The Adapted Practice Pattern addresses only tests and measures for that specific pattern; however, the cases in this chapter include examples of all 3 components of examination where appropriate. Chapter 4—Physical Therapist Examination and Evaluation: Focus on Tests and Measures of the *Guide*[32] provides an overview of the 3 components of examination. History involves collection of data/information (past and present) related to why the individual is coming to physical therapy. Table 6-3 lists the categories and data collected as part of the history.

Data are collected from the patient/client and/or caregivers when appropriate. This is the first piece of information that informs the physical therapist about the general status and abilities; possible limitations or restrictions; as well as possible health, wellness, and fitness needs of the patient/client. A brief review of systems is included in the history to identify any possible concerns that may necessitate referral for additional medical evaluation.[33] The systems review is a brief examination of the 4 body systems (cardiovascular/pulmonary, integumentary, musculoskeletal, neuromuscular) and communication ability, affect, cognition, language, and learning style. Table 6-4 lists the specific areas included in the systems review.

Tests and measures are selected based on the information obtained in the history and systems review and assist the physical therapist to begin to hypothesize the patient's/client's reason for seeking intervention. Table 6-5 lists the test and measure categories.

TABLE 6-3. HISTORY USED IN THE *GUIDE 3.0* (EXCLUDING SYSTEMS HISTORY AND REVIEW)

ACTIVITIES AND PARTICIPATION
- Current and prior role functions (eg, self-care and domestic; education; work; community, social and civic life)

CURRENT CONDITIONS
- Concerns that led the patient/client to seek the services of a physical therapist
- Concerns or needs of the patient/client that require the services of a physical therapist
- Current therapeutic interventions
- Mechanisms of injury or disease, including date of onset and course of events
- Onset and pattern of symptoms
- Patient/client, family, significant other, and caregiver expectations and goals for the therapeutic intervention
- Patient/client, family, significant other, and caregiver perceptions of patient's/client's emotional response to the current clinical condition
- Previous occurrence of current condition(s)
- Prior therapeutic interventions

FAMILY HISTORY
- Familial risk factors

GENERAL DEMOGRAPHICS
- Age and sex
- Education
- Primary language
- Primary ethnicity

GENERAL HEALTH STATUS (SELF-REPORT, FAMILY REPORT, CAREGIVER REPORT)
- General health perception
- Mental functions (eg, memory, reasoning agility, depression, anxiety)
- Physical functions (eg, mobility, sleep patterns, restricted bed days)

GROWTH AND DEVELOPMENT
- Developmental history (including hand dominance)

LIVING ENVIRONMENT
- Assistive technology (eg, aids for locomotion, orthotic devices, prosthetic requirements, seating and positioning technology)
- Living environment and community characteristics
- Projected destination at conclusion of care

continued

TABLE 6-3. HISTORY USED IN THE *GUIDE 3.0* (EXCLUDING SYSTEMS HISTORY AND REVIEW) (CONTINUED)

MEDICATIONS
- Medications for current condition, previously taken for current condition, or for other conditions

OTHER CLINICAL TESTS
- Laboratory and diagnostic tests; review of other clinical findings (eg, nutrition and hydration)
- Review of available records (eg, medical, education, surgical)

SOCIAL/HEALTH HABITS (PAST AND CURRENT)
- Behavioral health risks (eg, tobacco use, drug abuse)
- Level of physical fitness

SOCIAL HISTORY
- Cultural beliefs and behaviors
- Family and caregiver resources
- Social interactions, social activities, and support systems

Adapted from the American Physical Therapy Association. *Guide to Physical Therapist Practice 3.0.* Alexandria, VA: American Physical Therapy Association; 2014. http://guidetoptpractice.apta.org/.

Chapter 4 of the *Guide 3.0* provides a listing of the 26 tests and measures categories, and each category is linked to a page that includes[32]:
➤ A general definition and purpose
➤ Examples of clinical indications
➤ Examples of what tests and measures may characterize or quantify
➤ Examples of data-gathering tools
➤ Examples of data used in documentation

The clinical indications provided in each test and measures category are examples of specific findings of the history and system review, which may indicate the need for use of that category. Clinical indications are provided in the following disablement-enablement areas: risk factors; health, wellness, and fitness; pathology or health condition; impairments of body functions and structures; activity limitations; and participation restrictions.

The examples of what tests and measures may characterize or quantify include bullets that provide links to PTNow for summaries of specific tests and measures and, when available, links to specific tools.[24,31] When the tests and measures categories are accessed, a complete list of all the summaries of specific tests and measures for the bulleted area is provided. When the tests and measures from the examination area in the Adapted Practice Pattern are accessed, one will see only the summaries of the specific tests and measures appropriate for that pattern. The summaries of specific tests and measures are updated on a regular basis.

It should be noted that with pediatric patients/clients or any patient/client who cannot appropriately respond independently, the *Guide 3.0* assumes the parent/guardian or caregiver would be the responsible party to respond on behalf of the patient/client. The parent's/guardian's or caregiver's abilities to manage the child also may be appropriate to assess. If in the process of examining the caregiver's abilities the physical therapist determines that the caregiver has issues that may require his or her own episode of care, a separate examination of the caregiver should be recommended.

TABLE 6-4. HISTORY USED IN THE *GUIDE 3.0* (SYSTEMS HISTORY AND REVIEW)

MEDICAL/SURGICAL HISTORY

- Cardiovascular
- Endocrine/metabolic
- Gastrointestinal
- Genitourinary
- Gynecological
- Integumentary
- Musculoskeletal
- Neuromuscular
- Obstetrical
- Psychological
- Pulmonary
- Prior hospitalizations, surgeries, and preexisting medical and other health-related conditions

REVIEW OF SYSTEMS

- Cardiovascular/pulmonary
- Endocrine
- Eyes, ears, nose, and throat
- Gastrointestinal
- Genitourinary/reproductive
- Hematologic/lymphatic
- Integumentary
- Neurologic/musculoskeletal

Adapted from the American Physical Therapy Association. *Guide to Physical Therapist Practice 3.0*. Alexandria, VA: American Physical Therapy Association; 2014. http://guidetoptpractice.apta.org/.

Evaluation, Diagnosis, and Prognosis (Including Plan of Care)

These components of the patient/client management model are grouped together in each pattern. Readers are directed to Chapter 2—Principles of Physical Therapist Patient and Client Management[33] for more information. During the evaluation, examination data are analyzed, taking into consideration the patient's/client's expectations and potential for remediation or accommodation. Begin by looking for a clustering of impairments to body functions and structures that appear to be affecting the activity; participation; and health, wellness, fitness, and prevention needs of the patient/client. Most pediatric patients/clients will have conditions/pathologies that are lifelong. As a result, they always will have impairments in these areas. The key to evaluation is to determine which impairments to body functions and structures are the ones that are affecting the patient/client for this episode of care.

TABLE 6-5. TESTS AND MEASURES CATEGORIES

- Aerobic capacity/endurance
- Anthropometric characteristics
- Assistive technology
- Balance
- Circulation (arterial, venous, lymphatic)
- Community, social, and civic life
- Cranial and peripheral nerve integrity
- Education life
- Environmental factors
- Gait
- Integumentary integrity
- Joint integrity and mobility
- Mental functions
- Mobility (including locomotion)
- Motor function
- Muscle performance (including strength, power, endurance, and length)
- Neuromotor development and sensory processing
- Pain
- Posture
- Range of motion
- Reflex integrity
- Self-care and domestic life
- Sensory integrity
- Skeletal integrity
- Ventilation and respiration
- Work life

The diagnosis is determined at this point in the patient/client management process. The pattern title is the diagnostic classification for the pattern. The specific diagnosis should be determined and the primary impairments of body functions and structures that will drive the interventions identified. Remember, the diagnosis is not the pathology; it is the impairment(s) to body functions and structures you have identified that is(are) affecting the patient's/client's activities and participation abilities. You then determine whether your patient/client can be managed in this pattern with or without modifications, if another pattern is needed in addition to this pattern, or if a different pattern is more appropriate.

A prognosis statement identifies the optimal level of improvement in impairments of body functions and structures, activity abilities, and/or participation abilities, as well as the amount of time needed to attain them.[33] The Adapted Practice Patterns no longer have prognosis statements; however, for patterns that include individuals with lifelong conditions, the prognosis statement should provide for improvement within the context of the impairments, activity limitations, and participation restrictions[1] as there always will be some level of impairment in these areas.

> ## TABLE 6-6. INTERVENTION CATEGORIES
>
> - Airway clearance techniques
> - Assistive technology: prescription, application, and, as appropriate, fabrication or modification
> - Biophysical agents
> - Functional training in self-care and in domestic, education, work, community, social, and civic life
> - Integumentary repair and protection techniques
> - Manual therapy techniques
> - Motor function training
> - Patient/client instruction
> - Therapeutic exercise

Factors That May Require New Episode of Care or That May Modify Frequency of Visits/ Duration of Care[9] are included in each Adapted Practice Pattern. A listing of individual and environmental factors that may increase or decrease the frequency or expected range of visits is provided for consideration when determining the prognosis and plan of care.

The plan of care describes the goals and outcomes as well as types of interventions and frequency and duration of visits to attain the goals and outcomes and discharge plans.[33] The plan of care is developed with the patient/client and appropriate family members, caregivers, or other identified individuals. Coordination of care, communication and collaboration with other providers, documentation of patient/client status and response to intervention, and documentation of initial and changing functional status are performed throughout the patient/client management process.[33]

Intervention

Intervention can be provided throughout the patient/client management process. Chapter 5— Interventions describes the 9 intervention categories in detail. Each intervention category includes general definition and purpose, types of interventions, and goals and outcomes (Table 6-6).[34]

Each intervention category has a separate page that identifies the above information specific to that intervention. The goals and outcomes of each intervention are further delineated to address the disablement-enablement model through the impact on[34]:

- Pathology or condition
- Impairments in body functions and structures
- Activity limitations
- Participation restrictions
- Risk reduction and prevention
- Health, wellness, and fitness
- Societal resources
- Patient/client satisfaction

The Adapted Practice Patterns provide a listing of the intervention categories that are appropriate for that specific pattern. Examples provided on a specific intervention's page in Chapter 5—Interventions can be used to assist the therapist in determining whether the patient/client can be managed in this pattern and in selecting goals and outcomes. The specific interventions will vary based on the patient's/client's goals, health status, intellectual status, caregiver consistency and expertise, environment, and ability to follow through on a home program.

Reexamination

Reexamination can be performed at any time after the initial examination in the episode of care and may show the following results:

> Modification of the goals and outcomes, frequency, or duration of care
> Reclassification of the patient/client to a different pattern, addition of another pattern, or concluding the episode care
> Referral to another provider

Outcomes for Patients/Clients

Outcomes for patients/clients in this pattern are measured during the episode of care and measure the impact of physical therapy service on the plan of care. Outcome measurements are tests and measures used to determine change over time and may address a number of factors[33]:

> Pathology/pathophysiology
> Impairment
> Functional limitation
> Disability
> Risk reduction/prevention
> Health, wellness, and fitness
> Societal resources
> Patient/client satisfaction

These are the same domains for the goals and outcomes identified in the interventions. Goals and outcomes need to be meaningful to the individual, measurable, and time specific. Measurement of outcomes occurs at all levels of the disablement-enablement model; however, the *Guide 3.0* states: "Outcome measurements at the level of activity and participation demonstrate the value of physical therapy in helping individuals achieve their identified goals and, therefore, are most meaningful."[35] Keeping this in mind helps us focus on what is important to the patient/client rather than the health condition and impairments of body functions and structures.

Concluding an Episode of Care

Concluding an episode of care is based on how the patient/client is functioning in the plan of care. The episode of care may be concluded when the individual has met the goals of the plan of care, is not able to make progress toward the goals of the plan of care, decides to end the episode of care, or the physical therapist determines the individual no longer benefits from continued physical therapy.[34]

CASE STUDY #1: JASON

> *Practice Pattern 5C:* Impaired Motor Function and Sensory Processing Associated With Nonprogressive Disorders of the Central Nervous System—Congenital Origin or Acquired in Infancy or Childhood

> *Medical Diagnosis:* Cerebral palsy, right hemiparesis

> *Age:* 24 months

> *How does the patient/client management model help you determine what is going on with Jason and what you need to do? During the examination how did you know which specific tests and measures to use? How did you know to place Jason in Practice Pattern 5C? This case is an example of how to use all of the elements in the patient/client management in the* Guide 3.0.

Examination

History

The first information you received about Jason is from his history. You received his previous medical information, physical therapy chart/notes, and information provided to you by his parents. You interview Jason's mother and father to complete the information from the history section of the examination. Based on the information in his history, you began to form a picture of what his parents' concerns are and what impairments may be affecting Jason's functioning as well as his ability to do what he wants to do. You now have an overview of his medical status and how that may affect your examination today as well as how it may affect Jason's prognosis and plan of care.

> *Activities and Participation:* Jason is a son, brother, and grandchild. He enjoys age-appropriate play activities, but becomes frustrated that he cannot keep up with or make himself understood to his brother or peers. His parents report Jason is just beginning to assist with dressing and undressing activities. He also is beginning to show some interest in toilet training. He is a "messy" eater. He is very active but has difficulty keeping up with his brother. The family is very active in the community and enjoys outdoor activities. Jason participates in an early intervention program through his local school district.

> *Current Conditions:* His parents are concerned about general developmental delay and lack of use of his right side for play and self-care. Currently he is receiving home-based services consisting of weekly visits from the local school district alternating between teacher and occupational therapist. Parents would like to see him walk without falling, keep up with his brother, and be able to communicate with others.

> *Family History:* Noncontributory.

> *General Demographics:* Jason is a 24-month-old boy who is English speaking.

> *General Health Status (Self-Report, Family Report, Caregiver Report):*
>   ○ General health perception: Jason has been healthy other than the usual childhood illnesses, such as colds and flu.
>   ○ Mental functions: Jason's mom reports a happy, healthy child with delayed expressive language, who relies on gestures for communication and appears to learn by watching his brother.
>   ○ Physical functions: Jason began walking at 15 months and sleeps through the night.

> *Growth and Development:* At age 6 months there were definite asymmetries in stretch reflexes and voluntary use of his extremities.

> *Living Environment:* He lives in a split-level home. There is a small play area in the backyard and a community park 2 blocks away.

> *Medical/Surgical History:* Jason was the first born of nonidentical twins with a birth weight of 1660 grams. His Apgar was 7 at 1 minute and 9 at 5 minutes. He did not require mechanical ventilation and was discharged from the neonatal intensive care unit (NICU) after 40 days on caffeine-citrate for bradycardia with feedings. Initial follow-up at 2 months of chronological age was nonremarkable. At his follow-up at 6 months of chronological age definite asymmetries in stretch reflexes and voluntary use of his extremities were noted. Jason was referred for early intervention services. No medications or surgical procedures.

> *Other Clinical Tests:* Jason is on an Individualized Family Service Plan (IFSP). *You will need to review the IFSP to address potential overlap in goals and objectives (see Chapter 15).*

> *Review of Systems:* Jason is not demonstrating any need for further medical evaluation.

> *Social/Health Habits (Past and Current):*
>   ◦ Behavioral health risks: No members of immediate family smoke.
>   ◦ Level of physical fitness: Jason tires easily.
>   ◦ Physical function: Jason has limitations in mobility.

> *Social History:* Jason lives with his mother and father, who are the primary caregivers. He has a brother who is a nonidentical twin.

Systems Review

The systems review is a limited examination of the cardiovascular/pulmonary, integumentary, musculoskeletal, and neuromuscular systems. You next complete a review of Jason's systems by observing and taking measurements.

> *Cardiovascular/Pulmonary*
>   ◦ Blood pressure: 75/130
>   ◦ Edema: None observed
>   ◦ Heart rate: 100 bpm
>   ◦ Respiratory rate: 25 bpm

> *Integumentary*
>   ◦ Presence of scar formation: None
>   ◦ Skin color: Good
>   ◦ Skin integrity: Good

> *Musculoskeletal*
>   ◦ Gross range of motion: Within normal limits (WNL) on left, some limitation on right
>   ◦ Gross strength: Decreased on the right
>   ◦ Gross symmetry: Asymmetrical posture and positioning of right side

> *Neuromuscular*
>   ◦ Gross coordinated movements, irregular movements, difficulties with awareness, timing, and sequencing

> *Communication, Affect, Cognition, and Learning Style*
>   ◦ Delayed expressive language, relies on watching others and gestures
>   ◦ Mom reports she would prefer home program on video in addition to being written

Tests and Measures

Based on the findings of the history and systems review, you determine which specific tests and measures you will use. The history and systems review will identity clinical indicators for risk factors; health, wellness, and prevention needs; pathology or health conditions; impairments in body functions and structures; activity limitations; and participation restrictions that will assist you in ruling in or ruling out specific tests and measures. You can use the *Guide 3.0* to assist in identifying tests and measures categories, as well as specific tests and measures within a specific category. Using the Adapted Practice Patterns that are available online under the education tab,[10] you will be able to find and review specific tools as well as link to specific articles to help you determine which tools you will use for Jason. Based on Jason's findings, you select tests and measures from the following categories:

> *Anthropometric Characteristics:* Jason is noted to have a slightly smaller right upper extremity (noticeable only in the upper arm as compared with the right). He is of average height and weight for his age.

> *Assistive Technology* (observation of during testing): Determined orthotic device not beneficial at this time.

> *Education Life* (interview and review of records): Jason participates in an early intervention program receiving home-based services weekly with a teacher and occupational therapist alternating weeks. He receives private services from a speech-language pathologist and a physical therapist.

> *Environmental Factors* (observation, interview): Home has 6 steps between levels, ceramic tile floor in kitchen, and an upper level open to main level with a metal railing. Wood chips under swing set and wood timbers around sandbox. Community park has asphalt walking paths with irregular surfaces in grass. Mom reports Jason needs to be closely supervised because he falls frequently.

> *Integumentary Integrity* (observation, interview): Normal.

> *Mental Functions* (developmental inventory): Testing indicates that Jason's intellectual skills fall within the average range. He has delayed expressive language, using gestures to make needs known. During testing it was noted that tactile stimulation generally increased activity level.

> *Mobility (Including Locomotion)* (activities of daily living [ADL] scale, observation): Results of the Pediatric Evaluation of Disability Inventory—Computer Adaptive Test (PEDI–CAT) indicate that Jason has difficulty with transfers in and out of a bathtub, indoor locomotion in the areas of changing direction and carrying objects, outdoor locomotion on rough and uneven surfaces, and ascending and descending stairs in an upright position.

> *Motor Function* (ADL scales, observation): On the PEDI–CAT, Jason was able to initiate movement, but had difficulty modulating and stopping movement, especially with his right side. Difficulty with timing and sequencing of movement was noted when using his right arm and hand for self-care activities. He understands 2-step commands, but has difficulty completing the motor component of some tasks.

> *Muscle Performance (Including Strength, Power, Endurance, and Length)* (functional muscle test): Weakness is evident in the right upper extremity, particularly in the triceps and supinators of the forearm. Weakness also noted in right lower extremity, particularly in hip flexors, hip extensors, hamstrings, and plantar flexors.

> *Neuromotor Development and Sensory Processing* (Developmental Inventory): Gross motor skills range between 12 and 15 months. Just beginning to attempt running.

> *Pain* (interview): None reported.

> *Posture* (observation): Demonstrates asymmetrical posture in standing with excessive anterior tilt of the pelvis and excessive retraction of right shoulder. Tends to posture right arm in flexion at elbow, wrist, and fingers with forearm in pronation.

> *Range of Motion* (functional tests, observation): WNL for passive movement but demonstrates limitations in active movements on the right for reaching, grasping, extending hip, and rotating and flexing trunk. Limitations with active movement interfere with activities requiring 2 hands or use of right hand.

> *Reflex Integrity* (reflex tests): Hyperactive stretch reflexes are present to tendon tap at the ankle (plantar flexors), knee (quadriceps), and elbow (biceps) on the right. Normal stretch reflexes are evident on the left side of the body.

> *Self-Care and Domestic Life* (ADL scales, observation, interview): Results of the PEDI–CAT indicate difficulty with use of utensils, washing hands together, dressing, and toileting. Jason drools occasionally, especially when concentrating on an activity. He is a "messy" eater, often losing food out of his mouth. He does not seem to notice when food escapes his mouth.

> *Sensory Integrity* (observation): During administration of the PEDI–CAT, limited use and apparent lack of awareness of right arm for self-care activities were noted. Tactile defensive behaviors occasionally observed.

> *Ventilation and Respiration* (observation): Breathiness is noted during speech and consonants are limited in quantity and quality. He often gasps for breath after drinking.

> *Work Life* (ADL scales, observation, interview): Jason enjoys age-appropriate play activities and demonstrates typical behaviors for a 24-month-old child when his brother or other children are present. Results of the PEDI–CAT indicate difficulty with expressive communication, ability to report self-information (name), and safety within community. Parent reports difficulty with mobility in community park and backyard play areas.

Evaluation (Clinical Judgment)

You now organize the data from the examination to determine which impairments are affecting Jason's functional abilities. You determine whether the family's expectations for therapy are realistic, establish a diagnosis and a prognosis, and develop a plan of care.

Jason has impairments of motor function, weakness, and poor sensory appreciation on the right side. His gross motor skills are delayed, as is his expressive language. He relies on gestures for communication. He is a "messy" eater. Jason is starting to assist in dressing and has some interest in toilet training. He is walking; however, he has difficulty changing directions and stopping movement. He frequently falls. He has difficulty keeping up with his brother for play.

Diagnosis

Based on the evaluation, you determine that deficits in motor function and sensory processing are the primary impairments affecting Jason's functional abilities. The impairment of muscle performance as well as difficulty in communications appear to be secondary impairments.

The data collected helped determine the primary impairments of body functions and structures that will drive the interventions. Jason was placed in the practice pattern of 5C: Impaired Motor Function and Sensory Processing Associated With Nonprogressive Disorders of the Central Nervous System—Congenital Origin or Acquired in Infancy or Childhood.

Prognosis (Including Plan of Care)

Using Adapted Practice Pattern 5C, you review the Factors That May Modify Frequency of Visits/Duration of Care. You develop a prognosis for Jason that addresses his and his family's expectations with an agreed-on frequency and duration of services. As part of the plan of care, you determine the anticipated goals and expected outcomes with Jason's family.

Jason's plan of care statement: "Over the course of 12 months, Jason will demonstrate optimal motor function and sensory processing, and the highest level of function in the home and community within the context of his impairments, functional limitations, and disability. Jason will receive private physical therapy for 3 months, once weekly with family education for his home program. After that, physical therapy will decrease to 1 time every 2 weeks."

The family agreed to the program and the informed consent was signed. Jason will conclude this episode of care when the goals and outcomes have been met.

Interventions (for Clinical Consideration)

Using the goals and outcomes you developed as part of the plan of care, you review the interventions to determine which interventions will be appropriate. Two examples are (1) coordination, communication, and documentation, which are performed throughout the episode of care, and (2) patient-/client-related instruction, which is a required intervention for all patients/clients. You will need to select additional interventions to complete Jason's plan of care.

Coordination, Communication, and Documentation

> *Interventions:* Coordination and communication with school providers
> *Goals and Outcomes:* Family members will demonstrate enhanced decision-making skills regarding Jason's health and use of community resources.

Patient-/Client-Related Instruction

> *Interventions:* Jason and his family will receive instruction and education in a home program and updates. They will receive information on when it is appropriate to seek additional services.
> *Goals and Outcomes:* Jason's parents will have an increased understanding of goals and outcomes and demonstrate his home program independently.

Additional Interventions

You will need to select additional interventions from the intervention categories described in Chapter 5 of the *Guide 3.0* to complete Jason's plan of care. The Adapted Practice Patterns include a listing of examples for the pattern. You will need to use this information as well as information on all the interventions to determine the most appropriate interventions for Jason.

Reexamination

Reexamination is performed throughout the episode of care to assess the goals and outcomes. You will select the test and measure that best meets the goal and outcome. Remember to use the links in the selected test and measure to find tools for the specific area of the goal and outcome.

Outcomes for Patients/Clients

Outcomes for physical therapy services are measured by the impact of the interventions in the following areas:
> Pathology/pathophysiology (disease, disorder, or condition)
> Impairments in body functions and structures
> Activity limitations
> Participation restrictions
> Risk reduction and prevention
> Health, wellness, and fitness
> Societal resources
> Patient/client satisfaction

Concluding an Episode of Care

Concluding an episode of care is based on how the patient/client is functioning in the plan of care. The episode of care may be concluded when the patient/client has met the goals of the plan of care, is not able to make progress toward the goals of the plan of care, decides to end the episode of care, or the physical therapist determines the individual no longer benefits from continued physical therapy.[34]

CASE STUDY #2: JILL

> *Practice Pattern 5C:* Impaired Motor Function and Sensory Processing Associated With Nonprogressive Disorders of the Central Nervous System—Congenital Origin or Acquired in Infancy or Childhood

> *Medical Diagnosis:* Cerebral palsy, spastic quadriparesis, microcephaly, intellectual deficits, seizure disorder

> *Age:* 7 years

> This case is an example of how to use the Guide 3.0 *to transition from an episode of care to an episode of prevention.*

Examination

History

> *Activities and Participation:* Jill is not ambulatory and is unable to maintain her balance in any position. She is totally dependent on caregivers for self-care with the exception of assisting with arms through sleeves for dressing and weight-bearing for standing pivot transfers. She participates in a community sponsored adaptive aquatic class and therapeutic horseback riding (hippotherapy). Jill is in school in a special education classroom, mainstreamed with other children part of the day, and has a classroom aide available for assistance. She receives occupational, speech, and physical therapy. Her roles are daughter, granddaughter, and classmate.

> *Current Conditions:* Jill's parents are concerned about her ability to access their home. They would like to know about appropriate modifications, adaptations, or equipment to assist in managing Jill as she grows.

> *Family History:* Noncontributory.

> *General Demographics:* Jill is a 7-year-old white girl. English is the primary language spoken at home.

> *General Health:* Report gathered from patient, family or caregiver.
>   ○ General health perception: She is generally healthy, occasionally has seizures.
>   ○ Mental functions: Jill has very low intellectual abilities and low level of alertness.
>   ○ Physical functions: She is dependent on others for mobility, positioning, ADLs, and instrumental ADLs (IADLs).

> *Growth and Development:* Jill was born full term following a normal pregnancy. Her Apgar scores were 5 at 1 minute and 8 at 5 minutes. Jill had seizures during the neonatal period and had an abnormal electroencephalogram. She was on mechanical ventilation for several days and initially had feeding difficulties. She was discharged from the NICU on antiseizure medication. At the time of discharge, she was drinking well from a bottle. At the 4-month follow-up visit with her pediatrician, decreased head growth was noted. She had a normal eye exam and brainstem auditory evoked response. Jill has continued to have occasional seizures despite being on antiseizure medication.

> *Living Environment:* Jill has a manual wheelchair with a custom seating system. She lives in a ranch-style home; there are 3 steps to enter the home. Family is considering a ramp.

> *Medical/Surgical History:* Jill had orthopedic surgery (heel cord and adductor releases) at age 5 years.

> *Medications:* Antiseizure medications.

> *Review of Systems*
>   ◦ Integumentary: Jill has a mild irritation over ischial tuberosities and is at risk for skin breakdown because of limited movement and use of a seating device; no referral is needed at this time; further examination needed with ongoing monitoring and education of caregivers.

> *Social/Health Habits (Past and Current)*
>   ◦ Behavioral health risks: Noncontributory.
>   ◦ Level of physical fitness: Limited movement contributes to decreased cardiopulmonary and muscular fitness as well as increased risk for skin breakdown.

> *Social History*
>   ◦ Family/caregivers: Mother, father, aide at school.
>   ◦ Social activities: Aquatics class, horseback riding; enjoys watching videos and television.

Systems Review

> *Cardiovascular/Pulmonary*
>   ◦ Blood pressure: 78/128
>   ◦ Edema: None noted
>   ◦ Heart rate: 102 bpm
>   ◦ Respiratory rate: 25 bpm

> *Integumentary*
>   ◦ Presence of scar formation: Old scar on left arm, not necessary to assess
>   ◦ Skin color: Good
>   ◦ Skin integrity: Mild irritation on ischial tuberosities

> *Musculoskeletal*
>   ◦ Gross range of motion: Limited reach
>   ◦ Gross strength: Generalized weakness
>   ◦ Gross symmetry: Asymmetrical
>   ◦ Height: Fifth percentile
>   ◦ Weight: Fifth percentile

> *Neuromuscular*
>   ◦ Gross motor skills at 3-month level

> *Communication, Affect, Cognition, Language, and Learning Style*
>   ◦ Jill is able to make her needs known through variations in vocalized patterns to familiar listeners

Tests and Measures

Based on the information presented in the Chapter 5 case studies (in this text), you identify the risk factors; health, wellness, and fitness needs; pathology or health conditions; impairments in body functions and structures; activity limitations; and participation restrictions. Chapter 4—Physical Therapist Examination and Evaluation: Focus on Tests and Measures of the *Guide 3.0* provides examples of each factor for each test category. This information will help you in selecting the appropriate tests and measures as well as identifying impairments, activity limitations, and participation restrictions. Risk factors and health, wellness, and fitness needs also will be determined.

Selected Test Categories and Clinical Indications for Use

> *Mental Functions* (developmental inventory)
  - Risk factors: Slow rate of learning, difficulty attending, seizures, inability to understand and interpret environment, inability to communicate, vulnerability
  - Health, wellness, and fitness: Lack of awareness of need for fitness, inactivity, lack of education of caregivers on importance of health, wellness, and fitness
  - Pathology or health conditions: Neuromuscular (CP, seizures)
  - Impairments of body functions and structures: Arousal, cognition, distractibility, communication, motor function
  - Activity limitations and participation restrictions: Self-care, work, community/leisure (dependent in all areas, unable to participate without assistance, vulnerable)

> *Assistive Technology* (observation, reports)
  - Risk factors: Inactivity, contractures, skin breakdown, osteopenia, digestive function, bowel and bladder function, loss of standing ability
  - Health, wellness, and fitness: Inactivity, use of devices to address health, wellness, and fitness needs
  - Pathology or health conditions: Neuromuscular (cerebral palsy [CP], seizures) musculoskeletal (secondary to neuromuscular pathology)
  - Impairments of body functions and structures: Motor function (positioning), posture, range of motion, joint integrity and mobility, integumentary, gait, locomotion and balance, muscle performance, sensory integrity, ventilation and respiration
  - Activity limitations and participation restrictions: Self-care, work, community/leisure (dependent on devices to provide positioning; need for standing and assistive standing pivot transfers; ankle-foot orthotics needed to allow standing to complete role; dependent on devices to provide positioning for participation in activities)

> *Environmental Factors*
  - Risk factors: Decreased accessibility to home, work, community/leisure, evacuation plan
  - Health, wellness, and fitness: Caregiver's health, wellness, and fitness
  - Pathology or health conditions: Neuromuscular (CP, seizures)
  - Impairments of body functions and structures: Locomotion (wheelchair, assisted standing pivot transfers), caregiver's ergonomics and body mechanics (mother reports back injury from lifting)
  - Activity limitations and participation restrictions: Self-care, play, community/leisure (needs to use wheelchair for mobility, devices for positioning, dependent on caregivers, unable to control her environment)

> *Self-Care and Domestic Life* (ergonomics and body mechanics—examination of caregiver)
  - Risk factors: Repetitive stress, back injury of caregiver
  - Health, wellness, and fitness: Decreased understanding of importance of body mechanics and strength when lifting
  - Pathology or health conditions: None known
  - Impairments of body functions and structures: Muscle performance, body mechanics
  - Activity limitations and participation restrictions: Self-care (lifting, bathing, dressing, toileting); play and community (accessing environments, inability to care for daughter)

- *Integumentary Integrity* (observation, risk assessment scale)
  - Risk factors: Skin breakdown, inactivity
  - Health, wellness, and fitness: Caregivers need understanding of importance of positioning and devices to maintain skin integrity
  - Pathology or health conditions: Neuromuscular (CP, seizures)
  - Impairments of body functions and structures: Locomotion (inactivity), integumentary (redness on tuberosities), questionable circulation
  - Activity limitations and participation restrictions: Self-care, play, community/leisure (inactivity and inability to communicate discomfort, tolerance for sitting)
- *Motor Function* (observation, ADL scales)
  - Risk factors: Inactivity, safety, vulnerability
  - Health, wellness, and fitness: Inactivity, understanding of the importance of devices to provide stability for movement
  - Pathology or health conditions: Neuromuscular (CP, seizures)
  - Impairments of body functions and structures: Motor function (limited voluntary movement, poor head, ocular motor, and oral-motor control); locomotion (inactivity); range of motion; muscle performance; balance; posture
  - Activity limitations and participation restrictions: Self-care, work, community/leisure (dependent on others for participation in actions, tasks, and activities to fulfill required roles)
- *Range of Motion* (observation, goniometry, contracture test)
  - Risk factors: Contractures, skin breakdown, postural deviations, respiratory function
  - Health, wellness, and fitness: Importance of maintaining joint motion and muscle length for adequate positioning as Jill ages
  - Pathology or health conditions: Neuromuscular (CP), musculoskeletal (secondary to CP)
  - Impairments of body functions and structures: Range of motion, joint integrity and mobility, integumentary, posture, muscle performance, motor control
  - Activity limitations and participation restrictions: Self-care, work, community/leisure (dependent on others for movement and to participate in actions, tasks, and activities to fulfill required roles)

Evaluation

Using the information from the examination, what clustering of impairments, functional limitations, disability, risk factors, health, wellness, and fitness were identified?

In Jill's case the following clusters were identified:

- Risk factors: Inactivity, contractures, limited access to environment, skin breakdown
- Health, wellness, and fitness: Health and wellness of caregivers to assist Jill and prevent injury to caregivers; need for caregivers' understanding the importance of positioning and devices to maintain range of motion, skin integrity, joint integrity and mobility, muscle length, and stable positions to allow interaction with environment
- Pathology or health conditions: CP, severe intellectual impairment, seizures
- Impairments of body functions and structures: Motor function, range of motion, locomotion, cognition, caregiver body mechanics
- Activity limitations and participation restrictions: Mobility, accessing environments, and dependency on others in the areas of self-care, work, and community/leisure; dependence on others to meet roles of daughter, student, friend, child; barriers in home; evacuation plan

Diagnosis

Based on your evaluation, the impairment that will drive intervention for Jill is motor function. The most appropriate practice pattern is 5C: Impaired Motor Function and Sensory Processing Associated With Nonprogressive Disorders of the Central Nervous System—Congenital Origin or Acquired in Infancy or Childhood.

Prognosis (Including Plan of Care)

You also use the evaluation to determine the prognosis for Jill. An appropriate prognosis may be: "Jill will demonstrate optimal motor function and sensory integrity and the highest level of functioning in home, school, play, and community and leisure environments, within the context of her impairments, functional limitations, and disabilities."[3]

For Jill, the phrase "within the context of her impairments, functional limitations, and disabilities" has significance because she has a medical condition that you know is lifelong with impairments that will directly affect her ability to learn and move. Based on her age (7 years), cognitive level (severe intellectual impairment), rate of change (motor skills still at 3-month level), motor control (limited voluntary movement, poor head, ocular motor, and oral-motor control), and functional skills (dependence), you determine that her needs are for appropriate devices to provide positioning for her to access and interact with her environment. You also determine that her home environment requires modifications and adaptations, and that her caregivers should be trained to safely manage and assist Jill throughout her day.

Based on this prognosis you determine that Jill will benefit from an episode of care with the expected frequency to be 2 times per month the first month, then 1 time per month for the following 2 months. The goals and outcomes for this episode of care are to assess the home environment for modifications, equipment, and evacuation plan and to educate the caregivers in appropriate body mechanics, lifting, transfers, and use of devices. A home program will be developed to address Jill's risk factors and health, wellness, and fitness needs. Caregivers will demonstrate understanding and strategies used to implement her program.

Following achievement of the goals and outcomes, it is anticipated that Jill will be discharged from her episode of care and placed in an episode of prevention. During the episode of prevention, Jill will be monitored quarterly through phone contacts or visits for the next 6 months. Parents also may contact the physical therapist as needed. The purpose of this episode of prevention is to update the home program and evacuation plan, monitor orthotics and equipment, problem solve with caregivers, and advise family on community resources.

CASE STUDY #3: TAYLOR

> *Practice Pattern 5C:* Impaired Motor Function and Sensory Processing Associated With Nonprogressive Disorders of the Central Nervous System—Congenital Origin or Acquired in Infancy or Childhood

> *Medical Diagnosis:* Myelomeningocele, repaired L1-2

> *Age:* 4 years

This case is an example of using the Guide 3.0 *for reexamination and determination of a new diagnosis and need for a new or modified plan of care or when using the Adapted Practice Patterns, reclassification of the practice pattern. It also demonstrates how you can have 2 problems (diagnoses) that require use of 2 practice patterns at the same time.*

Taylor has been in an episode of care, classified into Adapted Practice Pattern 5C, because his primary impairments that were driving the intervention were motor function and sensory processing. Taylor was reexamined to determine whether his primary impairments have changed and if a new diagnosis is needed along with a new or modified plan of care or, using the Adapted Practice Patterns, if reclassification into another practice pattern is necessary.

Reexamination

Summary of History and Systems Reviews From Initial Examination

> *Activities and Participation:* Taylor attends a preschool program 3 mornings per week. Taylor is a son and classmate.
> *General Demographics:* Taylor is a 4-year-old boy.
> *General Health Status:* Parents report generally good health.
> *Living Environment:* Lives with parents in a ranch-style house.
> *Medical/Surgical History:* At birth a large myelomeningocele was found and closed surgically. A ventricular-peritoneal shunt was surgically inserted on day 5. Taylor had increased apnea and was on a respirator. He had questionable seizures, but his electroencephalogram was normal. He had a suspected Arnold-Chiari malformation that was treated by surgical release of the posterior fossa. He had equinovarus deformities and underwent serial casting beginning at age 2 weeks. He subsequently had surgery to correct bilaterally dislocated hips.

Reexamination Current Conditions

Taylor was seen by his physician, who requested an evaluation of Taylor's equipment needs as he will be entering kindergarten this fall. He has a skin breakdown on the sacrum that needs dressing changes 3 times per week.

Reexamination Tests and Measures

> *Assistive Technology* (observation, ADL and IADL scales): Taylor currently uses an anterior walker and a reciprocating gait orthosis. He self-propels in a manual wheelchair. He has an available loaner, manual wheelchair.
> *Balance* (observation): Balance reactions are slow in sitting and standing. He has good protective reactions in sitting, but not in standing.
> *Community, Social, and Civic Life* (observation, interview): Taylor is a sociable child who is interested in age-appropriate play and leisure activities. He is most interested in peer interaction in his home and in his classroom as he cannot keep up with peers outside or on the playground. He is enrolled in a Saturday karate class in the community.
> *Integumentary Integrity* (observation, palpation, classification): Taylor has an open wound that is draining, partial skin thickness, 0.5×0.3 cm, on sacrum (being followed by physician).
> *Mental Functions* (developmental inventory): Taylor has visual perceptual problems, which has made cognitive testing difficult. His performance suggests that his intellectual skills are in the average range. He has good attention skills and is usually cooperative and motivated in the classroom.
> *Mobility (including locomotion)* (ADL scales, observation, mobility skills, functional assessments): External support is necessary for standing. Taylor ambulates with a reciprocating gait orthosis and a walker, but is ready for long leg braces and crutches.
> *Motor Function* (observation, motor impairment tests, physical performance tests): Taylor has loss of motor function in his lower extremities. He has good head control in all positions and normal upper extremity coordination.
> *Muscle Performance (Including Strength, Power, Endurance, and Length)* (functional muscle tests, observation, palpation): Generalized weakness is noted in the upper extremities and trunk, especially in the abdominal muscles. Taylor tends to hold his breath when using

his upper extremities for weight bearing or strenuous tasks. He has inadequate abdominal strength to support sustained exhalation. He has poor active trunk extension. Overall endurance for physical activity is decreased compared with peers.

> *Neuromotor Development and Sensory Processing* (observation, motor function tests): Taylor rolls with poor leg dissociation. He can get in and out of sitting and onto all fours independently. He attempts to pull to kneeling. In sitting and on all fours he "hangs on his ligaments" rather than using muscle activity. He has normal grasp, manipulation, and release. He has visual acuity problems and wears glasses. He has particular difficulty with figure-ground discrimination, and bending his head to look at the floor disturbs his balance. He has an average sentence length of 3 to 4 words and sounds produced are within normal limits. He is being evaluated for speech and language services.

> *Posture* (observation): On all fours Taylor demonstrates a lordotic posture and "hangs" on his shoulder girdle. In sitting, he slumps rather than using muscle activity to sit upright. Caregivers have noticed his posture when sitting has declined.

> *Range of Motion* (contracture tests, observation, goniometry): Range of motion is within functional limits. Taylor has slightly tight hip flexors and hip adductors.

> *Self-Care and Domestic Life* (observation, barrier identification, physical performance tests, ADL and IADL scales): Taylor can put on and take off a T-shirt. He needs assistance for lower body dressing. Oral-motor skills are normal and there are no feeding problems. He needs assistance with other self-cares such as toileting.

> *Sensory Integrity* (sensory tests): Taylor demonstrates loss of cutaneous and proprioceptive sensation below L1-2.

Evaluation

Based on the reexamination you determine that Taylor's primary impairments are no longer motor function and sensory processing, but rather impaired muscle performance and integumentary. You review the Adapted Practice Patterns and determine that Taylor should be classified into Practice Pattern 4C: Impaired Muscle Performance and Practice Pattern 7C: Impaired Integumentary Integrity Associated With Partial-Thickness Skin Involvement and Scar Formation.

When determining the appropriate pattern, it is important to review the inclusion and exclusion or multiple-pattern classification sections. You will see by reviewing this page for Adapted Practice Pattern 4C that it includes conditions of chronic neuromuscular dysfunction and musculoskeletal dysfunction. You also will note that this Adapted Practice Pattern can be used with any patient/client regardless of the underlying pathology or condition as long as muscle performance is the primary impairment.

Taylor also is placed in Adapted Practice Pattern 7C to address the interventions for his skin breakdown. Placement in 2 patterns is appropriate when the interventions for the impairments cannot be address in only 1 pattern.

Diagnosis

The primary impairments that affect Taylor's functional abilities now fall into the Adapted Pattern of 4C: Impaired Muscle Performance and 7C: Impaired Integumentary Integrity Associated With Partial-Thickness Skin Involvement and Scar Formation.

Prognosis (Including Plan of Care)

When using 2 patterns it is important to use the Factors That May Require New Episode of Care or That May Modify Frequency of Visits/Duration of Care to determine the plan of care, including the range of number of visits for each pattern. In Taylor's situation, his prognosis statements would appear as: "In 3 months, Taylor will demonstrate muscle performance and the highest level of functioning in home, leisure, and community environments within the context of his impairments, functional limitations, and disabilities. In 4 weeks, Taylor will demonstrate optimal integumentary integrity and the highest level of function in home, school, and play."

CASE STUDY #4: ASHLEY

- ▸ *Practice Pattern 5B*: Impaired Neuromotor Development
- ▸ *Medical Diagnosis*: Down syndrome
- ▸ *Age*: 15 months

This case is an example of using the Guide 3.0 to select interventions based on the examination, evaluation, diagnosis, and prognosis.

Examination

History

- ▸ *Activities and Participation*: Ashley has a variety of movement patterns, but is slow and her postural reactions are delayed. She has poor oral-motor skills and does not assist in dressing. She observes other children but does not interact.
- ▸ *Current Conditions*: Ashley's parents are concerned about her motor skills at home. They are currently attending an early intervention class for parents and child 2 times per week with support services from physical therapy, occupational therapy, and speech therapy.
- ▸ *General Demographics*: Ashley is a 15-month-old girl.
- ▸ *General Health Status (Self-Report, Family Report, Caregiver Report)*:
  - ○ General health perception: Frequent colds.
  - ○ Mental functions: Intellectual delays.
  - ○ Physical functions: Movement is slow.
- ▸ *Growth and Development*: Ashley was discharged from the hospital at age 6 weeks. She was diagnosed with Down syndrome (DS) shortly after birth.
- ▸ *Living Environment*: She lives in a 2-level home with her bedroom on the second level.
- ▸ *Medical/Surgical History*: Ashley was a full-term infant born to a 26-year-old primipara mother who had experienced an uncomplicated pregnancy. Ashley was diagnosed with DS shortly after birth. She had esophageal atresia and primary repair was not possible. A gastrostomy was present for the first 6 months of age. She had a ventricular-septal defect that was surgically repaired at age 8 months. Ashley has a history of chronic otitis media with mild conductive hearing loss. Pressure-equalizing tubes were placed at age 12 months.
- ▸ *Medications*: None.
- ▸ *Social History*: Ashley lives with her mother and father, who are the primary caregivers. Ashley enjoys observing other children but does not interact with them.

Systems Review

- ▸ *Cardiovascular/Pulmonary*
  - ○ Heart rate: WNL
  - ○ Respiratory rate: WNL

- *Integumentary*
  - ○ Presence of scar formation: Scar present on chest from heart surgery, not available to assess
  - ○ Skin color: Normal
  - ○ Skin integrity: Normal
- *Musculoskeletal*
  - ○ Gross range of motion: Hypermobility is noted both in proximal and distal extremities
- *Neuromuscular*
  - ○ Gross coordinated movements: Ashley has good head control in all positions. She rolls independently, transitions in and out of sitting, and in and out of a hands-and-knees position. She also pulls to stand at furniture.
- *Communication, Affect, Cognition, Language, and Learning Style*
  - ○ Beginning verbal communication
  - ○ Parent requests written home program with diagrams

Tests and Measures

- *Anthropometric Characteristics* (scales, observation): Ashley's height and weight are within the normal range for children her age with DS. Facial features are characteristic of children with DS.
- *Community, Social, and Civic Life* (disability inventory, observation): Ashley observes other children but does not interact with them. She tends to fling objects or toys to dispose of them. Play is seldom goal directed.
- *Education Life:* Ashley and her mother attend a parent/caregiver-infant early intervention program twice weekly with consultative physical therapy, occupational therapy, and speech therapy available at each session. The family has declined home-based services.
- *Joint Integrity and Mobility:* Within normal range to passive movement.
- *Mental Functions* (developmental inventory): Formal IQ testing has not been completed on Ashley, although she has mild intellectual impairment associated with her medical diagnosis. She is a passive child, needing encouragement and stimulation to attend to motor and cognitive tasks. She has several words that she uses singly rather than in combination (eg, "more," "mama," "dada").
- *Mobility (Including Locomotion)* (ADL scales, observation): Ashley pulls to stand but is not yet attempting to cruise at furniture. She will walk with maximal assistance with 2 hands held. She has slow and usually ineffective protective and equilibrium reactions in sitting, all fours, and standing.
- *Motor Function* (ADL scales, observation): Although Ashley appears to have a typical variety of movement patterns, her movements are very slow and postural reactions are delayed. She needs multiple repetitions of cognitive and motor tasks for skill achievement and retention.
- *Muscle Performance (Including Strength, Power, Endurance, and Length)* (ADL scales, observation): Ashley has poor muscle definition throughout her body, particularly noticeable in the shoulders and hips. She tends to lock her elbows into extension and externally rotates her arms when making movement transitions. She has poor stability in weight-bearing positions (eg, all fours, kneeling).
- *Neuromotor Development and Sensory Processing* (developmental inventory, motor assessment, observation): Ashley has good head control in all positions. She rolls independently. She transitions in and out of sitting and in and out of a hands-and-knees position. She also pulls to kneeling and pulls to stand at furniture. She tends to use straight-line movements without using trunk rotation. She does not appear hypersensitive to tactile input. She generally is apprehensive about movement activities. She grasps objects but cannot release them with control. She cannot pick up pellet-sized objects.

> *Range of Motion* (observation): Hypermobility is noted in both proximal and distal extremities. She tends to keep her shoulders elevated with shortened capital extensor muscles.
> *Reflex Integrity* (reflex tests): Decreased tendon reflexes are present throughout the upper and lower extremities. Low muscle tone also is noted throughout the trunk.
> *Self-Care and Domestic Life* (physical performance tests): Ashley has poor oral-motor skills. She uses a suckling pattern in feeding. Her tongue is thick in contour and protrudes from her mouth. She drinks from a cup only at snack time. Solids are inconsistently presented. She tends to lose food from her mouth. She does not assist in any other self-cares.
> *Sensory Integrity:* Vision is normal. Mild hearing loss has been noted. Ashley tends to avoid movement-based activities.
> *Ventilation and Respiration:* Ashley has decreased respiratory-phonatory functioning. She is a mouth breather and occasionally drools.

Evaluation

The examination has taught you much about Ashley: Ashley has poor muscle definition throughout her body, with poor stability in weight-bearing positions. She has hypermobility in both proximal and distal extremities, and has low muscle tone. She is able to pull to standing at furniture but does not cruise. She has slow protective and equilibrium reactions in sitting, all fours, and standing. She grasps objects but cannot release them with control. She is a mouth breather and occasionally drools. She has a mild hearing loss.

Diagnosis

The data collected help determine the primary impairment that will drive the interventions, which is her impaired neuromotor development. You place Ashley in Adapted Practice Pattern of 5B: Impaired Neuromotor Development.

Prognosis (Including Plan of Care)

Ashley will demonstrate optimal neuromotor development and the highest level of functioning in the home and community, within the context of her impairments, activity limitations, and participation restrictions. The family declined home-based services but agreed to consultative services from occupational, physical, and speech therapy when Ashley and her mother attend an early intervention program provided 2 times per week. Ashley will be discharged when goals and outcomes have been met.

Interventions (for Clinical Consideration)

Coordination, Communication, and Documentation (Provided Throughout the Episode of Care)

> *Interventions:* Coordination and communication with occupational therapy, speech therapy, and early intervention program (teachers, classroom aides).
> *Goals and Outcomes:* Available resources are maximally utilized. Care is coordinated with family and any other caregivers.

Patient-/Client-Related Instruction

> *Interventions:* The family will receive instruction, education, and training in a home program and updates. They will receive information about when it is appropriate to seek additional services.

> *Goals and Outcomes:* Ashley's parents will have awareness of and use community resources. Parents and caregivers will have increased awareness of the impact of Ashley's diagnosis.

Additional Interventions

To assist Ashley in achieving her goals and outcomes, you select therapeutic exercise as one of her additional interventions. When selecting an intervention, you should review the information provided in the *Guide 3.0,* Chapter 5—Interventions, under the specific intervention.[34] Each intervention provides a definition and purpose; types of interventions with examples; and goals and outcomes as they affect pathology or condition; impairments in body functions and structures; activity limitations or participation restrictions; risk reduction and prevention; health, wellness, and fitness; societal resources; and patient/client satisfaction.[34] You can use this section to assist you in determining appropriate goals and outcomes.

For Ashley, you select therapeutic exercise as it addresses her needs for neuromotor development training, gait and locomotion training, and strength training.

Case Study #5: John

> *Practice Pattern 5B:* Impaired Neuromotor Development

> *Medical Diagnosis:* Developmental coordination disorder/attention-deficit hyperactivity disorder

> *Age:* 5 years

This case is an example of using the Guide 3.0 *for reexamination and concluding an episode of care.*

Reexamination

Summary of History and Systems Review From Initial Examination

> *General Demographics:* John is a 5-year-old boy.

> *Activities and Participation:* John attends full-day kindergarten, 5 days per week. He is a son, grandson, student, and friend.

> *General Health Status:* Stated prior health was excellent.

> *Medical/Surgical History:* John was a premature infant who spent a short time in the NICU before being discharged to home. He was noted to have slightly delayed motor milestones (sat at age 9 months; walked at age 18 months). He has always been considered to be a very active child. He is easily frustrated with motor tasks, and temper tantrums are frequent. He is noted to be "clumsy" and is unable to perform gross and fine motor tasks as well as peers (eg, cannot ride a bike without training wheels, has poor handwriting/printing). He was evaluated by a developmental pediatrician and neuropsychologist and received dual diagnoses of developmental coordination disorders/attention-deficit hyperactivity disorders.

Current Conditions

John has improved in his functional status in the areas of self-care and has learned to ride a bike without training wheels. He has not been cooperating in physical therapy, and his parents would like to discontinue physical therapy and occupational therapy and continue with a home program. They are interested in information on community resources.

Tests and Measures

> *Education Life:* John attends a full-day kindergarten program. He was assessed by the school and does not qualify for special education services.

> *Balance* (observation, functional assessment): John cannot walk a 4-inch (10 cm) balance beam without falling off and can maintain his balance on one foot for only 1 to 2 seconds.

> *Gait* (ADL scales, observation, functional assessment): John walks independently, but occasionally walks on his toes. John tends to walk with stiff legs and a decreased arm swing. He leans forward as he walks. He can walk with a heel-toe gait when reminded. He tends to walk too quickly with poor balance, often bumping into environmental objects or other people.

> *Mental Functions* (observation, safety checklist): John's attention span has improved since he began taking medication. He still has difficulty with selective attention and often has to be redirected to task. Formal IQ testing on the Stanford-Binet test suggests above-average intelligence. John has an expressive language delay, often omitting consonants in words and words in sentences.

> *Motor Function* (observation, coordination screens, movement assessment scales): John is consistently characterized as being "clumsy." He has difficulty varying the speed of movement and coordinating his upper and lower extremities, such as required when performing jumping jacks. He has motor planning problems and has difficulty learning new motor tasks. He requires increased practice to master each motor skill. Skills do not generalize easily.

> *Muscle Performance (Including Strength, Power, Endurance, and Length)* (timed activity tests, ADL and IADL scales): Upper extremity strength is decreased for his age. For example, he has difficulty supporting his weight on his arms to "wheelbarrow." Endurance for age-appropriate activities, such as soccer, is decreased compared with his peers.

> *Neuromotor Development and Sensory Processing* (activity index, motor function tests, neuromotor assessment): John ambulates independently. He can run, although he does so in a poorly coordinated pattern. He cannot skip, but gallops instead. He has difficulty with ball skills (eg, catching, throwing, dribbling) and eye-hand coordination. He uses a modified lateral pinch for coloring and printing. He occasionally demonstrates signs of tactile defensiveness.

> *Range of Motion:* WNL.

> *Self-Care and Domestic Life* (ADL and IADL scales, interview, observation): John has difficulty using utensils during meals and prefers finger foods. He is independent in dressing, but has difficulty with buttons, snaps, and zippers. He prefers Velcro closures, T-shirts, and sweatpants. He is independent in toileting, but needs to be monitored to do an adequate job bathing and tooth brushing.

Evaluation

John has been receiving physical and occupational therapy each 2 times per month from a private agency. He attends a half-day kindergarten program but does not qualify for special education. He has made progress in therapy, especially in self-care and gross motor skills; however, he is refusing to cooperate with therapy, and he has not met all his current anticipated goals and expected outcomes. His parents report that John enjoys and fully participates in a community-based circus program where he works on coordination and motor skills as part of the routines (Figures 6-2 through 6-5).

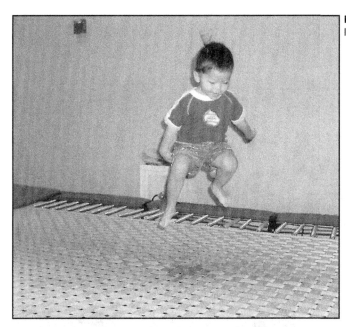

Figure 6-2. Child jumping on a trampoline during a circus gymnastics program.

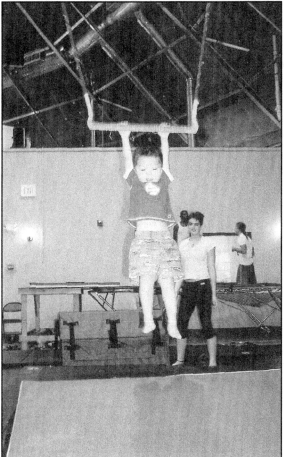

Figure 6-3. Child swinging on a trapeze and landing on a foam incline during a circus gymnastics program.

Figure 6-4. Child swinging on a trapeze and landing on a foam incline during a circus gymnastics program.

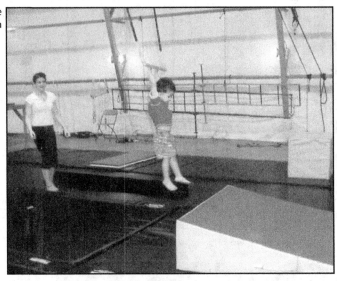

Figure 6-5. Assisted walking on a high wire during a circus gymnastics program.

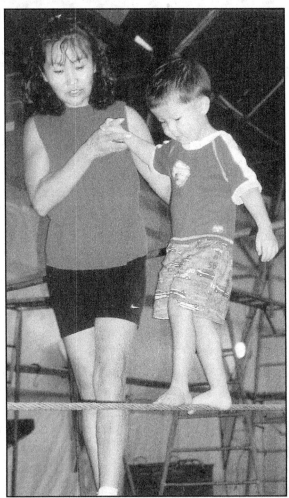

His parents report that staff members working with John are willing to incorporate ideas from therapists into his circus program activities. He also is participating in swimming classes in the community.

Diagnosis

The primary impairments that affect John's functional status continue to be consistent with Adapted Practice Pattern 5B: Impaired Neuromotor Development.

Prognosis (Including Plan of Care)

Should John's episode of care be concluded? The *Guide 3.0* provides the following criteria for concluding an episode of care[34]:

> ➤ The goals or outcomes for the individual have been achieved.
> ➤ The individual is unable to continue to progress toward goals.
> ➤ The individual chooses to conclude care.
> ➤ The physical therapist determines that the individual will no longer benefit from continued therapy.

Decisions about concluding any episode should be made in consultation with the client, family, and other appropriate individuals involved with the client. Remember: It is the client's episode of care, *not* the physical therapist's. Discussions with John and his family should include a review of current goals and outcomes, and John's activities and participation in home, community, and educational settings.

Based on John's lack of cooperation during therapy, his parent's request to end therapy, and John's involvement in a community-based children's circus program, you agree with the family that it is appropriate to conclude this episode of care. As part of the plan to conclude this episode of care, you recommend that you consult with the community-based circus staff and also establish a home program. Parents are in agreement with this plan. John will be seen 2 times per month for 2 months at his community circus site to consult with community-based staff. The parents will be provided a home program.

REFERENCES

1. American Physical Therapy Association. *Guide to Physical Therapist Practice 3.0.* Alexandria, VA: American Physical Therapy Association; 2014. http://guidetoptpractice.apta.org/. Accessed August 26, 2018.
2. American Physical Therapy Association. Guide to Physical Therapist Practice, Vol I: A Description of Patient Management. *Phys Ther.* 1995;75(8):707-764.
3. American Physical Therapy Association. Guide to Physical Therapist Practice. Second Edition. *Phys Ther.* 2001;81(1):9-744.
4. American Physical Therapy Association. Guide to Physical Therapist Practice. *Phys Ther.* 1997;77(11):1163-1650.
5. American Physical Therapy Association. Guide to Physical Therapist Practice. Revisions. *Phys Ther.* 1999;79(6):623-629.
6. American Physical Therapy Association. Guide to Physical Therapist Practice. Revisions. *Phys Ther.* 1999;79(11):1078-1081.
7. Appendix: History of Guide Development. *Guide to Physical Therapist Practice 3.0.* Alexandria, VA: American Physical Therapy Association; 2014. http://guidetoptpractice.apta.org/content/1/SEC41.body. Accessed August 26, 2018.
8. Updates and Summary of Revisions. *Guide to Physical Therapist Practice 3.0.* Alexandria, VA: American Physical Therapy Association; 2014. http://guidetoptpractice.apta.org/site/misc/revisions.xhtml. Accessed August 26, 2018.
9. Adapted Practice Patterns. Alexandria, VA: American Physical Therapy Association; 2014. Available at http://www.apta.org/Guide/PracticePatterns/. Accessed August 26, 2018.

10. Education Tools. *Guide to Physical Therapist Practice 3.0.* Alexandria, VA: American Physical Therapy Association; 2014. http://guidetoptpractice.apta.org/site/misc/education_tools.xhtml. Accessed August 26, 2018.

11. Introduction to the *Guide to Physical Therapist Practice.* Guide to Physical Therapist Practice 3.0. Alexandria, VA: American Physical Therapy Association; 2014. http://guidetoptpractice.apta.org/. Accessed August 26, 2018.

12. Nagi S. Some conceptual issues in disability and rehabilitation. In Sussman M, ed. *Sociology and Rehabilitation.* Washington, DC: American Sociological Association; 1965:100-113.

13. ICIDH. *International Classification of Impairments, Disabilities and Handicaps.* Geneva, Switzerland: World Health Organization; 1980.

14. National Advisory Board on Medical Rehabilitation Research. *Draft V: Report and Plan for Medical Rehabilitation Research.* Bethesda, MD: National Institutes of Health; 1992.

15. Nagi S. *Disability and Rehabilitation.* Columbus, OH: Ohio State University Press; 1969.

16. Nagi S. Disability concepts revisited: implications for prevention. In: Institute of Medicine. *Disability in America: Toward a National Agenda for Prevention.* Washington, DC: Institute of Medicine, National Academy Press; 1991.

17. ICIDH-2. *International Classification of Functioning, Disability and Health.* Geneva, Switzerland: World Health Organization; 2000.

18. Institute of Medicine. *Disability in America: Toward a National Agenda for Prevention.* Washington, DC: Institute of Medicine, National Academy Press; 1991.

19. Brandt EN Jr, Pope AM, eds. *Enabling America: Assessing the Role of Rehabilitation Science and Engineering.* Washington, DC: American Sociological Association; 1965:100-113.

20. Engle GL. The need for a new medical model: a challenge for biomedicine. *Science.* 1997;196(4286):129-136. https://www.ncbi.nlm.nih.gov/pubmed/847460. Accessed August 17, 2018.

21. Borrell-Carrió F, Suchman AL, Epstein RM. The biopsychosocial model 25 years later: principles, practice, and scientific inquiry. *Ann Fam Med.* 2004;2(6):576-582. doi:10.1370/afm.245.

22. *International Classification of Functioning, Disability and Health: ICF.* Switzerland: World Health Organization; 2001. http://www.who.int/classifications/icf/en/. Accessed August 11, 2018.

23. Glossary. *Guide to Physical Therapist Practice 3.0.* Alexandria, VA: American Physical Therapy Association; 2014. http://guidetoptpractice.apta.org/content/1/SEC42.body. Accessed August 26, 2018.

24. PTNow: Tools to Advance Physical Therapist Practice. Alexandria, VA: American Physical Therapy Association; 2018. https://www.ptnow.org/. Accessed August 26, 2018.

25. American Physical Therapy Association Board of Directors. Professionalism in Physical Therapy: Core Values (BOD P05-04-02-03). http://www.apta.org/uploadedFiles/APTAorg/About_Us/Policies/Judicial_Leagal/ProfessionalismCoreValues.pdf. Accessed August 28, 2018.

26. American Physical Therapy Association House of Delegates. Code of Ethics for the Physical Therapist (HOD S06-09-07-12). http://www.apta.org/uploadedFiles/APTAorg/About_Us/Policies/Ethics/CodeofEthics.pdf. Accessed August 28, 2018.

27. American Physical Therapy Association Judicial Committee. Guide for Professional Conduct. http://www.apta.org/uploadedFiles/APTAorg/Practice_and_Patient_Care/Ethics/GuideforProfessionalConduct.pdf. Accessed August 28, 2018.

28. American Physical Therapy Association House of Delegates. Standards of Practice for Physical Therapy (HOD S06-13-22-15). http://www.apta.org/uploadedFiles/APTAorg/About_Us/Policies/Practice/StandardsPractice.pdf. Accessed August 28, 2018.

29. American Physical Therapy Association Board of Directors. Criteria for Standards of Practice for Physical Therapy (BOD S03-06-16-38). http://www.apta.org/uploadedFiles/APTAorg/About_Us/Policies/Practice/CriteriaStandardsPractice.pdf. Accessed August 28, 2018.

30. American Physical Therapy Association House of Delegates. Standards of Ethical Conduct for the Physical Therapist Assistant (HOD S06-09-20-18). http://www.apta.org/uploadedFiles/APTAorg/About_Us/Policies/Ethics/StandardsEthicalConductPTA.pdf. Accessed August 28, 2018.

31. American Physical Therapy Association Judicial Committee. Guide for Conduct of the Physical Therapist Assistant. http://www.apta.org/uploadedFiles/APTAorg/Practice_and_Patient_Care/Ethics/GuideforConductofthePTA.pdf. Accessed August 28, 2018.

32. APTA. Physical Therapist Examination and Evaluations: Focus on Tests and Measurements. *Guide to Physical Therapist Practice 3.0.* Alexandria, VA: American Physical Therapy Association; 2014. http://guidetoptpractice.apta.org/content/1/SEC4.body. Accessed August 26, 2018.

33. APTA. Principles of Physical Therapist Patient/Client Management. Guide to Physical Therapist Practice 3.0. Alexandria, VA: American Physical Therapy Association; 2014. http://guidetoptpractice.apta.org/content/1/SEC2.body. Accessed August 26, 2018.

34. APTA. Intervention. *Guide to Physical Therapist Practice 3.0.* Alexandria, VA: American Physical Therapy Association; 2014. http://guidetoptpractice.apta.org/content/1/SEC31.body. Accessed August 28, 2018.

35. APTA. Measurement and Outcomes. *Guide to Physical Therapist Practice 3.0.* Alexandria, VA: American Physical Therapy Association; 2014. http://guidetoptpractice.apta.org/content/1/SEC3.body. Accessed August 26, 2018.

Physical Therapy in the Neonatal Intensive Care Unit

7

Roberta Gatlin, PT, DScPT, PCS

The neonatal intensive care unit (NICU) represents one of the most advanced and innovative environments for physical therapists in pediatrics. The team of NICU health care professionals with advanced training in neonatal development, pathophysiology, and related high-risk outcomes work diligently to provide life-saving interventions to neonates and their families from the critical time of admissions through the transitional period preparing for discharge. The NICU is an intense, fast-paced environment that promotes a family-centered care (FCC) model that is calm, quiet, and developmentally appropriate for neonates.[1,2] Medical and developmental interventions, equipment, and the environment all play an important role in neonates' maturation during NICU admissions and ultimately neurobehavioral and neurodevelopmental outcomes.

The neonate requires specialized care because of physiologic, behavioral, and neurodevelopmental vulnerabilities.[3] The physical therapist is instrumental in educating the family, NICU health care team members, and other professionals involved in the care of the neonate in the NICU and during preparation for the transition to home.

Clinical guidelines initially were published in 1999 that specified roles, competencies, and knowledge areas for physical therapists practicing in the NICU and updated in 2009.[4,5] Additionally, the guidelines recommended preceptor training. Part I of the guidelines addressed the concepts for developing training models, clinical competency training, and clinical decision-making algorithms.[5] Part II provided evidence and frameworks for supporting practices in the NICU. References were provided to assist physical therapists preparing for and practicing in the advanced subspecialty of neonatology.[4-6]

There are a number of competencies needed by the physical therapist in the NICU: (1) an advanced knowledge in neonatal neurobehavioral, neurodevelopmental, and multisystem embryological development; (2) the ability to perform an appropriate examination and evaluation; (3) an understanding of therapeutic interventions and how to incorporate the family into the plan of care; (4) experience in pediatric rehabilitative programming; (5) appropriate leadership skills to make positive changes in the NICU environment; and (6) proficiency in assisting the family and infant throughout their stay in the NICU, as well as preparing them for discharge

Connolly BH, Montgomery PC, eds. *Therapeutic Exercise for Children With Developmental Disabilities, Fourth Edition* (pp 177-210).
© 2020 Taylor & Francis Group.

home.[4-7] Competencies within these areas will enable the physical therapist to be a successful active team member and ensure protective, gestational-age developmental care.

THE NICU

The NICU is an environment where interventions are provided to a neonate born preterm or with medical complications. These complications may range from requiring assistance with feeding to specialized equipment for respiratory support, temperature control, or opioid withdrawal assistance. In 2012, The American Academy of Pediatrics proposed 4 levels of neonatal intensive care units (Table 7-1).[8]

The primary NICU team includes specialized medical professionals, the infant, and the family. The *neonatologist,* a pediatrician with specialized training in caring for preterm or critically ill newborns, coordinates the medical team and directs the overall care of the newborn. The *neonatal nurse practitioner,* a nurse with advanced training in providing medical interventions to neonates, works closely with the neonatologist to coordinate medical care. An instrumental team member is the *bedside nurse,* who has received education and training to care for this population. Depending on the NICU level and the association of the health care system with teaching programs, the unit may have a variety of medical residents from several different specialties, such as pediatrics, obstetrics, and family practice. Other instrumental health care members include: the *respiratory therapist,* who monitors the respiratory system of neonates requiring supplemental oxygenation or ventilation; the *medical social worker,* who provides supportive care to families and assists with discharge planning for infants and families during the transition to home; and the *neonatal dietician,* who ensures that the nutritional needs of premature or high-risk neonates are met.

Physical therapists, occupational therapists, and speech-language pathologists assist in examining, evaluating, and providing interventions for the neonate. Additionally, physical therapists develop in-service education programs for parents and nursing staff and provide orientation for resident physicians that include practical examples of intervention strategies as well as the theoretical basis for treatment. Physical therapists should provide consistent role modeling with proper positioning and handling techniques for the neonate. If in-service and orientation programs are successful, an increase in referrals to physical therapy may occur as staff members recognize the value of, and become comfortable with, requesting consultation.[9]

Other primary team members may include the lactation consultant, audiologist, chaplain or spiritual support, and a utilization review representative. These team members ensure there is supportive care in their areas of expertise.

The most important member of the NICU team is the family. Interventions the neonate receives while in the NICU and in preparation for home have increased positive outcomes when the family is actively involved in the child's care. Learning about, bonding with, and becoming an advocate for the child are crucial outcomes for the family and are reinforced by the FCC model.

THEORETICAL FRAMEWORKS TO GUIDE NEONATAL INTERVENTION

Theoretical frameworks help guide the physical therapist in providing services. There are 4 frameworks discussed in this section: (1) the *International Classification of Functioning, Disability and Health* (ICF) model,[10] (2) the FCC model,[11,12] (3) synactive theory,[13] and (4) dynamic systems theory (DST) of development.[4] All the models are representative of the interactive, complex relationships between a neonate's health and the environmental influences that assist the neonate to complete a functional task. For the neonate, this may be to maintain an alert, awake state for being able to take a bottle (PO feeding/taken by mouth, orally). These frameworks help practitioners

TABLE 7-1. LEVELS OF NEONATAL CARE

LEVEL I: BASIC NEWBORN NURSERY/WELL NEWBORN NURSERY

- Postnatal care and evaluation of the healthy newborn
- Neonatal resuscitation at delivery
- Stabilization and care for physiologically stable late preterm infants, born between 35 and 36.6 weeks' GA
- Stabilization of ill newborns until transfer to a facility where specialty neonatal care is provided

LEVEL II: SPECIALTY CARE NURSERY

Level I capabilities plus:

- Resuscitate and stabilize infants with medical needs or preterm infants prior to transfer
- Medical intervention to the infant > 32 weeks' GA and > 1500 g who has physiological immaturity, or who may be moderately ill with resolution of medical complication(s) within first 24 hours of life
- Provide mechanical ventilation or continuous positive airway pressure for short duration, < 24 hours

LEVEL III: SUBSPECIALTY UNIT/NICU

Level II capabilities plus:

- Provide medical intervention for the infant < 32 weeks' GA and weighing < 1500 g and infants at all GAs and birth weights with critical illness
- Provide a full range of respiratory support, including conventional mechanical ventilation, continuous positive airway pressure, high-frequency ventilation, and nitric oxide
- Provide access to advanced imaging, computed tomography, MRI, and echocardiography with interpretation for urgency
- Provide access to full range of pediatric medical subspecialists, pediatric surgical specialists, anesthesiologists, and ophthalmologists
- No major surgery
- Provide transport services for Level I and II NICUs

LEVEL IV: REGIONAL NICU

Level III capabilities plus:

- Location within an institution with the capability to provide on-site surgical interventions (eg, omphalocele repair, esophageal repair, bowel resection, or myelomeningocele repair)
- Provide access to full range of pediatric medical subspecialists, pediatric surgical specialists, anesthesiologists, and ophthalmologists
- Provide access to specialists for surgical repair of congenital heart anomalies that require cardiopulmonary bypass and/or ECMO
- Provide transport services for Level I, II, and III NICUs
- Provide training and educational outreach programs for medical professionals serving the neonatal and high-risk infant population

Abbreviations: ECMO, extracorporeal membrane oxygenation; GA, gestational age; MRI, magnetic resonance imaging; NICU, neonatal intensive care unit.

Adapted from the American Academy of Pediatrics Committee on Fetus and Newborn. Levels of neonatal care. *Pediatrics.* 2012;130(3):587-597.

develop and implement neurobehavioral and neurodevelopmental programs for the neonate, the family, and the medical team.[4,10-13]

International Classification of Functioning, Disability and Health

The ICF represents interactions between the health condition and the various components of the neonate's ability to function.[10] The ICF models an interactive, complex relationship between the neonate's health and the multifactorial components related to gestational age (GA), musculoskeletal system, the environment, and family dynamics that factor into the ability to function. The ICF model allows the physical therapist to organize information such as the pathologies, impairments, activity limitations and difficulties in participatory activities that are specific to the individual neonate (Figure 7-1). The advanced skills of the physical therapist in the NICU allow integration of the ICF model within the plan of care for the neonate while accounting for the multifactorial components that relate to a successful outcome.

Family-Centered Care

FCC promotes the family as a key member of the health care team and encourages active involvement in the care of the child while in the NICU or when undergoing medical care.[11,12] FCC recognizes family members as those who may profoundly influence the personal life of an individual over an extended period of time, and this model has influenced a change in providing medical services in the health care system (see Chapter 4). Today, FCC is considered the medical system's standard of care to achieve optimal health outcomes. FCC recognizes 9 principles: (1) respecting each child and the family, (2) honoring diversity, (3) recognizing and building on strengths of the family, (4) supporting and facilitating choices, (5) ensuring flexibility, (6) sharing honest and unbiased information, (7) providing support, (8) collaborating with the family, and (9) empowering and discovering the family's strengths.[11,12,14] Collaboration between the family and the NICU medical team reinforces the family's ability to participate in the care of their infant and prepares the family for life after the neonate's discharge. Implementing FCC principles ensures the medical team is respecting and recognizing the family's knowledge, strengths, and diversity. The collaboration between the medical team and the family helps support and facilitate family choices, as well as assists the family in empowerment to make informed decisions regarding their child.

Synactive Theory of Development

Als, a child psychologist, was instrumental in developing the synactive theory of development, which has changed the way the medical health care team interacts with the neonate (Figure 7-2).[13] The synactive theory encourages the NICU practitioner to recognize the neonatal subsystems that continually react and influence each other.[15-17] The 5 subsystems in synactive theory are organized as a set of hierarchical behaviors, but are closely interconnected and continually react to influence each other.[13,15-18] The least mature subsystem, the autonomic system, oversees the vital functions of the neonate, including the heart rate, respiratory rate, thermoregulation, and visceral functions. The second subsystem in this hierarchical model is the motor system, responsible for the neonate's postural muscle tone and movement patterns. The third and fourth subsystems are related to the infant's ability to sustain and transition between various states of alertness and maintain attention during an interactive session. The fifth and most mature subsystem is self-regulatory behavior, which is the ability of the neonate to maintain the stable and smooth interaction of the other 4 subsystems. Each subsystem relies on other subsystems' support for intactness and smooth progression. An example of synactive theory can be observed in the NICU. When a neonate is

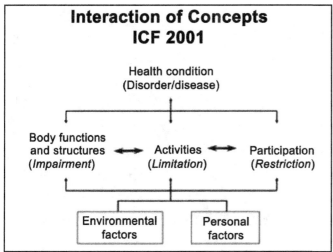

Figure 7-1. The *International Classification of Functioning, Disability and Health* model. (Reprinted with permission from the World Health Organization. *International Classification of Functioning, Disability and Health [ICF].* Geneva, Switzerland: World Health Organization; 2001.)

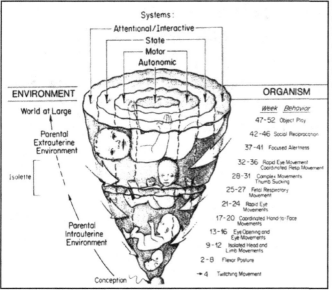

Figure 7-2. The Model of the Synactive Organization of Behavioral Development by Als. (Reprinted with permission from Als H. Toward a synactive theory of development: promise for the assessment and support of infant individuality. *Infant Ment Health J.* 1982;3[4]:229-243.)

newly admitted, he or she is functioning in the physiological subsystem, attempting to maintain homeostasis of vital functions. As the neonate stabilizes, he or she progresses with motor activity by presenting with postural muscle tone, actively moving an extremity to cover the face, or arching away from a stimulus. As the infant continues to mature, the next level of maturational subsystem behavior noted is his or her ability to alert, transition smoothly to an alert state, and transition back into periods of sleep. The fourth subsystem of behavioral maturation is engagement or interaction, often observed prior to discharge when he or she is able to attend to and interact with the caregiver. The most mature of the subsystems is noted when he or she is able to self-regulate or maintain a balance among the subsystems. The physical therapist uses these behaviors to assess the neonate and develop plans of care specific to reactions within these subsystems.

In the synactive theory, the infant provides cues to "tell us" how he or she is tolerating various stimuli.[13,15] These cues are protective mechanisms that allow the neonate to avoid interactions that become too stressful. The physical therapist uses these cues to guide interventions with the infant and to assist the family in recognizing the infant's behavioral communication strategies.

Figure 7-3. Approach cues.

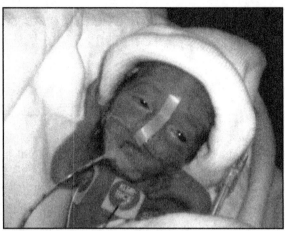

Figure 7-4. Coping cues.

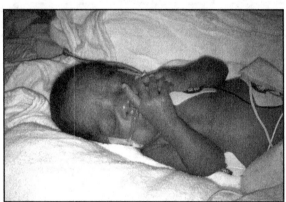

Some behavioral cues are categorized as approach behaviors; these behaviors say, "I am ready for interaction" or "I am engaging in this interaction" (eg, soft, relaxed limbs, quiet and alert state, smooth body movements, or soft relaxed facial expressions; Figure 7-3). The second type of behavioral cues are coping behaviors or warning behaviors; these behaviors say, "I am handling the interaction(s) but it is stressful to me" (eg, leg bracing, hands to face or mouth, sucking motions, grasping observed in the hands or feet, fisting, or moving away from the stimuli; Figure 7-4). The third category of behaviors are stress cues; these behaviors say, "I am not handling this input and I am about to shift back into a less mature subsystem if this stress continues" (eg, gaze aversion, 5-finger salute; Figure 7-5).

The therapist must be aware of the infant's approach and avoidance behaviors, as these behaviors will guide the amount, intensity, and timing to provide stress-free interventions. Table 7-2 presents a summary of self-regulatory behavioral cues that are approach, coping, or stress cues that may be observed.

Dynamic Systems Theory

DST is the fourth framework used to assess and establish care for the infant in the NICU (Figure 7-6).[4] DST recognizes the many interactions that occur among the infant's body systems (ie, ability to move and produce postural control for functional activities), and how the family, home, and community environments may influence participatory interactions and activities. The infant's subsystems include body structure, physiology, and behavior. Interactions among the infant's biological makeup, ability to move and sustain postural control, motor patterns, and

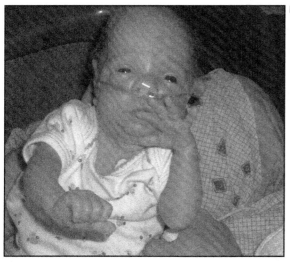

Figure 7-5. Stress cues.

TABLE 7-2. SELF-REGULATORY BEHAVIORAL CUES

APPROACH CUES	COPING CUES	STRESS CUES
• Quiet and alert state • Soft, relaxed facial expressions • "Ohh" face • Cooing • Relaxed extremities • Smooth body motions • Smile	• Purposeful shift to a drowsy or light sleep state • Extremity bracing hand to face • Sucking motions • Hand or foot clasping • Fisting • Bracing of body to support surface (searching for boundaries)	• Gaze aversion • Grimace/frowning, "worry wrinkles" • Tongue thrusting • Salute sign • Stretching or arching away • Finger splay • Yawning, burping, or gagging • Spitting up • Changes in vital signs, homeostasis

learned behavioral reactions will influence the ability to perform functional tasks and participate within the infant-family system.[4] The physical therapist must recognize how the infant's postural control and ability to move may directly impact the functioning of physiological and structural systems. DST recognizes the importance of how interventions with the infant and interactions within and around the environment of the infant may produce adverse stress. A change in the environment, such as a loud noise, or a handling technique that moves the infant too quickly may adversely affect the infant and elicit an atypical motor or behavioral response. DST acknowledges how an interruption of function in one system may be a stressor to the infant and adversely disrupt the ability to maintain stability of other systems. Emphasis in this theory is placed on the contributions of interacting environments in facilitating or constraining the functional performance of the infant. DST offers a model to the therapist for considering the many potential positive or negative influences on the infant, and how these influences may affect the child's stability.[4,19]

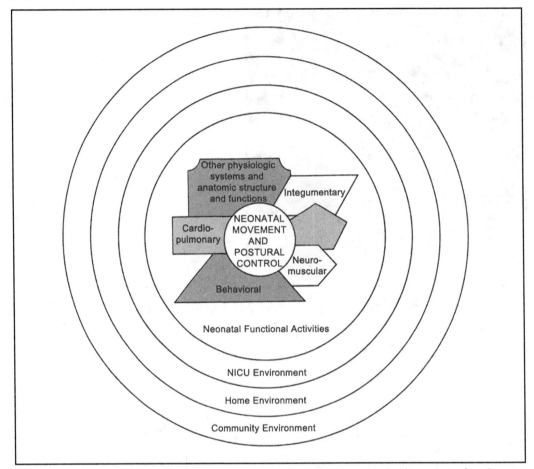

Figure 7-6. The dynamic systems theory in the neonatal intensive care unit. (Reprinted with permission from Sweeney JK, Heriza CB, Reilly MA, Smith C, VanSant AF. Practice guidelines for the physical therapist in the neonatal intensive care unit [NICU]. *Pediatr Phys Ther.* 1999;11[3]:119-132.)

All the theoretical frameworks reviewed in this section assist the therapist in designing and implementing an effective neurobehavioral and neurodevelopmental program for the infant and family to ensure the best outcomes possible.

Indications for Admission Into the NICU

Neonates admitted to the NICU often are very tiny and preterm; however, other infants admitted to the NICU are born close to term (referred to as the late preterm infant [LPI]), or are infants born full-term with a medical condition.

Gestational Age and Birth Weight

Knowledge of neonatal terminology is essential for the physical therapist in the NICU. GA refers to the length of time a baby was in the mother's womb, and is counted in weeks from the mother's last menstrual period to the birth of the baby. Term gestation is typically 40 weeks, but the infant is considered full term if born between 37 and 41 6/7 weeks. A baby born before 37 weeks' GA is considered preterm. A baby born after 42 weeks is considered post-term. The LPI infant is born between 34 weeks and 36 6/7 weeks' GA. Infants also are designated by their birth weight: low birth weight (LBW) weighing between 1501 and 2500 g; very low birth weight (VLBW) 1001 to 1500 g; and extremely low birth weight (ELBW) less than 1000 g. Infants admitted into the NICU also may have a diagnosis related to their size and GA, for example, appropriate for gestational age; small for gestational age (defined as weight less than 10th percentile at a given GA); and large for gestational age (LGA, defined as weight greater than the 90th percentile for the duration of gestation).[20] A diagnosis of intrauterine growth restricted is a rate of fetal growth that is less than typical for the gestational growth potential of that specific infant.[21,22] Infants born preterm or smaller than their GA expectation are at a high risk for multisystem concerns.

The Centers for Disease Control and Prevention reported an increase in preterm birth rates from 2014 to 2016 (ie, from 9.63% in 2014 to 9.85% in 2016). Many of the infants born preterm between 2014 and 2016 were LPI (ie, 6.82% in 2014 to 7.09% in 2016.) The early preterm birth rate was reported as unchanged (ie, 2.7% in 2016). Also reported was that the increase in LPI births was among women of all age groups and that multiple births had declined significantly across all age groups.[23] Trends reported for these key measures were due to a decline both in the general fertility rate and the number of multiple births. While no direct medical interventions were reported to have an effect on preterm birth epidemiology, health care professionals have noticed an increased availability of and improvement in neonatal medical and surgical interventions. Administration of advanced life support resuscitation, surfactant therapy, and positive pressure support has improved the ELBW and VLBW infant's survivability. However, associated poor neurodevelopmental outcomes in preterm infants of < 29 weeks' GA diagnosed with bronchopulmonary dysplasia, necrotizing enterocolitis (NEC), and severe neurological injury remain.[24]

Differentiation among preterm size, appropriate for gestational age, small for gestational age, and intrauterine growth restricted are important secondary to maternal causative factors that may lead to small or poor intrauterine growth. Maternal factors such as smoking, poor nutrition, prescription or recreational drugs and alcohol use, intrauterine infections, or placental insufficiency all may play a significant role in the size of the neonate at birth.

Medical Diagnoses

Common neonatal medical diagnoses are apnea and bradycardia; sepsis; respiratory distress syndrome, resulting in chronic lung disease; intracranial hemorrhage; hypoxic ischemic encephalopathy (HIE); NEC; and/or retinopathy of prematurity. Many of these diagnoses have long-term implications for the infant in addition to the often long-term hospitalizations required for medical management. The intensity of medical care and the high level of vigilance required by the family to meet the needs of their preterm child make it likely that having a preterm child adversely affects the quality of life of the parents and the family overall.[25] The physical therapist has an instrumental role in assessing familial-related predisposing factors that may affect bonding opportunities for the parents while the infant is hospitalized. Positive opportunities for the family to be involved with care of their baby should be provided. These opportunities will assist family members in understanding medical diagnoses, recognizing and interacting according to their infant's behavioral cues, and becoming advocates for the health care needs of their infant not only while in the NICU, but also after discharge.

With advances in neonatal care, survival of preterm neonates as young as 23 weeks' GA has been reported. However, along with improved survival rates, the risk of neurodevelopmental impairment increases with the degree of prematurity.[26] The cost of preterm births is financially as well as emotionally high and may result in irreparable damage to the structure of the family. In some cases, mothers of preterm infants may be young, have little financial or emotional support, and may have received little if any prenatal care.[27] Any of these factors place the infant at higher risk of a poor outcome.

TABLE 7-3. NEONATAL ABSTINENCE SYNDROME SIGNS AND SYMPTOMS

- High-pitched crying
- Shaking/jitteriness
- Fussiness
- Difficulty calming and sleeping
- Stiffness in extremities and trunk
- Tachypnea or rapid breathing
- Stuffy nose/sneezing
- Stomach cramping/gastrointestinal irritability
- Feeding difficulties/poor oral-motor coordination
- Poor weight gain
- Vomiting/diarrhea
- Integumentary breakdown/diaper dermatitis

Neonatal Abstinence Syndrome

Many NICUs have been inundated with admissions of neonates diagnosed with neonatal abstinence syndrome (NAS).[28] This occurs when infants are born having been exposed to opiates (such as morphine, methadone, buprenorphine, hydrocodone, and oxycodone) and experience withdrawal symptoms after birth. The dramatic rise in NAS has occurred in association with the increase in opioid use by pregnant women. These neonates often display signs and symptoms that are very different from the typical preterm neonate (Table 7-3).

NICU admissions for neonates with NAS increased from 0.6% in 2004 to 4.0% in 2013. The length of stay for these neonates rose from 13 days in 2004 to 19 days in 2013.[28] As more evidence accumulates, these numbers steadily are increasing. These neonates require a special environment and medical staff that recognize the neonates' irritability; inability to calm or transition between states of alertness, especially to obtain and maintain a sleep state; and feeding difficulties. Physical therapists offer strategies to assist the infant to transition to calm states of alertness, be positioned optimally for improved feeding, and to decrease hypersensitive and irritable behaviors. Physical therapists also play a critical role in providing individualized caregiver education, with the emphasis on assisting the family to understand their infant's behavioral cues. Teaching the family and caregivers strategies to assist the infant with transitioning and maintaining a calm state of alertness will improve infant-family interactions. When there are added issues of a young maternal age, maternal substance abuse, and/or an economically disadvantaged family situation, the health care providers face added concerns about the long-term outcomes of the infant.[27]

Hypoxic Ischemic Encephalopathy

Neonates presenting with HIE are typically full-term with resultant central nervous system cell death due to an inadequate supply of oxygen, prior to, during, or shortly after birth. These neonates may qualify for hypothermia intervention, which typically begins within 6 to 12 hours after HIE.[29,30] Evidence suggests that hypothermia administered to neonates with HIE results in reduction in mortality and neurological impairment. However, survival is associated with a risk of seizures, changes in tonicity, and poor motor control. In a follow-up assessment of children (age 5.5 years) who had moderate HIE, the children were found to perform significantly lower than the comparison group with respect to everyday motor, complex motor, and fine motor skills.[31] Thus, the infant with HIE should receive developmental follow-up with physical therapy after discharge from the NICU.

Genetic Syndromes

Neonates with syndromes and/or congenital anomalies, including chromosomal abnormalities (eg, Down syndrome [DS]); birth defects (eg, myelomeningocele and cleft palate); congenital heart defects; limb deficiencies secondary to known and unknown maternal risk factors; and/or musculoskeletal asymmetries related to lack of intrauterine space (eg, congenital torticollis or positional clubfoot), may be seen by physical therapists. These neonates usually require therapeutic intervention in the NICU, parental counseling regarding long-term implications, and a variety of therapy services and referrals following discharge. Neonates with specific medical diagnoses and identified risks for developmental delay are the easiest to assess and implement intervention plans in the NICU and after discharge. However, there are other neonates at risk for developmental problems who may not be admitted to the NICU (eg, neonates with brachial plexus injuries or healthy children with DS). Physical therapists should be available to all levels of NICUs, including the Level I, Well-Baby Nursery, as they can play an instrumental role in educating the health care team in care-related issues and, when appropriate, ensure proper referrals to local community agencies for therapy services and/or community early intervention programs.

The Role of the Physical Therapist in the NICU

As previously noted, neonatal physical therapy is a highly specialized area of practice within the field of pediatric physical therapy and encompasses many areas of advanced practice. It is recommended that the physical therapist in the NICU use the American Physical Therapy Association's Hypothesis-Oriented Algorithm II.[32] This algorithm guides the therapist in clinical decision making across all age groups. The algorithm components are the examination, evaluation, establishment of a physical therapy diagnosis and prognosis, and determination of the most appropriate intervention(s) with the inclusion of a prevention component. Examination in the NICU is best performed through observation, conversation, and coordination with other team members and includes appropriate tests and measures designed for use with the fragile and preterm infant. Evaluation of the examination data allows the therapist to make clinical judgments based on medical stability, GA, diagnoses, and environmental and family needs. The therapist then determines an appropriate physical therapy diagnosis and prognosis, reflective of any neurobehavioral and neurodevelopmental concerns. Establishing a prognosis for the infant in the NICU is extremely difficult and often may change depending on the infant's frequent changes in medical status, changes in developmental maturation, and development of secondary chronic diagnoses that may interfere with the infant's future participation in functional activities. Intervention requires coordination, communication, documentation, and instruction of all team members working collaboratively to promote positive interactions with the infant. Physical therapy intervention may include, but is not limited to, proper positioning, promotion of maturational motor patterns and behaviors, individualized handling and participatory interactions, fabrication of splints, or assistance in wound care. All interventions should promote positive changes in the infant's condition. A key role of the therapist is related to understanding and accepting the family as part of the NICU team. Engaging the family to assist in the care of their infant is an instrumental part of the physical therapist's plan of care. Through appropriate family education and instruction, the family can be actively involved with their infant's daily care needs and be able to carry over recommended interventions. Evidence has shown that active interactions of the family with their infant help to reduce later feelings of social isolation, lessen financial burden, improve home safety, and increase enrollment in early intervention programming, all of which lessen the family burden of having a preterm or high-risk infant.[25] Dynamic coordination and communication among NICU team members with the family is imperative to ensure ease of transition to a home environment.

NICU Environment

The physical therapist providing services in the NICU must be aware of the highly sensitive environment and how it plays a crucial role in neonatal development. For example, environmental stressors that may negatively affect the infant can include high sound levels, bright lighting, excessive unsupported movements of the infant, or sensory input that disrupts the neonate's sleep cycles. The therapist should be able to offer suggestions such as making changes to reduce sound levels, offering cyclic lighting, or promoting postural positioning support, and suggesting intervention protocol changes, such as initiating infant-driven feedings that may eliminate or lessen the impact of neonatal stressors (see Oral-Motor Facilitation/PO Feeding). Adopting and implementing new practices (eg, FCC or interventions such as infant-driven feeding) may be difficult for some team members, and the therapist may play a crucial role by providing evidence-based research and practice guidelines.

Equipment in the NICU

The physical therapist must be familiar with specialized equipment particular to the NICU, recognize and understand why certain equipment is being used, and provide input to the team about the infant's response during interventions. Table 7-4 contains a list of common equipment found in a NICU.

Knowledge Base

The physical therapist assessing and working with neonates should understand the typical physiological presentation of neonates at each GA, and how subsequent months of development are crucial for development of postural tone, motor patterns, and behavioral stability. With neonates surviving as early as 23 to 24 weeks' GA, the therapist must have mastery of the expected developmental maturation of these ELBW infants.[33] The LPI neonates born between 34 and 36.6 weeks' GA have a very different course of development. The therapist must be able to differentiate the presentation of neonates born at a specific gestational week. Even within a gestational week the infant may present differently and, depending on the medical diagnoses, the therapist must be able to examine, evaluate, and determine an intervention plan that is best for that infant at that point in time.

Previous experiences with full-term newborns, older infants with medical diagnoses post-NICU, and infants with movement impairments will aid the physical therapist in the examination, evaluation, and development of treatment plans that assist the NICU team and, most important, families in the care of the infants.[4] For example, the therapist must recognize and understand that the physiological flexion observed in full-term infants is not a postural pattern of preterm infants. Infants born at 32 weeks' or less GA often present with fewer flexor patterns and an appearance of hypotonia. Neonates born preterm typically present in more of an extended posture with the inability to bring their extremities to midline or into flexed positions.[34,35] Knowledge that typical 32-week GA infants present with this lack of flexion is key to understanding the developmental needs over the next 2 months as infants mature to 40 weeks' GA or newborn adjusted age. The therapist must develop interventions for proper positioning and handling to promote the development of physiological flexion (Figure 7-7).

Therapists must have experience with healthy, full-term infants from birth through age 6 months to understand typical postures, movement patterns, behaviors, and functional skills. Infants admitted into the NICU with NAS or HIE are typically full term or close to 40 weeks' GA. However, these diagnoses may affect the infant's ability to present with typical newborn developmental functioning. The therapist must recognize these differences, which will assist in making a proper physical therapy diagnosis.

TABLE 7-4. COMMON MEDICAL EQUIPMENT IN THE NEONATAL INTENSIVE CARE UNIT

RADIANT WARMER	An open bed for stabilizing an infant's body temperature with an overhead heat source and specialized lighting for examination and hyperbilirubinemia.
ISOLETTE	An enclosed incubator providing environmental-controlled temperature and humidity. Access to the infant is through port holes on each side of the plastic box.
OPEN CRIB	Open bassinet bedding without a heat source.
VENTILATOR	
IPPV	Intermittent positive pressure ventilation applies to whole-spectrum ventilation modes that deliver pressure-limited, time-cycled ventilation.
SIMV	Synchronized intermittent mandatory ventilation similar to IPPV that delivers a predetermined number of breaths per minute.
HVOF	High-frequency oscillatory ventilator employs supraphysiological ventilation rates and tidal volumes frequently less than dead space.
CPAP-Binasal Cannula	Continuous positive airway pressure forces high pressures of air into the nasal passages to overcome any obstructions in the airway and stimulate breathing.
UMBILICAL LINES	
UVC	Umbilical venous catheter is placed into the vein of the umbilical cord, allowing access to the central circulation of the newborn for the administration of fluids, nutrition, and medications.
UAC	Umbilical arterial catheter is placed into the artery in the umbilical cord of the newborn. It allows the team to draw blood samples, continuously monitor blood pressure, and sample blood gas.
PICC	Peripherally inserted central catheter is a long, slender catheter inserted into a peripheral vein and advanced until termination in a large vein in the chest near the heart. The PICC serves as a central line and may stay in place for weeks, which is less invasive and has decreased complications in neonates who require long-term nutritional and medication needs.
PIV	Peripheral intravenous line is a short-term access through the peripheral vein used to administer fluids, nutrition, or medications.
PHOTOTHERAPY	
Overhead Bili Lights	Overhead ultraviolet lights called phototherapy administered to infants with hyperbilirubinemia or jaundice.
Bili Blanket	A bilirubin blanket or phototherapy blanket provided with an ultraviolet light the infant with jaundice can lie on.
NEONATAL SNUGGLEUP	Positioning aid that provides support and maintains a physiological flexed position for the premature or medically ill infant.

continued

TABLE 7-4. COMMON MEDICAL EQUIPMENT IN THE NEONATAL INTENSIVE CARE UNIT (CONTINUED)	
DANDLE ROO	Positioning aid that supports and maintains a physiological flexed position for the premature or medically ill infant.
WEIGHTED BLANKETS	A froggy or Dandle PAL are smaller, plastic pellet–filled positional blankets that provide proprioceptive input around the boundaries and/or over the pelvis. Must never be used over the thoracic spine or lungs, where the weight may restrict the breathing of the infant.
WEE THUMBIE PREEMIE PACIFIER	A specialized pacifier designed for the ELBW or VLBW premature infant.
WEE SOOTHIE PREEMIE PACIFIER	A specialized pacifier designed for premature infants of LBW or typically between 30 and 34 weeks' GA.

Abbreviations: ELBW, extremely low birth weight; GA, gestational age; LBW, low birth weight; VLBW, very low birth weight.

Figure 7-7. Physiological flexion.

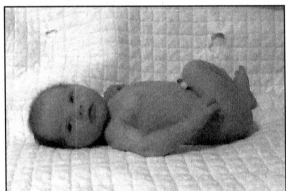

NEONATAL NEUROLOGICAL EXAMINATION AND EVALUATION

History/Chart Review

The neonatal examination begins with a thorough chart review of the infant's admission history and maternal medical history. The chart review will provide the admission medical diagnosis or diagnoses, the GA, day of life or chronological age, current medical interventions and medications, special tests or procedures, and the social worker's report. The physical therapist will need to gather additional information from multiple sources in the NICU, such as current medical status of the neonate, the need for supplemental respiratory support (such as oxygen or supplemental ventilator support), medications, parenteral nutrition, intravenous access, baseline vital signs, and individualized behavioral cues. Other information gathered should include socioeconomic, environmental, and family needs. The gathering of all pertinent information about the admission history assists the therapist in developing the best strategies for beginning hands-on assessment, evaluating the examination results, developing plans of care, and determining discharge readiness.

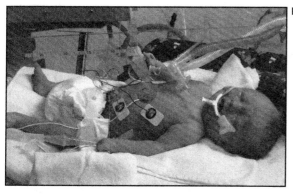

Figure 7-8. Medically fragile infant.

Medical Stability

The physical therapist must recognize the primary medical instability or stability of the infant. As physical therapists, we strive to practice under the principle of beneficence—"Above all, do no harm"—to our patients.[9,36] The therapist must recognize the vulnerability of the neonate and use careful, skilled observations to recognize changes in physiological stability.

The neonate's GA alone does not determine medical stability. The ability to maintain homeostasis depends on the medical diagnosis and GA. For a neonate who is medically fragile or unstable, the physical therapist uses observational skills for identifying stimuli that compromise physiological stability and elicit stressful behavioral cues (Figure 7-8).

As the therapist begins the examination, it is important to recognize the nursing care schedule of the infant. Typically, medically fragile neonates have a 1:1 or 1:2 ratio for nursing care. The physical therapist and nursing staff can assist each other in gathering pertinent information about the neonate's stability and self-regulatory behavior using "cluster care."[37] The clustering of care provides that all interventions occur during a set time period, such as when changing diapers, drawing labs, administering medications or feedings, or any other hands-on interventions. Cluster care provides the fragile neonate with longer undisturbed periods between interventions. Undisturbed periods of rest promote deep sleep patterns and, possibly, may facilitate opportunities for neuronal growth and maturation.[37] Examination of the medically fragile neonate is primarily observation, noting changes in homeostasis/physiological stability and signs/behavioral cues of stress. Intervention then concentrates on priorities for the neonate, such as positioning and environmental changes to decrease excessive stress. Interactions with the neonate depend on medical stability. Working closely with nursing staff provides a less stressful interaction with the neonate and allows team members to gather information about the neonate's medical status and ability to maintain stability during interventions by eliciting self-regulatory behaviors.

Examining the medically stable infant may be more hands-on, letting the infant be the safety monitor. The physical therapist observes the infant's self-regulatory ability, postural and motoric activity presentation, interactive capabilities, and functional activities. During the hands-on examination, the therapist continues to monitor the infant's behavioral cues, which communicate the child's ability to tolerate the interaction. Many medically stable infants are on a steady path, progressing with feedings, gaining weight, and maturing. These infants often are termed "feeder growers." Although these infants typically are quiet and progressing well, just needing time to learn to take nutrition by mouth (PO feeding), to grow and develop, they continue to benefit from cluster care interactions. Cluster care intervention also may offer these infants periods of longer deep sleep, during which neuronal proliferation may be undisturbed.

TABLE 7-5. STATE-RELATED BEHAVIORS
• State 1: Deep sleep—eyes closed, regular respirations, no active movements
• State 2: Light sleep—eyes closed, rapid eye movements, small motor movements, no gross body movements
• State 3: Drowsy—eyes open or closed, quiet, diffuse movements but no gross motor movements
• State 4: Alert—eyes open, gross movement, not crying, able to focus on stimulation, taking in information
• State 5: Active awake—eyes open/closed, infant awake/aroused, fussy but not crying, not taking in information
• State 6: Crying—intense cry
Adapted from Brazelton TB. *Neonatal Behavioral Assessment Scale. Clinics in Developmental Medicine No. 50. Spastics International Medical Publications.* Philadelphia, PA: JB Lippincott Co; 1973.

Examination of the infant should occur when the infant is in a calm, awake state. Components of the examination include systems review, observation of posture at rest, quality and quantity of active movement patterns, reflexive patterns, passive range of motion, sensory processing, habituation patterns, tolerance to stress and self-regulatory patterns, oral-motor or PO readiness, and any special tests and measures.

Behavioral States of Alertness

During evaluation, the neonate's alertness and ability to transition between alert states should be noted. Brazelton defined 6 states of behavior in relation to wakefulness and sleep[38] (Table 7-5). Neonates less than 36 weeks' GA may not possess the ability to smoothly transition between the states of alertness.

As the neonate matures, the ability to sustain periods of alert and sleep behaviors increases and improved transitions may be noted between the various states. Assessed during interventions with the neonate are individual variability, what time of day is best for intervention, what procedures the neonate had prior to the examination, and whether there are any medical concerns that may alter the alert state.[36]

Systems Review

After gathering and organizing information from the chart on the history and current medical status, the physical therapist may begin the "hands-on" component of the examination. The system review may be a brief or limited examination but should include the following components:

> *Cardiovascular:* The assessment of heart rate, respiratory rate, oxygen saturations, blood pressure, and edema

> *Integumentary:* The assessment of risk for skin breakdown, skin condition, pliability (texture), presence of bruising or mottling, skin color, and skin integrity, potential equipment risks to skin

> *Musculoskeletal:* The assessment of symmetry, gross active and passive range of motion, gross strength, length, and weight

> *Neuromuscular:* A general assessment of gross movement patterns and appropriate gestational developmental motor function

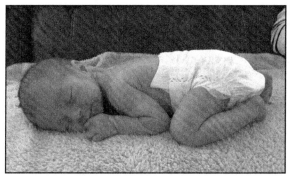

Figure 7-9. Full-term physiological flexion.

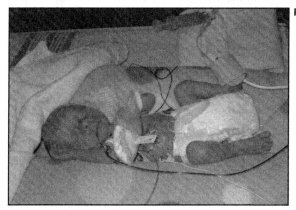

Figure 7-10. Supportive physiological flexion.

The systems review assists the physical therapist in identifying concerns and developing a plan of care that may require consultation with or referral to another health care team member. As the examination progresses, the physical therapist may identify additional concerns not uncovered by the history and systems review and may conclude that other specific tests and measures or portions of other specific tests and measures are required to obtain sufficient data to perform an evaluation, establish a diagnosis and a prognosis, and select interventions. The examination, therefore, must be dictated by the medical stability of the neonate.

Positioning

As mentioned previously, premature infants are born with immature muscle tone and present with less physiological flexion.[34,35] A full-term infant typically presents flexed with the arms close to midline, shoulders adducted and in neutral internal-external rotation, with elbows flexed and hands near the mouth. The hips are typically externally rotated and abducted with knees flexed and ankles dorsiflexed. The head, neck, trunk, and pelvis are tucked into flexion as well (Figure 7-9). When examining a preterm infant, the physical therapist assesses the child's ability to maintain flexion against gravity. Infants of younger GA will benefit from positioning to facilitate boundaries and supportive nesting into patterns of physiological flexion. Positioning should include supporting the proximal joints into flexion, adduction, and neutral internal/external rotation; hands close to the mouth; and ankles in dorsiflexion with supportive boundary for the feet to push off (Figure 7-10). If the infant is positioned in prone, the knees should be tucked under the pelvis so the infant is weight bearing through the knees and is not in excessive external rotation at the hips. In supine, the infant's head should be in midline to promote posterior occipital weight bearing, which assists in off-loading the parietal and temporal areas of the skull to facilitate rounding of the infant's head. Examining and evaluating an infant's ability to elicit and sustain physiological flexion is key to the ongoing assessment. Providing boundaries allows small ranges of resistive movements, simulating the movement opportunities that would have taken place in the intrauterine environment.

Commercial products are available that provide positioning into physiological flexion but have associated costs that depend on the hospital system's contractual agreements. These products provide a supportive "nesting" blanket for the infant while in any type of bed and are available in various sizes for positioning the ELBW infant, as well as the full-term infant. Baby blankets available in all NICUs may be used to provide unique positional support for any body part and can offer the supportive "nesting" boundaries for facilitation of physiological flexion. The physical therapist must assess the needs of the infant for body support both at the initial examination and throughout the stay in the NICU.

Another positional assessment is of the shape of the infant's head. The therapist may use the *cranial index ratio*, which is the caliper measurement of the widest transverse diameter of the head over the length of the head.[39] The cranial index or a visual observation of the cranium can be used to document any asymmetries. Preterm infants typically do not have the strength to rotate their head from side to side; therefore, they often spend long periods of time in side-lying with their head in a lateral position. With the weight of the head and the pressure of gravity, the infant's head may become bilaterally flattened on the lateral skull.[40] This cranial shape is referred to as *dolicho-cephaly*, which evidence has demonstrated causes an elongated anterior-posterior axis of the head. Dolichocephaly has been associated with delayed reaching skills, torticollis, and asymmetrical motor development.[39] Infants in the NICU also can develop an asymmetrical cranial shape, such as *plagiocephaly*, or asymmetrical posterior flattening, termed *brachycephaly*. The most common cranial molding concern of the less than 32 weeks' GA infant is dolichocephaly.[39] In 2017, McCarty et al[39] reported that the use of a commercial midliner positioning system was associated with fewer cranial molding concerns of dolichocephaly. Thus, in addition to facilitating physiological flexion in the infant, the therapist should recognize postural requirements and supportive boundaries for midline positioning of the head.

Reflexes, Muscle Tone, and Motor Patterns

Saint-Anne Dargassies[34] described neurological characteristics of fetal maturation from 20 to 41 weeks' GA, and considered muscle tone as the fundamental feature of the preterm infant's neurological assessment. Therapists and many other health care professionals continue to rely on her documentation of fetal resting posture and passive and active muscle tone for assessment of the neurological presentation of the infant. The Neurological Examination of the Preterm and Full-Term Infant provides the physical therapist a developmental framework to approach the assessment of reflexes, tonicity, and motor patterns in relation to each specific week in gestation. As each week of gestational maturation occurs, primitive reflex patterns emerge, muscle tonicity in relation to extensibility and consistency matures, physiological flexion develops, and active motor patterns become more purposeful.[34,35] The infant born before 32 weeks' GA presents with lower extremity flexor tone, flexor recoil, and primitive reflex patterns as compared with the upper extremities. Presentation of tone, reflex patterns, and deep tendon reflexes evolve in the lower extremities, then mature in a caudal-cephalic direction. Many reflex patterns, such as the asymmetrical tonic neck reflex (ATNR), may be observed in the lower extremities prior to the upper extremities. The preterm infant's inability to grow within the mother's uterus places the child at a disadvantage for developing physiological flexion. During the last month within the mother's uterus, the infant develops a flexion posture and experiences smaller resistive ranges of motions. The preterm infant developing outside the uterus is exposed to gravitational forces, has immature muscle tone, and is moving more frequently in an unrestricted environment, all factors that predispose the child to atypical postural and less functional motor patterns.[36,40]

When assessing the infant's posture, tone, and movements, it is best for the therapist to first observe the infant at rest, progressing to an interactive quiet, alert state, then make observations during routine cares, social interactions, and at feeding time.[4,5,15,16,18,39] The infant's presentation of muscle tone, posture, and motor patterns will be related to physiological stability. If an infant is struggling to maintain homeostasis, then resting posture and motor activity will be negatively affected, causing the infant to appear hypotonic, flaccid, or lethargic. The infant's tone and motor patterns also may be related to the state of alertness, previous interactions, and other stressors that may have occurred prior to the assessment.

As an infant awakens and interactions occur for scheduled care, the physical therapist observes the infant's nonvolitional and volitional movement patterns. Nonvolitional movement patterns are primitive reflex patterns, such as an ATNR or rooting reflex. To manually move an infant through a primitive reflex pattern assessment is too stressful for the premature or high-risk infant. "Handling" may cause the infant to "shut down" or possibly transition into a lower state of physiological functioning, such as dropping oxygen saturations or becoming bradycardic. Primitive reflex patterns are best observed when independently *generated* by the infant. Volitional movements of the infant are noted as well, such as hands to mouth, and pushing or extending the extremities. The therapist should note whether the volitional movements are cues by the infant for handling toleration or warning or stress cues. Any movement observed in the infant is assessed for quality and quantity. The reflexive patterns are documented using the reflex name and elicitation of side. Volitional movements are documented by what the movement pattern is, which side, and whether the movement is a self-regulatory pattern, warning cue, or stress cue. The therapist continually assesses the infant's maturation of muscle tone and motor patterns with each interaction, assessing for developmental progression and presence of consistent typical or atypical patterns and responses.

Tests and Measures

Tests and measures available for assessing the infant in the NICU are used to gather information about neurobehavioral and neurodevelopmental functioning. The neuromotor examination requires the infant to be in a calm, alert state prior to the administration of the test. Objective information gathered from tests and measures are used to assess an infant's change in motor function over time, to justify the need for developmental intervention, to determine intervention outcomes, and to identify the need for developmental follow-up and intervention after discharge from the NICU.[36,41] Tests and measures are available for data collection on pain, GA presentation, and neurological and neurobehavioral functioning. One examination tool is available for predicting motor behavior after discharge.

Pain Assessment

The Joint Commission requires assessment of neonatal pain with a standardized assessment scale.[36] Multiple tools are available for the assessment of pain in the neonate, with the most common being the Neonatal Infant Pain Scale; Neonatal-Pain, Agitation Sedation Scale; Scale of Face-Legs-Activity-Cry-Consolability; and Crying, Requirement of O_2, Increased Vital Signs, Expression, and Sleeplessness.[19,36,41-43] These scales provide the therapist an objective way to document the suspected pain level of the infant by observing facial and activity presentation, motor activity, and behavioral state. The pain level should be documented prior to, during, and after any examination or therapeutic intervention. The pain levels during each phase of the therapeutic intervention and the ability of the infant to soothe him- or herself or exhibit self-regulatory behavior provide the therapist crucial information about the child's ability to function within the environment related to his or her GA, medical status, and developmental activities.

One tool available to assess the neonate with NAS is the Finnegan,[44] which provides a comprehensive way to collect objective data on the infant's withdrawal symptoms. This tool divides the neonatal systems into 3 categories of system responsiveness to the opioid withdrawal: (1) the central nervous system; (2) the metabolic, vasomotor, and respiratory systems; and (3) the gastrointestinal and integumentary systems. (See Video 7-1.)

Preterm/Full-Term Tests and Measures

Standardized tools for preterm infants available include the Neurological Examination of the Preterm and Full-Term Infant; Neurobehavioral Assessment of the Preterm Infant; Neonatal Behavioral Assessment Scale (NBAS); Newborn Behavioral Observation System; Newborn Individualized Developmental Care and Assessment Program; Assessment of Preterm Infant Behavior; Assessment of General Movements; Hammersmith Infant Neurological Examination; and the Test of Infant Motor Performance.[19,36,41,45] These assessments all include handling of the infant, and it must always be determined whether the infant will be tolerant of the test administration.

Of the testing tools available, it is important to choose one that provides an objective measure of an infant's functioning over time; justification for the need for physical therapy services; assessment of the outcomes of intervention services; and identification of need for developmental or physical therapy follow-up programming, which will assist the infant and family post-NICU discharge.[19,36,41] The physical therapist may decide to use one, more than one, or portions of several specific tests and measures as part of the examination, based on the purpose of the examination, the complexity of the condition, and the clinical decision-making process. When administering a test, the therapist always considers the behavioral cues of the infant, asking: "Is this infant able to tolerate the handling required to complete this assessment?" The reader is referred to Chapter 2, which presents detailed information on several of these tests and measures that can be used in the NICU.

THERAPEUTIC INTERVENTIONS

Physical therapy interventions in the NICU typically are designed around 4 goals: (1) provide an appropriately sensory modulated environment, (2) encourage proper positioning postures for neuromusculoskeletal maturation, (3) offer movement opportunities for future participatory interactions, and (4) encourage infant-family interactions.[46-49] Therapeutic interventions should follow the team approach of cluster care and be reinforced during all interactions with the infant. Therapeutic interventions often include positioning, facilitative movement, skin-to-skin holding, massage, and specialized interventions such as feeding, splint fabrication, and wound care. The overall goal for physical therapy intervention is to promote positive sensorimotor interactions that will foster the self-regulatory behaviors required by the infant during maturation in the NICU, as well as those required for future participatory interactions.

When beginning an intervention with an infant, the physical therapist must adhere to the basic principle: When in doubt, do no harm.[9,36] The desired outcome of the intervention must be assessed for any potential undue stress to the infant. The therapist continuously assesses the infant's capability to self-regulate during the intervention, and monitors any delayed reactions from an intervention. For example, an infant may demonstrate apnea or bradycardia 30 to 60 minutes after an intervention. This delayed response of gestationally premature infants is commonly seen in the NICU population.

Physical therapy interactions begin with the concept of providing individualized care. As the therapist intervenes with the infant and family, observation and documentation of the infant's vital signs, state of alertness, pain level, positioning and postures, and self-regulatory behaviors before, during, and after the intervention are important. Documentation of objective data also may provide analyses of interventions and responses of the infant that might offer insight into evidence-based practices within the NICU.

Ross et al[48] reported that early therapy services in the NICU might optimize the outcome of infants admitted to a Level IV NICU. They reviewed occupational therapy, physical therapy, and speech-language pathology services to describe predictors of early therapy usage and to test the hypothesis that more NICU-based therapy would relate to better neurobehavioral outcomes. Of the 79 infants reviewed (born ≤ 32 weeks' GA), 100% received occupational and physical therapy and 51% received speech-language services.[48] The infants received 56 different therapeutic interventions. Whereas more therapy was not directly related to improved neurobehavioral outcomes, the researchers reported that infants with more complex medical issues received more therapy services. This descriptive study provided preliminary data for the identification of neonatal therapeutic interventions currently being implemented in a Level IV NICU; however, there were insufficient data to support specific therapeutic interventions.[48]

Specific Interventions

Therapeutic interventions of positioning, facilitated movement, skin-to-skin holding, and massage are 4 of the most typically implemented interventions and are used to assist the infant for participatory interactions, such as oral-motor readiness and feeding. Physical therapy interventions may play a key role in providing wound care and splint fabrication.

Positioning

The musculoskeletal system of a neonate in the NICU is placed under extreme forces by gravity, presents with generalized hypotonia, and has lost uterine constraints.[19,36,40] Positioning of the neonate is a standard of care that is implemented by all NICU team members. Sweeney and Gutierrez[40] reported fundamentals for musculoskeletal implications of preterm infant positioning. The authors state, "The primary goals of positioning are to support postures and movements, optimize skeletal development and biomechanical alignment, provide a controlled exposure to varied proprioceptive, tactile, and visual stimuli, and promote a calm, regulated behavioral state."[40] In addition to addressing generalized positional needs to reinforce postures of physiological flexion, physical therapists may be consulted regarding specialized positional needs for the infant who presents with a postural anomaly. Additional examples are to provide support during use of medical equipment or for behavioral patterns of unrest, as often occurs with the infant with NAS. Generally, positioning of the infant has a regular alternating pattern; prone, right side-lying, supine, and left side-lying. The alternating patterns are intended to prevent skin breakdown, promote development of the musculoskeletal system, improve head rounding, and aid in gaseous exchange in all lung fields.[36]

Therapists must be cautious when using positional devices that inhibit movement. An infant within the uterus experiences small resistive ranges of motion. The intrauterine infant has the ability to move the arms and legs within small ranges of flexion and extension patterns, and these movements are resisted by the amniotic fluid and uterine wall. Reproducing the small ranges of resistive motions may assist in the development of mechanoreceptors in the joint capsules and contribute to the proprioceptive sensory input. Offering movement opportunities may influence maturational joint shaping and facilitate future motor control required for participatory interactions during the first years of life and after.[19,36,40]

Facilitated Movement

Therapists may provide facilitated movement opportunities for infants, such as providing cephalocaudal input or facilitated tucking, and assistive range of motion patterns. The cephalocaudal input may be used during stressful procedures or during transitional periods of alert states.

Figure 7-11. Cephalocaudal proprioceptive input.

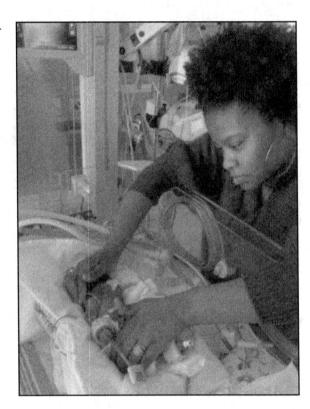

Hands are placed over the infant's cranium and the pelvis or lower part of the body to facilitate a tucked or flexed posture. The deep proprioceptive sensation offered through the cephalocaudal input is reported by experienced NICU caregivers to calm the infant. This handling technique may be provided during any phase of an infant's stay in the NICU and is often the first type of touch parents are shown with their baby (Figure 7-11). Another facilitated motion is providing assistive ranges of motion in specific patterns for promotion of self-regulation. Assisting the infant to move his or her hand to mouth for oral-motor stimulation will promote the ability to self-regulate. Any facilitation or assistive motor pattern may be taught to the family for carryover.[45,46] Spittle and colleagues,[47] in a Cochrane Review, reported that early interactions of the parents in active participation in the care of their infant may improve the infant-parent bond and improve child cognitive outcomes.

Skin-to-Skin Holding

Another intervention is "kangaroo care" or "skin-to-skin holding," which supports maternal bonding, milk production, and improved breastfeeding.[49,50] The practice of skin-to-skin holding involves placing the infant onto the mother or father's bare chest. The infant is placed prone between the breasts, and the parent holds the infant in a flexed posture, typically with 1 or 2 heated blankets over the infant. Research has shown that infants who are offered skin-to-skin holding demonstrate improved thermoregulation, respirations, and oxygenation; a decrease in apneic and bradycardic events; improved self-regulatory patterns; and an overall decrease in length of hospitalization.[49,50] Hospitals may have their own skin-to-skin protocols. Implementation of skin-to-skin holding may be dependent on the GA and the medical stability of the infant, and whether an infant is intubated or on continuous positive airway pressure. One benefit of skin-to-skin holding is the opportunity for the family to become more aware of the infant's physiological, behavioral, and motor responses. Parents who were offered skin-to-skin holding during their infant's NICU admission were reported to be more sensitive to the infant's behavioral cues and to feel more

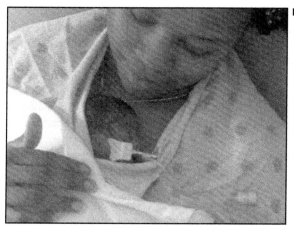

Figure 7-12. Skin-to-skin kangaroo care.

prepared to take care of him or her following discharge.[51] The physical therapist can foster skin-to-skin holding in the NICU by discussing benefits with team members and developing protocols for implementation (Figure 7-12).

Infant Massage

Infant massage is a widely used therapeutic intervention in the NICU. Studies conducted to evaluate the effectiveness of massage have suggested it promotes positive effects on the infant's ability to gain weight and on the immune system, improves tolerance to painful stimuli, improves self-regulatory behaviors, decreases hospital length of stay, and improves developmental outcomes.[52] A systematic review of massage with preterm infants by Niemi[53] revealed many of these studies were too small to determine a direct correlation, and further evidence is needed. However, many therapists working in the NICU report that infant massage fosters improved parental interactions and decreases parents' anxiety levels related to caring for the infant following discharge.

Implementation of infant massage always should begin with asking: "What is the desired outcome of the massage?" The goals may include facilitating calming behaviors, providing a specific massage for a restriction of motion, or a whole-body massage to assist the infant with transitions between states of alertness. Whatever the primary goal of the infant massage, the physical therapist must monitor the primary behavioral responses of the infant while implementing the massage. General guidelines for providing infant massage include (1) not massaging an infant prior to a PO feeding attempt because massage may induce a deeper sleep pattern and (2) allowing adequate time between the massage and feeding time because the gastric mobility facilitated by massage may lead to an emesis. Overall, there are many proposed positive effects of infant massage, and although many outcomes are not evidence based, negative effects have not been reported. Infant massage is a wonderful way for parents to provide hands-on care for their infant and allows them to participate in and learn their infant's behaviors for communication. These cues between the infant and parent will assist in child-parental bonding and thereby facilitate improved interactions after discharge.

Oral-Motor Facilitation/PO Feeding

One of the most important participatory goals for the infant in the NICU is to obtain nutrition through breastfeeding or nipple feeding with a bottle system. In the NICU, successful feeding by mouth is when the infant sucks, swallows, breathes, and maintains alertness to successfully ingest the required nutrition by breast or bottle system within a set time frame. An infant's ability to PO feed requires considerable oral-motor control and energy expenditure.

At 34 weeks' GA, the neurological system responsible for the controlled motor action of sucking-swallowing-breathing is just beginning to mature. Preterm infants born prior to 34 weeks' GA typically do not exhibit the oral-motor coordination or the endurance required to efficiently ingest the amount needed for nutritional support in a timely manner. Most infants younger than 35 to 36 weeks' GA will have a nasogastric or oral gastric tube inserted for nutritional intake. Infants in the NICU are offered oral-motor activity described as non-nutritive sucking (NNS) or sucking on a pacifier. Depending on the GA of the infant, NNS may facilitate oral-motor readiness for nipple feeding. Early NNS or oral-motor intervention should be included in the plan of care, but cautiously assessed in infants younger than 32 weeks' GA, as NNS may be stressful and elicit behavioral signs of instability. The NNS should be offered during infants' gavage feedings so they will associate the sucking motion (NNS) with stomach fullness. As the infants reach 35 to 37 weeks' GA, many receive bottle or breastfeeding at each scheduled feeding time. The physical therapist should coordinate intervention times around feedings.

Oral-motor control has been directly linked to neurodevelopmental outcomes.[54,55] Jadcherla et al reported that infants discharged on full PO feedings were associated with fewer long-term neurodevelopmental impairments as assessed with the Bayley Scales of Infant Motor Development at age 18 to 24 months.[56]

When the neonate reaches 32 to 34 weeks' postconceptual age, the physical therapist may provide therapeutic interventions in conjunction with a PO feeding. The therapist offering a PO feeding should have experience in feeding full-term medically stable infants and have received sufficient mentoring for feeding preterm infants. Knowledge of the normal progression of oral-motor maturational patterns and signs of feeding dysfunction is important and, when appropriate, referrals to a feeding specialist can be made.

Physical therapists play an integral role with oral-motor readiness and feeding activities. Feeding is an important time for fostering successful interactions between parents and infants. Early support to parents coping with infants having feeding difficulties increases parental competence in caregiving and commitment to participate in outpatient developmental monitoring. Parents of infants with feeding dysfunction have been reported as experiencing higher rates of anxiety. Physical therapists can assist in providing parents with positive intervention techniques during NNS and PO feeding. Assistance may be offered for proper positioning, handling, and oral-motor activities to promote a successful PO attempt. By reinforcing successful parental interactions during feeding, anxiety levels may lessen and feelings of competence increase. Evidence-based studies for infant-driven feedings are continuing to grow; however, the key to providing a feeding protocol must be embraced by all team members.[54,55] Infant-driven feedings are focused on the quality of the feeding experience by offering an oral feeding when the infant presents with oral-motor readiness cues.[54] The rehabilitative team, along with nursing, the lactation consultant, and the physician, should implement the infant-driven feeding program, which has been shown to improve feeding outcomes, lessen parental anxiety, and improve long-term neurodevelopmental outcomes.

Specialized Therapeutic Interventions

Physical therapists may provide additional interventions, such as wound care and splint fabrication. These interventions are considered to be advanced practice areas within the NICU. Working closely with a mentor or having access to a mentor to assist in clinical decision making for wound care and splinting options is recommended. Partnerships with the health care team members to develop skin integrity assessments, wound care interventions, and extremity splinting or taping techniques will help encourage evidence-based studies.

DISCHARGE PLANNING

Identifying postural needs, facilitating motor activities, fostering infant-parent education and interactions, and assessing the infant for future needs, as well as family needs, are key components of the physical therapist's role in the NICU. The physical therapist considers all the information about the infant and family from the time of admission throughout the NICU stay. To provide appropriate discharge recommendations, the therapist reviews the infant's history while in the NICU and assesses the infant prior to discharge in the following areas: postural and motor patterns, self-regulatory behaviors, GA, appropriate developmental presentation, participatory interactions such as PO feeding, and medical diagnoses. The neonate admitted to the NICU may qualify for state or federally funded programs, such as Social Security Administration, Medicaid, and/or early intervention programming through the Individuals with Disabilities Education Act. The medical social worker often is responsible for providing the family this information and obtains authorization for referrals prior to discharge. The physical therapist may recommend individualized physical therapy services to immediately follow discharge. Some diagnoses obtained during the NICU admission, such as intraventricular hemorrhage, HIE, NEC, or retinopathy of prematurity place the infant at a high risk for developmental delays. The key goal of discharge preparation is to offer the family educational information about their infant throughout the NICU admission and to reinforce the positive reasoning behind referrals. For example, many families do not fully understand the implications of an intraventricular hemorrhage diagnosis until closer to discharge. Working as a team to offer the family consistent, accurate, and meaningful information about their infant will reinforce understanding and importance of the many discharge referrals and future appointments that may be necessary.

NICU FOLLOW-UP CLINIC

Infants who have spent time in a NICU are at a high risk for developmental delays or disabilities. Studies have documented negative outcome diagnoses of high-risk infants, including tonicity changes, developmental delays, and behavioral concerns.[33,57,58] Most NICUs are associated with a neonatal follow-up program and offer an interdisciplinary approach to assessing the NICU graduate. NICU follow-up programs typically gather data for monitoring the outcomes for high-risk infants to determine the outcomes of NICU interventions and to determine whether referral for developmental intervention programming has taken place for the infant and family. Harris and Welch reported the typical neonatal criteria for the child to receive follow-up[9]:

> LBW (this can mean anything from below 2000 g to below 1250 g)
> Perinatal asphyxia, often determined by Apgar scores
> Infants requiring mechanical ventilation (the length of time on a respirator varies)
> Intrauterine growth retardation
> Neurological abnormality (seizures, abnormal muscle tone, intracranial hemorrhage, congenital or acquired hydrocephalus)
> Documented sepsis or meningitis
> Congenital anomalies, birth defects, and chromosome abnormalities
> Vision and hearing defects
> NAS or narcotic withdrawal
> Gastrointestinal abnormalities or prolonged feeding difficulties, which may lead to failure to thrive
> High-risk indicators of potential HIV infection

Physical therapists bring a unique strength to NICU follow-up programming by providing expertise in movement analysis and pediatric GA development to assist in identifying concerns and referral needs. The therapist offers specialized understanding of movement patterns and the identification of changes over time that may indicate the need for further intervention. Specific tests and measures to obtain developmental functional levels may be administered to determine appropriate referrals to early intervention programs or to recommend individualized therapy needs. Therapists participating in NICU follow-up programming may identify related community resources appropriate for the family and infant.

SUMMARY

The NICU is a wonderful environment where a physical therapist has the opportunity to assist with the growth and maturation of fragile infants born too soon. The therapist practicing in the NICU must recognize the NICU as an advanced practice area, and seek the mentoring and education needed to ensure competence in the required skills and knowledge for providing services to high-risk infants and their families. The therapist may examine, evaluate, intervene, and recommend specialized programming for infants and their families and is a key member of the neonatal health care team. The NICU team ensures that infants and families receive the most current evidence-based care to optimize outcomes. Being a part of the team that assists with the growth and maturation of these fragile infants, the physical therapist experiences relationships that will have a lifelong impact on the children, families, and therapist.

CASE STUDY #1: JASON

> *Medical Diagnosis:* Cerebral palsy, right hemiparesis
> *Gross Motor Function Classification System:* Level I
> *Age:* 24 months

History

Jason was the first born of nonidentical twins delivered by cesarean birth 8 weeks prematurely, (ie, 32 weeks' GA). His Apgar scores were 7 at 1 minute and 9 at 5 minutes. His birth weight, head circumference, and length were appropriate for GA. He did not require any mechanical ventilation at birth. A cranial ultrasound at age 3 days showed a left-sided germinal matrix hemorrhage with normal-sized ventricles. A follow-up ultrasound 1 week later, however, revealed complete reabsorption of the clot and normal ventricular size bilaterally.

Jason received physical therapy services throughout his NICU stay designed to facilitate physiological flexion (ie, "nesting"). Before oral-motor coordination for PO feeding developed, oral stimulation and NNS on a pacifier were provided during gavage feedings.

The NBAS initially was performed when Jason was age 3 weeks (35 weeks' postconceptional age). At that time, Jason demonstrated few self-calming strategies, such as NNS or hand-to-mouth activities, and his tendon reflexes generally were brisk. Jason's disorganized movement did not support his attempts at self-calming, such as hand to mouth and hand to face. He also had difficulty with positioning while in the NICU because of these diffuse disorganized movements, which were extensor dominant. He maintained his head tilted to the right, which placed him at risk for neck muscle tightness. Trunk incurvation was diminished slightly on the right. There was significant ankle clonus bilaterally, and he was jittery. He was on caffeine citrate, which was being used to control apnea and bradycardia spells that occurred, particularly during feeding. This medication has been noted to result in some generalized jitteriness and increased muscle tone in infants. Jason's visual focusing was minimal because of his apparent overstimulation in the NICU environment.

Jason was reevaluated by the physical therapist at age 7 weeks (39 weeks' postconception). At that time, the asymmetry was no longer apparent, but he continued to be difficult to calm and was jittery. Jason was discharged at age 40 days on caffeine citrate. No specific interventions were recommended at discharge, even though there were early, subtle, transient findings of asymmetry and jitteriness. The use of caffeine citrate creates difficulty in accurately assessing the neurological status. The majority of children who present with a history like Jason's develop normally. However, there have not been comprehensive long-term studies conducted to evaluate the outcome of therapeutic doses of caffeine.

The twins were seen in follow-up clinic at age 4 months (2 months' corrected GA). Jason had decreased strength in his flexor muscles and tended to overuse his extensor muscles, but this was felt to be due to his "prematurity." He continued to be irritable and preferred to hold his head to the right, but his examination was otherwise "normal."

The next visit was scheduled at Jason's 6-months-adjusted chronological age (8 months' true chronological age). At this time his mother remarked that Jason was "left handed." She also noted that Jason did not kick his right leg as frequently as his left. His mother remarked that Jason was more difficult to hold than his twin and that he didn't seem to mold to her body as easily. Jason's neurological examination was markedly asymmetrical, with a persistent ATNR to the right, fisting of the right hand with the thumb flexed in the palm, and 5 to 7 beats of ankle clonus on the right. The Bayley Scales of Infant Motor Development were administered by the physical therapist at this visit, but Jason was age appropriate when adjusted for prematurity.

The abnormal neurological findings were discussed with his parents, and a more complete neurological examination was recommended. Jason was referred for physical therapy intervention in their local community. Neurological abnormalities in children like Jason may not become obvious before age 6 to 9 months. For this reason, it is important for NICU follow-up clinics to monitor closely such infants and refer them for services as soon as abnormalities become apparent.

CASE STUDY #2: JILL

> *Medical Diagnosis:* Cerebral palsy, spastic quadriparesis, microcephaly, intellectual deficits, seizure disorder
> *Gross Motor Function Classification System:* Level V
> *Age:* 7 years

History

Jill was the product of a full-term, uncomplicated pregnancy. She was the first child for her 30-year-old mother. The delivery was very rapid and Apgar scores were 5 at 1 minute and 8 at 5 minutes. There were no initial problems and Jill was placed in the Well-Baby Newborn Nursery. The nurses in the nursery noted some unusual eye movements and occasional stiffening of Jill's extremities when she was age 4 hours. Jill was immediately transferred to the NICU and given a loading dose of phenobarbital. Her seizures continued, and several other antiseizure medications were added following an examination by the pediatric neurologist. The increase in medication resulted in respiratory depression, and Jill was placed on a respirator at age 12 hours (Figure 7-13). The electroencephalogram (EEG) was markedly abnormal at this time. Over the next several days, the seizures gradually subsided, medications were decreased, and Jill was weaned from the respirator. However, Jill had overall decreased responsiveness to her environment. Her alertness was poor as well as her orientation to stimuli. She exhibited a general startle response that included whole-body extension.

Figure 7-13. Jill on respirator.

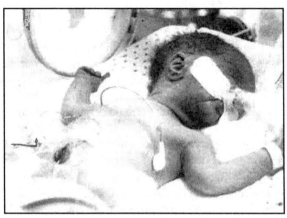

Initial physical therapy evaluation at age 5 days, using the NBAS and Dubowitz scales, revealed a sleepy child with generalized hypotonicity, absent suck, and diminished gag response. Over the next week, the speech-language pathologist developed a PO feeding plan of care with the physical therapist assisting the family during PO feeding attempts as well. Feeding techniques recommended by the physical therapist to the mother and nursing staff included allowing Jill a transitional period between alerting and bedside care needs, and the oral-motor attempt to either breastfeed or PO feed by bottle. During the intervention readiness time (ie, changing diaper, obtaining vital signs, and swaddling in blanket), the readiness cues were observed. The physical therapist recommended Jill be swaddled in a blanket with her hands in midline at the oral area, positioned in side-lying for PO feeding by bottle, and with no secondary sensory stimuli present. The recommendation was to use a pacifier between feedings to strengthen the oral-motor structures and endurance of NNS, as well as offering positioning in upright postures when Jill was alert. As Jill's PO feeding improved, her mother began working with the lactation consultant and was sent home breastfeeding and PO feeding as needed.

The physical therapist met with the parents, the pediatric neurologist, and the neonatologist to discuss long-term prognosis and program planning. A brainstem auditory evoked response test was administered because of neonatal seizures, and the response time was slightly delayed. An eye exam was recommended at age 2 months because Jill required assisted ventilation.

Prior to discharge, Jill's parents were instructed in positioning and handling techniques. Jill initially presented as a child with low muscle tone, but with potential for increased tone with time, which mandated close monitoring of her home program. The parents were given a handout discussing the use of toys to enhance visual and auditory skills. Jill's stay in the NICU was short, but she will need long-term programming. It is extremely important for the physical therapist working in the NICU to maintain good communication with community agencies providing therapy services. Because of her history of prolonged seizures and early feeding problems, Jill was referred for home-based physical therapy services when she was discharged.

When seen initially in follow-up clinic at age 4 months, Jill was a very irritable child, with generalized increased muscle tone. The parents reported Jill was difficult to hold because of her strong extensor pattern. Her extensor tone with a possible tongue thrust also made sucking on a bottle or on her pacifier frustrating for Jill and her parents. Jill also tended to keep her hands fisted with poor hands-to-face and hands-to-midline movements. Overall, she had decreased active movement in her head, trunk, and extremities. Jill's visual orientation and ability to focus were poor. At this visit, a decrease in her head growth was noted. The eye exam and a repeat brainstem auditory evoked response were normal. The need for continued therapy services as well as future needs were discussed, and the parents were referred to the local agency for early intervention and family support services.

Case Study #3: Taylor

> *Medical Diagnosis:* Myelomeningocele, repaired L1-2
> *Age:* 4 years

History

Taylor was born at full term and delivered by cesarean section because of fetal distress, breech presentation, and a lumbar myelomeningocele, which had been diagnosed prior to birth. At birth, he immediately was transferred to the NICU. After examining Taylor, the neurosurgeon explained to his parents the long-term implications of myelomeningocele, including paralysis, potential intellectual impairments , hydrocephalus, bowel and bladder dysfunction, and the need for long-term care, and many surgical procedures. They were given the option of an immediate operation, and they chose to have primary closure of the myelomeningocele.

Taylor was examined by the physical therapist prior to the surgery. He had 90-degree hip flexion contractures and knee flexion was limited to 60 degrees. He also had severe equinovarus deformities of both feet. There was no response to sensory input of touch, pressure, or pin prick on either lower extremity.

Following primary closure of the myelomeningocele, the physical therapist met with the parents to discuss the long-term rehabilitation goals for Taylor, including the good potential for assisted ambulation. The parents were instructed in range of motion techniques and advised regarding skin precautions because of the sensory loss. Emphasis was placed on developing good head and trunk control, upper extremity skills, maintaining lower extremity mobility, and intellectual skills. They were given a list of books on typical development that were available in the hospital parent library. They were encouraged to be aware of the positive aspects of Taylor's development and not concentrate solely on his diagnosis. Referral was made, with their permission, to the local spina bifida association, which had an excellent parent-to-parent support network. Referral also was made to early intervention and state services for children with special needs.

Three days following primary closure of the myelomeningocele, a bulging fontanelle was noted. Cranial ultrasound revealed enlarged ventricles, and a ventricular-peritoneal shunting was performed on day 5. Taylor continued to have severe apnea spells and was placed on a respirator. The neurosurgeon recommended an EEG to rule out seizures, and fortunately the EEG was normal. An Arnold-Chiari malformation was suspected as causing compression of the brainstem and the resultant apnea spells. At age 2 weeks, a surgical decompression of the posterior fossa was performed. The apnea improved and the respirator was discontinued, but Taylor continued to have apnea several times a day requiring stimulation to resume breathing.

Because of the medical concerns, little attention was paid to rehabilitation services. However, the foot deformities were being treated with serial casting by the orthopedist. During this time the physical therapist performed passive range of motion to Taylor's lower extremities and instructed parents and the nursing staff on range of motion and prone positioning to reduce hip flexion contractures. On the Infant Neurological International Battery, Taylor had an overall score that was in the abnormal range because of his hypotonic lower extremities. Suggestions for toys were given to the family to encourage them to address Taylor's need for normal sensory input.

The apnea spells continued and Taylor remained in the NICU for 4 months. Every attempt was made to provide a variety of sensorimotor experiences appropriate for his age that would not compromise his medical status (Figure 7-14).

Additionally, infant massage was taught to the parents and the nurses to increase tactile input. A specialized water mattress was used with Taylor to provide vestibular input that may have been lacking because of decreased movement in utero as well as in the external environment. Discharge plans were eventually made, with a cardiorespiratory monitor for home use. The

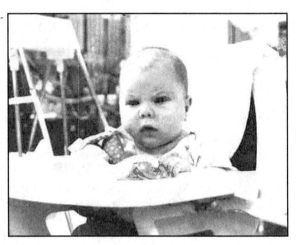

Figure 7-14. Four-month-old child in NICU experiences normal upright positioning.

need for continuing range of motion activities and observing Taylor's skin integrity was reviewed with the parents. He was referred to a physical therapist for home services once per week and to the myelomeningocele clinic at the local children's orthopedic hospital outpatient department. Because so many community services were available to this family, Taylor was not scheduled to return to the NICU follow-up clinic.

CASE STUDY #4: ASHLEY

- › *Medical Diagnosis:* Down syndrome
- › *Age:* 15 months

History

Ashley was the first child born to a 26-year-old woman. The pregnancy was uncomplicated, and Ashley was born full term. Characteristics of DS were noted in the baby at the time of delivery. She was transferred to the NICU because of a heart murmur. Cardiac echogram revealed a rather large ventricular septal defect. On further examination, an esophageal atresia was noted. Primary repair of the esophageal atresia was not possible, and a gastrostomy was performed. No oral feedings were permitted. However, Ashley had a fair suck on a pacifier, and this was encouraged.

Activities suggested to Ashley's parents included positioning in various ways: skin-to-skin in prone and other upright positions with as little support as necessary to enhance head and trunk control, prone to encourage head control and upper extremity weight bearing, and side-lying to encourage hands together and hand-to-mouth activities (Figure 7-15).

There is no contraindication to prone positioning in a child with a gastrostomy. After the first week postoperatively, these children can be positioned safely in prone. Most children do not require any special devices for prone positioning, but for those who do, a small cutout in a foam rubber block or wedge to accommodate the tube is sufficient. The earlier these children are placed in prone positioning, the easier it is for them, their parents, and the nursing staff. Other suggestions given to Ashley's parents included wrist rattlers and bells on her hands and feet to encourage movement, water toys to encourage movement against the resistance of water, holding her while in a rocking chair, use of a baby swing for vestibular input, and olfactory input with pleasant odors (cinnamon, cherry) during NNS.

Ashley was discharged from the hospital at age 6 weeks. Because of concerns regarding medical complications, the family refused to become involved with an early intervention program. They

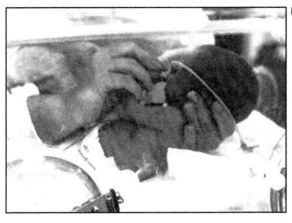

Figure 7-15. Facilitating hand to mouth.

were unwilling to follow a program of activities suggested to enhance motor development. They had many toys for Ashley, but these were used generally to provide visual and auditory stimulation and not movement.

At age 6 months, the esophageal atresia was repaired. At age 8 months, the heart defect was surgically corrected. At age 10 months, the family consented to become involved with an early intervention program. When Ashley finally was evaluated by the physical therapist, she was age 10 months and very hypotonic even for a child with DS. She was prop-sitting momentarily (ie, using upper extremities for support), had moderate head lag when pulled to sit, and would bear minimal weight on her legs. Ashley had many ear infections and finally received pressure equalizing tubes at 12 months of age. She had a mild conductive hearing loss.

In children such as Ashley, with complex medical problems, the family may not be willing or able to participate even in nonstressful therapeutic activities. All their energy is concentrated on the child's acute medical needs. Experience has shown that these families will eventually recognize the need for physical therapy services, as the child's developmental delays becomes more apparent and the child grows larger as well as more difficult to handle. It is important to continue to reinforce the need for physical therapy services for the child. Often the best way to do this is for the primary physician or a specialist (eg, cardiologist) to suggest programming to the family, because they will continue to see these children on a regular basis. The physical therapist in the NICU as well as those in the community must keep physicians informed regarding the need for developmental physical therapy services and their availability.

CASE STUDY #5: JOHN

> *Medical Diagnosis:* Developmental coordination disorder/attention-deficit hyperactivity disorder
> *Age:* 5 years

History

John was born at 36 weeks' GA to a 34-year-old mother. His Apgar scores were 8 at 1 minute and 10 at 5 minutes. He spent a short time in the NICU before being discharged to home, but with no major medical problems noted at the time of birth or after birth. Many children who are later diagnosed with developmental coordination disorder have a history of prematurity but no abnormal neurological signs as infants. He was not referred for early intervention services at the time of discharge from the NICU.

REFERENCES

1. Lawson K, Daum C, Turkewitz G. Environmental characteristics of a neonatal intensive care unit. *Child Dev.* 1977;48(4):1633-1639. doi:10.1111/j.1467-8624.1977.tb03974.x.

2. Avery ME. Pioneers and modern ideas. Neonatology. *Pediatrics.* 1998;102(1 pt 3):270-271.

3. Academy of Pediatric Physical Therapy. Neonatal physical therapy practice: roles and training. http://pediatricapta.org/includes/fact-sheets/pdfs/13/20Neonatal/20Fact/20Sheet.pdf. 2013. Accessed March, 2018.

4. Sweeney JK, Heriza CB, Reilly MA, Smith C, VanSant AF. Practice guidelines for the physical therapist in the neonatal intensive care unit (NICU). *Pediatr Phys Ther.* 1999;11(3):119-132. doi:10.1097/00001577-199901130-00002.

5. Sweeney JK, Heriza CB, Blanchard Y; American Physical Therapy Association. Neonatal physical therapy. Part I: clinical competencies and neonatal intensive care unit clinical training models. *Pediatr Phys Ther.* 2009;21(4):296-307. doi:10.1097/PEP.0b013e3181bf75ee.

6. Sweeney JK, Heriza CB, Blanchard Y, Dusing SC. Neonatal physical therapy. Part II: practice frameworks and evidence-based practice guidelines. *Pediatr Phys Ther.* 2010;22(1):2-16. doi:10.1097/PEP.0b013e3181cdba43.

7. Rapport MJ. A descriptive analysis of the role of physical and occupational therapists in the neonatal intensive care unit. *Pediatr Phys Ther.* 1992;4(4):172-178. doi:10.1097/00001577-199200440-00003.

8. American Academy of Pediatrics Committee on Fetus and Newborn. Levels of neonatal care. *Pediatrics.* 2012;130(3):587-597. doi:10.1542/peds.2012-1999.

9. Harris MH, Welch R. Physical therapy in the neonatal intensive care unit. In: Connolly BH, Montgomery PC, eds. *Therapeutic Exercise for Children with Developmental Disabilities.* 3rd ed. Thorofare NJ: SLACK Incorporated; 2005:157-188.

10. Steiner WA, Liliane R, Huber E, Uebelhart D, Aeschlimann A, Stucki G. Use of the ICF model as a clinical problem-solving tool in physical therapy and rehabilitation medicine. *Phys Ther.* 2002;82(11):1098-1107. doi: 10.1093/ptj/82.11.1098.

11. Malusky SK. A concept analysis of family-centered care in the NICU. *Neonatal Netw.* 2005;24(6):25-32. doi:10.1891/0730-0832.24.6.25.

12. Institute for Patient and Family Centered Care. Principles of the FCC model. www.ipfcc.org. Accessed January 2018.

13. Als H. Toward a synactive theory of development: promise for the assessment and support of infant individuality. *Infant Ment Health J.* 1982;3(4):229-243. doi:10.1002/1097-0355(198224)3:4<229::AID-IMHJ2280030405>3.0.CO;2-H.

14. Cleveland LM. Parenting in the neonatal intensive care unit. *J Obstet Gynecol Neonatal Nurs.* 2008;37(6):666-691. doi:10.1111/j.1552-6909.2008.00288.x.

15. Als H. A synactive model of neonatal behavioral organization: framework for the assessment of neurobehavioral development in the premature infant and for support of infants and parents in the neonatal intensive care environment. *Phys Occup Ther Pediatr.* 1986;6(3-4):3-53. doi:10.1080/J006v06n03_02.

16. Als H, Lawhon G, Duffy FH, McAnulty GB, Gibes-Grossman R, Blickman JG. Individualized developmental care for the very low-birth-weight preterm infant. Medical and neurofunctional effects. *JAMA.* 1994;272(11):853-858. doi:10.1001/jama.1994.03520110033025.

17. Als H, Gikerson L. Developmentally supportive care in the neonatal intensive care unit. *Zero to Three.* 1995;15(6):1-10.

18. Als H, Butler S, Kosta S, McAnulty G. The assessment of preterm infants' behavior (APIB): furthering the understanding and measurement of neurodevelopmental competence in preterm and full-term infants. *Ment Retard Dev Disabil Res Rev.* 2005;11(1):94-102. doi:10.1002/mrdd.20053.

19. Sweeney JK, Gutierrez T, Beachy JC. Neonates and parents: neurodevelopmental perspectives in the neonatal intensive care unit and follow-up. In: Umphred DA, Lazaro RT, Roller ML, Burton GU, eds. *Neurological Rehabilitation.* 6th ed. St. Louis, MO: Mosby Elsevier; 2013:271-316.

20. Engle WA; American Academy of Pediatrics. Age terminology during the perinatal period. 2004;114(5):1362-1364. doi:10.1542/peds.2004-1915.

21. Glass H, Costarino AT, Stayer SA, Brett C, Cladis F, Davis PJ. Outcomes of extremely premature infants. *Anesth Analg.* 2015;120(6):1337-1351. doi:10.1213/ANE.0000000000000705.

22. Sharma D, Shastri S, Sharma P. Intrauterine growth restriction: antenatal and postnatal aspects. *Clin Med Insights Pediatr.* 2016;10:67-83. doi:10.4137/CMPed.S40070.

23. Centers for Disease Control and Prevention. *Births in the United States, 2016. NCHS Data Brief.* 2017;287.

24. Asztalos EV, Church PT, Riley P, Fajardo C, Shah PS; Canadian Neonatal Network and Canadian Neonatal Follow-up Network Investigators. Neonatal factors associated with a good neurodevelopmental outcome in very preterm infants. *Am J Perinatol.* 2017;34(4):388-396. doi:10.1055/s-0036-1592129.

25. Lakshmanan A, Agni M, Lieu T, et al. The impact of preterm birth <37 weeks on parents and families: a cross-sectional study in the 2 years after discharge from the neonatal intensive care unit. *Health Qual Life Outcomes.* 2017;15(1):38. doi:10.1186/s12955-017-0602-3.

26. Craciunoiu O, Holsti L. A systematic review of the predictive validity of neurobehavioral assessments during the preterm period. *Phys Occup Ther Pediatr.* 2017;37(3):292-307. doi:10.1080/01942638.2016.1185501.

27. Johnson SH. *High-Risk Parenting: Nursing Assessment and Strategies for the Family at Risk.* Philadelphia, PA: JB Lippincott; 1979.

28. Tolia VN, Patrick SW, Bennett MM, et al. Increasing incidence of the neonatal abstinence syndrome in U.S. neonatal ICUs. *New Engl J Med.* 2015;372(22):2118-2126. doi:10.1056/NEJMsa1500439.

29. Jia W, Lei X, Dong W, Li Q. Benefits of starting hypothermia treatment within 6 h vs. 6-12 h in new-borns with moderate neonatal hypoxic-ischemic encephalopathy. *BMC Pediatr.* 2018;18(1):50. doi.10.1186/s12887-018-1013-2.

30. Higgins RD, Shankaran S. Hypothermia: novel approaches for premature infants. *Early Hum Dev.* 2011;87(suppl 1):S17-S18. doi:10.1016/j.earlhumdev.2011.01.004.

31. Natarajan G, Pappas A, Shankaran S. Outcomes in childhood following therapeutic hypothermia for neonatal hypoxic-ischemic encephalopathy (HIE). *Semin Perinatol.* 2016;40(8):549-555. doi:10.1053/j.semperi.2016.09.007.

32. Rothstein JM, Echternach JL, Riddle DL. The Hypothesis-Oriented Algorithm for Clinicians II (HOAC-II): a guide for patient management. *Phys Ther.* 2003;83(5):455-470. doi:10.1093/ptj/83.5.455.

33. Glass HC, Costarino AT, Stayer SA, Brett C, Cladis F, Davis PJ. Outcomes for extremely premature infants. *Anesth Analg.* 2015;120(6):1337-1351. doi:10.1213/ANE.0000000000000705.

34. Dargassies SS. *Neurological Development in the Full-Term and Premature Neonate.* Amsterdam, Netherlands: Experta Medica; 1977.

35. Prechtl H, Beintema D. *The Neurological Examination of the Newborn Infant.* Clinics in Developmental Medicine, 12. London, UK: Heinemann Educational Books; 1964.

36. Versaw-Barnes D, Wood A. The infant at high risk for developmental delay. In: Tecklin JS, *Pediatric Physical Therapy.* 5th ed. Baltimore, MD: Lippincott Williams & Wilkins; 2015:103-186.

37. Coughlin M. Guidelines for protective sleep. In: *Trauma-Informed Care in the NICU: Evidence-Based Practice Guidelines for Neonatal Clinicians.* New York, NY: Springer; 2017:137-161.

38. Brazelton TB. *Neonatal Behavioral Assessment Scale. Clinics in Developmental Medicine No. 50. Spastics International Medical Publications.* Philadelphia, PA: JB Lippincott Co; 1973.

39. McCarty DB, O'Donnell S, Goldstein RF, Smith PB, Fisher K, Malcolm WF. Use of a midliner positioning system for prevention of dolichocephaly in preterm infants. *Pediatr Phys Ther.* 2018;30(2):126-134. doi:10.1097/PEP.0000000000000487.

40. Sweeney JK, Gutierrez T. Musculoskeletal implications of preterm infant positioning in the NICU. *J Perinat Neonatal Nurs.* 2002;16(1)58-70. doi:10.1097/00005237-200206000-00007.

41. McManus B, Blanchard Y, Dusing S. The neonatal intensive care unit. In: Palisano RJ, Orlin M, Schreiber J. *Campbell's Physical Therapy for Children.* 5th ed. St. Louis Missouri: Elsevier; 2017:672-702.

42. Hillman BA, Tabrizi MN, Gauda EB, Carson KA, Aucott SW. The neonatal pain, agitation and sedation scale and the bedside nurse's assessment of neonates. *J Perinatol.* 2015;35(2):128-131. doi:10.1038/jp.2014.154.

43. O'Neal K, Olds D. Differences in pediatric pain management by unit types. *J Nurs Scholarsh.* 2016;48(4):378-386. doi:10.1111/jnu.12222.

44. Maguire D, Cline GJ, Parnell L, Tai CY. Validation of the Finnegan Neonatal Abstinence Syndrome Tool-short form. *Adv Neonatal Care.* 2013;13(6):430-437. doi:10.1097/ANC.0000000000000033.

45. Dusing SC, Murray T, Stern M. Parent preferences for motor development education in the neonatal intensive care unit. *Pediatr Phys Ther.* 2008;20(4):363-368. doi:10.1097/PEP.0b013e31818add5d.

46. Pineda R, Guth R, Herring A, Reynolds L, Oberle S, Smith J. Enhancing sensory experiences for very preterm infants in the NICU: an integrative review. *J Perinatol.* 2017;37(4):323-332. doi: 10.1038/jp.2016.179.

47. Spittle AJ, Doyle LW, Boyd RN. A systematic review of the clinimetric properties of neuromotor assessments for preterm infants during the first year of life. *Dev Med Child Neurol.* 2008;50(4):254-266. doi:10.1111/j.1469-8749.2008.02025.x.

48. Ross K, Heiny E, Conner S, Spener P, Pineda R. Occupational therapy, physical therapy and speech-language pathology in the neonatal intensive care unit: patterns of therapy usage in a level IV NICU. *Res Dev Disabil.* 2017;64:108-117. doi:10.1016/j.ridd.2017.03.009.

49. Anderson G. Kangaroo care and breastfeeding for preterm infants. *Breastfeeding Abstracts.* 1989;9(2):7.

50. Nunes CRDN, Campos LG, Lucena AM, et al. Relationship between the use of kangaroo position on preterm babies and mother-child interaction upon discharge. *Rev Paul Pediatr.* 2017;35(2):136-143. doi:10.1590/1984-0462/;2017;35;2;00006.

51. Feldman R, Weller A, Sirota L, Eidelman AI. Testing a family intervention hypothesis: the contribution of mother-infant skin-to-skin contact (kangaroo care) to family interaction, proximity, and touch. *J Fam Psychol.* 2003;17(11):94-107. doi:10.1037/0893-3200.17.1.94.

52. Porreca A, Parolin M, Bozza G, Freato S, Simonelli A. Infant massage and quality of early mother-infant interactions: are there associations with maternal psychological wellbeing, marital quality, and social support? 2017;7:2049. doi:10.3389/fpsyg.2016.02049.

53. Niemi AK. Review of randomized controlled trials of massage in preterm infants. *Children (Basel).* 2017;4(4). doi:10.3390/children4040021.

54. Ross ES, Philbin MK. Supporting oral feeding in fragile infants: an evidence-based method for quality bottle-feedings of preterm, ill, and fragile infants. *J Perinat Neonatal Nurs.* 2011;25(4):349-357; quiz 358-359. doi:10.1097/JPN.0b013e318234ac7a.

55. Philbin MK, Ross ES. The SOFFI Reference Guide: text, algorithms, and appendices: a manualized method for quality bottle-feedings. *J Perinat Neonatal Nurs.* 2011;25(4):360-380. doi:10.1097/JPN.0b013e31823529da.

56. Jadcherla SR, Khot T, Moore R, Malkar M, Gulati IK, Slaughter JL. Feeding methods at discharge predict long-term feeding and neurodevelopmental outcomes in preterm infants referred for gastrostomy evaluation. *J Pediatr.* 2017;181(2):125-130.e1. doi:10.1016/j.jpeds.2016.10.065.

57. Nwabara O, Rogers C, Inder T, Pineda R. Early therapy services following neonatal intensive care unit discharge. *Phys Occup Ther Pediatr.* 2007,37(4):414-424. doi:10.1080/01942638.2016.1247937.

58. O'Shea TM, Allred EN, Kuban KC, et al. Intraventricular hemorrhage and developmental outcomes at 24 months of age in extremely preterm infants. *J Child Neurol.* 2012;27(1):22-29. doi:10.1177/0883073811424462.

The Influence of Oral, Pharyngeal, and Respiratory Functions

Rona Alexander, PhD, CCC-SLP, BCS-S, C/NDT

All pediatric therapists must recognize the influence that oral, pharyngeal, and respiratory processes have on the functional activities an infant or child participates in each day. The earliest coordination of oral, pharyngeal, and respiratory function will keep an infant from aspirating when swallowing during bottle drinking and breastfeeding. What if an infant or child has a chronic pulmonary system disease; neuromuscular system impairments that limit or restrict oral movements, pharyngeal movements, or respiratory musculature activity; or structural and alignment issues of the mouth, pharynx, upper airway, or thoracic cage? What if sensory system impairments limit awareness of food, liquid, or saliva in the oral cavity or pharynx during feeding or the child exhibits overresponsiveness of the tongue, jaw, or cheeks/lips to texture or temperature changes in food, liquid, or feeding utensils brought to or into the mouth? Any of these primary neuromuscular, musculoskeletal, respiratory, and sensory systems impairments can lead to secondary impairments that may result in functional limitations and participation restrictions in a wide variety of activities including eating, drinking, sound/speech production, communication, walking, running, dressing, reaching for toys, climbing stairs, and play.

This chapter will present information specifically relevant to the evaluation and treatment of oral, pharyngeal, and respiratory activity during feeding/swallowing and respiratory-phonatory-sound production functions because of their intimate relationship to and effect on general movement development. However, it is important to recognize that comprehensive evaluation and treatment of children in the areas of receptive language, expressive language, cognition, and oral, pharyngeal, and respiratory coordination functions for feeding/swallowing and speech production/communication also may be needed. This type of comprehensive intervention requires the specialized knowledge and experience of a qualified speech-language pathologist to develop an appropriate plan of care.

Connolly BH, Montgomery PC, eds. *Therapeutic Exercise for Children With Developmental Disabilities, Fourth Edition* (pp 211-238).
© 2020 Taylor & Francis Group.

Typical Oral, Pharyngeal, and Respiratory Development

To provide comprehensive pediatric evaluation and treatment services, the pediatric therapist must understand the changes that occur in typical oral, pharyngeal, and respiratory function during the first year of life as the baby participates in feeding and swallowing, respiratory-pho-natory-sound production, and general movement activities.[1-8] From birth, the typical full-term infant uses the oral, pharyngeal, laryngeal, esophageal, and respiratory mechanisms for feeding, swallowing, breathing, crying, sound production, and sensory exploration. Liquids presented by breast or bottle are ingested using a negative-pressure sucking pattern. This sucking pattern, composed of negative pressure both in the oral and oropharyngeal areas, is created by a combination of jaw, tongue, and cheek/lip activity. This oral and pharyngeal activity is directly related to the newborn's physiological flexion, body alignment, small intraoral space, short and more limited in diameter pharyngeal area, the elevated and close approximation of the structures in the pharynx, the short length of the head/neck musculature, and the elevated and compact thoracic cage (ie, rib cage and shoulder girdle complex). The newborn can breathe through the nose and suck simultaneously, as liquids are pumped back through the nipple passing around the sides of the epiglottis and directly into the esophagus. During the swallowing process, upper airway protection is provided by brief closure of the vocal folds in the high-positioned laryngeal area, which is protected by the hyoid cartilage, pharyngeal musculature, and the close approximation of the uvula and epiglottis (Figure 8-1).

As the infant begins to turn and lift the head with extension against gravity, the influence of physiological flexion on the mouth is reduced and the jaw biomechanically opens, resulting in wider ranges of jaw and tongue activity. Suckling now becomes the active oral pattern of the infant and is composed of large up/down and forward/backward movements of the jaw and large, rhythmical, forward and backward movements of a thin, cupped tongue. As the sucking pads in the cheeks provide stability to the cheek musculature, there is minimal muscle activity occurring in the cheeks and lips. Oral movements for sucking still will occur when the infant is held with his or her head in a more stable, flexed position by the feeder during breastfeeding or bottle drinking.

The newborn's respiratory function at rest is characterized by obligatory nasal breathing and an open pharyngeal airway. There is close approximation of the back of the tongue to the soft palate. The thoracic cage (ie, rib cage and shoulder girdle complex) is elevated within the trunk with the upper ribs (ribs 1 to 6), which are directly connected to the sternum anteriorly and the thoracic vertebrae posteriorly, at almost a 90-degree angle to the spine. This elevated thoracic cage and the shortened neck musculature provide stability, supporting the musculature of the oral, pharyngeal, and laryngeal mechanisms.

The skeletal framework of the rib cage is limited in its joint mobility (ribs to thoracic vertebrae, ribs to sternum, and within the sternum and the thoracic spine) and range of active movements (Figure 8-2). Although its skeletal framework is cartilaginous, the rib cage of the newborn generally must serve as a more stable structure to support the activity of the muscle fibers of the diaphragm, which attach within the lower rib cage during respiration. The rib cage stability comes from the newborn's physiological flexion, elevated thoracic cage alignment, lack of joint mobility, and shortened musculature, both within the rib cage (eg, intercostals and levatores costarum) and surrounding the rib cage through the chest wall musculature (eg, anterior chest wall muscles, neck muscles, shoulder girdle musculature, and the latissimus dorsi).

On inhalation, abdominal or belly breathing occurs as the muscle fibers of the diaphragm contract and its central tendon lowers, causing expansion of the abdominal wall and expansion and lifting up of the lower ribs. With effortful crying, movement, or stress, strong contraction of the diaphragm may pull the cartilaginous anterior ribs and sternum downward and posteriorly

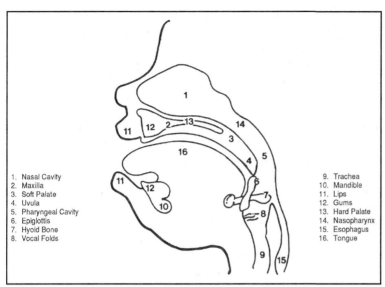

Figure 8-1. Diagram of the full-term newborn's oral and pharyngeal areas.

1. Nasal Cavity
2. Maxilla
3. Soft Palate
4. Uvula
5. Pharyngeal Cavity
6. Epiglottis
7. Hyoid Bone
8. Vocal Folds
9. Trachea
10. Mandible
11. Lips
12. Gums
13. Hard Palate
14. Nasopharynx
15. Esophagus
16. Tongue

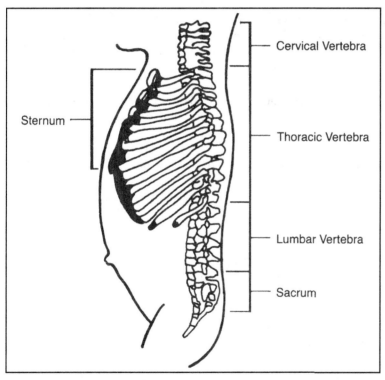

Figure 8-2. Diagram of the full-term infant's rib cage.

Cervical Vertebra

Sternum

Thoracic Vertebra

Lumbar Vertebra

Sacrum

toward the spine while expanding the abdominal wall and pulling the lower ribs upward and outward. This active lower rib expansion often is referred to as "rib flaring" and is seen with belly breathing.

A direct relationship exists between phonation/sound production and body movement starting at birth and continuing until approximately age 8 to 9 months. Sounds are produced spontaneously on expiration, and crying is nasal in quality. Short-duration and low-intensity vegetative sounds are produced by the young infant, especially during feeding when oral and pharyngeal sensory and movement experiences are being stimulated.

The infant's development of greater postural control, alignment, and movement throughout the first year of life establishes a foundation on which a greater variety of oral, pharyngeal, rib cage/respiratory, phonatory, and sound production activities can be experienced. These changes in oral, pharyngeal, and rib cage/respiratory function influence not only feeding, swallowing, sound production, and communication, but have direct influences on general movement and shoulder girdle/upper extremity development and function. This is apparent in the development of neck elongation as the thoracic cage descends and elongates in the trunk and in the development of well-controlled head and neck flexion, which depends on the active use of the suprahyoid and infrahyoid muscles that have primary control of jaw, tongue, and hyoid movements.

Developmental changes in the respiratory system have a profound effect on general movement, as well as on oral, feeding/swallowing, and respiratory-phonatory function. As the child of age 3 to 5 months begins to use the abdominal musculature in supine, starting with the rectus abdominus, and is supported passively upright against gravity in sitting, the ribs are drawn downward, creating an angle between the ribs and spine of less than 90 degrees. The contour of the rib cage also changes, allowing the scapulae to stabilize on the posterior rib cage and the shoulder girdle complex to begin to change in its alignment on the upper rib cage. Greater joint mobility and elongation and stabilization of the rib cage by the abdominals (ie, internal and external abdominal obliques) in a more downward direction will gradually modify the 3-dimensional contour and alignment of the rib cage. The intercostals and levatores costarum will be prepared for future active use in more adult abdominal/thoracic respiratory functioning. Abdominal, pelvis, and hip musculature activities will provide the musculature of the head, neck, shoulder girdle, mouth, and pharynx with a base of stability from which more integrated, controlled movements can be developed.

As the rib cage angles downward and then begins to elongate and increase in its mobility, the diaphragm within the lower rib cage begins to change in its alignment and activation. Full activation of the muscle fibers of the diaphragm occurs as the muscle fibers of the diaphragm elongate and then activate as the infant learns to move in sagittal, frontal, and transverse planes of movement.

Oral and pharyngeal movement development is affected by a variety of factors, including growth, contour, and alignment changes; the introduction of new varieties of oral and pharyngeal sensory stimulation (eg, pureed foods, solids, new tastes, toys, and feeding utensils); the child's new active coordinated movements in supine, prone, side-lying, and sitting; and changes in rib cage and respiratory function. The 6-month-old child reflects the interaction of these factors in the use of the cheeks, lips, and tongue in bottle drinking or breastfeeding for more active coordinated negative-pressure sucking. However, the wider range of movements that comprise suckling continue to predominate in spoon feeding and the introduction of cup drinking, facial expression, and phonation/sound production. Although solid food generally will be handled using sucking or suckling movements of the tongue, jaw, and cheek/lips, some new movements of the tongue and jaw may appear as a munching pattern develops and as biting and holding on solid foods using the biting surfaces of the gums or new teeth may occur. Sound production will modify to include a greater variety of vowels and consonants with changes in duration, loudness, intonation, and vocal quality.

By age 10 to 12 months, the child has grown in height and weight and has developed more highly coordinated and controlled general movement abilities incorporating this changing body size and alignment. This new level of postural control, alignment, and movement primarily reflects the multisystem interactions of the neuromuscular, musculoskeletal, and sensory body systems. However, interactions with changes in the child's respiratory, gastrointestinal, cardiovascular, and perceptual/cognitive systems also have a great influence on the child's body movement experiences and development.

These changes in postural control, alignment, and movement establish the foundation from which more coordinated and efficient oral, pharyngeal, and rib cage/respiratory musculature activity can be produced and integrated into function. Isolated, controlled movements of the jaw, tongue, cheeks, and lips for sucking and fine coordination of these movements with breathing are now predominant in bottle drinking, breastfeeding, and spoon feeding. Greater sucking activity is evident in cup drinking, although large vertical ranges of jaw activity often are compensated for by use of tongue protrusion under the cup or by biting on the cup rim for stability. Some children may use a cup with a short, attached straw to drink liquids with varying abilities in the organization of their oral, pharyngeal, and respiratory activity with the speed and volume of the liquid flow. The tongue exhibits lateral movements as it transfers and maintains food on the side biting surfaces in coordination with lip and cheek musculature activity during chewing. The jaw uses a variety of up and down, diagonal, and circular-diagonal movements as it breaks up the solid food in preparation for swallowing; however, the strength of the child's biting and chewing still affects the types of solids that can be eaten safely. Greater abdominal, lower back, pelvic, and hip musculature activity to connect the lower rib cage to the pelvis and hips now results in greater instances of rib cage expansion on inhalation without lower rib flaring. Longer, more sustained exhalation to support changes in sound production and in respiratory coordination with all general movement and feeding activities also results.

Impairments That Affect Oral, Pharyngeal, and Respiratory Function

Infants who begin life with a suspected or diagnosed pathophysiology often will exhibit issues that influence their oral, pharyngeal, and respiratory function. The types and severity of involvement will result in impairments of the neuromuscular, musculoskeletal, sensory, perceptual/cognitive, respiratory, cardiovascular, or gastrointestinal systems. The oral and pharyngeal mechanisms are structurally within the respiratory and gastrointestinal systems and can therefore be directly influenced by impairments anywhere within these systems or resulting from the interactions of these systems. Impairments in the neuromuscular, musculoskeletal, or sensory systems may directly or indirectly influence oral and pharyngeal sensory responsiveness and movement activities. These impairments also may influence upper and lower respiratory system alignment, musculature activity, and coordination with the gastrointestinal and cardiovascular systems.

When infants with impairments begin moving in supine or in prone, they may attempt to lift, turn, and hold the head by obtaining stability at the head, neck, mouth, and shoulder girdle through the use of head and neck hyperextension, tongue retraction (ie, pulling back and holding of the tongue body in a more posterior position in the oral mechanism behind the gums), and humeral hyperextension with adduction and internal rotation. With the head and neck in a hyperextended position, the cheeks and lips will be drawn back in retraction, shortening the muscles of the cheeks and lips, and the jaw will depress (or thrust open) and retract. Compensatory shoulder elevation with internal rotation and compensatory oral movements such as lip pursing (ie, pursestring positioning of the lips and cheeks), tongue thrusting (ie, strong forward pushing of a thickly bunched tongue), tongue retraction with anterior tongue elevation against the hard palate, jaw thrusting with protrusion, or exaggerated jaw closure may develop. These compensations create greater functional limitations for the infant when fed, producing sounds/crying, and with general movement activities.

When infants exhibit head and neck hyperextension, jaw depression with retraction, and tongue retraction during feeding, the tongue is usually thick in contour. The tongue is unable to thin and cup around the nipple as it is placed in the mouth, limiting the infant's ability to efficiently pump the milk out of the nipple using rhythmical tongue and jaw activity. As liquid moves back to the pharyngeal area for swallowing, adequate sustained closure of the airway may not be elicited, thereby increasing the infant's risk for aspiration. Some infants may attempt to use greater head and neck hyperextension with asymmetry and tongue protrusion or tongue thrusting, which may result in instances of choking, coughing, or gagging. When children exhibit excessive jaw depression or thrusting and exaggerated jaw closure as a spoon is brought toward the mouth, the jaw instability or poor jaw grading that occurs often will lead to an excessive loss of food from the mouth and limited control of the small amount of food as it falls back into the pharyngeal area.

Feeding is an activity that infants and children participate in many times a day. The issues in body alignment, oral and pharyngeal activities, and respiratory coordination for airway protection that an infant or child with impairments may experience are being repeated on a daily basis. These experiences may negatively affect not only their feeding and swallowing but also all functional activities they attempt to participate in throughout their day.

Respiratory-phonatory-sound production coordination will be affected directly by impairments that directly influence head, neck, shoulder girdle, rib cage, respiratory, jaw, and tongue musculature activity. When children exhibit limitations in their ability to coordinate breathing with oral and pharyngeal activities for phonation and sound production, the underlying impairments may result from limited diaphragm musculature activity; elevation and immobility of the ribs at the sternum and thoracic vertebrae; shortened and weak abdominal musculature; limited vocal fold activity in the larynx; and specific activities of the jaw, tongue, or cheeks/lips.

Postural Considerations

Compensatory shoulder elevation and use of a shortened rectus abdominus for stability in supine, prone, or sitting may result in retraction of the sternum and anterior ribs with excessive lateral flaring of the lower ribs. This will negatively affect diaphragm activity for inhalation and abdominal musculature activity for exhalation. Coordination of breathing with general movement activities will be limited, often resulting in breath-holding and restrictions in attempts at movement in the sagittal, frontal, and transverse planes.

When lumbar hyperextension with hip flexion, abduction, and external rotation is maintained for stability, the hip flexors remain in a shortened position. This posture places the pelvis in an anterior tilt and does not allow for active abdominal muscle activity. Therefore, a shallow belly breathing pattern will be used. Changes in the contour and alignment of the structures of the rib cage as well as activity of its musculature will be limited, giving the thoracic area a more barrel-shaped appearance. Longer, controlled exhalations for sound production and speech cannot be developed. If compensatory humeral hyperextension with adduction is used to reinforce spinal extension in prone, sitting, or standing, additional compensations at the head, neck, and mouth may result.

When adequate thoracic and lumbar extension and abdominal muscle activity do not develop, some children attempt to stabilize the trunk using the hip adductors and hamstrings. To shift the center of gravity forward in sitting and standing, compensatory humeral extension with adduction, upper trunk flexion, and compensatory head and neck hyperextension are used. Limitations in the expansion of the upper thoracic area and shortening with contraction of the rectus abdominus may occur. Rib cage mobility as well as rib cage and abdominal musculature activity for respiratory coordination with feeding, phonation, and sound production activities will be restricted. When limitations in oral, pharyngeal, and respiratory coordination activities exist during feeding/swallowing and respiratory-phonatory-sound production, it is essential to look for the influences that postural alignment, control, and movement have on these functional activities. When limitations in postural control, alignment, and movement exist, multisystem interactions are influencing not only general movement activities, but also feeding, swallowing, and sound production. Pediatric therapists always must look at the influences that a child's oral, pharyngeal, and respiratory function may have on the child's overall participation, especially when neuromuscular, musculoskeletal, and sensory system impairments exist.[9-11]

The Assessment Process

When clinically evaluating a child's oral, pharyngeal, and respiratory functioning, information should be obtained during feeding, swallowing, sound production, communication, and general movement activities. The quality and coordination of oral movements and the effect of postural control, alignment, movement, and sensory stimulation on oral, pharyngeal, and respiratory-phonatory-sound production also should be assessed. In addition, the coordination of respiration with feeding, sound production, and general movement activities must be observed. The child's use of different modes of communication during movement, play, and feeding activities are important components of the examination process. This information is gathered through careful questioning of the parent or caregiver, observation of the child with the caregiver during various activities, and, when appropriate, direct testing by the evaluator.[12-18]

Observations During Functional Activities

A comprehensive clinical evaluation of oral, pharyngeal, and respiratory function requires observation during a variety of functional activities. It is important to observe the child and the child-caregiver interactions before and after any mealtime feeding activities. How a child uses his or her mouth in play will be different from how he or she uses it when drinking from a cup or biting on a toy. How a child uses the mouth when in standing while playing with a toy will be different from when supported in sitting and laughing with the parent.

Relevant questions include the following: Is congestion (ie, wet, gurgling noises) heard in the throat, in the nose, in the chest while the child is playing and are there attempts at trying to clear the congestion? Is there congestion heard as the child is in supine, in prone, in supported sitting, or in standing and interacting with a parent/caregiver? Some children exhibit congestion in all activities with limited attempts at clearing the congestion. Other children sound congested only in play and not during feeding activities. Congestion is of particular concern because it may indicate reduced pharyngeal sensory awareness that can result in aspiration or other health issues.

Observation of a child's respiratory function and coordination during play and general movement activities is as important as observations made during feeding. Does the child exhibit instances of breath-holding during rolling on the floor or rising to stand from sitting? Is the child's respiratory rate so high that it is difficult for him or her to have the energy to move to get a toy or the ability to protect the airway when swallowing saliva, food, or liquids? The influences of a child's respiration on all attempted functional activities is an essential aspect of every pediatric evaluation.

Observations During Feeding

Analysis of the child's oral, pharyngeal, and respiratory coordination during feeding/swallowing activities is a significant part of the evaluation process. Questions should be posed to the caregiver to obtain information on feeding and respiratory history as well as on mealtime length, nutritional intake, preferred food textures, feeding utensils, positioning used, and the child's feeding activity. Often the information gathered from caregivers helps the evaluator to discover factors that may be influencing a child's function, especially in feeding and swallowing, that may not be evident during observation of a mealtime feeding activity.

Careful observation of the interactions of the caregiver and child, the procedures used, and the child's oral, pharyngeal, and respiratory function during feeding are essential components of the evaluation process. Special emphasis should be placed on describing the initial body alignment of the child for feeding and any changes that occur in this alignment over time. How food and liquid are presented, the child's response to these presentations, the oral movements used during feeding, and the coordination of respiration with oral movements also are noted.

Observations During Handling

After observing the child and caregiver, the evaluator may want to analyze movements already observed or try to modify oral, pharyngeal, or respiratory function through changes in handling and positioning or non-nutritive oral activities. Handling to stimulate more active postural control and movement as well as modifications to a child's body alignment/positioning during a specific functional activity may help to assess the child's future potential for changes in oral, pharyngeal, respiratory-phonatory-sound production, and general communication functions. Special care must be taken by the evaluator when considering the introduction of changes in food texture or food presentations during the evaluation process, especially when pharyngeal issues are suspected.

Instrumental Examinations of Swallowing

If pharyngeal movement or sensory issues are suspected based on the child's history and observations during the clinical examination, a videofluoroscopic evaluation of swallowing (VFSS; eg, video swallow study, modified barium swallow, or oral-pharyngeal motility study) or a fiber-optic endoscopic evaluation of swallowing may be conducted. These studies more directly evaluate if, when, and under what conditions aspiration or problems with controlling the food/liquid bolus and protecting the airway may be occurring. The findings of these instrumental evaluations will be important to obtain prior to implementing significant changes in the child's mealtime feeding whenever pharyngeal issues are suspected.[19-21]

Effect of Primary Gastrointestinal Issues

A child's oral and pharyngeal function, as well as body alignment, actually may reflect primary gastrointestinal issues. When gastrointestinal issues exist, such as gastroesophageal reflux, constipation, slow stomach emptying, and esophageal motility issues, the child may be resistant to changes in body alignment and resistant to body movements and activities that cause discomfort. When primary pulmonary and respiratory issues exist, the child often will be resistant to oral activities (eg, feeding, toothbrushing). The child also may resist movement activities that require changes in shoulder girdle, rib cage, diaphragm, and pelvis/hip alignment, as well as musculature activity, especially through frontal and transverse planes of movement. When gastrointestinal and pulmonary system impairments exist, the child's oral, pharyngeal, and respiratory function as well as general movement for all functional activities will be challenged.

Development of Plan of Care

Subsequent to the completion of a thorough clinical examination and evaluation of a child's oral, feeding/swallowing, and respiratory coordination function, recommendations are made regarding the need for other medical evaluations, the appropriateness of the procedures being used for nutritional intake, the need for instrumental assessment of the swallowing process because of suspected pharyngeal issues, and the need for future treatment programming. A comprehensive plan of care will include delineation of participation restrictions, functional activity limitations, and systems impairments, as well as goals and objectives both for direct patient treatment by the therapist and carryover activities, such as mealtime feeding and toothbrushing.

During mealtime feeding, the primary goal always will focus on adequate nutritional intake and hydration and its presentation in the safest manner possible for the child. The implementation of new strategies to modify a child's oral function or body alignment during mealtime may initially lead to reduced nutritional intake. This often will result in the caregiver's rejection of these new strategies. Further investigation of the child's oral, pharyngeal, and general movement activities; coordination with respiration; and other factors that may be influencing the child's activity as a component of the child's plan of care is essential prior to making changes in procedures being used in mealtime feeding. New strategies can be introduced during direct treatment and carried over into mealtime when the child's response does not negatively impact the primary mealtime feeding goal.

Direct patient treatment should improve function through active handling, movement, and sensory strategies based on knowledge of typical and atypical developmental processes, body systems and their interactions, and the influences of single and multisystem impairments on function. Treatment must reflect understanding of the relationship between general movement, oral function, pharyngeal function, and respiratory coordination development. We must recognize as well the importance of repetition for learning and the ability to analyze the specific movements required for task accomplishment. Once specific functional outcomes begin to be accomplished in direct treatment, they can be incorporated into carryover activities.

TREATMENT PROGRAMMING

See Videos 8-1 through 8-3. Treatment to improve oral, pharyngeal, and respiratory coordination must address functional outcomes and strategies, which help the child develop the motor components required to more successfully use the oral, pharyngeal, laryngeal, esophageal, and respiratory mechanisms. These mechanisms are essential for feeding/swallowing, crying, sound/speech production, and communication, as well as coordination with general movements and upper extremity activities. Emphasis must be placed on developing functional activity of the cheeks, lips, tongue, jaw, and pharynx as well as their coordination with respiration. Strategies for direct treatment services leading to progressive improvement in function may not be immediately incorporated into activities such as mealtime feeding if their use initially interferes with overall nutritional intake. Therefore, a well-coordinated plan of care for improved function both through direct treatment and carryover activities must be designed.[22-33]

Postural Control and Alignment

Underlying all treatment for improved oral, pharyngeal, and respiratory coordination is the relationship among active movements in these specific areas and their coordination with the child's postural control, alignment, and movement. Dynamic therapeutic handling during direct treatment is essential to facilitate more active movements of the head, neck, mouth, shoulder girdle, spine, rib cage, pelvis, hips, and upper and lower extremities. Appropriate handling strategies will lead to the development of active functional movements, which can be repeated and integrated into a wide variety of functional activities that will expand the child's potential for participation in the home and community.

Proper body alignment through positioning may provide a base of central stability for better oral, pharyngeal, and respiratory function during carryover activities such as mealtime feeding. This alignment alone will not provide a foundation for the generalized integration of these new movements to other activities (eg, general movements, sound and speech production). Dynamic therapeutic handling, which facilitates the integration of musculature activity through movement, and proper body alignment through positioning play important roles in the child's overall treatment program.

When pharyngeal and gastrointestinal issues are not primary issues for a child, there are strategies that may be implemented more successfully during mealtime feeding to support the primary goal of nutritional intake. These strategies often include the establishment of proper positions for feeding (for both the child and the caregiver), the modification of sensory characteristics of the foods/liquids (eg, texture, taste, smell), feeding utensils being used, and the incorporation of other methods or procedures for food presentation. There is not one piece of equipment or one way to

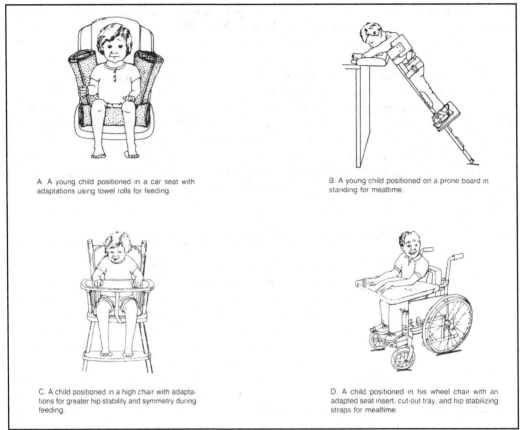

A. A young child positioned in a car seat with adaptations using towel rolls for feeding.

B. A young child positioned on a prone board in standing for mealtime.

C. A child positioned in a high chair with adaptations for greater hip stability and symmetry during feeding.

D. A child positioned in his wheel chair with an adapted seat insert, cut-out tray, and hip stabilizing straps for mealtime.

Figure 8-3. Examples of proper body positioning for improved oral-motor and respiratory functioning during mealtime.

adapt equipment that is successful in establishing good feeding positions. However, positioning for better oral and pharyngeal function at mealtime requires good body alignment. For children who are age 8 to 10 months and older, this includes neutral, symmetrical head flexion with neck elongation; symmetrical, stable shoulder girdle depression; and symmetrical trunk elongation. Also included are neutral positioning of a stable, symmetrical pelvis with several degrees of anterior tilt; symmetrical hip stability with neutral abduction and rotation; and stable, symmetrical positioning of the feet flat on a surface with a few degrees of dorsiflexion (Figure 8-3). Any deviation from this central base of good body alignment due to physical deformity or inappropriate equipment will restrict the positive effects of positioning with good body alignment on function during mealtime.

Sensory Experiences

Although proper body alignment will have a significant effect on mealtime feeding, the wide variety of sensory experiences that occur during mealtime may continue to make feeding difficult. Modifications in the food or liquid texture, taste, smell, or temperature may provide sensory information that stimulates more active oral or pharyngeal functioning. The selection of appropriate feeding utensils can be essential to the encouragement of greater functional activity of the cheeks, lips, tongue, and jaw during mealtime. The presentation of food and liquid by the feeder must be modified so visual, auditory, and tactile input do not result in overresponsiveness that results in atypical body alignment and activity. Atypical body alignment may reduce nutritional intake and restrict or limit oral activity and coordination with respiration.

Strategies directed toward mealtime feeding are important but narrow in focus. Strategies for direct treatment are of primary significance to the modification of overall oral, pharyngeal, and respiratory coordination. As function is modified through direct treatment, changes will be made in postural control and alignment as well as procedures used during mealtime feeding.

Therapeutic Handling

Preparation through therapeutic handling is necessary for developing the motor components required for coordinated oral, pharyngeal, and respiratory functions. Therapeutic handling is combined with specific strategies to facilitate the development of active, controlled neutral head flexion with neck elongation and stable shoulder girdle depression on a mobile, downwardly angled and elongated rib cage. Activities to encourage sustained abdominal musculature activity in sagittal, frontal, and transverse planes of movement are essential. Additionally, handling should integrate the facilitation of active lip closure; rounding and spreading as well as active up and down, forward and backward, diagonal, and circular-rotary jaw movements; and up and down, lateral, and forward and backward movements of a thin, contoured tongue during feeding, swallowing, and sound/speech production activities.

Special emphasis in treatment must be placed on handling, which enhances respiratory coordination with oral and pharyngeal function. Facilitation of active thoracic and lumbar spinal extension in supine, prone, and during transitional movements will help elongate and activate shoulder girdle and abdominal musculature. As frontal plane (lateral) and transverse plane (rotation) movements are experienced with weight shifting, greater rib cage mobility and lower rib cage stability are developed. As the child begins to sit and move in and out of sitting and standing, the abdominals actively stabilize the rib cage from below. This results in elongation of the musculature between each rib and between the ribs and spine. Thus, the rib cage can begin to expand on inhalation and the abdominals can begin to provide a foundation for longer controlled exhalation. This allows more mature abdominal/thoracic respiratory function to occur. In addition, active shoulder girdle and upper rib cage stability, along with active abdominal musculature, provide the postural foundation for coordinated oral and pharyngeal movements.

Sensory Intervention

Modifying oral tactile sensory awareness is another important aspect of treatment. Deep pressure tactile stimulation presented on the face and within the oral area can prepare the mouth for more typical sensory-based movement activity. Deep pressure stroking on the face toward and through the lips can help to elongate cheek and lip musculature, preparing the child for the initiation of more active cheek, lower lip, and upper lip movements. Cup drinking, bottle drinking, spoon feeding, or stimulation for bilabial sound production can now be introduced to encourage the activation and organization of these new sensory and movement experiences into functional activities.

A consistent sensory program of deep pressure input through the biting surfaces of the gums or teeth is another important aspect of treatment. Input through the biting surfaces assists in providing sensory input, which encourages graded movements of the jaw that are essential for cup drinking, spoon feeding, toothbrushing, speech, and all biting and chewing tasks.

The range, direction, and quality of tongue movements can be modified through the integration of sensory information and the presentation of feeding activities to the mouth. The use of rhythmical, well-graded, moderate pressure stroking to the lateral surfaces of the tongue body prior to feeding and sound production stimulation allows the child to begin to move the tongue laterally toward the teeth/gums or toward a toy or solid food placed on the lateral biting surfaces. Gradually, sensory input can be presented on the lateral, upper surface of the tongue, stimulating changes in tongue shape, contour, and movement. This tactile input to the tongue can have influences on respiratory function as well as on head, neck, and shoulder girdle activities and alignment.

SUMMARY

Treatment of oral, feeding/swallowing, respiratory-phonatory-sound production mechanisms will promote functional skill development in the child. These treatments strategies are based on our knowledge of the motor components required and our understanding of the influences that body system impairments have on function. Strategies for direct treatment and carryover activities in the child's plan of care must be well coordinated if the child is to function effectively and efficiently in the oral, feeding/swallowing, respiratory-phonatory, and speech/communication areas as the child expands participation at home, school, and within the community.

CASE STUDY #1: JASON

- ► *Medical Diagnosis:* Cerebral palsy, right hemiparesis
- ► *Gross Motor Function Classification System:* Level I
- ► *Age:* 24 months

Examination

A clinical examination of Jason's oral-motor, feeding/swallowing, and respiratory coordination function was conducted at his home. He was observed during play, communication, gross motor activities, and mealtime. His parents reported that he has had 2 ear infections in his right ear over the past 12 months.

At rest, Jason exhibits subtle cheek/lip retraction on the right, an asymmetrical contour to his tongue, and a slight lateral pull of his jaw to the right. During play and gross motor activities, cheek/lip retraction and lateral jaw deviation to the right increase, and some asymmetry of the tongue is evident. Drooling, which increases with gross motor and upper extremity activities, is noted from the right side of the mouth.

Jason relies heavily on gestures and movement for communication. As with many children his age, he has a small number of real single words. His overall use of vocalizations and jargon with gestures for communication is limited, especially when he is ambulating. His vocalizations are nasal in quality and reveal minimal variety in intonation and inflectional patterns, unlike what would be expected at his age.

Jason produces a variety of vowel sounds while his consonants are limited in quantity and have some distortions. He is unable to produce good-quality lip activity for bilabial productions (/m/, /b/, /p/) because of his cheek/lip retraction and lateral jaw deviation to the right.

Jason eats a limited variety of foods. He chews easily dissolvable solids, such as cookies or crackers, only on the left side of his mouth and uses his hand to move pieces initially placed on the right to the left. His tongue lateralizes more to the left than to the right. He often loses crumbs and small pieces of solids from his mouth while chewing. His lips surround the spoon for food removal, but he cannot clear all the food from the spoon with his lips. Food remains on his lips, especially on the right, during spoon feeding. When drinking from a cup, Jason places the cup far back between his teeth and uses slight head/neck hyperextension to compensate for his cheek/lip retraction. He occasionally loses some liquid when the cup is removed. After swallowing, some residual food/liquid is evident on the right side of his tongue and inner cheek cavity.

Jason exhibits problems in his coordination of breathing with oral and pharyngeal activity. He holds his breath during and gasps for breath after drinking liquid from an open cup. His vocalizations are limited in length. His rib cage is somewhat elevated with asymmetry and greater flattening of the upper anterior thoracic area on the right. Rib flaring is evident, revealing limited elongation of the rib cage and a lack of good consistent abdominal musculature activity.

Participation Restrictions

Jason eats a very limited variety of foods, which affects his participation in snacks and lunch at day care. This limitation also makes it difficult for his parents when they are invited over to friends' homes for playdates. He is a "messy" eater, and often chooses to sit by himself and not socialize with his peers while eating. He is resistant to toothbrushing activities at home, especially for brushing on the right side of his mouth.

Activity/Functional Limitations

Jason has difficulty using speech to communicate with others and relies on gestures more than other children his age. He is a "messy" eater, often leaving food on his lips and cheeks and losing food from his mouth as he chews. He has difficulty eating foods with increased texture and often spits pieces out. He frequently has food remaining in the right side of his mouth after swallowing and shows little awareness of the food being there. He uses breath holding during cup drinking and often gasps for breath and coughs after drinking several sips in a row from an open cup.

Impairments

Jason demonstrates poor sensory awareness on the right side of his body, on his face, and within his oral mechanism. He demonstrates poor lip closure with retraction of the cheeks and lips, greater on the right. He has difficulty moving his tongue laterally, especially to the right, and generally exhibits a thickened tongue contour. His jaw deviates to the right when opened and during closure. He has difficulty coordinating breathing with oral, pharyngeal, and some general movement activities.

Goals

Jason has a number of treatment goals:
1. Increase sensory awareness of the right side of his body, face, and within the oral mechanism.
2. Increase lip closure with reduced cheek and lip retraction during eating, drinking sound/ speech production, and upper extremity and gross motor activities.
3. Increase use of up/down, forward/backward, and lateral tongue movements with thinning of the tongue contour during eating, drinking, sound/speech production, and upper extremity and gross motor activities.
4. Increase use of graded jaw movements with reduced jaw deviation during eating, drinking, sound/speech production, and upper extremity and gross motor tasks.
5. Improve the coordination of respiration with oral and pharyngeal activity during eating, drinking, and sound/speech production tasks.

Participation/Functional Outcomes

After 3 months of intervention, Jason will be able to accomplish the following:
1. Take 3 or 4 sips of liquid from an open cup before pausing to breathe with no gasping or choking.
2. Produce the consonant sounds for /b/ and /m/ spontaneously with good symmetrical lip closure.
3. Initiate and maintain symmetrical lip closure on the cup rim while drinking 4 ounces of liquid from an open cup.

4. Eat soft meats using lateral tongue movements to keep food on the side biting surfaces without losing food or saliva from his mouth.

5. Remove food from the spoon using symmetrical lip closure and graded jaw activity.

6. Use a greater number of single words when communicating with others.

Intervention

To determine the appropriateness of strategies being used in treatment and to assess the progress being made toward achieving specific functional outcomes, measurable objectives should be established. These measurable functional objectives will be used as pretest and posttest activities at the start of and conclusion of each treatment session depending on the functional activities focus for that specific session. Jason's intervention program will include measurable functional objectives:

1. While sitting in his adapted toddler seat, Jason will bring an open cup of water or milk to his mouth, symmetrically close his lips on the cup, and take 1 or 2 sips from the cup 3 times without losing any liquid from his mouth. The adapted seat should have a cutout tray at an appropriate height to assist in maintaining symmetrical neutral head flexion, neck elongation, shoulder girdle depression, and trunk elongation. Additionally, the seat should position Jason with a few degrees of anterior tilt to the pelvis, at least 90 degrees of hip flexion, 90 degrees of knee flexion, and feet flat and in contact with a stable surface.

2. While sitting in his adapted toddler seat, Jason will lower his jaw, keeping his tongue contour flat and positioned just behind his lower front teeth as the therapist brings a spoon to his mouth. He will elevate his jaw and close his lips symmetrically on the spoon as it enters his mouth, and keep his lips symmetrically closed as the spoon is moved forward out of his mouth 5 times without any head/neck hyperextension.

3. While sitting in his adapted toddler seat, Jason will chew a small piece of soft chicken presented to his lateral biting surfaces using up/down and some lateral-diagonal jaw movements as well as lateral tongue movements to the side where the food is located 3 times without losing any of the food from his mouth before swallowing.

4. While straddling the therapist's leg (therapist sitting on a small bench) with his feet flat on the floor and the therapist providing him with stability through his trunk and pressure input at his pelvis/hips down into the surface as well as proprioceptive input symmetrically down through his feet, Jason will repeat specific vowel-consonant-vowel combinations or single words with the consonants /b/ and /m/ presented by the therapist using symmetrical lip closure while looking in a mirror 5 times using 1 inhalation-exhalation cycle for each vowel-consonant-vowel combination/single-word production.

An essential component of intervention with Jason is to combine movement facilitation with appropriate tactile and pressure input directed through the rib cage, shoulder girdle, and pelvis/hips to increase sensory awareness. This will assist him in establishing a more symmetrical foundation of postural control and alignment prior to and in coordination with interventions presented more directly to the face and in the oral mechanism. Well-graded input to elongate the chest wall musculature of the anterior rib cage, as well as to increase rib-to-spine and rib-to-sternum mobility within the rib cage in coordination with frontal plane movements on a stable base of support with weight shifting, will encourage elongation on the weight-bearing side and lateral flexion on the non–weight-bearing side. This intervention will provide a foundation from which shoulder girdle depression, rib cage mobility and elongation, and abdominal musculature activity through the internal and external abdominal obliques can be facilitated. While on a moveable surface (eg, ball, peanut roll, bolster), Jason is encouraged to play using transitional movements (eg, supine to side-lying to sitting or prone to side-lying to sitting), while tactile and proprioceptive input is presented through the rib cage, shoulder girdle, pelvis/hip, and abdominals directed toward the base of support. Longer and more varied sound productions, including vowel-consonant-vowel combinations, can be stimulated through movement activities especially in frontal and transverse planes, combined with singing and other sound play games.

Jason is given the opportunity to take sips of liquid by cup, with his lips symmetrically closed on the cup rim, periodically during treatment as his respiratory function appears to be increasing in its inhalation depth and his sounds are longer in duration. When drinking, he is assisted in maintaining a symmetrical upright posture with his feet weight bearing on a stable surface. This may be in sitting initially and later, as he gains more postural control, in standing.

Well-graded oral sensory stimulation directed at the cheeks and lips, through the biting surfaces of the teeth/gums, on the hard palate, and to the lateral surfaces of the tongue, may be presented in conjunction with general movement facilitation activities as well as prior to more specific sound production, eating, and drinking activities. Jason's caregivers are instructed in oral sensory stimulation procedures so they can be encouraged to implement them as part of his daily toothbrushing routine and periodically during his day with play.

Following oral sensory activities presented during a treatment session, more specific eating or drinking activities can be introduced with modifications in the sensory characteristics of the food/liquid or feeding equipment or changes in the presentation of the food/liquid by the therapist. Thickened liquid that provides greater tactile information or cold liquid to increase sensory awareness may be presented by open cup, thus stimulating greater cheek, lip, and tongue activity. Pieces of crunchy cereal can be placed on the biting surfaces of the teeth/gums, more often on the right, while encouraging active lateral tongue movements in response to this tactile input. Active symmetrical lip closure and jaw grading may be stimulated with the presentation of yogurt with a more distinctive taste and texture using a spoon with greater tactile surface input. Jason's caregivers are encouraged to follow similar procedures for food presentation during meals at home only when these procedures or changes in food/liquid/equipment are found to be successful in treatment. Special care must be taken in helping caregivers to integrate changes in the mealtime routine so nutritional intake and hydration are not compromised.

CASE STUDY #2: JILL

- ▸ *Medical Diagnosis:* Cerebral palsy, spastic quadriparesis, microcephaly, intellectual deficits, seizure disorder
- ▸ *Gross Motor Function Classification System:* Level V
- ▸ *Age:* 7 years

Examination

A clinical examination of Jill's oral-motor, feeding/swallowing, and respiratory coordination functions was conducted. She was observed during activities in and out of her wheelchair.

Jill uses head/neck hyperextension with shoulder girdle elevation and internal rotation, tongue retraction, severe cheek/lip retraction, and jaw thrusting with retraction in all her attempts to move, communicate, eat, and drink. A minimum of 1 hour is needed to feed Jill a meal. Her nutritional intake is primarily composed of pureed food by spoon and water or milk by cup.

Her rib cage generally is immobile. The sternum is fixed in retraction by her shortened, tight rectus abdominus. Although the lower ribs appear flat in contour, the upper ribs appear rounded in the front and flat laterally. Jill has a shallow belly-breathing pattern with retraction of the sternum and anterior ribs on inhalation. Greater retraction of the anterior rib cage with severe rib flaring is evident as she attempts to move, communicate, and eat.

Jill sits in a wheelchair with adaptations for feeding. She continues to exhibit asymmetry, head/neck hyperextension, humeral extension/adduction/internal rotation, hip extension/adduction/internal rotation, and significant problems with coordinating her respiratory function in this position. Therefore, her body alignment in her adapted wheelchair does not provide an optimal foundation for oral, pharyngeal, and respiratory functioning.

While feeding, Jill remains in some degree of head/neck hyperextension with humeral extension/adduction/internal rotation and shoulder girdle elevation. Her tongue is thick in contour and retracted, with only a small range of forward/backward movement noted during spoon feeding and cup drinking. Cheek/lip retraction is noted during all feeding activities, although she inconsistently attempts to compensate with lip pursing at the initiation of cup drinking. Initially when food is presented, jaw thrusting with retraction occurs. She uses some exaggerated jaw closure on the spoon and cup rim for stability. Small horizontal shifts of the tongue are noted to the left with solid food presentation, which is very limited. Generally, Jill uses her head/neck hyperextension and small-range, suckling movements of the tongue to move food and liquid back for swallowing. Respiratory coordination during cup drinking is poor with much coughing and choking.

Jill attempts to say a few words such as "bye," "hi," and "mom." However, her attempts to say these words are greatly restricted by the body hyperextension she uses to initiate sound.

Recommendations from the clinical examination included requests for additional medical evaluations in the areas of nutrition as well as gastrointestinal and pulmonary function. Jill's history of upper respiratory infections, coughing and choking during cup drinking, oral-motor dysfunction, poor muscle bulk development, and poor postural alignment during eating and drinking tasks support the need for an instrumental evaluation of her swallowing process such as a VFSS evaluation of swallowing (ie, video swallow study, modified barium swallow, oral-pharyngeal motility study). The study should provide more specific information related to her oral and pharyngeal function, especially in regard to her posterior tongue activity and her ability to protect her airway during swallowing. Prior to making any changes in her head/neck and body position during feeding, it will be important to have the information from the VFSS evaluation of swallowing. Information from the study also will help in the further development of appropriate functional outcomes and treatment goals and strategies.

Participation Restrictions

Jill's antiseizure medication often results in sleepiness and lethargy, which limits her ability to stay alert and be involved in many of her school and family activities. Jill requires assistance by a caregiver for all her self-care needs and to participate in any of her school activities. She is extremely susceptible to respiratory infections, which greatly limits the variety of activities in which she can participate.

Activity/Functional Limitations

Jill coughs and chokes often during feeding because of the poor coordination of her breathing with oral and pharyngeal function and questionable sensory awareness in her oral and pharyngeal mechanisms. She eats a very limited variety of food textures because of her poor oral, and probably pharyngeal, function. Jill is resistant to toothbrushing, which puts her at higher risk for dental problems, ear infections, and upper respiratory infections. Jill can produce only a few single-syllable words and performs this using excessive hyperextension of her body. Her communication generally consists of vocalizations with some variations in loudness and intonation.

Impairments

Jill demonstrates overresponsiveness to oral tactile stimulation. Her rib cage lacks mobility and her respiratory pattern is shallow, asynchronous, and poorly coordinated with oral and pharyngeal function. She exhibits severe cheek/lip retraction, severe jaw thrusting with retraction, and severe tongue retraction with a thick tongue contour. Jill's postural alignment and control do not provide a foundation that can be supportive of coordinated oral, pharyngeal, and respiratory function.

Goals

The following treatment goals will need to be modified subsequent to further evaluation of Jill's feeding/swallowing function through instrumental testing and the gathering of additional medical information related to her pulmonary and gastrointestinal function, as well as her nutritional status. No functional outcomes/goals related to her feeding and swallowing or mealtime feeding will be implemented until further evaluation information has been collected, especially pertaining to her oral and pharyngeal function for feeding, swallowing, and her pulmonary function.

Jill has a number of treatment goals:

1. Improve coordination of respiration with oral and pharyngeal activity during eating, drinking, sound/speech production, and gross motor tasks.
2. Increase forward/backward, up/down, and lateral tongue movements with reduced tongue retraction and reduced thickness in tongue contour during feeding and sound/speech production tasks.
3. Increase cheek and lip activity with reduced cheek/lip retraction during cup drinking, spoon feeding, sound/speech production, and upper extremity and gross motor tasks.
4. Increase active jaw movements and graded jaw closure during feeding, sound/speech production, and gross motor tasks.
5. Increase tolerance for oral tactile stimulation on her face, to her inner cheek/lip surfaces, through her teeth/gums, and on her hard palate.

Participation/Functional Outcomes

Prior to further evaluation of Jill's oral and pharyngeal function for feeding and swallowing, her pulmonary status and gastrointestinal function, and her nutritional status, emphasis will be placed on functional outcomes #1 and #4. Subsequent to further evaluation information gathering, additional outcomes listed will be modified or implemented.

After 3 months of intervention, Jill will be able to accomplish the following:

1. Initiate the production of vowel sounds without hyperextension of her body.
2. Close her lips on the cup rim on presentation of the cup.
3. Use forward/backward tongue movements with a thinner tongue contour to move pureed foods back in the oral cavity during spoon feeding.
4. Handle having a toothbrush brought into her mouth providing input through the biting surfaces of her teeth/gums and on her hard palate without increased cheek/lip retraction.

Intervention

To determine the appropriateness of strategies being used in treatment and to assess the progress being made toward achieving specific functional outcomes, measurable objectives should be established. These measurable functional objectives will be used as pretest and posttest activities at the start of and conclusion of each treatment session depending on the functional activities focus for that specific session. Jill's intervention program prior to implementing any tasks focused on feeding/swallowing tasks includes measurable functional objectives:

1. While sitting on a bench with her hips in contact with the base of support, her trunk supported by the therapist from behind, and without her feet in direct contact with the surface of the mat/floor, Jill will easily initiate 2 mid-vowel sounds of 2 to 4 seconds in length during or subsequent to sitting 3 times without eliciting greater head/neck/trunk hypertension or lower extremity hyperextension/adduction.

2. While sitting on a bench or straddling a bolster with her hips in contact with the base of support, her body supported by the therapist/caregiver, and without her feet in contact with the floor surface, Jill will participate in toothbrushing/oral sensory activities focusing on her facial musculature (cheeks/lips), the inner cheek/lip musculature, the biting surfaces of teeth/ gums, and the surface of her hard palate one time for each area of her face/mouth without eliciting greater head/neck/trunk hypertension or lower extremity hypertension with adduction.

Treatment activities need to combine facilitation strategies directed toward increased mobility of the ribs at the spine and at the sternum with tactile and proprioceptive input to stimulate greater overall postural musculature activity and sensory readiness. In sitting, slowly graded frontal (lateral) plane and transverse (rotational) plane trunk and pelvis/hip movements are facilitated while providing moderate pressure input inward and downward on a diagonal through the lateral rib cage toward the weight-bearing hip. This will increase rib cage mobility and improve alignment of the rib cage within the trunk. As rib cage mobility increases, input is moved to the area at which the lower anterior-lateral rib cage meets the abdominal area to encourage elongation of the rib cage and abdominal musculature activity. Jill may be sitting on a bench or straddling a bolster between the legs of the therapist with her pelvis and hips in contact with the base of support. Activities to stimulate mid-vowel sounds then can be presented.

In side-lying, facilitating slow, graded movements in and out of side-lying with moderate pressure input inward and downward on a diagonal through the upper rib cage toward the base of support can assist in stimulating greater rib cage and scapulohumeral mobility, as well as preparing the trunk musculature for greater activity. This may be performed on a mat, large wedge pillow, or a large ball. Activities to stimulate longer mid-vowel sounds then can be implemented.

Well-graded, moderate-pressure input combined with elongation through the musculature of the cheeks and lips helps to establish a better sensory base for cheek and lip activity. This input can be combined with movement facilitation in side-lying and sitting to better organize Jill's cheek and lip activity with head, neck, and trunk activity. Other oral sensory activities within the oral mechanism are combined with well-graded body movements to assist Jill in tolerating tactile input using a soft brush through the inner cheek/lip musculature surfaces, the biting surfaces of her teeth/gums, and on her hard palate. Jill's caregivers will be shown procedures for oral sensory stimulation at home and are encouraged to provide input for brief periods of time throughout her day and prior to mealtimes, whenever possible.

Special attention must be placed on increased saliva production that will occur in response to these oral sensory strategies. Jill may require time to swallow her saliva during or immediately after each strategy being implemented.

Oral sensory input is followed by spoon feeding of a thickened pureed food, encouraging more sustained closure of the lips on the spoon on presentation and more rhythmical forward/ backward tongue movements with a thinner tongue contour to move the food back for swallowing. Closure of the lips on the cup rim on presentation of the cup will help Jill organize her oral mechanism for cup drinking. (Goals and strategies directed toward feeding/swallowing activities will be modified or implemented as originally stated after the review of additional instrumental evaluation information.)

Case Study #3: Taylor

➤ *Medical Diagnosis:* Myelomeningocele, repaired L1-2
➤ *Age:* 4 years

Examination

Taylor's oral-motor activity during spoon feeding, cup drinking, and solid food intake appears to be within normal age limits. He uses a variety of communication modes, including speech. His mean sentence length of 3 to 4 words, and the sounds he produces during spontaneous speech appear to be within normal age limits.

Taylor does not have adequate abdominal activity to support sustained exhalation and good respiratory coordination. He appears to run out of air after about 3 words and can sequence only about 3 sips from a cup before stopping to breathe.

Taylor should have a thorough evaluation of his language functioning by a qualified speech-language pathologist. Children with myelomeningocele and hydrocephalus often appear to have normal language functioning according to tests of intelligence and vocabulary comprehension that require specific verbal responses. Many speak excessively using clichés and phrases learned by rote. These children may be unable to identify words during testing that they produce in spontaneous speech. This suggests the existence of very specific expressive and receptive language deficits.

Participation Restrictions

Taylor is unable to keep up with peers outside or on the playground, limiting his opportunities for social interactions. His physical endurance is limited, which makes it difficult for him to participate in more strenuous activities. As he fatigues, his abdominal support for speech is more challenged.

Activity/Functional Limitations

Taylor cannot speak in sentences of more than 3 or 4 words in length because of his inadequate breath support for sustained exhalation. He can sequence up to only 3 sips of liquid from a cup before he has to stop to breathe.

Impairments

Taylor exhibits generalized weakness through his upper extremities and trunk, especially in his abdominal musculature. Rib flaring is evident on inhalation due to abdominal musculature weakness, restrictions in rib to spine mobility, and limited elongation of musculature between the ribs and spine and between the ribs themselves. Limited sustaining of respiratory musculature activity impacts speech, endurance, and respiratory coordination with upper extremity activities.

Goals

Taylor has a number of treatment goals:
1. Improve coordination of respiration with oral and pharyngeal activities during speech and other communication tasks.
2. Improve coordination of respiration with oral and pharyngeal activities during cup drinking, straw drinking, and blow toy activities.

Other goals will depend on results from an evaluation of Taylor's language function.

Participation/Functional Outcomes

After 3 months of intervention, Taylor will be able to accomplish the following:

1. Produce sentences of 3 or 4 words on 1 exhalation without running out of breath support.
2. Drink 3 or 4 sips of liquid from a cup before stopping to breathe.

Intervention

To determine the appropriateness of strategies being used in treatment and to assess the progress being made toward achieving specific functional outcomes, measurable functional objectives should be established. These measurable objectives will be used as pretest and posttest activities at the start of and conclusion of each treatment session depending on the functional activities focus for that specific session. Examples of measurable functional objectives for Taylor's intervention program include the following:

1. While sitting in his wheelchair with trunk elongation and his pelvis/hip alignment providing a good base of support, his lower extremities properly aligned, and his feet in dorsiflexion, Taylor will talk with the therapist about school or other activities he likes, producing sentences of 3 to 5 words in length without running out of breath support a minimum of 2 to 3 times per session.
2. While sitting in his wheelchair with trunk elongation and his pelvis/hips providing a good base of support, his lower extremities properly aligned, and his feet in dorsiflexion, Taylor will drink a sequence of 3 to 5 sips of liquid of his choosing (water, milk, or juice) before stopping to breathe 5 times during each treatment session.

Increasing Taylor's respiratory support for speech and other oral/pharyngeal activities will require the incorporation of activities suggested by his physical and occupational therapists. These activities will focus on the stimulation and strengthening of the muscles of Taylor's upper extremities and trunk, especially his abdominals and back extensors. Tasks to encourage speech production on a more sustained exhalation can be incorporated into these activities.

While in supported sitting on a bench or roll, Taylor can come forward over his hips while pushing with extended arms and hands on the wall. While pushing through his arms, he is asked to repeat sentences of 3 to 4 words in length presented by the therapist during 1 exhalation. Subsequent to activities encouraging greater trunk and abdominal activity, Taylor will drink a sequence of 4 sips from a cup before lowering the cup from his lips to breathe.

Taylor may benefit from the use of an abdominal binder made of neoprene or spandex or a specially designed compression shirt and shorts that can provide 3-dimensional compression input and downward alignment to the lower ribs (especially ribs 7 to 10) extending downward to his hips. When he is in sitting on a bench with his hips in contact with the base of support or when he is standing, this additional sensory compression and alignment should assist in providing a foundation from which he can stimulate greater use of his abdominal musculature. He can engage actively in tasks such as singing, playing with easily initiated blow toys, or talking with the therapist or caregivers. The focus should be on expanding his respiratory support for longer, more sustained speech or longer sequencing of sips from a cup or from a straw. Use of such a compression garment/binder easily may be incorporated at home and at school to assist Taylor in being able to use his speech more effectively and efficiently and to coordinate his breathing with eating and drinking tasks.

Case Study #4: Ashley

> ➤ *Medical Diagnosis:* Down syndrome
> ➤ *Age:* 15 months

Examination

A clinical examination of Ashley's oral-motor, feeding/swallowing, and respiratory coordination function was conducted. She was observed during play, communication, gross motor activities, and mealtime.

According to her mother, Ashley had esophageal atresia and required a gastrostomy tube for feeding for the first 6 months of her life. She has a history of chronic otitis media with a mild conductive hearing loss. Pressure equalization tubes were placed at age 12 months. Consultative speech services are provided as part of a mother-infant early intervention program that Ashley and her mother attend 2 times per week.

Ashley has generally low muscle tone, which provides a poor base for oral, pharyngeal, and respiratory-phonatory functioning. A suckle pattern is used in all feeding activities. The tongue is thick in contour and always protrudes from the mouth. The hole in the nipple has been slightly enlarged to allow for greater liquid intake during bottle drinking. She has to pause quite often to breathe during bottle drinking.

Cup drinking has been introduced, but only during snack time. Ashley likes only stage 2 baby foods by spoon. She has been given some solids (crackers, cookies), but her lack of positive response to them has not encouraged their consistent presentation. She takes a maximum of 3 to 4 ounces of food by spoon per meal.

Ashley's mother reports that Ashley spit up quite often when she was fed by gastrostomy tube. Since the tube was removed and her cardiac defect was repaired, she does not spit up during or after a meal.

During spoon feeding, it was noted that some food remains in her mouth between her gums and cheeks even after several swallows of one spoonful. If she is not presented with another spoon of food immediately, some of the remaining food residual drools out of her mouth. She shows no sensory awareness of the food remaining in her mouth.

Ashley's rib cage is flat, yet high in position. Retraction of the anterior rib cage, especially at the sternum during belly breathing, increases in severity with effortful crying, movement, and attempts at vocalization. Her vocalizations are breathy, nasal, soft, and short. She is a mouth-breather and struggles for breath if her mouth is held in a closed position. This is not unusual for children with Down syndrome. Their small oral mechanism size does not appear to provide enough space for the tongue to sit in the oral cavity without closing off the oropharyngeal and nasopharyngeal areas when the mouth is closed.

A thorough prelinguistic/cognitive/language evaluation needs to be conducted because of Ashley's present lack of goal-directed play activities and her history of chronic otitis media with a mild conductive hearing loss. She should have periodic reevaluations of her hearing status by a qualified audiologist.

Participation Restrictions

Ashley does not easily engage in play activities and shows no interest in interacting with peers. She requires assistance in all movement activities because of her ineffective balance and protective reactions. She has limited ways to communicate with caregivers or other children her age.

Activity/Functional Limitations

Ashley takes limited amounts of food by spoon at a meal. She has shown no interest in crackers or cookies. She uses a suckle pattern with a thickened tongue contour and excessive tongue protrusion in all feeding activities. Bottle drinking is her primary means of liquid intake. Liquid and food are lost from her mouth during all feeding activities. Her vocalizations are breathy, nasal, soft, and short in duration. She has only a few words (eg, "more," "mama," "dada") and uses them separately but not in combination to communicate.

Impairments

Ashley demonstrates poor oral sensory awareness and poor oral-motor activity. Her tongue movements are limited to the forward/backward dimension. Poor lip closure is evident. Her mouth is always in a somewhat open position with some jaw depression. She reveals no awareness of food remaining in her mouth after swallowing or when she drools. Problems in respiratory coordination with oral and pharyngeal activity are evident during bottle drinking, spoon feeding, sound production, and general movement activities.

Goals

Ashley has a number of treatment goals:
1. Improve coordination of respiration with oral and pharyngeal activity during feeding and sound/speech production tasks.
2. Increase active use of the cheeks and lips during feeding and sound/speech production tasks.
3. Increase active up/down and lateral movements of the tongue during feeding and sound/speech production tasks.
4. Increase oral sensory awareness during feeding and sound/speech production activities.

Participation/Functional Outcomes

After 3 months of intervention, Ashley will be able to accomplish the following:
1. Bring her lower lip up and out, stabilizing under the cup rim with her tongue back behind her lower front teeth when the cup is presented for drinking.
2. Move her tongue laterally to touch solids and objects placed on the biting surfaces of her side gums/teeth.
3. Produce vocalizations of 3 to 5 seconds in length with reduced nasality and increased loudness.
4. Position her tongue back within her oral cavity with reduced protrusion during nonfeeding activities when in supported sitting and when supported in standing.
5. Eat an easily dissolvable solid at every meal as dessert.

Intervention

To determine the appropriateness of strategies being used in treatment and to assess the progress being made toward achieving specific functional outcomes, measurable objectives should be established. These measurable functional objectives will be used as pretest and posttest activities at the start of and conclusion of each treatment session depending on the functional activities focus for that specific session. Examples of measurable functional objectives for Ashley's intervention program include the following:

1. While sitting in her adapted toddler seat with cutout tray and her feet flat on the floor, her hips against the seat bottom as a base of support, her trunk symmetrical and elongated with shoulder girdle depression, her head in neutral flexion, and her neck elongated, Ashley will eat 6 spoonfuls of food from the spoon with her tongue behind her lower front teeth and her lips closing on the spoon 3 times during each treatment session.

2. While sitting in her adapted toddler seat, Ashley will drink a minimum of 3 ounces of milk or water from a cutout cup with her lower lip under and in contact with the bottom cup rim, her upper lip in the liquid, and her tongue back behind her lower front teeth during a 1-hour treatment session.

3. While sitting on a bench or straddling an anteriorly angled bolster with her feet flat on the floor and the therapist behind her providing assistance to keep her hips on the surface, her pelvis slightly forward with her trunk elongated and supported from behind, and her head in neutral flexion with neck elongation, Ashley will bite, chew, and use tongue lateralization while having easily dissolvable cookies/crackers/dry cereal when presented to her lateral biting surfaces 1 to 2 times per treatment session.

4. Ashley will produce vocalizations that are 3 to 5 seconds in length and increased in loudness at least 5 times while engaged in activities focusing on increased rib cage mobility and elongation, greater diaphragmatic activity for deeper belly breathing, and greater exhalation with abdominal musculature activity during her 1-hour treatment session.

In treatment, it will be essential to combine appropriate somatosensory, vestibular, visual, or auditory sensory input with the facilitation of active movements using therapeutic handling focusing on greater trunk, shoulder girdle, and lip musculature activity. Combining moderate pressure input through the lower rib cage and abdominals with the facilitation of transitional movement (eg, side-lying to sitting, sitting to quadruped, kneeling to standing) activities can assist Ashley in developing a postural foundation for improved breath support. Activities to stimulate louder and longer vocalizations can be presented in conjunction with these movement activities to engage Ashley in some vocal interactions.

At brief intervals during movement facilitation activities, well-graded oral sensory input to the cheeks and lips, through the biting surfaces of the gums/teeth, to the hard palate, and to the tongue can be provided. Once Ashley begins to exhibit greater postural activity and increased active responses to the oral sensory input, some feeding experiences can be presented. Cup drinking can be introduced with a thickened liquid or pureed food. Easily dissolvable solids can be placed on the lateral biting surfaces for chewing. Food can be presented by spoon while encouraging active lip closure on the spoon for food removal.

Introducing different food textures (thick purees, grainy purees, cereal, crackers), tastes, smells, and temperatures can be performed as part of play. While performing active transitional movements, hands, feet, trunk, face, and mouth can be brought in contact with different food textures to encourage increased tolerance for these new tactile experiences. Different smells, tastes, and temperatures of food can be introduced to determine those that elicit the most active and positive responses of the oral and pharyngeal mechanisms. These can be incorporated into Ashley's mealtime routine.

Strategies and procedures found successful in treatment may be incorporated into Ashley's daily routine as long as they have a positive impact on her nutritional intake. Ashley's caregivers will need to view such recommendations as beneficial if they are to be carried over by them into daily activities. This will be especially important when introducing new experiences with solid foods and cup drinking.

Case Study #5: John

> *Medical Diagnosis:* Developmental coordination disorder/attention-deficit hyperactivity disorder

> *Age:* 5 years

Examination

John's kindergarten teacher expressed concerns regarding his speech to the school's speech-language pathologist. The speech-language pathologist arranged to observe John in his kindergarten classroom to determine whether more formal testing will need to be scheduled.

Prior to this classroom observation, John's parents were contacted by telephone to obtain some background information related to his speech and language development and function.

John's mother reports that she and John's dad understand most things that he says, although other adults have trouble understanding him, especially when he is excited and talking quickly. John becomes frustrated when not completely understood. For a long while, he primarily communicated using facial expressions, gestures, pointing, and by producing grunts and some vowel sounds. His speech became more intelligible about 1 year ago. He still has problems sitting for long periods of time to play games or to color, although this has improved since he started taking Ritalin (methylphenidate).

John's mother noted that he has always been a picky eater. He drank from a bottle until he was about age 3 years and still does best when drinking from his lidded sipper cup. He enjoys eating crackers, cold cereal without milk, peanut butter and jelly or grilled cheese sandwiches cut in quarters, cheese cubes, raisins, Rice Krispies Treats, macaroni and cheese, and Spaghetti-Os. He likes to drink only milk, not juices or water. He refuses to open his mouth for fruits. He will eat french fries and mashed potatoes and has occasionally eaten some cooked carrots. John's mother assists him at dinner, which is when he appears to have more trouble feeding himself if he needs to use a spoon or fork. John's mother noted that he still puts some objects in his mouth for biting, especially when he is very tired. Although she is pleased that the neuropsychologist said John appears to have above normal intelligence, she is very concerned about his temper tantrums, his speech, and the diagnosis of development coordination disorder.

During the classroom observation, it was noted that John prefers to play with toys he has already experienced. He tends to be a loner and does not initiate conversations or play with other children in his class. He does willingly interact if another child initiates the activity.

John uses gestures to supplement his speech when communicating with others. He often takes an adult's arm to show what he wants at the same time he is speaking. The other children in his class do not generally like it when he does this to them.

During snack time, he showed no interest in the juice that everyone else was drinking. He drank the milk that his mother sent along for him. He appears to initially bite on the sipper cup's spout when starting to drink. He ate the graham crackers, exhibiting some rhythmical vertical jaw movements and tongue lateralization. He refused to try Jell-o and insisted on having more graham crackers instead.

His speech reveals expressive language delays. He often omits consonants, especially those in the middle or at the end of a word. It was noted that he also omitted words from sentences during his spontaneous speech productions. It was recommended that John be referred for a comprehensive speech and language evaluation. His parents will be contacted to obtain additional information related to nutrition, eating, and drinking.

Participation Restrictions

John avoids physical activities and group sports, preferring to play video games by himself. He requires more time to practice new motor skills than his peers because of his motor planning problem, which is frustrating and may result in temper tantrums. He uses gestures and physical directions when communicating, which is not always acceptable to his peers. John has very specific likes and dislikes related to what he will eat and drink and related to the equipment he will use for eating and drinking.

Activity/Functional Limitations

The intelligibility of John's speech is variable, resulting in his consistent use of gestures and pointing to help communicate what he wants. When not understood, he may become extremely frustrated. He has problems attending to a task for an extended period of time. John is a "picky" eater and frequently refuses drinks, foods, and utensils offered to him. He has greater problems using his spoon and fork later in the day as he is more fatigued. He does not always brush his teeth completely and this activity needs to be monitored by his parents.

Impairments

John demonstrates difficulties initiating, coordinating, and sustaining his jaw, tongue, and lip movements for consistently intelligible speech production. He exhibits problems in the somatosensory area as well as in his ability to modulate visual and auditory information in the environment. Respiratory coordination with oral and pharyngeal activities and with gross motor and upper extremity activities is restricted.

Goals

John has a number of treatment goals:
1. Improve the coordination of respiration with oral and pharyngeal activity during eating, drinking, sound/speech production, blowing, and upper extremity and gross motor tasks.
2. Improve the initiation and coordination of lip, tongue, and jaw movements during speech, eating, and drinking tasks.
3. Increase oral sensory awareness and sustained muscle activity and strength of the tongue, lips, and jaw.

These goals will be modified based on the findings of a comprehensive speech and language evaluation.

Participation/Functional Outcomes

After 3 months of intervention, John will be able to accomplish the following:
1. Attend to an activity while sitting at a table without being distracted by other visual and auditory stimulation in the environment for 5 minutes.
2. Blow a toy horn or whistle, sustaining a sound for 3 to 5 seconds.
3. Produce the consonants /t/ and /d/ when they appear at the end of a word in 3- to 4-word sentences or phrases.

Intervention

To determine the appropriateness of strategies being used in treatment and to assess the progress being made toward achieving specific functional outcomes, measurable objectives should be established. These measurable functional objectives will be used as pretest and posttest activities at the start of and conclusion of each treatment session depending on the functional activities focus for that specific session. Examples of measurable functional objectives for John's intervention program include:

1. While sitting in his classroom chair with his feet flat on the floor and his arms supported on a table, John will read a kindergarten-level book with the therapist or his caregiver. He will attend to each word/picture in the book, appropriately turn the pages, and, when requested, read/say a word that ends in /t/ or /d/ for a minimum of 5 minutes without being distracted by other visual/auditory stimulation in his environment.

2. While in standing and using sustained pushing with his arms extended and his hands flat on a wall that has no additional visual stimulation, John will repeat vowel-consonant combinations and short single words ending in /t/ and /d/ presented verbally and visually by the therapist or his caregiver for a minimum of 5 minutes.

3. John will use his toothbrush with a small amount of his preferred toothpaste, dipping it in water, and brushing his teeth, inner cheeks, and hard palate while standing at the sink with his feet flat on the floor and his arms supported so he can stand up straight with little physical effort, spit out in the sink, and take sips of water from a cup within a 5-minute period of time.

Before presenting activities that involve changes in oral and pharyngeal function, it is necessary to engage John in activities that prepare his overall sensory foundation. Activities that stimulate greater shoulder girdle/upper extremity or hip/lower extremity strength with sustained muscle activity will help to establish a base for improved oral and pharyngeal activity. Activities that assist John in modulating and integrating somatosensory information generally in his body as well as specifically within his oral and pharyngeal areas also help to establish a readiness for more specific speech/sound production tasks. A number of activities can be developed from which John and the speech-language pathologist can choose a few to perform prior to focusing on more speech specific tasks. These same sensory preparation activities can be used at home and at school to keep John in a state that allows him to attend to tasks longer and to be able to handle more challenging tasks such as speech.

Activities that are more directly related to oral, pharyngeal, and respiratory coordination function must accommodate John's motor planning, motor learning, and somatosensory issues. Practice of specific sounds and the specific sound combinations subsequent to providing tactile, visual, and auditory cues will be essential. Repetition of these tasks will be required for John to maximize his potential for learning. Combining /t/ and /d/ with vowels into vowel-consonant combinations and then into single syllable words will provide a starting point from which further expansion into phrases and sentences can occur. Finding the combinations of sensory cues that work best for John will be a primary initial focus so the same framework can be used for the learning of other consonants and words for speech.

Blowing activities using musical instruments and blow toys will be useful in helping to increase John's respiratory depth, ability to sustain exhalation, and overall endurance. The focus should be on the length of the sounds, rather than the loudness, to increase support for exhalation. Cues provided prior to blowing into the toy will assist John in expanding his anterior chest wall on inhalation so greater respiratory depth is stimulated. It may be necessary to start with some movement activities that encourage greater mobility within the rib cage in lateral, diagonal, and rotational dimensions (ie, frontal and transverse planes) prior to presenting cues that focus on the expanding inhalation/exhalation. Consistent practice as part of a daily routine will be an essential part of any intervention program in which John is expected to be successful.

Increasing the foods and liquids that John will eat/drink will require careful analysis of the sensory characteristics (eg, texture, taste, smell, temperature, auditory, visual) of his present diet, the utensils he presently uses, the environment in which he eats best, and at what times of the day he eats his greatest volume of food in the least amount of time. A specially designed program to expand his food choices combined with a focus on his overall sensory needs should help expand his mealtime choices for school, home, and family outings to a restaurant.

REFERENCES

1. Alexander R, Boehme R, Cupps B. *Normal Development of Functional Motor Skills: The First Year of Life*. Austin, TX: Hammill Institute on Disabilities, PRO-ED, 1993.
2. Boliek C, Hixon T, Watson P, Morgan W. Vocalization and breathing during the first years of life. *J Voice*. 1996; 10(1):1-22.
3. Gregory A, Tabain M, Robb M. Duration and voice quality of early infant vocalizations. *J Speech Lang Hear Res*. 2018;61(7):1591-1602. doi:10.1044/2018_JSLHR-S-17-0316.
4. Hixon T, Weismer G, Hoit J. *Preclinical Speech Science: Anatomy, Physiology, Acoustics, Perception*. 2nd ed. San Diego, CA: Plural Publishing, 2014.
5. Morris SE, Klein MD. *Pre-Feeding Skills*. 2nd ed. Austin, Texas: PRO-ED; 2000:59-95.
6. Redstone F. *Effective SLP Interventions for Children with Cerebral Palsy*. San Diego, CA: Plural Publishing, 2014.
7. Ross E. Development of feeding progression. In: Van Dahm K, ed. *Pediatric Feeding Disorders: Evaluation and Treatment*. Framingham, MA: Therapro; 2012:35-53.
8. Scarborough D, Brink KE, Bailey-Van Kuren M. Open-cup drinking development: a review of the literature. *Dysphagia*. 2018;33(3):293-302. doi:10.1007/s00455-017-9871-6.
9. Alexander R. Transitioning to cup drinking. In: Van Dahm K, ed. *Pediatric Feeding Disorders: Evaluation and Treatment*. Framingham, MA: Therapro; 2012:171-188.
10. Alexander R. Feeding and swallowing. In: Best S, Heller K, Bigge J, eds. *Teaching Individuals with Physical or Multiple Disabilities*. 6th ed. Upper Saddle River, NJ: Pearson; 2010:257-288.
11. Stamer M. *Posture and Movement of the Child with Cerebral Palsy*. 2nd ed. Austin, TX: PRO-ED; 2015.
12. Arvedson JC. Oral-motor and feeding assessment. In: Arvedson JC, Brodsky L, eds. *Pediatric Swallowing and Feeding: Assessment and Management*. 2nd ed. Albany, NY: Singular Publishing Group; 2002:247-291.
13. Beecher R, Alexander R. Pediatric feeding and swallowing: clinical examination and evaluation. *Perspectives on Swallowing and Swallowing Disorders (Dysphagia)*. 2004;13(4):21-34. doi:10.1044/sasd13.4.21.
14. Gross RD, Trapani-Hanasewych M. Breathing and swallowing: the next frontier. *Semin Speech Lang*. 2017;38(2):87-95. doi:10.1055/s-0037-1599106.
15. Hixon T, Hoit J. Physical examination of the diaphragm by the speech-language pathologist. *Am J Speech Lang Pathol*. 1998;7(4):37-45. doi:10.1044/1058-0360.0704.37.
16. Hixon T, Hoit J. Physical examination of the abdominal wall by the speech-language pathologist. *Am J Speech Lang Pathol*. 1999;8(4):335-346. doi:10.1044/1058-0360.0804.335.
17. Hixon T, Hoit J. Physical examination of the rib cage wall by the speech-language pathologist. *Am J Speech Lang Pathol*. 2000;9(3):179-196. doi:10.1044/1058-0360.0903.179.
18. Morris SE, Klein M. *Pre-Feeding Skills*. 2nd ed. Austin, TX: PRO-ED, 2000:157-186.
19. Arvedson JC, Lefton-Greif MA. *Pediatric Videofluoroscopic Swallow Studies: A Professional Manual with Caregiver Guidelines*. San Antonio, TX: Communication Skill Builders; 1998.
20. Delaney A. Special considerations for the pediatric population relating to a swallow screen versus clinical swallow or instrumental evaluation. *Perspectives on Swallowing and Swallowing Disorders (Dysphagia)*. 2015; 24(1):26-33. doi:10.1044/sasd24.1.26.
21. Willging JP, Miller CK, Link DT, Rudolf CD. Use of FEES to assess and manage pediatric patients. In: Langmore SE, ed. *Endoscopic Evaluation and Treatment of Swallowing Disorders*. New York, NY: Thieme; 2001:213-234.
22. Alexander R. Pre-speech and feeding development. In: McDonald E, ed. *Treating Cerebral Palsy: For Clinicians by Clinicians*. Austin, TX: PRO-ED; 1987:133-152.
23. Alexander R. Oral-motor treatment for infants and young children with cerebral palsy. *Semin Speech Lang*. 1987;8(1):87-100. doi:10.1007/BF00341263.
24. Arvedson J, Clark H, Lazarus C, Schooling T, Frymark T. Evidence-based systematic review: effects of oral motor interventions on feeding and swallowing in preterm infants. *Am J Speech Lang Pathol*. 2010;19(4):321-340. doi:10.1044/1058-0360(2010/09-0067).
25. Bierman J, Franjione MR, Hazzard C, Howle J, Stamer M. *Neuro-Developmental Treatment: A Guide to NDT Clinical Practice*. New York, NY: Thieme; 2016.
26. Kelly B, Huckabee ML, Jones R, Frampton C. Integrating swallowing and respiration: preliminary results of the effect of body position. *J Med Speech Lang Pathol*. 2007;15(4):347-355.

27. Lazarus C. History of the use and impact of compensatory strategies in management of swallowing disorders. *Dysphagia.* 2017;32(1):3-10. doi:10.1007/s00455-016-9779-6.

28. Morris SE, Klein MD. *Pre-Feeding Skills.* 2nd ed. Austin, TX: PRO-ED; 2000.

29. Pinder GL, Faherty AS. Issues in pediatric feeding and swallowing. In: Caruso AJ, Strand EA, eds. *Clinical Management of Motor Speech Disorders in Children.* New York, NY: Thieme; 1999:281-318.

30. Redstone F. *Effective SLP Interventions for Children with Cerebral Palsy: NDT/Traditional/Eclectic.* San Diego, CA: Plural Publishing; 2014.

31. Solomon NP, Charron S. Speech breathing in able-bodied children and children with cerebral palsy: a review of the literature and implications for clinical intervention. *Am J Speech Lang Pathol.* 1998;7(2):61-78. doi:10.1044/1058-0360.0702.61.

32. Steele C, Alsanei W, Ayanikalath S, et al. The influence of food texture and liquid consistency modification on swallowing physiology and function: a systematic review. *Dysphagia.* 2015;30(1):2-26. doi:10.1007/s00455-014-9578-x.

33. Van Dahm K. *Pediatric Feeding Disorders: Evaluation and Treatment.* Framingham, MA: Therapro; 2012.

Sensory Considerations in Therapeutic Interventions

9

David D. Chapman, PT, PhD

Studies suggest that learned movements can be performed in the absence of sensory input.[1,2] Sensory input and feedback are essential, however, during learning or relearning motor skills. Many children with developmental disabilities (DD) face the challenge of learning and performing movements with diminished or discrepant sensory information. The multitude of neuroanatomical pathways communicating afferent information to the motor control centers of the central nervous system (CNS) supports the critical nature of sensory input. Therefore, therapists rely on theoretical models, such as dynamic systems theory, that enable us to examine and evaluate multiple factors, including sensory processes that influence how children learn to move.

The sensory systems provide a primary media through which therapists can influence the motor behavior of a child with DD. Our touch, voice, and way of moving a child provide the CNS a multitude of sensory data to be received, processed, and acted on. The effectiveness of our handling techniques depends in part on our orchestration of the sensory information reaching the child's CNS. Our intervention techniques are based on the manipulation of sensory input through one or more sensory systems.

The information in this chapter addresses the broad general category of DD. An assumption has been made that the movement problems of children are of central origin and that the mechanics of processing and responding to sensory information are affected. These problems are discussed from a dynamic systems perspective to illustrate how contemporary theory, when coupled with basic knowledge of anatomy and neuroanatomy, can be used to guide therapeutic interventions. The premise is that although different treatment approaches may be needed for children with a peripheral nerve lesion or lower motor neuron dysfunction, the theoretical basis for treatment remains consistent.

Connolly BH, Montgomery PC, eds. *Therapeutic Exercise for Children With Developmental Disabilities, Fourth Edition* (pp 239-269).
© 2020 Taylor & Francis Group.

Figure 9-1. Specially designed infant seat for infants with lumbar or sacral spina bifida. (Reprinted with permission from David D. Chapman, PT, PhD.)

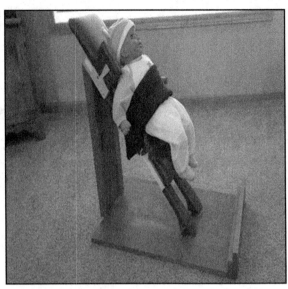

DYNAMIC SYSTEMS THEORY

Principles and concepts from dynamic systems theory can be used to guide interventions with children to move more effectively.[3] Proponents of this approach suggest that new motor skills emerge through the process of *self-organization* rather than by prescribed or hard-wired neural templates.[4] This means the movements children produce are the result of the "real-time" interactions between their multiple intrinsic subsystems, such as the quality of sensory information, perceptions of the task, and fat-to-muscle ratio in the legs, as well as extrinsic factors including handling techniques and available assistive device(s).[3,5]

Additional principles and concepts from dynamic systems theory that are used to guide treatment sessions include control parameters, rate-limiters, and attractors. A *control parameter* is a component or factor that helps the child move differently in more functional and effective ways. For example, when infants with lumbar or sacral spina bifida are placed in a specially designed infant seat, they flex and extend their legs at their hips and knees (eg, kick) significantly more often than when they are seated in a conventional infant seat (Figure 9-1).[3,6] Kicking is an important behavior because babies who kick their legs more often begin to walk earlier in life than infants who kick less frequently.[7] This example shows that the environmental context, an extrinsic factor, may be a control parameter that is used to facilitate specific movement patterns.

Additionally, as this example illustrates, the context for movement also may function as a *rate-limiter*. A rate-limiter is an element that limits the ability of the child to demonstrate a given movement. In this case, the conventional infant seat inhibited the ability of the infant with limited or absent sensory information to kick with flexion and extension at the hips and knees. As a result, this environmental context can be viewed as a rate-limiter for leg and knee kicks—one that may contribute to the delays these infants experience in learning to kick and then learning to walk.[6]

Control parameters and rate-limiters are not always located in the treatment environment or movement context. Instead, they may be found within the child. For instance, Ulrich et al[5] found that when infants with Down syndrome were held over a pediatric-sized treadmill over several months of time, they produced more alternating steps when they showed an increased rate of weight gain and a decrease in their thigh and calf skin-fold measures. These researchers suggested a relationship existed between these 2 variables. They stated that an increase in lower extremity strength was sufficient enough to enable the infants to produce more alternating steps on the treadmill when their rate of weight gain was less and/or their thigh and calf skin-fold measures were larger.

Attractors are the final concepts from dynamic systems theory that are presented as constructs to help design effective treatment strategies. Within a dynamic systems approach, attractors are thought of as stable behavioral patterns or, in this case, movement patterns.[8-10] Attractors are perceived to be preferred, but not obligatory, movement patterns that result from the cooperation of the child's intrinsic subsystems within a given environment.[9,11] Within a particular context at a given point in development (or time), the child will "settle into" preferred and perhaps limited range of movement patterns.[9] This means that certain behaviors are more likely to occur than others given the demands of the task, the status of the child and multiple subsystems, and the movement context.[10,12] For example, young typically developing infants between ages 7 and 11 months when held over a pediatric-sized treadmill seem to prefer producing alternating steps vs other types of stepping patterns, such as single or parallel steps.[5,11,13,14]

An attractor represents a stable movement pattern for a child at a given point in time within a specified context. Over time and with intervention, the stability of a specific attractor is expected to change. This loss of stability can be viewed as an increase in variability.[9] Therapists can measure this by monitoring the variability (eg, standard deviation) for that movement pattern. For example, the relative consistency or variability of a child's step length with each lower extremity may provide insight into how "stable" the child's gait pattern has become in a given context (eg, on a smooth, level indoor surface with a reverse walker). The child's progress then can be evaluated by comparing the consistency of the step length on a level surface without the reverse walker to the consistency of the step length when walking on a similar surface with the reverse walker.

The loss of a stable attractor should not be interpreted as an inherently negative event in the therapeutic process. Clearly children with DD need to develop stable movement patterns to function effectively. However, these children also need to develop adaptability in their movement patterns if they are going to successfully confront changes in environments and the expectations that come with different contexts. Thus, an increase in variability should simply be viewed as a sign or indicator that children are trying out new ways of moving or trying to develop new ways of coping with change within their internal systems or within a given environment. The therapist's responsibility is to discover what has changed (ie, the control parameter), thereby facilitating children to develop new more functional, yet stable, ways of moving within a given environment.

Motor control theory principles and concepts from the dynamic systems perspective enable therapists to appreciate how important sensory information is to children as they seek to move more effectively and efficiently. Conceptual models of motor learning also highlight the significant function that sensory information plays in the production of functional movement patterns. For example, sensory feedback, in Adams' closed-loop theory of motor learning, is necessary for the ongoing production of skilled movement.[15] Schmidt, in his schema theory, suggested that the sensory consequences of a movement—how it felt, looked, and sounded—play an important part in learning to move in an effective manner.[16] More recently, Newell, in his attempts to interface perception with action in an ecological theory of motor learning, emphasized the significant role that perception of sensory information plays as the mover seeks to find (learn) optimal movement strategies given selected task and environmental constraints.[17]

None of these theories alone can explain the complex task confronting children with DD who seek to move effectively and efficiently. Each theory, however, reinforces how dependent children are on the quality and quantity of sensory information available to them as they learn to generate well-controlled, coordinated movements.

Sensory Information

Within the normal process of motor learning, the ability to use sensory information appropriately is a critical component—an important subsystem—that affects how children learn to perform coordinated movements. Edelman suggested in his theory of neuronal groups selection that when movements in a given category (eg, kicks) repeatedly are performed, the information generated from the efferent activations that result from these movements and the afferent sensory consequences are continuously and temporally correlated within and between local neuronal groups.[18,19] Thus, when movement patterns are repeated over time this ongoing multimodal flow of information strengthens the neural connections between localized groups of neurons within the motor cortex. More recently, researchers have described these types of neuronal changes as *neuroplasticity.*[20-22] That is, neurons alter their structure and function in response to internal factors (eg, neuron excitability, dendritic arborization, increased spine density, synaptogenesis) and external factors (eg, training, rehabilitation experiences, and learning opportunities). As such, neuroplasticity can be thought of as continuous neural remodeling that results in short-term changes in strength or efficiency of synaptic connections and long-term structural changes in the organization and number of connections and neural maps.[20-22] In addition, Edelman suggested that connections among related groups of neurons in other areas of the CNS, such as the visual and somatosensory areas, also are strengthened as the child moves in real time.[18,19] These ideas and concepts imply that movement patterns that are repeated frequently generate stronger neural connections that provide the basis for stable movement patterns.

Experimental support for Edelman's theory, as well as neural plasticity, was provided by Ulrich and colleagues,[7] who found that infants with and without Down syndrome who kicked more often walked significantly earlier in life than similar infants who kicked less often. These results suggest the infants experienced neural plasticity as the neural connections within the CNS that supported the stable action pattern of walking were strengthened when they repeatedly produced a pattern of movement that was similar to the walking pattern (ie, kicked their legs). As a result, they were able to walk earlier in life than babies who kicked their legs less often.

Therapists create a therapeutic environment through their touch, voice, equipment, and home programs in which the child can perform certain movement patterns. For example, having the child practice alternating steps, consistently from session to session and between sessions, will help strengthen the neural connections that support these movements. This will lead to the development of a stable attractor for alternating steps. In other words, the child will be more likely to produce alternating steps in the future given similar sensory input to the system. Alternatively, the therapist who disregards the need for consistent sensory information being available to the child and the CNS will, in effect, interfere with the child developing the stronger neural connections that support stable movement patterns. This will force the child into a situation in which he or she is required to learn or "relearn" how to produce a given pattern of movement.

During movement, the CNS must differentiate between movement-related and nonmovement-related information. When considering the processing of sensory information, keep in mind that the CNS is analyzing sensory input available prior to the movement as well as the data generated as the result of the movement (feedback). Figure 9-2 diagrams the categorization of sensory information.

As discussed in Chapter 1, intrinsic and extrinsic feedback in the form of knowledge of results and knowledge of performance are critical variables in motor learning. Peripheral feedback helps to strengthen neural connections and provides the CNS information about the results of movement. Was the movement of the arm successful in positioning the hand to grasp the cup? Was the speed of movement of the protective extension reaction sufficient to stop the displacement of the child's center of gravity? The child gains knowledge of the results of his or her movements from internal and external sources. Internal sources of feedback include information from the sensory receptors, such as the muscle spindles and Golgi tendon organs (which contribute to our "feel" of

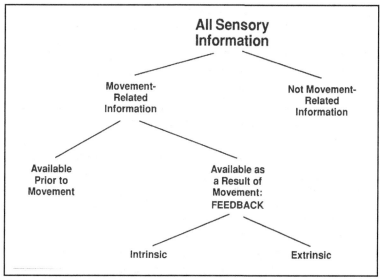

Figure 9-2. Utilization of sensory information in the process of motor control. (Adapted from Schmidt RA. *Motor Control and Learning.* 2nd ed. Champaign, IL: Human Kinetics Publishers; 1988.)

the movement), and the vestibular receptors (which contribute to our sense of position in space). External sources of information include visual and auditory input. Depending on the characteristics of the visual and auditory input, the information may be used as intrinsic feedback in which the information is compared with a learned reference of correctness. This comparison process provides an error-detection mechanism or serves as extrinsic feedback, which supplements or augments the intrinsic feedback.[2] Internal and external feedback help strengthen the neural connections that support stable movement patterns.[18,19]

The therapist can act to augment intrinsic or extrinsic feedback, or both. If the therapist provides a guiding resistance to the movement pattern, intrinsic proprioceptive information is increased. Extrinsic feedback can be increased by the therapist providing verbal commentary on the quality of the movement task—"Good hold!" (knowledge of performance) or commentary on the outcome of the movement—"Good step!" (knowledge of results).

Whereas peripheral feedback plays a role in learning movement, once movements are learned, central monitoring of the movement increases in importance. As you first learn a motor pattern, such as playing a piano, multiple sources of peripheral feedback inform you of the results of your finger movements. You attend to the feel of the movement, the sound produced by the movements, or the scowl of your teacher as you hit the wrong key. Once the movement is learned, the movements flow into each other without the need for delayed internal or external verifications of correctness of one movement before the next movement is made. Therapeutic handling techniques are designed to lead to this progression of motor learning and control.

Before developing balance within a posture, the child must have the sensory experience of being in the posture. Proprioceptive, vestibular, tactile, and visual information received by the CNS are unique to each particular posture. No amount of practice of head control in prone on elbows can provide an equivalent sensory picture of the responses necessary for head control in sitting or standing (see discussion of Transfer of Learning in Chapter 1). As the therapist handles the child within postures and when moving between postures, the handling techniques should not interfere with the experience of being in the posture. The therapist's role is to assist the child in producing an appropriate movement response. Incorrect sensory feedback due to overcontrol or undercontrol of the child by the therapist will act as a rate-limiter and weaken the supporting neural connections. This will result in altered or inappropriate postural alignment and movement.

In either case, the therapist must correct or compensate for the problem to assist the child in learning to produce the most efficient and effective movements possible.

Multiple mechanisms are available within the normally functioning CNS to protect higher centers from bombardment of sensory information. Some receptors, particularly the exteroceptors, demonstrate adaptation to a maintained stimulus. Awareness of a bandage on your finger fades quickly after it is placed on the skin, as the cutaneous receptors adapt to the continuous stimulation. With other receptors, it is crucially important that adaptation does not occur. Imagine the difficulties we would have moving if the vestibular macula did not inform us continuously of our position in relation to gravity.

With the magnitude of divergence of sensory information, a system of inhibition is necessary for the cortex to receive a clear representation of sensory input. The systems of feedforward, feedback, and local inhibition ensure that a clear sensory message ascends through the long ascending pathways and synaptic connections to the cerebral cortex and other motor control centers. If these inhibitory mechanisms are not functioning appropriately, the cortex may receive a confused sensory picture, resulting in an inappropriate movement.

Sensory pathways have not only ascending but also descending connections with the higher centers of the CNS. The descending connections allow the higher centers to support or shut down ascending information from receptors. The CNS can attend selectively to or enhance a particular set of sensory information while ignoring or suppressing another set. This ability of the CNS allows the student to concentrate on the teacher's instructions despite the noise of other children in the hallway. Deficits with the complex mechanism of selectively attending to particular avenues of sensory information present major problems for a child attempting to learn in an unstructured school environment.

Characteristics of Sensory Systems

No sensory system should be classified as inherently facilitatory (control parameters) or inhibitory (rate-limiters). Each system has the potential for increasing or decreasing the level of activity of the CNS, as well as strengthening or weakening the neural connections that support stable movement patterns, depending on the manner in which the sensory stimulus is delivered. Rood formulated general guidelines that assist in predicting the types of motor response that will be elicited based on the characteristics of the delivery of the sensory input.[23] A quick, brief stimulus results in a burst of motor activity. One can predict that a light stroke to the arm of a child may elicit a phasic burst to withdraw from the stimulus. Rapid, repetitive stimulation results in a more maintained response. Repetitive tapping or mechanical vibration of a muscle are techniques that have been used to induce a sustained contraction of the muscle.

Slow, rhythmical, repetitive stimuli decrease the level of responsiveness of the individual. Parents instinctively rock fussy infants to calm them. Monotone, droning instructors have deactivated the minds of students for centuries. A maintained stimulus, such as gravity, should elicit a maintained response. The influence of gravity continuously should elicit the automatic responses necessary to maintain a posture. When considering the response to a maintained stimulus, therapists must evaluate the potential adaptation of the receptor to the stimulus. A maintained cutaneous input should result in accommodation of the receptors and therefore a decreased rate of firing of these sensory pathways.

The therapist should consider additional influences on a child's response to sensory input. The set point of the autonomic nervous system is a potential rate-limiter. For example, a child who is tense and sympathetically dominated may respond to a friendly pat with a startle and withdrawal. Variations in the sympathetic or parasympathetic set point of the child result in variations in the response to a particular handling technique. The technique that was a control parameter and effective yesterday may be a rate-limiter today and produce less optimal responses because the child's autonomic nervous system is activating sympathetic responses.

Past experiences also influence the interpretation of sensory data. A particular cologne or aftershave may elicit parasympathetic responses if associated by the child with the scent of a loving parent. The same scent could elicit sympathetic responses if it were associated with the scent of an abusive parent.

The therapist must evaluate the number of sensory channels being stimulated by a particular handling technique. Depending on the functional and maturational level of the CNS, the child may not be able to respond appropriately to techniques or environments that provide multimodal stimulation. The child may be able to attend to controlling the position of his or her head when sitting with the therapist controlling the position of his or her pelvis, only if there are no other distractions such as the therapist talking. Gradually, and in a controlled manner, the therapist should introduce additional sources of input so the child can function within a more typical environment. Responsibility to control the amount and type of sensory input requires the therapist to constantly analyze the stimuli the child is receiving to avoid inappropriate stimulation.

Motor responses are specific to the environmental context of the moment. It is input from sensory systems that provides the CNS with the internal and external information necessary to assess the constraints under which the movement is to be performed. Gentile's Taxonomy of Motor Tasks provides therapists a system for analyzing the complexity of different movement tasks.[24] Inherent in understanding the complexity of the movement is an analysis of the spatial and temporal attributes of the environment and the body's movement. From the perspective of the child's CNS, the larger the quantity and diversity of sensory information that must be received and processed, the more difficult the process becomes—a rate-limiting process for the child who needs to move more efficiently and effectively. Walking and chewing gum at the same time is a more complex task than either performed independently. The addition of an object to carry or manipulate while walking further complicates the task. As treatment progression is planned for a particular child, one must remember to consider the potential rate-limiting aspect of the amount of sensory information that must be analyzed to produce the appropriate movement pattern under a given set of environmental constraints.

SELECTION OF SENSORY INPUT

Each intervention technique should be selected to facilitate or act as a control parameter for the child in producing an adaptive response. A response is considered to be adaptive if it indicates a higher level of function than the previous behavior of the child. Farber defined an adaptive response to sensory stimuli as a "behavior of a more advanced, organized, flexible, or productive nature than that which occurred before stimulation."[23] We attempt to assist the child to produce higher level, more appropriate, and functional movement(s). This is the measurement tool used to determine if the appropriate intervention techniques were selected. How consistently the child produces a more functional movement is an indicator of how stable that attractor or movement pattern has become.

The concept of using sensory input to provide guidance as a teaching technique to assist the individual in learning to perform a specific movement pattern was introduced in Chapter 1. Remember that the strongest effect of guidance is to alter the performance of the movement pattern during a specific trial. When the child is unable to execute a movement pattern that is effective and efficient, the physical therapist is responsible for selecting the control parameter (ie, treatment technique) that will enable the child to make a better response. Guidance in the form of therapist-enhanced sensory input is reduced as the child takes more responsibility for producing an adaptive response and moves independently.

The process of selecting an appropriate technique can seem overwhelming to the inexperienced clinician. The following general guidelines may assist in the process of selecting sensory techniques to be used as an intervention:

1. The therapist should select sensory stimuli that are more naturally occurring in preference to those that are artificial. An electric vibrator may elicit the contraction of a muscle, but is not the type of stimulus to which the child will respond in a typical movement situation. Preferentially, the activation of muscles can be achieved by weight-bearing, vestibular input, or cutaneous facilitation. These are the types of sensory information that the child will be required to respond to outside of the therapeutic setting and that can be administered by a parent or other caregiver.

2. Interventions should be developmentally appropriate for the child. Appropriateness must be considered in terms of physical, intellectual, and social development. Working on locomotion in quadruped may be perceived as demeaning by a teenager with a DD. Although quadruped may be therapeutically appropriate for the movement problems, the therapist must either convince the teenager to accept the rationale or select another posture.

3. The type of sensory stimulation should be appropriate to the activity. The postural neck muscles respond to vestibular input and to proprioceptive information, such as approximation through the cervical spine. Rapid, quick stretch is not a stimulus to which these muscles routinely are subjected. Intervention techniques based on approximation or vestibular input would be more appropriate to activate these muscles than a quick stretch.

4. The quality of the adaptive response frequently is enhanced if the child can respond to sensory cues other than cortically processed verbal commands. In our daily activities, many postural movements are made in response to intrinsic sensory cues. We hold our heads erect in response to vestibular, proprioceptive, and visual information, not in response to being told to pick up our heads and tuck our chins. Therapists should attempt to elicit automatic postural adjustments in response to the demands of the situation or the desire to accomplish the task. The more automatic the movement becomes (a function of strengthened neural connections), the more likely it will be incorporated in the child's repertoire of movements outside the therapeutic setting (a stronger or more stable attractor).

5. The therapist should use the least amount of control or sensory input necessary to elicit an adaptive response. Throughout the intervention process, the therapist must remember that a primary goal is to lessen and eventually to remove the intervention. The therapist must assess constantly whether components of the intervention strategy can be withdrawn. If the child is working on head control in sitting with the therapist controlling the position of the pelvis in all planes, the therapist could challenge the child by gradually relinquishing control in movements requiring flexion. As this control is beginning to be mastered by the child, control of extension gradually is relinquished by the therapist. As long as the therapist retains total control, the child will not have the opportunity to actively strengthen the neural connections that support the appropriate movements and, as a result, will be less likely to learn the appropriate movements in response to incoming sensory messages.

EXAMINATION AND EVALUATION

In examining the status of sensory systems in children with DD, the therapist basically is evaluating the perception of sensation. The therapist is looking for indications that the information is being received and processed, thus producing appropriate motor responses or providing correct feedback for internally produced movement. This intent is different from the purpose of sensory testing in children with peripheral nerve or spinal cord lesions. In these cases, the therapist is more concerned with the presence of sensation rather than the interpretation of sensory information.

The goal of the examination is to determine which sensory systems are functionally intact. The therapist then can design intervention strategies based on these systems. For example, if the child does not respond to vestibular input or responds inappropriately, techniques that use other sensory systems should be the primary focus in the initial interventions.

The therapist should guard against overtesting of the sensory systems. A complete neurological sensory examination can be time consuming, fatiguing, and tedious for the child. Before beginning a comprehensive evaluation, try to target specific sensory systems on which your examination and evaluation should focus. If the physician's neurological examination is available, review the results to identify areas that should be explored further. Interviews of parents, teachers, or other caregivers may provide indications of sensory dysfunction. Does the child seem to attend to visual or auditory input consistently? Does the child explore or attempt to explore objects with his or her mouth or with both hands equally? Does the child withdraw from touch, which could indicate tactile defensiveness? How does the child react to being moved through space? Does the child appear to enjoy movement or is the child fearful? How accurate is the child in reaching for objects? Answers to questions such as these will provide the therapist insight into how the various sensory systems are functioning. Additionally, the use of standardized sensory profiles such as the Sensory Processing Measure or the Sensory Profile 2 allows the therapist to determine the child's responses in a "natural environment" and to compare the child's responses with peers (see Chapter 2).

Therapists can gather similar information by examining the child's movements. Does the child orient appropriately to gravity? Does the child seem to correctly perceive the relation of his or her body parts? Can the child accurately place the extremities for support or for reaching? From this process, the therapist should be able to target specific sensory systems for further evaluation. Examples of examining and evaluating each sensory system within a therapeutic framework will be discussed in combination with intervention strategies.

The sensory examination and evaluation should not only establish the level of integrity of a particular sensory system, but also must attempt to determine the child's sensory preferences. A child might enjoy vestibular input while being less comfortable with cutaneous/proprioceptive input. The therapist must investigate whether this indicates a like/dislike or represents a dysfunction within a system. Although the determination may be difficult to make, the therapist should attend to behavioral cues. For example, consistent increases in activity level and aversion responses to tactile input may indicate tactile defensiveness.

Examination and evaluation of function of the sensory systems should encompass more than examining each system in isolation. The child may attend preferentially to a particular input or to input on one side of the body when presented with multiple inputs. In the presence of auditory distractors (a potential rate-limiter), the child may be unable to process visual input. The child with hemiplegia may be able to attend to cutaneous input on the involved side only if presented in isolation. If the child is touched on both sides simultaneously, only the touch on the uninvolved side (cortical inattention or bilateral extinction) may be reported. Preferential attending to certain sensory modalities may account for the difficulties a child has in making the transition from a controlled therapeutic environment to a more typical environment with its multitude of simultaneous, competing information.

Postural control or balance requires the integration of sensory input to construct an awareness of the location of the body's center of gravity in relation to the base of support as well as the ability to perform an appropriate musculoskeletal response. Visual, vestibular, and somatosensory information are combined in the perception of one's orientation in relationship to gravity, the support surface, and surrounding objects.[25] Deficits in any of these systems will affect balance control, particularly in situations in which the remaining alternative sensory inputs are not available or are in conflict. A child with reduced vestibular function may increase the reliance on visual references to maintain postural control. For this child, the performance of balance tasks will be increasingly difficult as the level of illumination is decreased or the eyes are closed. The therapist must monitor the child's responses throughout the assessment process for indications of difficulties with intersensory integration in relationship to postural control (see Chapter 10).

Intertwining Examination and Intervention Strategies

In this section, examples of treatment techniques based on input via the major sensory systems are presented. Methods of examining and evaluating the child's response to the sensory input are discussed. Examination, evaluation, and intervention are integrated in this section because therapists frequently conduct these processes simultaneously. The therapist may use the child's responses during intervention to evaluate the function of one or more sensory systems.

Cutaneous Input

Receptors located in the skin are responsible for touch and temperature information. Therapists can stimulate touch receptors to either inhibit or facilitate motor activity. Static, maintained contact of a surface with the child's skin should result in adaptation of touch receptors and inhibition of the muscles underlying the skin.[26] Therapists use this technique by resting their hands on the skin overlying spastic muscles to inhibit the muscles. Care must be taken to maintain constant, even pressure on the child's skin. Changing pressures could result in an increase in the activity of the underlying muscle. This concept is used in the construction of splints.[24] The static surface should be in contact with the surface overlying the spastic muscle. Straps are placed preferentially over the antagonists to the spastic muscles. The therapist assesses the success of inhibitory, maintained touch by the response of the child. Has the muscle relaxed? If the child is able to make more functional movements, then the inhibitory, maintained touch has functioned as a control parameter enabling the child to move more effectively.

When the therapist attempts to facilitate a muscle, manual contacts should be placed over the muscle belly. A changing, nonstatic pressure is used. Cutaneous receptors make spinal cord-level synaptic connections with gamma motoneurons.[27] Cutaneous input may enhance the sensitivity of the muscle spindle and, therefore, positively influence the response of the muscle. Just as with inhibitory touch, the effectiveness of the technique is assessed by evaluating changes in the child's response.

Temperature receptors increase their rate of firing as the skin temperature changes. The concept of "neutral warmth" can be used when the therapist attempts to decrease the overall level of the child's activity or stiffness in a limb. The therapist attempts to create an environment in which neither the temperature nor cutaneous receptors are being stimulated to fire above the base firing rate. This environment is created by wrapping the child or the body part in lightweight toweling or a sheet blanket (Figure 9-3).

The neutral environment is maintained until the desired response occurs. If the child is wrapped for too long, the increase in skin temperature may result in an increase in activity rather than a decrease. This is analogous to the restlessness created when you become too warm while sleeping and attempt to kick off the covers. Therapists should attend to the temperature of the room in which they are working with a child. In the optimal setting, the temperature would be adjusted to meet the needs of each child. A child with limited body fat and low activity level would be treated in a warmer room. In selecting the appropriate room temperature, the therapist should consider the baseline skin temperature of the child. The baseline skin temperature will vary with the child's health and the temperature of the child's previous environment. Remember that the temperature receptors are reporting deviations from baseline. It is important, therefore, to consider whether the child has been in a warm, muggy environment or a windy, cold environment prior to therapy. This may affect the baseline of muscle activity and the type of temperature input the therapist chooses to use. When considering the effects of temperature changes on the child, remember to consider your hand temperature. Therapist-child rapport can quickly be disturbed by a cold hand placed on a warm abdomen.

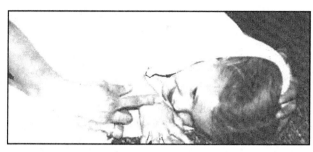

Figure 9-3. Child positioned in side-lying with sheet blanket for neutral warmth to decrease overall level of activity. Note the therapist's control of the hand position of the child and use of approximation to control head position. (Reprinted with permission from William D. Porter.)

In general, sensory inputs that evoke a withdrawal response or that are interpreted by the child as noxious or painful are functioning as rate-limiters and will be counterproductive to the goal of learning to make adaptive movements. A child with DD may demonstrate an aversive response to light touch, which may be described as tactile defensiveness. The therapist can help the child prepare for the therapy session by allowing him to desensitize the skin by vigorous rubbing with various textures and media. The child may tolerate the process better if he or she is allowed to control the input. When the therapist uses cutaneous input to guide the child through a movement pattern, a firm touch should be employed.

Vestibular Input

Vestibular input can either arouse or depress the level of activity of postural extensors and the level of alertness of the child, depending on the characteristics of the stimuli. Slow, rhythmical, repetitive rocking, rolling, or swinging movements typically relax and calm the child. Parents combine the concepts of neutral warmth and repetitive vestibular input by wrapping a fussy baby in a blanket and slowly rocking the child to sleep. Rapid, nonrhythmical stimulation with stops, starts, and changes in direction of movement is arousing and increases postural tone. Encouraging a child to move prone on a scooter board requires the use of postural extensors, while allowing vestibular input to reinforce the activity of the postural muscles (Figure 9-4).

Inversion is a technique used by therapists to stimulate the vestibular receptors to elicit a response similar to the Landau response or pivot prone posture. Infants who have had limited exposure to being placed in prone (as may occur when parents avoid any time in prone as a misinterpretation of the "Back to Sleep" campaign) may require additional stimulation to develop the postural extensors to work against gravity. According to McGraw, the child progresses through 4 developmental stages in response to inversion.[28] Initially, the infant responds to inversion with increased flexion and emotional arousal. The next stage is the extension response, which is the response sought when inversion is used as a therapeutic intervention. Crying seldom is heard during this phase. Later, inversion of the infant results in attempts to appropriately right the head to the horizon. Crying is frequent because these attempts are not successful. In the final stage, the child seems to recognize the futility of reversing the inverted position and hangs relaxed. Therapists should be aware of these developmental stages. If a child responds to inversion with a flexion response rather than the expected extension response, inversion may not be a developmentally appropriate technique. The therapist may need to use other forms of sensory stimulation to activate extension and introduce inversion later.

Some therapists have used the postrotatory nystagmus test developed by Ayres as an indicator of the integrity of the vestibular system.[29] The duration of nystagmus is measured following 10 rotations of the child in a 20-second period. The head of the child must remain flexed at 30 degrees during the duration of the rotation. Other sensory stimuli, particularly visual, should be controlled during the rotations because they may influence the results. This test indicates the integrity of the vestibulo-ocular connections, but does not necessarily provide information concerning the multiple diverse connections between the vestibular system and other parts of the CNS.

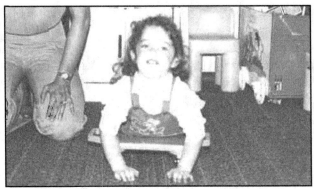

Figure 9-4. Use of a scooter to facilitate postural extension. The child can control the amount of vestibular stimulation being provided. (Reprinted with permission from William D. Porter.)

Proprioceptive Input

Proprioceptive or, more generally, somatosensory input is provided by almost every handling technique used by therapists. Many techniques have used the concept of reciprocal innervation to affect spasticity. The antagonist of the spastic muscle is activated (a potential control parameter) to achieve inhibition of the spastic muscle (a likely rate-limiter). A therapist might use a quick stretch to the triceps brachii (Figures 9-5 through 9-7). The quick stretch elongates the equatorial region of the muscle spindle, increasing the discharge rate of the Ia fiber. The Ia fiber monosynaptically connects with an alpha motoneuron innervating a motor unit in the triceps resulting in a contraction of those fibers. Resistance helps maintain the contraction response of the muscle, so the phasic burst following the quick stretch becomes a maintained or tonic response.

Activation of the triceps should result in reciprocal inhibition of the spastic biceps. If the therapeutic goal is to facilitate a particular muscle, a quick stretch followed by resistance can be used to attempt to activate the hyporesponsive muscle. A mechanical vibrator with the appropriate characteristics will produce a muscle contraction. The vibrator should have an amplitude of 1.0 to 2.0 mm[30] with a frequency of 100 to 125 Hz (cycles per second).[26] The vibration increases the discharge rate of the Ia fiber from the muscle spindle, resulting in a contraction of the muscle being vibrated. Although the technique may be effective in producing a contraction, it is difficult to use a vibrator within the context of producing functional, adaptive behaviors. Because vibration is not a stimulus that evokes movement responses in a normal framework of movement patterns, it should be reserved for occasions when other techniques are not effective.

Joint receptors appear to influence the type of contraction produced by the muscles crossing the joint. Approximation, or compression of the joint space, seems to elicit a holding contraction, particularly in the joint alignment typical for weight bearing (see Figure 9-7). Traction or separation of the joint spaces assists with movement. As the therapist assists the child with movement between postures, traction can be added to an extremity to facilitate the transition. Once the child has assumed a posture, traction can be added through the extremities in weight-bearing positions or through the vertebral column to reinforce the holding contraction necessary to maintain the position.

The therapist may alter the child's proprioceptive input (and to some extent, other sensory input) by using guidance assistance/resistance to facilitate movement. The purpose of the guidance assistance/resistance is to enable the child to experience movement within the environmental context in which the response should occur. This technique is employed when the child has been unable to use trial-and-error learning to refine a movement pattern.

Tests for proprioception frequently are not appropriate for the child with DD. The young child or a child with marked limitations cannot reproduce the postures with one extremity that a therapist has created with the opposite extremity. This represents deficits in position sense,

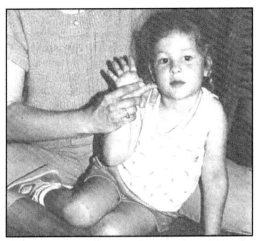

Figure 9-5. The therapist applies a quick stretch to the triceps brachii. (Reprinted with permission from William D. Porter.)

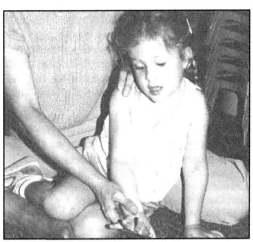

Figure 9-6. The therapist applies resistance to extension to augment the contraction of the triceps brachii. (Reprinted with permission from William D. Porter.)

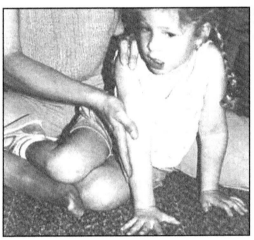

Figure 9-7. This demonstrates the target posture with the activated triceps being used in a support response. (Reprinted with permission from William D. Porter.)

which is a common rate-limiter in children with DD. The child may not understand or be able to communicate when the therapist moves a toe or finger up or down (kinesthesia or movement sense). In these cases, the therapist must evaluate how the child moves and uses the extremities to gain an understanding of the child's ability to act on proprioceptive information. A child may allow an extremity to lag behind when moving between postures, or fail to appropriately position the extremity when assuming a resting position, despite having the ability to move the extremity. In this case, the therapist would suspect that the child has difficulty in processing the proprioceptive input to know the location of the extremity. The therapist's observational skills will be the primary tool to evaluate proprioception in the majority of children with DD.

Visual Input

As discussed previously, visual information is one of the critical elements for maintaining postural control, particularly in individuals with vestibular system deficits. Assessment of static and dynamic balance tasks with and without vision will provide clues to the child's reliance on visual input. Woollacott reported that young infants commit more errors in their responses to perturbations when visual information also is being processed.[31] Apparently infants learn to use the visual input in conjunction with other sensory information over time, as motor control is mastered in various postures.

When children have difficulty maintaining appropriate vertical alignment in sitting or standing, some therapists use positioning in front of a mirror to provide visual cues on alignment. This tactic encourages the substitution of visual information for attention to internal cues (eg, somatosensory and vestibular input) indicating appropriate alignment. Attention to internal cues is necessary to remain aligned when the mirror is removed. The reversal of movements that occurs when viewing actions in a mirror may function as a rate-limiter and cause some children initially to hesitate in moving, resulting in errors in moving toward a target. Therapists should consider the effects of substituting visual information for proprioceptive/vestibular cues when deciding to use mirrors in teaching maintenance of vertical alignment postures or movements.

Auditory Input

If a child has difficulty processing multiple sensory inputs selectively, extraneous sounds from the environment often are distracting. If a child has this problem, the therapist should select a treatment environment that limits or eliminates extraneous auditory inputs. As the child masters a particular task, background noises should be added. The goal should be to progress the child to performing the task within a nonisolated environment.

The therapist's voice is an important therapeutic tool. Tone, volume, rate, and rhythm of speech must be modulated to meet the needs of the child. A child who is easily upset would respond best to a soothing, slow-paced, repetitive speech pattern. The child who is lethargic may need more authoritative, brisk verbal cues. Therapists should not confuse the need to be authoritative with being loud. Therapists can apply general rules of sensory input discussed previously to the therapeutic use of their voices.

SUMMARY

The most effective therapists engage in constant analysis of the child's response to handling and the environment. This analysis includes consideration of all the sensory input the child is receiving. Therapists should note the conditions under which appropriate and inappropriate responses are made. Evaluation of these observations can help therapists identify control parameters and rate-limiters, which will lead to the construction of more effective intervention programs.

As examination, evaluation, and interventions are discussed in other chapters of this text, consider the type and quality of sensory input that underlies the technique. For example, in Chapter 10, the types of sensory stimuli that elicit postural reactions are presented. If the child cannot appropriately process one type (or types) of sensory input, the response may not be demonstrated or the response may be degraded. This represents a very different problem from the child who cannot demonstrate the appropriate response because of muscle weakness. Just as the CNS must integrate input from multiple sensory systems, the reader is encouraged to integrate the information from this chapter with other concepts throughout this text.

CASE STUDY #1: JASON

- *Medical Diagnosis:* Cerebral palsy, right hemiparesis
- *Gross Motor Function Classification System:* Level I
- *Age:* 24 months

Examination

In observing Jason's play, the therapist notes that Jason does not spontaneously use his right upper extremity to assist in manipulating objects. This observation plus others made during the initial intervention session leads the therapist to conclude that Jason is demonstrating sensory neglect of the involved extremities, particularly the right upper extremity. Jason will turn his head to look at an object that touches him on the right. However, if the therapist touches both the right and left sides simultaneously, Jason seems to notice only the contact on the left. This observation reinforces the therapist's conclusion that Jason demonstrates sensory neglect. Jason's mother reports that he does not like to snuggle on her lap. He cries or fidgets when she tries to kiss his neck. Jason grimaces, fusses, or pulls away when the therapist lightly touches him on the right side. The therapist concludes that Jason is tactilely defensive on the right side. When objects are placed in Jason's right hand, he grasps them tightly and cannot control release.

Jason is able to come to standing independently from the floor by assuming a bear stance (support on hands and feet) and rising. The therapist notes that when Jason stands, he has a slight anterior tilt of his pelvis with pelvic retraction on the right. His standing posture improves when the therapist controls the position of the pelvis and approximates through the right lower extremity to reinforce weight bearing through the heel. The therapist observes that contact of the ball of the foot with the floor results in a plantar grasp response. During gait, Jason demonstrates a short stride length on the right due to backward rotation of the right pelvis with genu recurvatum and a valgus foot position during stance. Jason's mom reports that he frequently falls, has difficulty keeping up with his peers, and usually falls when he tries to run. The results of testing for righting and equilibrium reactions suggest that the vestibular system information is being interpreted appropriately; however, motor control dysfunction interferes with a complete response on the right side.

Participation Restrictions

Jason is unable to effectively manipulate some toys or move as quickly as peers during gross motor activities, limiting social interaction and development of play skills. He cannot eat some of the same foods as his peers and may not participate in snack time. He tends to avoid activities and other children to his right side of space, limiting learning experiences and movement exploration of his environment.

Activity/Functional Limitations

Jason does not use his right arm and hand effectively for self-care tasks or for manipulation of toys during play. He does not protect himself well when falling backward or to the right side in sitting or in standing and frequently bumps his head. He demonstrates poor coordination during gross motor tasks. He falls frequently when walking, and cannot run and keep up with peers. Jason is a "messy" eater, frequently losing food out of his mouth. He has difficulty eating food with texture and often spits it out or chokes on it.

Impairments

Jason demonstrates poor sensory awareness on the right side of his body. He has poor motor control of the right upper extremity and slow protective reactions. He demonstrates poor lip closure, difficulty in moving his tongue laterally, and an immature chewing pattern. He does not seem to notice when food is escaping from his mouth. Jason's balance in standing is poor, and he relies on his left side to control initiation and propulsion during gait.

Goals

Jason has a number of treatment goals:

1. Increase sensory awareness of the right side of his body, especially the right upper extremity and right side of his mouth.
2. Increase speed and effectiveness of upper extremity protective reactions.
3. Improve lip closure and tongue control.
4. Improve balance reactions, especially in standing.
5. Improve coordination during gross motor tasks, such as running.
6. Improve coordination during fine motor tasks, such as manipulation of toys.

Participation/Functional Outcomes

After 3 months of intervention, Jason will be able to accomplish the following:

1. Use both hands to take off socks.
2. Use both hands to catch and throw a 12-inch (30.5-cm) ball to an adult.
3. Fall fewer than 3 times per day.
4. Use his arms to catch himself when he falls.
5. Eat soft meats without losing food out of his mouth.
6. Run 10 to 20 feet (3 to 6 m) and keep up with his peers.
7. Enjoy cuddling with his parent.

Intervention

To assess the progress being made toward meeting the general treatment goals, the therapist establishes several measurable functional objectives for Jason. Jason's ability to perform the tasks will be evaluated at the conclusion of each intervention session and at the initiation of the subsequent session to determine changes in performance as well as motor learning. After treatment, Jason will be able to accomplish the following:

1. In sitting, lift an 8-inch (20-cm) diameter ball 5 inches (13-cm) from the table top using both upper extremities (with the therapist assisting the right extremity). Jason must be seated in an appropriate chair to permit his feet to rest on the floor. The table height should be adjusted to provide a comfortable working surface. The therapist can use approximation through the right lower leg to reinforce a flat position of the foot.
2. In sitting, with his right hand placed on an 8-inch (20-cm) diameter ball placed 12 inches (30.5 cm) in front of him, he will roll the ball from side to side 5 times without losing contact with the ball.

3. Tolerate contact of the handler (his therapist or one of his parents) on his right upper extremity for 1 minute without signs of emotional distress.

4. In spontaneous play, attempt to use the right upper extremity in an appropriate manner 5 times during a 3-minute observation period.

5. In standing at a table, maintain a neutral foot flat position of the right lower extremity for 1 minute while playing with a toy.

6. In standing, will use 2 hands (with therapist assistance for the right arm/hand) to throw a 6-inch (15-cm) diameter lightweight playground ball at a target that is 8 to 10 feet (2 to 3 m) away while stepping forward with his right foot. (The therapist will need to emphasize heel contact through visual or auditory cues.)

7. Practice walking on different types of surfaces (eg, level, single-thickness tumbling mat, double-thickness tumbling mat, up/down a 10-foot [3 m] ramp) using different types of stepping patterns, such as long steps, marching, or running with minimal handheld assistance.

To help Jason progress toward meeting these objectives, the therapist could include the following activities as part of the intervention program. The session should begin with Jason, one of his parents, or the therapist rubbing different textures or materials over the left and right sides of his body. The contact with Jason's skin should be steady and continuous. Materials with rougher textures, such as toweling or cotton sheet blankets, should be used initially (Figure 9-8). The handlers also should use their hands to rub his skin so that Jason is comfortable with the touching that will follow during the session. The therapist can assist Jason in rubbing body lotion over his extremities as a reward for tolerating the contact (Figure 9-9).

With Jason appropriately seated at the table, the therapist should position Jason's right arm so he is weight bearing through the elbow with his hand flat on the table. Jason is allowed to play in this position for a few minutes. Then he is encouraged to participate in activities such as water play or finger painting with his right arm. These activities are designed to increase his awareness of his right arm and to decrease tactile defensiveness. Following inhibition of inappropriate upper extremity posturing, Jason should engage in 2-handed activities with an 8-inch (20-cm) diameter ball.

With the therapist controlling the position of the right extremity and the weight of the ball, Jason should push the ball away from his chest and pull it back. After several repetitions, Jason should be guided to lift the ball from the support surface and return it (Figures 9-10 through 9-12). The therapist should attempt to reduce the amount of external control required to keep Jason's right hand in contact with the ball. The therapist also should assist Jason in pronation and supination movements (Figure 9-13). This is a developmentally advanced activity; therefore, more control by the therapist will be necessary. The activity is included to work toward appropriate range of motion and to promote inhibition of inappropriate movements.

Chapter 12 addresses developing ambulation skills. The weight-bearing activities presented in the treatment sequence are effective activities in inhibiting the influence of the plantar grasp reflex. When an appropriate weight-bearing posture is achieved, approximation through the pelvis reinforces maintenance of the position. Throwing the ball at a target is included to promote forward rotation of the right side of his pelvis along with a more normal heel contact with his right foot while giving Jason experience with a gross motor skill that he can perform with his peers. Practicing walking in a variety of ways on multiple surfaces is designed to increase his movement repertoire, as well as improve his dynamic balance and motor control.

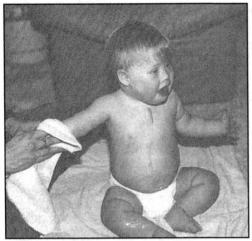

Figure 9-8. Use of toweling to increase the child's tolerance for the therapist's manual contacts with the extremity during the treatment session. (Reprinted with permission from William D. Porter.)

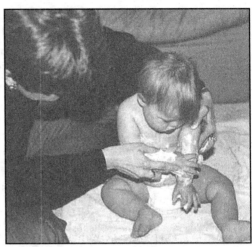

Figure 9-9. Participation of the child in activities such as spreading foam over the trunk and extremities may increase the child's tolerance for these types of interventions. (Reprinted with permission from William D. Porter.)

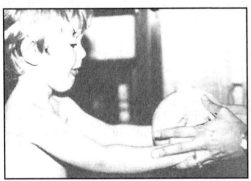

Figure 9-10. Ball activities to promote inhibition of inappropriate overflow in the right upper extremity and to promote 2-handed activities. (Reprinted with permission from William D. Porter.)

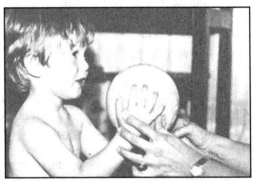

Figure 9-11. Ball activities to promote inhibition of inappropriate overflow in the right upper extremity and to promote 2-handed activities. (Reprinted with permission from William D. Porter.)

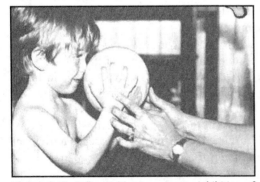

Figure 9-12. Ball activities to promote inhibition of inappropriate overflow in the right upper extremity and to promote 2-handed activities. (Reprinted with permission from William D. Porter.)

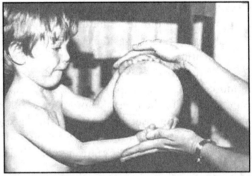

Figure 9-13. Use of ball to promote supination range of motion of right forearm and inhibition of inappropriate posturing. (Reprinted with permission from William D. Porter.)

CASE STUDY #2: JILL

> ▸ *Medical Diagnosis:* Cerebral palsy, spastic quadriparesis, microcephaly, intellectual deficits, seizure disorder
> ▸ *Gross Motor Function Classification System:* Level V
> ▸ *Age:* 7 years

Examination

Jill's parents report that she does not like to be moved between positions. Her therapist notes that movement through space results in signs of autonomic distress, such as increased respiration and heart rate, perspiration, stiffness, and crying. Righting reactions are not present beyond her ability to maintain her head in neutral when she is held vertical; however, the assessment of her ability to respond to vestibular input is complicated by the pattern of muscle tightness. She typically postures with her head extended and her mouth open with her lips and tongue retracted. Any touch to the lips or skin overlying the oral musculature results in increased lip retraction and head extension.

Participation Restrictions

Jill cannot maintain sustained visual contact for effective social interactions with adults or peers. She has difficulty maintaining attention to classroom activities, limiting opportunities for peer interactions as well as academic/cognitive learning. Her poor tolerance for movement results in limited exposure to movement-based play activities. She has limited ability to control her environment, interfering with the development of independence and exploration of physical space.

Activity/Functional Limitations

Jill is nonambulatory and unable to maintain her balance in any position. She demonstrates poor head control in all positions, except when held vertically, during which she can maintain a neutral head position. Jill requires physical support to sit and cannot roll over. She presents with no independent floor mobility. Her protective and equilibrium responses to movement are absent. It is difficult for Jill to voluntarily grasp and release objects. Jill has difficulty eating and drinking. Her ocular control is poor.

Impairments

Jill has limited cognitive ability and demonstrates poor selective attention. Her motor control is diminished secondary to generalized muscle weakness, especially for trunk, head, and neck control. She presents with a kyphotic posture in the upper back with a mild scoliosis and an indented sternum. Jill responds to movement through space with autonomic distress and shows hypersensitivity in the oral area.

Goals

Jill has a number of treatment goals:

1. Increase her ability to attend to visual and auditory stimuli.
2. Improve her strength and motor control, especially of her head, neck, and trunk muscles.
3. Improve her ability to tolerate movement through space with little to no autonomic distress.
4. Decrease her sensitivity to stimulation in the oral area.

Participation/Functional Outcomes

After 3 months of intervention, Jill will be able to accomplish the following:

1. Hold her head erect for 5 minutes when positioned in her vertical stander to watch a classroom activity or video.
2. Tolerate being lifted out of her wheelchair and carried during movement transitions without signs of distress.
3. When positioned in her adapted wheelchair, maintain lip closure for 1 minute with no more than one assist from the handler during feeding.
4. When positioned in her adapted wheelchair, maintain jaw closure for 1 minute with no more than one assist from her handler during feeding.
5. When positioned in her adapted wheelchair, appropriately close lips and jaw on the rim of a drinking glass with no assistance from the handler other than to position and hold the glass.
6. Tolerate being pushed around classroom by classmate while positioned side-lying in a wagon.
7. Hold head erect for 2 minutes while seated in wheelchair to maintain eye contact for social interaction with peer.

Intervention

Jill's intervention program must include a systematic introduction of activities to stimulate the vestibular system to increase her tolerance for movement. Positioned securely in supine in a hammock, she can be rocked gently in an anterior-posterior direction. The initial excursion of the swing would be small. The amplitude and frequency of swings gradually will increase as Jill's tolerance increases. Given the autonomic signs of distress Jill displayed during the examination, the therapist will take baseline measurements of pulse, respiration rate, or blood pressure to determine Jill's response to intervention. Other vestibular activities would include anterior-posterior rocking with Jill positioned in her wheelchair and moving through space while positioned side-lying in a wagon. It is important that Jill experience movement in a variety of positions. It is equally important that Jill feel secure while she is being moved.

As Jill's tolerance for anterior-posterior movement increases, movements in other directions would be added. Movements to be introduced would include medial-lateral, cephalocaudal, nonrepetitive rotation about the body axis (as in rolling prone to supine to prone), diagonal, and finally rotatory movements. Tolerance of each new movement would be carefully assessed.

As Jill's control of her head and trunk position improve (see Chapter 10), problems with control of the oral musculature can be addressed. Maintained jaw closure will be difficult to achieve as long as Jill continues to posture with her head and neck extended. The skin overlying the oral musculature can be desensitized by the therapist's use of maintained manual contact around the mouth (see Chapter 8). This should assist in decreasing withdrawal responses. The therapist must be sure to approach Jill's face carefully so a visual startle or withdrawal is not elicited.

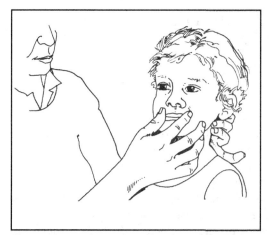

Figure 9-14. Quick stretch to orbicularis oris to facilitate lip closure.

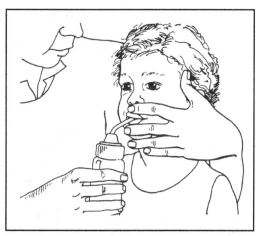

Figure 9-15. Therapist facilitation of jaw and lip closure to assist Jill in drinking through a straw.

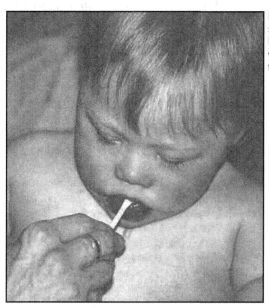

Figure 9-16. Introduction of an oral hygiene swab for stimulation of intraoral muscles. Note that the child's head is positioned in flexion to counter the tendency to withdraw from the stimulus. (Reprinted with permission from William D. Porter.)

Jaw and lip closure can be facilitated by a quick stretch (Figure 9-14) or fingertip vibration of the appropriate musculature. The therapist should desensitize the skin prior to application of these techniques. Functional activities such as drinking from a straw will assist Jill in consolidating her gains (Figure 9-15). The therapist can use finger pressure to the orbicularis oris to facilitate lip closure or can construct a mouthpiece as suggested by Farber to provide a similar response.[20]

The therapist should attend to stimulation of intraoral muscles as well as extraoral musculature. Oral hygiene swabs can be used to stroke the gums, to stretch the insides of the cheeks, or to resist tongue motions (Figure 9-16). The therapist must select an instrument that will not harm the child in case a bite reflex is triggered.

Jill's progress in control of her mouth and tongue will be linked with her progress in developing head and trunk control. Activities in these 2 areas will reinforce her attempts at oral-motor control.

Case Study #3: Taylor

▸ *Medical Diagnosis:* Myelomeningocele, repaired L1-2
▸ *Age:* 4 years

Examination

The examination of Taylor related to his sensory problems reveals a loss of cutaneous and proprioceptive sensation below the level of L1-2. Decreased proprioceptive information from hips, knees, ankles, and feet presents difficulties in Taylor's attempts to maintain a challenged sitting posture, static all fours position, or standing posture in long leg braces.

Taylor's visual acuity problems necessitate the wearing of eyeglasses at all times. Taylor has figure-ground discrimination difficulties and has difficulty locating small objects on a visually distracting background. In standing, when he bends his head to look at the floor through his glasses, his balance is disturbed. This presents difficulty in correct placement of his crutches among objects on the floor. The therapist must extrapolate information from the overall examination to suggest the origin of the balance deficit when Taylor looks down in standing. Because somatosensory information from the lower extremities is lacking, Taylor has an increased reliance on vestibular and visual information for balance. Normal head righting and protective extension reactions in sitting suggest that vestibular responses are within normal limits. The therapist concludes that visual perceptual problems are the primary contributors to balance problems in standing with head movement. Taylor must learn to produce the appropriate compensatory movements when his center of gravity is displaced by motion of the head.

Participation Restrictions

In play activities on the floor with peers, Taylor has difficulty visually locating and manipulating toys. He is unable to make movement transitions to keep up with his peers as they move around the classroom play area. These 2 factors limit social interactions, development of play and cognitive skills, and opportunities for visual-motor exploration of his physical environment.

Activity/Functional Limitations

Taylor requires external support to stand and ambulates using long leg braces and a walker, but is ready to begin using crutches. Although he attempts to pull to kneeling, Taylor demonstrates poor sitting and standing balance. Taylor requires assistance for lower body dressing. Taylor has difficulty placing his crutches in the correct location on the floor.

Impairments

Taylor demonstrates loss of cutaneous and proprioceptive sensation below L1-2. Taylor has visual acuity and perceptual problems, especially figure-ground discrimination, with slow balance reactions in sitting and standing. He experiences frequent skin breakdowns and has loss of motor function in his lower extremities. Taylor shows generalized muscle weakness and lack of endurance in his upper extremities and trunk, particularly his abdominal muscles.

Goals

Taylor has a number of treatment goals:

1. Improve his visual perceptual skills, especially figure-ground discrimination.
2. Improve his balance reactions in sitting and standing.
3. Decrease the frequency of skin breakdowns.
4. Improve the strength and endurance of upper extremity and trunk muscles, especially abdominals.

Participation/Functional Outcomes

After 3 months of intervention, Taylor will be able to accomplish the following:

1. Correctly don his shoes and socks, eliminating potential pressure areas every time.
2. Maintain correct body alignment in his long leg braces while reciprocally lifting his crutches 10 times in 30 seconds.
3. Maintain standing balance in his long leg braces for 15 seconds with his eyes closed (with crutches).
4. Maintain standing balance in his long leg braces for 1 minute while moving his head up, down, right, and left (with crutches).
5. In standing, identify numbers placed on shapes on the floor with 80% accuracy. (This outcome assumes that Taylor can visually identify numbers and shapes on a plain background.)
6. In floor sitting, during play with peers, be able to discriminate and locate small toys on a patterned carpet background.
7. In his wheelchair, be able to move around classroom areas to join in group activities with peers.

Intervention

Included in Taylor's intervention program would be education of Taylor and his parents on techniques for providing good skin care. Taylor and his parents will learn to monitor the condition of the skin with each change of his shoes or orthoses. The therapist should evaluate the consistency of the parents' visual inspection of Taylor's legs at each preschool session they attend. If the behavior is established at school, it should generalize to other situations. The objective would be stated as follows: Taylor's parents will visually inspect his lower extremities for indications of skin irritation or pressure following every removal of shoes and socks or orthoses.

Activities addressing balance and figure-ground training should be conducted in standing with his long leg braces and crutches. Taylor eventually can learn to maintain his balance while hitting a ball with one crutch. A variety of floor backgrounds can be used, progressing from plain to visually distracting patterns. Initially, he should be stationary with the ball position being varied for different trials (Figure 9-17).

As Taylor increases his balance and skill, the ball can be rolled to him so he can bat it with his crutch. Objects of varying heights can be placed around Taylor with the goal of touching the top of each object with his crutch without knocking over the object (Figure 9-18).

Taylor may benefit from activities such as a wheelchair obstacle course. Manipulation of his chair will increase upper extremity and trunk strength and endurance. Successful completion of the course requires good visual perceptual skills and motor planning. This activity can be a fun reward for successful completion of more difficult tasks during the therapy session.

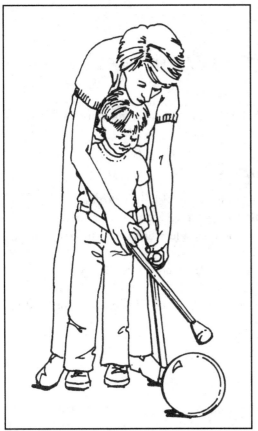

Figure 9-17. Balance activities in standing while hitting a stationary ball with one crutch.

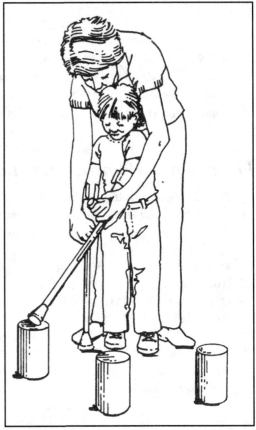

Figure 9-18. Trunk rotation in standing promoted by touching objects placed in a semicircle around Taylor.

CASE STUDY #4: ASHLEY

> *Medical Diagnosis:* Down syndrome
> *Age:* 15 months

Examination

Ashley demonstrates a lack of stability in all positions as well as generalized hypotonia (Figure 9-19). During her examination, she was noted to respond to rapid, irregular vestibular input with more appropriate postural tone and stability. Proprioceptive and cutaneous input also improved her ability to maintain postures.

Ashley was noted to be generally apprehensive about movement. Discussion with the parents indicates that Ashley's ongoing series of medical problems have resulted in her being treated by the family as a "fragile" child. Ashley has not had the opportunity to experience motion as a part of typical games parents play with infants. The therapist must not only introduce Ashley to the fun of movement activities, but also reassure her parents that the activities are appropriate for her.

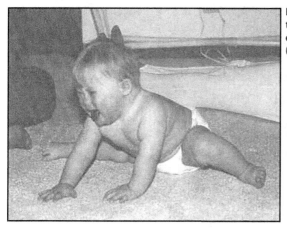

Figure 9-19. Ashley's posture in moving from prone to sitting indicates the exaggerated flexibility present in the hips due to her generalized hypotonia. (Reprinted with permission from William D. Porter.)

Participation Restrictions

Ashley avoids physical contact with adults and peers and appears to be anxious about being pushed or bumped. She prefers to limit her personal space, thereby decreasing opportunities for peer play and social interactions. Owing to poor fine motor and oral-motor skills, Ashley often becomes fussy during snack time and does not want to participate with the group. Her limited motor skills and apprehension about movement limit her ability to explore her physical environment.

Activity/Functional Limitations

In general, Ashley avoids movement, demonstrates slow movements, and has delays in postural reactions. She relies on a wide base of support with lumbar lordosis, knee hyperextension, and foot pronation when she stands. Ashley is not attempting to cruise at furniture at this time. She has difficulty performing grasp and release tasks and shows limited oral-motor skills.

Impairments

Ashley presents with hypermobile joints, low muscle tone (hypotonia), a mild hearing loss, and intellectual challenges associated with her medical diagnosis.

Goals

Ashley has a number of treatment goals:
1. Increase her stability in all positions, especially at the shoulder and hip joints.
2. Increase strength and endurance in all positions, particularly in sitting and standing.
3. Reduce her and her parents' apprehension regarding movement activities.
4. Increase the frequency of self-initiated movement through space.

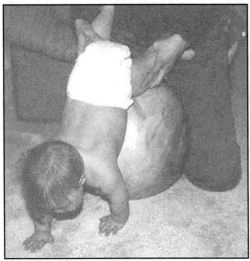

Figure 9-20. Inversion over a ball to promote shoulder girdle stability with weight-bearing through upper extremities. (Reprinted with permission from William D. Porter.)

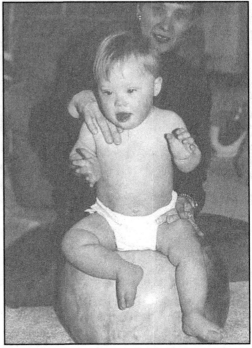

Figure 9-21. Bouncing on ball with the therapist assisting in maintaining appropriate postural alignment. (Reprinted with permission from William D. Porter.)

Participation/Functional Outcomes

After 3 months of intervention, Ashley will be able to accomplish the following:

1. Maintain appropriate alignment in quadruped position during play for 30 seconds with no more than one cue from the handler.
2. Maintain appropriate alignment in standing with upper extremities on a support for one minute with the handler providing no more than 2 cues.
3. Move from standing to sitting to all fours position with no indications of apprehension.
4. Tolerate therapist-assisted movements between various developmentally appropriate postures with no indications of apprehension.
5. Tolerate other children bumping into her without becoming upset.
6. Remain seated close to a peer for 5 minutes during snack time.

Intervention

Intervention activities are designed to increase postural stability and decrease apprehension regarding movement. Ashley can be inverted on a ball leading to weight-bearing support through her arms (Figure 9-20). Sitting on the ball, she can be bounced. This provides vestibular stimulation and approximation through the vertebral column (Figure 9-21). Ashley should be encouraged to rock in an all fours position while the therapist approximates through the head or pelvis in the long axis of the vertebral column (Figure 9-22).

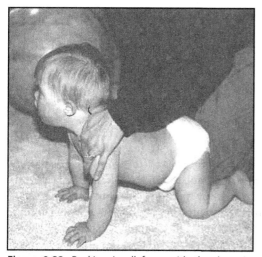

Figure 9-22. Rocking in all fours with the therapist approximating through the long axis of the vertebral column to reinforce postural alignment. (Reprinted with permission from William D. Porter.)

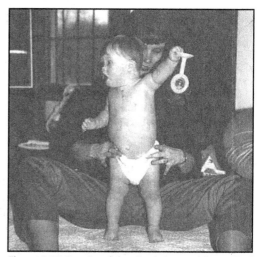

Figure 9-23. Practice of standing balance while involved in upper extremity play activities. (Reprinted with permission from William D. Porter.)

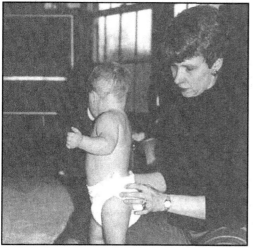

Figure 9-24. Practice of standing balance while involved in upper extremity play activities. (Reprinted with permission from William D. Porter.)

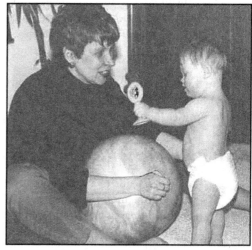

Figure 9-25. Practice of standing balance while involved in upper extremity play activities. (Reprinted with permission from William D. Porter.)

The therapist may approximate through the long axis of the upper extremities or the femurs to reinforce postural holding contractions through the extremities. Following the inversion activity on the ball, Ashley could be moved into a standing position. Approximation through the pelvis with the force vector through the correct alignment of the lower extremities should improve Ashley's standing posture. Ashley should be involved in upper extremity play activities as the therapist reinforces correct standing alignment (Figures 9-23 through 9-25). This should assist Ashley in integrating the control she is learning in situations outside therapy.

Following inversion or other vestibular facilitation techniques, the therapist should assist Ashley in moving through a variety positions. The therapist is assisting Ashley in using the increased postural control developed during the intervention session.

CASE STUDY #5: JOHN

> *Medical Diagnosis:* Developmental coordination disorder/attention-deficit hyperactivity disorder
> *Age:* 5 years

Examination

In observing John's play and after conferring with his parents, it became apparent that John changes activities very quickly for someone his age, usually after just 1 to 2 minutes. His parents indicate that his short attention span also is a concern at school, as is his reluctance to participate in any structured gross motor activities. John tends to move by walking or jogging. When provided a demonstration, John was able to gallop but had difficulty with single-leg balance as well as hopping and skipping. John attempted to catch an 8-inch (20-cm) lightweight ball, but after 2 tries he simply moved to another area of the gym and began to play with small toy animals.

John's parents report he does not ride a bike independently and does not seem to like to play on playground equipment at the neighborhood park. During the examination, John completed an obstacle course by playing Simon Says with the therapist in which he completed each obstacle separately rather than linking each task into a complete series of movement challenges. The series of tasks revealed John has normal range of motion in his extremities, but has difficulty supporting his body weight with just his upper extremities.

Participation Restrictions

John limits his physical activities and interactions with peers during recess at school and at the neighborhood playground. These limitations reduce opportunities for social interactions, as well as opportunities to improve his motor planning, gross motor skills, and physical fitness.

Activity/Functional Limitations

In general, John tends to avoid physical activity and is described as "clumsy." He is unable to perform gross and fine motor tasks as well as his peers, such as skipping, throwing and catching a ball, using utensils during meals, and manipulating buttons, snaps, and zippers. He also has difficulty with maintaining balance when standing still, walking on a 4-inch (10-cm) balance beam, and climbing over and under barriers.

Impairments

John has difficulty with selective attention and demonstrates an expressive language delay. His motor planning ability is poor, and he has difficulty generalizing motor skills from one situation to another. John has decreased upper extremity strength and lower than normal cardiovascular endurance.

Goals

John has a number of treatment goals:
1. Improve his motor planning ability.
2. Increase the fluidity of his movement sequences.
3. Use his motor skills in multiple settings.

4. Increase his upper body strength.
5. Increase his cardiovascular endurance.
6. Participate in structured gross motor games with his peers.

Participation/Functional Outcomes

After 3 months of intervention, John will be able to accomplish the following:
1. Use 2 hands to throw and catch a 10-inch (25-cm) ball with an adult.
2. Participate in directed physical activities in the physical therapy gym, during recess at school, and in the neighborhood playground.
3. Use 2 hands to hit a stationary ball with a lightweight bat or racquet.
4. Participate in physical activity for 15 to 20 minutes without undue fatigue.
5. Move in a variety of ways (eg, skipping, galloping, hopping, running) in the treatment gym, as well as at school and in the neighborhood playground.

Intervention

Initially, John should be treated in a well-controlled 1:1 setting with limited interruptions and distractions. The equipment used with John from session to session should remain consistent in the early phases of therapy. Over time and with experience, the therapist will need to gradually introduce different pieces of equipment (eg, different sized and colored balls) as well as people into the treatment sessions.

Timing of activities and sequencing of activities will be crucial to John's success. The therapist will need to be sensitive to John's "rhythms" during early treatment sessions. This will necessitate having equipment ready and the treatment area well controlled so the therapist can transition between activities according to John's needs/schedule rather than some external or fixed factor (eg, time or someone else needing a piece of equipment). This will maximize John's ability to succeed when moving, which will facilitate his attention to the movement task as well as his motivation to keep moving, both of which will be critical to helping him learn that it is fun to move in different ways and in different environments. As John's skills develop and his ability to complete movement tasks successfully are established, the therapist should move to more of an "on-demand" approach so John develops the ability to attend to and comply with requests that come from outside his internal schedule/rhythms. This can be accomplished by having John help develop a schedule of events for his treatment sessions by offering John structured choices from a preselected array of activities.

As John progresses with his skill development and his ability to attend to the task, the therapist will need to introduce "controlled" distractors. These distractors might be a sibling or friend who participates in therapy with John or moving to a treatment area that has windows or a door that John must learn to ignore. Moving to a more open treatment setting will be the next step in advancing John's skills. Communication and coordination with the physical therapist in John's school district is essential. At this point, John will begin to transition to school services and community activities designed to build on his progress and to continue to expand his motor planning skills.

During the final phase of this episode of care, John should be expected to participate in various physical activities for increasingly longer periods of time. The therapist should set expectations that are similar to what other 5-year-old children can meet successfully. For example, 10 to 15 minutes of active gross motor movement is not uncommon for most 5-year-olds. This expectation may need to be developed in the more controlled therapeutic setting initially before being applied in more open environments, such as the school or a public playground.

Acknowledgment

The editors wish to express appreciation to Rebecca E. Porter, PT, PhD, FAPTA for contributions to earlier editions of this chapter.

References

1. Polit A, Bizzi E. Characteristics of motor programs underlying arm movements in monkeys. *J Neurophys.* 1979;42(1 pt 1):183-194. doi:10.1152/jn.1979.42.1.183.

2. Schmidt RA. *Motor Control and Learning.* 2nd ed. Champaign, IL: Human Kinetics Publishers; 1988.

3. Chapman D. Context effects on spontaneous leg movements of infants with spina bifida. *Pediatr Phys Ther.* 2002;14(2):62-73.

4. Kamm K, Thelen E, Jensen JL. A dynamical systems approach to motor development. *Phys Ther.* 1990;70(12):763-775. doi:10.1093/ptj/70.12.763.

5. Ulrich BD, Ulrich DA, Collier DH, Cole EL. Developmental shifts in the ability of infants with Down syndrome to produce treadmill steps. *Phys Ther.* 1995;75(1):14-23. doi:10.1093/ptj/75.1.14.

6. Chapman D. The influence of position on leg movements and kicks in older infants with spina bifida. *Pediatr Phys Ther.* 2016;28(4):380-385. doi:10.1097/PEP.0000000000000299.

7. Ulrich BD, Ulrich DA. Spontaneous leg movements in infants with Down syndrome and nondisabled infants. *Child Dev.* 1995;66(6):1844-1855. doi:10.1111/j.1467-8624.1995.tb00969.x.

8. Abraham RH, Shaw CD. *Dynamics—The Geometry of Behavior. Part 1: Periodic Behavior.* Santa Cruz, CA: Aerial Press; 1982.

9. Thelen E. Self-organization in developmental processes: can systems approaches work? In: Gunnar G, Thelen E, eds. *Systems in Development: The Minnesota Symposia in Child Psychology.* Hillsdale, NJ: Erlbaum; 1989:77-117.

10. Ulrich BD, Ulrich DA. Dynamic systems approach to understanding motor delay in infants with Down syndrome. In: Savelsbergh GJP, ed. *The Development of Coordination in Infancy.* Holland: Elsevier Science; 1993:445-459.

11. Thelen E, Ulrich BD. Hidden skills: a dynamic systems analysis of treadmill stepping during the first year. *Monogr Soc Res Child Dev.* 1991;56(1):1-98; discussion 99-104. doi:10.2307/1166099.

12. Thelen E, Smith L. *A Dynamic Systems Approach to the Development of Cognition and Action.* Cambridge, MA: The MIT Press; 1994.

13. Thelen E. Treadmill-elicited stepping in seven-month-old infants. *Child Dev.* 1986;57(6):1498-1506. doi:10.1111/j.1467-8624.1986.tb00474.x.

14. Chapman D, Angulo-Kinzler R. Mechanisms for the initiation of infant treadmill steps. Paper presented at: North American Society for the Psychology of Sport and Physical Activity; 1995; Clearwater, FL.

15. Adams JA. A closed-loop theory of motor learning. *J Motor Behav.* 1971;3(2):111-150. doi:10.1080/00222895.1971.10734898.

16. Schmidt RA. A schema theory of discrete motor skill learning. *Psychol Rev.* 1975;82(4):225-260. doi:10.1037/h0076770.

17. Newell KM. Motor skill acquisition. *Annu Rev Psychol.* 1991;42(2):213-237. doi:10.1146/annurev.ps.42.020191.001241.

18. Edelman GM. *Neural Darwinism: The Theory of Neuronal Group Selection.* New York, NY: Basic Books; 1987.

19. Edelman GM. *The Remembered Present.* New York, NY: Basic Books; 1989.

20. Stein D. Concepts of central nervous system plasticity and their implications for recovery after brain damage. In: Zasler ND, Katz DI, Ross DZ, Arciniegas DB, Bullock MR, Kreutzer JS, eds. *Brain Injury Medicine: Principles and Practice,* 2nd ed. New York, NY: Demos Medical Publishing; 2012:162-174.

21. Kleim J. Neural plasticity and neurorehabilitation: teaching the new brain old tricks. *J Comm Disord.* 2011;44(5):521-528. doi:10.1016/j.jcomdis.2011.04.006.

22. Warraich Z, Kleim JA. Neural plasticity: the biological substrate for neurorehabilitation. *PM R.* 2010;2(12 suppl 2):S208-S219. doi:10.1016/j.pmrj.2010.10.016.

23. Farber SD. *Neurorehabilitation—A Multisensory Approach.* Philadelphia, PA: WB Saunders; 1982.

24. Gentile AM. Skill acquisition: action, movement, and neuromotor processes. In: Carr JH, Shepherd R, Gordon J, Gentile AM, Held JM, eds. *Movement Science Foundations for Physical Therapy in Rehabilitation.* Rockville, MD: Aspen Publishers; 1987:155-177.

25. Nashner LM. Sensory, neuromuscular, and biomechanical contributions to human balance. In: Duncan PW, ed. *Balance: Proceedings of the APTA Forum.* Alexandria, VA: American Physical Therapy Association; 1990:5-12.

26. Umphred DA. Classification of treatment techniques based on primary input systems. In: Umphred DA, ed. *Neurological Rehabilitations.* 3rd ed. St. Louis, MO: CV Mosby; 1995:118-178.

27. Noback CR, Strominger NL, Demarest RJ. *The Human Nervous System.* Malvern, PA: Lea & Febiger; 1991:160.

28. McGraw MB. Neuromuscular mechanism of the infant. *Am J Dis Child.* 1940;60(4):1031-1042. doi:10.1001/archpedi.1940.02000050015003.

29. Ayres AJ. *Southern California Postrotatory Nystagmus Test.* Los Angeles, CA: Western Psychological Services; 1975.

30. Hagbarth KE, Eklund G. The muscle vibrator—a useful tool in neurological therapeutic work. In: Payton O, Hirt S, Newton R, eds. *Therapeutic Exercise.* Philadelphia, PA: FA Davis; 1978:138.

31. Woollacott MH. Postural control and development. In: Whiting HTA, Wade MG, eds. *Themes in Motor Development.* Boston, MA: Martinus Nijhoff; 1986.

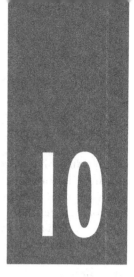

Developing Postural Control

Patricia C. Montgomery, PT, PhD, FAPTA
Susan K. Effgen, PT, PhD, FAPTA

Postural control is a broad term encompassing a variety of processes, functional movements, and skills. During the first 2 years of life, the child achieves head and trunk control and gross motor skills, such as independent sitting, kneeling, and standing. (See Video 10-1.)

Functional mobility, whether by rolling, crawling, or walking, requires a variety of active movements and postural adjustments. Postural adjustments are necessary if a child is to move freely and efficiently and respond rapidly to the demands of the environment. As children mature, they display a number of distinct movements, some anticipatory and some reactive, which orient the head and body in space, protect them when they fall, and assist them in attaining and maintaining balance. These postural and extremity movements fall under the broad description of postural control. The term *postural control* often is used interchangeably with the terms *balance* or *stability*. Postural control involves regulating relative positions of the parts of the body and of the whole body with respect to a frame of reference.[1] One major goal is to keep the center of mass (COM) within the margins of the support surface. Stability and orientation are 2 distinct goals of the postural control system. Some tasks, needing a particular orientation, are accomplished at the expense of stability. An example is riding a bicycle around a tight corner, thereby leaning into the curve. The child would have orientation against gravity, but would be vulnerable to instability. The demands of stability and orientation change with individual tasks.

SYSTEMS APPROACH TO POSTURAL CONTROL

Multiple intrinsic systems, as well as cultural and environmental influences,[2] play a role in the development of postural control. Merzenich et al[3] reviewed the large body of science demonstrating that expressive behaviors are the product of complex, multilevel recurrent networks ("reverse hierarchy theory") in the central nervous system (CNS; see Chapter 1). Neural mechanisms, however, do not exert their influence in a vacuum, but rather through children's musculoskeletal systems. Range of motion (ROM) must be adequate to allow postural control, such as upper extremity protective reactions and lower extremity hip or ankle strategies in standing, to occur. Limited

Connolly BH, Montgomery PC, eds. *Therapeutic Exercise for Children With Developmental Disabilities, Fourth Edition* (pp 271-303).
© 2020 Taylor & Francis Group.

ROM in children with developmental disabilities (DD) may have adverse effects on postural control. For example, a significant proportion of children with juvenile idiopathic arthritis affecting the lower extremities have impaired static and dynamic balance.[4]

Herskind and colleagues[5] demonstrated through ultrasonography of the medial gastrocnemius muscle that bone length increased with age similarly in young typically developing (TD) children and children with cerebral palsy (CP). However, by age 15 months muscle volume was significantly decreased in children with CP compared with their TD peers. The lack of muscle growth relative to bone growth may be a contributing factor for development of limitations in motion and contractures in this population. The interaction of neural and musculoskeletal mechanisms is complex, and reflex-mediated muscle stiffness is difficult to distinguish clinically from changes in passive muscle stiffness that are already present from at least age 3 years in children with CP.[6]

Children must have sufficient muscle strength to resist the forces of gravity and environmental perturbations. Neural elements that may contribute to weakness in children with CP include possible reduced central drive, insufficient and disorganized motor recruitment, impaired voluntary control, and impaired reciprocal inhibition (ie, cocontraction).[7] Musculoskeletal elements contributing to weakness may include selective atrophy of fast fibers, changes in length-tension curves, reduced elasticity, and impoverished tissue development. In a study of 2- to 6-year-olds with CP (Gross Motor Function Classification System Levels II and III), a significant predictor of independent walking was functional strength, such as the ability to get up and down from sitting.[8]

Sensory systems provide crucial information for motor control throughout development. Even newborn infants process sensory information for use in modifying movements and organizing the postural control system in relation to task demands.[9] Sensory organization can be evaluated in children during standing by using a visual enclosure and moveable platform that allows computerized measurements of postural stability and the strategies used to maintain balance. Testing usually is completed in 6 conditions: 1) eyes open, 2) eyes closed, 3) sway-referenced visual surround, 4) sway-referenced support surface, 5) eyes closed and sway-referenced support surface, and 6) sway-referenced support surface and visual surround referenced. Rine et al[10] used this protocol to compare the performance of 23 TD children (age 3.5 to 7 years) and 11 adults. Results indicated that children demonstrated adult-like use of somatosensory information between age 4 to 6 years. Measures of vestibular and visual effectiveness in postural control, however, were not similar to adults by age 7.5 years, indicating that sensory integrative mechanisms were still maturing.

Lui et al[11] used these 6 sensory conditions to compare the performance of 12 children with Tourette syndrome with 12 TD control individuals. Children with Tourette syndrome had more difficulty in maintaining postural stability, especially when vestibular information was challenged (conditions 5 and 6). This suggests possible deficits in processing vestibular information related to postural control in children with Tourette syndrome.

Twenty-five children between age 8 and 10 years with unilateral cochlear implants and bilateral vestibular hypofunction were tested on a force plate during different balance tasks.[12] Performance was improved when the cochlear implants were turned "on" compared with when they were "off," demonstrating that auditory information improved postural stability in these children.

Hatzitaki and colleagues[13] examined the relationship between specific perceptual and motor skills and static and dynamic balance performance in 50 TD children between age 11 and 13 years. Correlation analysis suggested that balancing (one-legged tasks) under static conditions was associated with the ability to perceive and process visual information (suggesting the use of feedback-based control). Under dynamic balancing conditions, however, the ability to respond to destabilizing hip abductions/adductions was associated with motor response speed (suggesting use of a descending, feedforward control strategy). The authors concluded that 11- to 13-year-old children have the ability to select varying balance strategies depending on task constraints.

Children, as well as adults, must have accurate information regarding their position in space as well as the position of their body parts and be able to process this information efficiently for optimal motor control. Because perception is preparatory to movement, sensory functions are an integral part of the examination of children with deficits in motor control. Sensory systems and examination and intervention strategies are discussed in Chapter 9.

Cognitive processes involved in looking, attention, memory functions, and motor organization and sequencing are neural processes underlying postural control. If 2 tasks can be performed as well simultaneously as individually, then at least one does not require attention ("automatic"). However, if one task is performed less well with a secondary task, both are thought to require some attention. Dual-Task methodology and performance of TD children at various ages have been described.[14-16] Boonyong et al[17] investigated development of postural control in younger (age 5 to 6 years) and older children (age 7 to 16 years) and a group of healthy young adults during 2 gait tasks paired with an auditory Stroop test (verbal reaction time: "high" vs "low"/"high" vs "low" pitch). Gait performance decrements in dual-task conditions were greater in the younger vs older children, and younger children were slower and less accurate on the Stroop test. Results supported the idea that there is a developmental trend in attentional resources used to control gait in typical development.

EARLY MOTOR BEHAVIOR

Now that the hierarchical reflex model is not considered an adequate framework for the development of postural control, does that mean children no longer demonstrate a Moro response, primitive stepping, or an asymmetrical tonic neck "reflex"? No, of course not. Early motor behavior has not changed, but how we conceptualize what that motor behavior represents has changed.

"Primitive Spinal Reflexes" (Patterns of Movement)

Consider the "primitive spinal cord reflexes" described in the reflex model. Included in this category are "flexor withdrawal," "positive supporting," "placing," and "stepping."[18] Multiple studies have demonstrated the presence of central pattern generators [CPGs] consisting of neurons and interneurons in the spinal cord and brainstem that can spontaneously generate a motor pattern or movement without peripheral sensory or higher brain center input.[19-21] The CPG for stepping in many animals has been demonstrated to be located in the spinal cord. A similar CPG is proposed in the spinal cord of the human infant. This hypothesis is based on studies of fetal and early infant stepping,[22,23] as well as the ability of children with anencephaly to produce stepping movements.[24]

Studies of TD infants stepping in different directions on a treadmill,[25] as well as comparisons of upper and lower limb kinematics of forward and backward walking in primary school-aged children,[26] support the idea that the same locomotor CPG controls different directions of stepping in humans.

One hypothesis, then, is that movements historically described as "spinal reflexes" are present in a CPG located in the spinal cord and can be elicited through sensory input or used actively by the child for early kicking, supported stepping, and later for independent ambulation. CPGs for stepping, however, are not sufficient to generate a mature gait pattern. Supraspinal influences are necessary for transformation to a normal, mature gait pattern (eg, transition from digitigrade to plantigrade, development of upright balance). Ivanenko and colleagues[27] used imaging to map motor neuron activity in the lumbosacral spinal cord during stepping to study the development and function of pattern-generation networks in the spinal cord in newborn stepping and walking in toddlers and adults. Their research demonstrated development of human locomotion from the neonate to adult starts from a rostrocaudal excitability gradient and involves a gradual functional reorganization of the pattern-generation circuitry. A subsequent study compared electromyography (EMG) activity profiles from simultaneously recorded muscles onto anatomical locations of motor neurons pools in the spinal cord of 35 children with CP compared with 33 TD controls (age 1 to 12 years).[28] A significant difference was noted between the groups, with TD children showing progressive reduction of EMG burst duration and gradual reorganization of spatiotemporal motor neuron output with increasing age. However, children with CP showed very limited age-related changes. These findings are consistent with the hypothesis that early injuries to developing motor regions of the brain substantially affect maturation of the spinal locomotor output and consequently future locomotor behavior.

"Tonic Neck and Labyrinthine Reflexes" (Patterns of Movement)

Another example of how we conceptualize what "reflex" patterns represent is how we view tonic neck reflexes and labyrinthine righting reflexes. A close examination of the effects on the extremities of the tonic neck reflexes and the labyrinthine righting reflexes demonstrates that these 2 postural mechanisms represent exactly opposite changes in postural tone or movement patterns (Figure 10-1).[29]

In the classic studies of Magnus and DeKleijn,[30] side-down tilting of decerebrate cats resulted in a decrease in extensor tone of the limbs toward which the chin pointed. In the decerebrate cats without labyrinths, rotation of the head with the body upright resulted in an increase in extensor tone of the limbs toward which the chin rotated. The common description of the asymmetrical tonic neck reflex (ATNR) as producing increased extensor tone on the face side and increased flexor tone on the skull side is not technically correct. A more precise definition would be that increased extensor tone or an extensor movement pattern is produced on the face side, and less extensor tone is elicited on the skull side, with resulting flexion.

In animals that do not have a neck (eg, fish), the vestibular apparatus is sufficient for determining body position. In animals that have developed the ability to move the head on the body, vestibular input is no longer sufficient to monitor body position. For example, in Figure 10-2, if the CNS has information only from the labyrinthine receptors, it cannot tell whether the head has moved on the body or the body has moved in space, as the vestibular input is the same. In Condition A, neck receptors inform the CNS that the head has moved on the body (not the body through space). In Condition B, the neck receptors inform the CNS that the head has not moved on the body, therefore, the body must have moved through space. In a normal situation, changes in somatosensory information related to weight shift (or the absence of weight shift) and visual information also provide information to the CNS regarding movement of the body, head, and extremities.

Although the role of the ATNR in eye-hand coordination has face validity, the relationship between movements associated with labyrinthine and neck inputs suggests a role in postural control.[29,31-32] In 1974, Kornhuber[29] stated that Magnus,[30] who initially described the neck "reflexes," failed to appreciate the functional relationship with labyrinthine responses and his erroneous interpretation of the neck reflexes as "static" or "attitudinal" persists.

The human infant learns to differentiate various combinations of head movement on the body in relation to movement of the body in space as he creeps on hands and knees (ie, quadruped). If the infant creeps onto an unstable surface and tips to the left side, increased weight bearing must occur on the down side of the tilt and less weight bearing must occur on the up side of the tilt to prevent a fall. If the infant were to continue to bear weight symmetrically when tipping, he or she would fall off the surface. If the infant is creeping on a stable surface and turns his or her head to look to the right, he or she must bear weight equally on both arms and not produce asymmetrical weight bearing as on the moveable surface. If the degree of tilt in the first example (unstable surface) results in the same labyrinthine information as active head turning to the right on a stable surface, the infant has to use somatosensory information from the neck receptors (as well as somatosensory information from the extremities and visual input) to determine whether he or she has moved through space or the head has moved on the body or both.

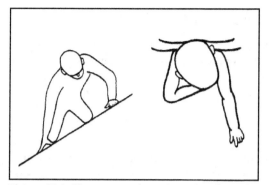

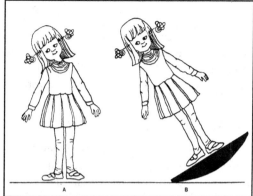

Figure 10-1. The asymmetric tonic neck reflexes (to the right in a child) are the antagonistic partners of the labyrinthine tilting reflexes (to the left). When the head is turned with the nose toward the left, the neck reflex induces extension of the left arm and the right arm flexes. Rapid lateral tilt with the nose to the left, however, causes extension of the right with flexion of the left arm. Labyrinthine tilting reflexes prevent falling during rapid tilt; neck reflexes prevent falling due to labyrinthine reflexes when only the head is moved. (Reprinted with permission from Kornhuber HH. The vestibular system and the general motor system. In: Kornhuber HH, ed. *Handbook of Sensory Physiology.* Heidelburg, Germany: Springer-Verlag; 1974.)

Figure 10-2. If the body is tilted (B) or the head moved on the trunk (A) in the same plane of motion with identical excursion and rate of movement, the labyrinths receive the same stimulus. Information from neck receptors provide the CNS with information to determine whether the body has moved in space or if the head has moved on the body. Body proprioception, signaling the presence or absence of weight shift, and visual input also contribute to the orientation process. (Reprinted with permission from the Haworth Press, Inc. Birmingham, NY. From Montgomery PC. Vestibular processing in children. *Phys Occup Ther Pediatr.* 1985;2/3:33-55.)

Reflexes and Medical Diagnosis

Physical therapists who work in neonatal intensive care units or who are responsible for the examination of young infants need to have a working knowledge of early motor responses to sensory stimulation. Reactions to sensory stimulation that, for example, elicit a palmar grasp, rooting reflex, sucking reflex, walking reflex ("stepping"), or Moro, and startle responses are used in the neurological assessment of preterm and full-term newborn infants[18,33] and to determine gestational age.[34]

Hamer and Hadders-Algra[35] reviewed studies on the prognostic significance of neurological signs in high-risk infants. Data indicated that in early infancy, absent Moro or plantar grasp responses may be predictive of adverse developmental outcome. After early infancy, persistence in the Moro response and ATNR was clinically significant. Abnormal performance on the pull-to-sit maneuver and vertical suspension had predictive significance throughout infancy.

In a study of 87 high-risk infants assessed with the General Movement Assessment and for the presence of "fidgety" movements at 3 months postterm and followed until age 2 years, the risk of motor problems increased with extent of negative results on the assessment and was 10 times higher when fidgety movements were absent at 3 months.[36] Thus, this lack of fidgety movements at 3 months' corrected age was predictive of the development of CP.[37]

In summary, persistence of early motor patterns and reduced variability of movements are suggestive of pathology to the motor control areas and functions of the CNS. If neuromodulary influences from higher brain centers do not occur during development, motor synergies will not be used efficiently for meaningful movement and early appearing movements may not be modified and more complex motor performance will be limited (see Chapter 1).

Developmental Motor Skills

During the first 2 years of life, the child achieves basic motor skills. Learning to roll over, crawl, sit, and walk are frequently learned through trial and error experimentation.[38] Monumental gains in motor skills often are accidental, the result of random movements. For example, in prone on elbows infants may follow something of interest with their eyes until, to their surprise, they roll over.

Nature Versus Nurture

Early studies in typical postural development suggest 2 general principles. The first principle is Edelman's concept of Neuronal Group Selection, which emphasizes variability in motor development and a repertoire of strategies.[39] The second principle is that postural control is organized into 2 functional levels. The most basic level is direction specificity, which suggests some level of innate ability. If balance is threatened by forward sway of the body, for example, muscles on the dorsal side are primarily activated. The opposite would occur with backward sway, with muscles on the ventral side activated. The second level would be "fine-tuning" of these direction-specific adjustments to the specifics of the situation. This might include the number, order of activation, and strength of muscles that are activated. In Edelman's theory there are genetically predetermined neuronal groups that are not precisely "wired." Development is "tuning" of the innate circuits driven by experiences and mediated by synaptic modifications of the neuronal group response.

One view is that the human CNS solves the problem of multiple motor possibilities for postural control through functional organization of basic direction-specific synergies adapted to specific biomechanical constraints.[40-43] Thelen et al[44,45] proposed an alternative view of postural development, mainly that self-organization occurs as a result of "learning by doing." They rejected the application of the term *CPGs* to infant muscle patterns and reviewed evidence that peripheral input can modulate movement patterns at birth. They also cited the high variability and number of possible combinations of movements that infants demonstrate. The dynamic systems approach views postural control as emerging from the interaction of the system's components within a particular task and environmental context.

Studies have demonstrated that practice or experience plays a role in developing "automatic" postural responses, as TD infants have exhibited a positive training effect of platform perturbations on movement patterns in sitting[46] and standing.[47,48] In a study of 6- to 9-month-old TD children, sitting and controlling posture on forward and backward slopes also was associated with experience.[49]

The debate on the "nature" vs "nurture" contributions to motor development is an old one and has not been resolved. Dynamic systems theorists recognize "the fact that infants are born with a species-typical neuronal anatomy, and that this anatomy forms the basis for further epigenetic changes."[45(p512)] Theorists adhering to the importance of genetically predetermined repertoires of direction-specific responses acknowledge that "experience plays an obvious role and probably helps to find the best connections among the myriad options provided by genetic information."[46(p297)]

Clinical Implication

Dynamic systems theory suggests that motor development is driven mainly by practice. This has obvious implications for pediatric intervention as physical therapists contribute to decisions regarding what motor behaviors are to be practiced and where and how children will practice (eg, direct intervention, home programs, community-based activities). On the other hand, it is unclear how amenable the child who has damage to genetic motor programs and CNS structures will be to motor interventions, and, in the presence of pathology, what neural mechanisms are available for achieving postural control. Our knowledge will continue to expand as researchers document ontogenetic changes that occur in the development of postural control, the variables that contribute to this process, the neuroplastic features of the brain, and the effects of various interventions.

Types of Postural Control

Pavão et al[50] described methods used to assess postural control in children with CP and reviewed studies of "steady-state" postural control (ie, quiet sitting and standing), "reactive" postural control (ie, recovery from an unexpected threat to balance), and "anticipatory" postural control (ie, activation of postural muscles prior to an action).

Postural Responses to Perturbations

A child's responses to being moved while on an unstable surface often are used clinically to assess postural control. Hedberg and colleagues[41] studied the ontogeny of postural adjustments during sitting in TD infants. Because infants at age 1 month showed direction-specific muscle activation when balance was perturbed in sitting by horizontal forward and backward displacements of the support surface, an innate model of origin for the motor response patterns was suggested. Presumably, the children had not "practiced" sitting for the skill to be dependent on experience alone.

Hadders-Algra et al[51] assessed 21 TD children ages 1.5 to 4.5 years, noting their postural responses in sitting following platform movements. Comparable data were obtained for 11 infants seen 3 times between ages 5 and 10 months. There was a transient period between ages 9 to 10 months to 2.5 to 3 years during which perturbations in sitting resulted in high activity in the direction-specific agonist muscles as well as the antagonist muscles. With maturation, agonist activity became more variable and antagonist activity disappeared.

Hadders-Algra and colleagues,[52] in a separate study, assessed postural responses in sitting on a moveable platform in 3 groups of children (age 1.5 to 4.5 years). One group consisted of 13 preterm infants who had lesions of the periventricular white matter (PWM) of the brain that occurred in the neonatal period. The second group consisted of 13 preterm infants with normal neonatal brain scans, and the third group consisted of 13 healthy children born at term. The children whose history included PWM lesions demonstrated a limited repertoire of response variation to platform movement. Preterm birth without PWM lesions was related to a decreased ability to modulate postural responses (ie, higher sensitivity to platform velocity and difficulty modulating EMG amplitude with respect to the initial sitting position). The authors proposed 2 hypotheses to account for the differences in postural adjustments between preterm children without PWM lesions and age-matched children born at term. One hypothesis was that the neural circuitries producing direction-specific responses were not developed in the preterm infants. The second hypothesis was that sensory pathways may not have been integrated sufficiently to elicit activity in the necessary synergies. They noted that variation in development of postural control is important to selection of the most appropriate response pattern.

Studies comparing children with CP with age-matched TD children have documented basic difficulties tuning postural adjustments to task-specific conditions in sitting[53] as well as standing.[54,55] Infants with motor delay compared with TD infants not only had delayed postural stability at all stages of sitting, but increased look time (eg, a measure of visual attention).[56] Decreased look time, a measure of cognitive processing, is a positive sign indicating the need for less time to extract and process information received from a visual stimulus. Thus, delays in sitting postural control may indicate delays in cognitive processing.

The performance of children with attention-deficit hyperactivity disorder when placed on a balancing platform and compared with the performance of TD peers suggested difficulties in dynamic balance.[57] Children with autism spectrum disorder also are reported to have significant motor impairments in motor coordination, gait, and postural stability when compared with controls.[58]

Postural Adjustments Before and During Active Movement

Scientists also study the development of postural movements or "adjustments" that accompany active movements, as well as "anticipatory" movements that are essential in feed-forward motor control. Van der Fits and Hadders-Algra[59] discussed reaching movements in adults that are accompanied by complex postural adjustments controlled by spatial, temporal, and quantitative parameters. They studied the development of postural adjustments during reaching over time in infants age 3 to 18 months when placed in supine and sitting positions. The data suggested that by age 4 months reaching patterns were accompanied by complex postural adjustments with features similar to adults. There was a transient period of less extensive postural activity at 6 to 8 months, the age at which mobility skills such as rolling, sitting up, and crawling develop. In a similar study, Van der Fits et al[60] described 2 transition periods. The first was at age 6 months (as previously noted) when postural muscles were infrequently activated during reaching. At age 8 months postural activity reappeared, and infants were able to adapt postural adjustments to task-specific constraints, such as arm movement velocity or initial sitting position. The second transition occurred at age 12 to 15 months. Consistent "anticipatory" postural activity was not present before age 15 months, but became consistent after that age, particularly in the neck muscles. Refer to Chapter 13 for more information on the development of reaching and upper extremity control.

Van Balen et al[61] studied postural adjustments in sitting in a longitudinal study of TD and high-risk infants at corrected age 4, 6, and 18 months. Postural activity was similar for both groups at age 4 months. However, at 18 months, infants at high risk demonstrated less direction specificity, longer latencies for trunk muscle activation, and less anticipatory activation than the TD children.

Dinkel et al[62] compared postural control strategies of TD infants, 19 with normal weight and 10 who were overweight. Center of pressure was measured during sitting using a force platform at onset of sitting and 1 month post onset. The infants who were overweight adopted different postural control strategies than the infants with normal weights, although whether this limits exploration in early development or whether longitudinal differences emerge was unclear.

Hedberg et al[63] evaluated 4 TD infants at age 8, 10, 12, and 14 months standing with or without support. In both conditions, children exhibited direction-specific postural adjustments before they could stand independently. Great variation in postural adjustments early with fine tuning with increasing age and experience was present.

The development of anticipatory postural adjustments was studied in TD children age 4 to 8 years in a task that required maintaining the stabilization of forearm position despite imposed or voluntary unloading of the forearm.[64] A clear developmental sequence was noted. First, the selection of an efficient EMG pattern underlying forearm stabilization occurred, followed by mastery of timing adjustments. Shiratori et al[65] compared performance in catching a load from a prespecified height in children with hemiparesis or diplegia CP with TD control subjects. In children with CP the magnitudes of anticipatory postural adjustments were smaller, and onset was delayed in dorsal (agonist) postural muscles. Children with hemiplegia or diplegia were noted to use different postural strategies.

Grasso and colleagues[66] studied the emergence of anticipatory head orienting strategies during goal-directed locomotion in children. Eight children ranging from age 3.5 to 8 years walked along a 90-degree right-corner trajectory to reach a goal, in light and in darkness. The results demonstrated that predictive head-orienting movements occurred, even in the youngest children. The authors suggested that feedforward control of goal-directed locomotion appears very early in the development of gait.

Simple arm movements can occur 150 to 200 msec following an external "go" signal. If a standing individual is asked to suddenly lift both arms up and forward, the shift in gravity would cause a loss of balance forward. However, EMG recordings demonstrate these movements require "anticipatory" muscle contractions of the legs and trunk prior to the prime movers of the shoulders to prevent loss of balance. Girolami et al[67] studied TD children between ages 7 to 16 years while performing various arm movements while standing on a force platform. By at least age 7 years,

TD children demonstrated patterns of anticipatory muscle activation and suppression in leg and trunk muscles along with center of pressure changes similar to those reported in healthy adults.

Anticipatory postural adjustments in standing were studied in children with CP and compared with those of TD peers (ages 8 to 12 years).[68] The task was to reach forward and touch a target on the wall. Posterior center of pressure shift was frequently observed in both groups of children before arm movement; however, the children with CP showed greater variability and significantly shorter amplitude of the anticipatory postural adjustments compared with controls. Chen et al,[69] in a similar reaching study, demonstrated that children with Down syndrome (DS) used more postural adjustment strategies and inefficient strategies. These included increased reaction and execution times, and decreased amplitude of COM displacement compared with TD controls.

Another study of children with spastic diplegia CP (age 12 to 22 years) measured muscle activation when flexing both shoulders and lifting a load under 2 different load conditions.[70] Anticipatory activation of erector spinae and medial hamstring muscles was similar to control participants; however, the gastrocnemius muscle group fired significantly later in the children with CP. Children with CP often have difficulty recruiting distal musculature and prefer to initiate movements with larger proximal muscles.

In a study of 64 children (age 8 to 10 years), the performance of 32 children with developmental coordination disorder (DCD) was compared with the performance of 32 TD children during a rapid, voluntary, goal-directed arm movement.[71] The children with DCD demonstrated altered activity in postural muscles, including early activation of shoulder muscles and postural trunk muscles with anterior trunk muscles demonstrating delayed activation. In children with DCD, anticipatory function was not present in 3 of the 4 anterior trunk muscles studied. The authors hypothesized that altered postural muscle activity may contribute to poor proximal stability and poor upper extremity control for goal-directed movement in children with DCD. Another study used electromyography to compare frequency of anticipatory postural adjustments for 3 bilateral trunk and unilateral tibialis anterior muscles between children with and without DCD (age 7 to 14 years).[72] Tasks were kicking a ball, stepping onto a step, and standing on one foot. Children with DCD used anticipatory postural adjustments one-half to one-quarter less often as the TD controls.

Postural Strategies

"Postural strategies" initially described in healthy adults[73,74] have been studied in children. One example is an "ankle strategy" (swaying around the ankles with knees and hips extended) that typically is used when perturbations are small and the support surface is firm. In contrast, a "hip strategy" controls COM by large rapid motions at the hip joints with antiphase rotations of the ankles. A hip strategy typically is used when larger, faster perturbations are present or when the support surface is compliant or small, such as standing on a foam cushion or a balance beam. With larger perturbations that displace the COM outside the base of support (BOS), a series of steps or hops ("stepping strategy") is used to bring the BOS back into alignment under the COM. Roncesvalles et al[75] studied the ability to use a step for balance recovery in 25 TD children between age 9 and 19 months. New walkers (up to 2 weeks' walking experience) used a step infrequently and ineffectively when balance was threatened. Intermediate walkers (1 to 3 months' walking experience) showed an increasing tendency to step and a significant improvement in execution compared with new walkers. Advanced walkers (greater than 3 months walking experience) did not fall during backward support-surface translations and maintained balance with their feet in place or by using a step response. The authors concluded there was a significant developmental transition in the emergence of compensatory stepping with 3 to 6 months of experience being required for an effective step response to develop.

Figure 10-3. Vertical neck righting reaction in an infant when suspended upright and tilted laterally.

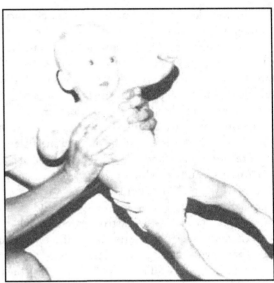

Examination and Evaluation Principles

As therapists, we are concerned with several aspects of postural control. These are the "responses" that occur to maintain balance following a perturbation (eg, being bumped in a crowd); the ability to maintain steady postures in various positions (eg, sitting, kneeling, standing); the postural "adjustments" that occur during active movement; and the "anticipatory" muscle activity that occurs in feedforward planning of movement. These functional components of postural control are not, however, proposed to be exclusive and, of course, are interrelated. They are intended to serve as a framework for physical therapy examination, evaluation, and intervention as our understanding of the mechanisms contributing to postural control evolves.

Examination of Righting, Protective, and Equilibrium Reactions

Postural reactions are divided traditionally into 3 groups: (1) righting, (2) protective, and (3) equilibrium or balancing reactions. They are not, however, separate distinct entities because they are interdependent and represent interactive subsystems.

Righting Reactions

Righting reactions orient the head in space so the eyes and mouth are in a horizontal plane or the body parts are restored to a normal alignment following rotation to any position in space. Righting reactions have been classified according to the receptor stimulated, the proposed regulating area of the brain, or the response. Righting reactions depend on a number of different stimuli, including visual, vestibular, and somatosensory. (See Video 10-2.)

VERTICAL-RIGHTING REACTIONS

Vertical-righting reactions refer to the ability to orient the head to vertical in a number of different positions. If a child is held upright and tilted 30 to 45 degrees in a lateral, anterior, or posterior direction (Figure 10-3), alignment of the head to vertical with the mouth horizontal is the expected response. Maintaining the head in alignment with the body is a partial response. The child should be able to right his or her head by age 2.5 to 6 months.[76-78] If visual input is eliminated

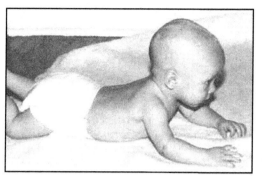

Figure 10-4. Head righting reaction in prone position.

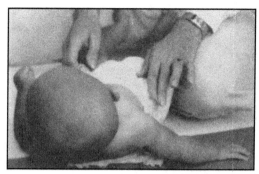

Figure 10-5. Head righting reaction seen in the supine position.

by blindfolding the child, the head still should right to vertical (in response to vestibular and somatosensory input). This response also has been called labyrinthine righting.[75]

Vertical-righting reactions in prone occur when the child extends his or her head. These are present by age 1.5 to 4 months (Figure 10-4).[77,79,80] Lifting the head to 45 degrees is considered a partial response. Capital hyperextension frequently is observed in the child with CNS dysfunction. By age 3 to 10 months, a TD child should be able to extend his or her entire trunk and pelvis when suspended in prone so an upward concavity is observed.[79] This posture is referred to as the Landau reaction or prone extension. The ability to achieve antigravity extension and to display a response to prone suspension is an excellent example of the complex interaction among multiple systems. By age 6 months, an infant has the cognitive ability to cooperate (or not cooperate) in movement. If the infant is unhappy or tired, he or she may choose not to extend the body when suspended in prone. An overweight infant may not be able to produce enough muscle force to volitionally lift his or her body against gravity. In a comprehensive study of 51 low-risk infants, Touwen[79] found the "Landau response" was highly inconsistent and a definite developmental sequence could not be established.

In supine, the child should be able to lift his or her head from the supporting surface by age 5 months (Figure 10-5). This is not a frequent spontaneous activity, and gently pulling the child up to sitting and observing for chin tuck may be necessary for testing. Haley[77] reported that, when testing in this manner, a complete chin tuck throughout the entire movement did not occur in a sample of infants without disabilities until age 8 to 10 months.

Head righting also should be present in side-lying and other positions. If the child can sit or stand with proper head position, it can be assumed the righting reactions have developed and do not have to be tested.

ROTATIONAL-RIGHTING REACTIONS

The rotational-righting reactions[81] or body-righting reactions[82] have many different, confusing, and contradictory names. It is best to describe the stimulus and response to avoid misleading terminology. The rotational-righting reactions restore the body parts to normal alignment following rotation of some body segment. In the neonate, when the head is turned or the leg is flexed and adducted, he or she rotates like a log (nonsegmentally). This nonsegmental roll can be seen as late as age 6 to 12 months,[76,83] after which it is considered an immature response. A mature response occurs when the head is turned or the leg is flexed and adducted and the child rolls showing distinct rotation between the pelvis and shoulder girdle with head and trunk rotation around the central body axis. Somatosensory input results from asymmetrical body contact, joint proprioception, and muscle stretch, and, as the head turns, vestibular and visual inputs also occur.

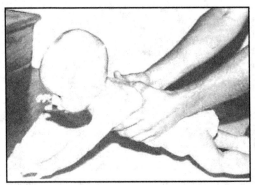

Figure 10-6. Protective reaction when infant is moved forward toward the ground.

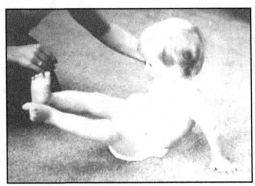

Figure 10-7. Backward protective reaction noted in sitting.

Protective Reactions

Protective reactions, also called parachute or propping reactions,[84] consist of extension movements of the extremities generally in the same direction of a displacing force that shifts the body's COM past the limits of stability. These reactions can be facilitated by vestibular input caused by movement in space, somatosensory input to the weight-bearing skin surfaces and changes in joint angles, and visual or auditory input from the impending displacing force.

Protective reactions can be elicited in many different positions. If the child's body is thrust downward, feet first from the upright vertical position, leg extension and abduction are expected by age 4 months. If adduction and internal rotation occur, a pathological condition might be suspected. When a child is moved forward toward the ground head first, arm extension and abduction should be observed by age 6 to 7 months (Figure 10-6).

In sitting, a child can be pushed gently in all directions to facilitate protective reactions of the arms. Protective reactions in sitting are related to experience and are context dependent. Progression in development is thought to be laterally or sideways by age 6 to 11 months, then forward, and finally backward by age 9 to 12 months (Figure 10-7).[77,79] A study by Touwen[79] indicated that lateral protective reactions improved along with a parallel increase in sitting duration.

The amount, speed, and point of application of force, as well as the child's anticipation, will affect the protective reaction observed. For example, less force is needed at the shoulder than at the pelvis to shift COM. If the child anticipates the stimulus, he or she may prepare his or her body and an equilibrium reaction might occur instead of a protective reaction. If the speed of the force is too rapid, and there is not enough time for a protective response, a fall will occur. If the speed of the force is too slow, an equilibrium reaction may occur. Facilitating a protective reaction in a child who already has developed equilibrium reactions is difficult. The child usually will employ equilibrium movements initially and display a protective reaction only when pushed past the limits of stability.

Equilibrium Reactions and Balance

Numerous terms have been used to describe the ability of an individual to maintain an upright posture, and a distinction is made between shifts of posture on a stable or unstable BOS. The terms *postural fixation* and *balance* have been used to describe reactions on a stable base, where the body moves over the support surface.[80] Equilibrium reactions,[77] tilting reactions, and balance[85] have been used to describe movements on an unstable BOS (eg, tilt-board, ball, foam rubber surface, or moving platform), where the supporting surface moves under the body.

Clinical observations consist of noting counter-movements of the head, neck, trunk, or extremities to displacement of the body's COM. The movement generally is in a direction opposite the opposing force, unlike protective reactions, which are in the same direction as the force.

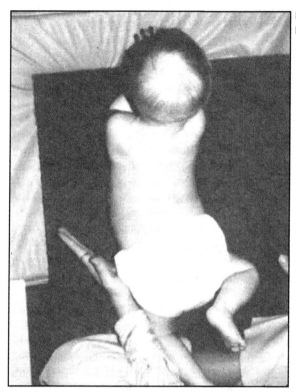

Figure 10-8. Equilibrium reactions seen in prone position.

When pushed or tilted laterally, the response can include a spinal concavity on the side pushed or elevated. Rotation of the upper trunk and head toward midline and counter-rotation of the lower trunk may occur.[81] Extension and abduction of the extremities on the elevated side or side being pushed may occur to help bring the body alignment back to center. Abduction and extension of the extremities on the depressed side or in the direction of a push also might occur in preparation for a protective reaction if the limits of stability are surpassed. When pushed or tilted forward so the anterior support surface is lowered, extension of the legs and trunk occurs. When pushed or tilted in a posterior direction, hip and trunk flexion occur. The amount of flexion or extension will depend on numerous factors, such as the position of the child, the amount of sensory input, and the ability of the child to respond. Reactions also can be tested in diagonal planes and should result in rotational responses. Balance reactions are tested by pushing the child gently while he or she is supported on a stable BOS or with the child on an unstable BOS, such as a ball, bolster, moving platform, or adult's lap. Speed of tilt and length of time allowed for a response are important variables that determine the movement patterns observed.

Generally, balance reactions develop on a stable BOS before an unstable BOS in that position. Equilibrium reactions usually occur first in prone (age 5 to 9 months; Figure 10-8), then supine (age 7 to 11 months), sitting (age 7 to 8 months), quadruped (age 8 to 12 months), and standing (age 12 to 21 months).

Haley[77] suggested that equilibrium reactions in sitting might occur before those in prone and supine. The age of achievement of these reactions is related to the achievement of motor skills in that position and interaction with the environment. Therefore, variability can be expected.

Examination of Postural Adjustments and Anticipatory Movements

Most physical therapists do not use EMG or computer-controlled platforms in their examination of children. We rely on our clinical observation skills as we watch children move or attempt to move in various environments to accomplish specific gross and fine motor tasks.

Where do we start? One determinant will be the age and expected motor competency of the child. What we observe and expect in a 3-month-old infant certainly will be different from what we observe and expect in a 13-year-old child. One framework for evaluation of postural control in children has been to examine "static" and "dynamic" balance abilities. Static balance, although never really static since there are always shifts in the center of pressure, refers to maintaining balance in a specific posture, such as sitting or standing. Maintaining balance while actively moving is categorized as dynamic balance.

In the infant and young child, trunk control develops starting from the cervical/thoracic area followed by the lumbar/pelvic regions.[86] Development of postural control in sitting is interrelated to reaching. Segmental assessment of trunk control is a clinical measure of trunk control. Manual support is provided at various levels (following a top-down sequence) and is used to assess static sitting ability.[87,88]

The child's performance on sections related both to static and dynamic postural control on standardized tests that have good reliability and validity (see Chapter 2) can be used to determine the skill level of the child and whether the skill level falls below the expected competency for the his or her age. Even if a child can accomplish expected motor skills, he or she still may have problems with postural control. This is especially applicable to children with mild motor delays, motor planning problems, or DCD who accomplish age-appropriate motor skills, but who are considered "clumsy."

An observational examination of postural control is accomplished by observing the child as he or she spontaneously moves through his or her environment, whether this is by rolling, crawling, scooting on his or her bottom, or walking. Specific observations should be made: Are the child's movements smooth and controlled? How is each body part moving? Is he or she steady or unsteady? Can he or she navigate obstacles in the path? Can the child make transitions in and out of positions with control, or does he or she "fall" into positions assisted by gravity? Can the child maintain his or her balance in various positions including sitting, all fours, kneeling, and standing?

The types of postural strategies used by the child (eg, ankle, hip, or stepping) should be determined (Table 10-1).

The more strategies the child has available, the more flexibility he or she has when selecting the most efficient movements required by various environmental contexts. The child may rely primarily on one strategy to maintain balance. For example, a child may not be able to "stand still" but can maintain balance by continually "stepping" or bringing his or her BOS under his or her COM. The child with stiff ankles or who wears fixed ankle-foot orthoses will be prevented from using an ankle strategy and will have to rely on a hip or stepping strategy to maintain upright balance.

Observing "anticipatory" components of postural control is particularly difficult. Is the child able to lift his or her arm in sitting, kneeling, or standing without falling or leaning forward? If the child consistently falls forward, he or she may not be "anticipating" the load of his or her arm in front of him or her and is not presetting back extensor muscles in anticipation of a load. Can the child stand in place and swing a bat without losing his or her balance? Does the child demonstrate clumsiness or loss of balance when lifting objects off a table or from the floor?

There may be a cognitive component to postural difficulties in some children. For example, if the child does not accurately judge the anticipated weight of the object to be lifted, he or she cannot efficiently preset his or her back extensor muscles in anticipation of counteracting a specific

TABLE 10-1. ACTIVITIES TO PROMOTE VARIOUS POSTURAL STRATEGIES

ANKLE STRATEGY

- In standing, with hips and knees straight, raise both arms slowly up in front of the body and hold 5 seconds, return arms to sides; extend both arms slowly behind body and hold 5 seconds, return arms to sides.
- In standing, with hips and knees straight, sway like trees in a breeze (forward/backward) or dance/sway to music.
- Standing on tilt-board with hips and knees straight, sway forward and backward very slowly.

HIP STRATEGY

- Balance on tiptoes.
- Walk forward and backward on tiptoes; stop on verbal command and maintain balance.
- Walk on narrow balance beam or 4-inch- (10-cm-) wide elastic band placed on floor (pretend the child is walking a tightrope in the circus); start and stop on verbal command without stepping off the beam or band.

STEPPING STRATEGY

- March to music (forward, backward, sideways).
- Twirl to the left 3 times, then twirl to the right 3 times—vary speed.
- Walk on uneven terrain outside (eg, grass, gravel, pea rock).

HIP AND STEPPING STRATEGIES

- In standing on a tilt-board, tip board faster until hip or stepping strategy demonstrated.
- Play "statue" or "freeze" (ie, child moves spontaneously then attempts to maintain posture when the adult says "freeze").
- Bounce a ball to the child outside his or her base of support.

load. Can the child maintain balance when asked to talk or when distracted (ie, dual-task/cognitive interference)? Can the child imitate unfamiliar positions and maintain balance (ie, motor planning)?

The therapist should note any additional variables that might affect the child's postural control. For example, what is the health status of the child? Are his or her levels of arousal and attention appropriate for the task? Is the child on any type of medication (eg, antiseizure medication) that might affect arousal states or balance?

The child should be observed during daily activities or the parents or other caregivers should be interviewed to determine functional anticipatory movements and control. For example, does the child judge the height of curbs and steps to successfully clear the obstacles with his or her foot without tripping? Can he or she step on and off an escalator or a moving walkway and maintain balance? For the ambulatory child who is considered "clumsy," ask the parent or teacher to describe the specific situations or tasks in which the child is observed to have difficulty.

An observational analysis can be helpful in determining postural control during basic movements such as rolling, batting at a ball from a hands-and-knees position, putting pellets in a bottle, or completing a pencil-and-paper task in a sitting position.[89] For example, during rolling, does the child spontaneously lift his or her head off the floor in all positions, or does the head touch or

Figure 10-9. Task: Rolling. Scoring key: 1 = most atypical performance, 5 = typical performance. Head righting: Score (1) head touches floor in prone. Antigravity extension: Score (1) flexed posture when prone (hips, knees, arms). (Reprinted with permission from Richter EW, Montgomery PC. *Sensorimotor Performance Analysis.* Stillwater, MN: PDP Press; 1989:97-133.)

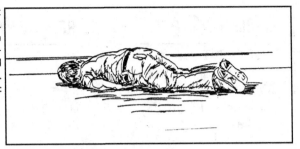

Figure 10-10. Task: Pellets in bottle. Scoring key: 1 = most atypical performance, 5 = typical performance. Trunk stability: Score (1) leans on table. Head position: Scores (3) rotates, (3) flexed-eyes close to table. Grasp adequate for age: Score (5). Changes hands at midline: Score (1). Inconsistent hand usage: Score (1). (Reprinted with permission from Richter EW, Montgomery PC. *Sensorimotor Performance Analysis.* Stillwater, MN: PDP Press; 1989:97-133.)

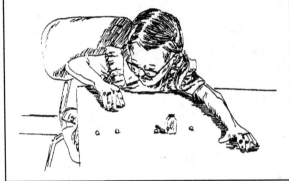

remain on the floor (Figure 10-9); does the child assume antigravity extension when prone and antigravity flexion when supine? In a fine motor task while sitting, does the child need to adjust his or her posture often, or does he or she appear secure during the task? Does the child need to lean on the table to stabilize him- or herself (Figure 10-10)? Are extraneous, nonessential movements obvious during the task? Does the child use optimal upper extremity positions and control for the fine motor task? Because it is difficult to simultaneously direct the child, observe, and document performance, video recording may be used to provide a permanent record that can be replayed and objectively analyzed.

INTERVENTION CONSIDERATIONS

Areas to be considered in physical therapy intervention have been discussed previously in this chapter and include sensory processing, cognitive functions, musculoskeletal issues, practice, and experience. In addition, other issues may become evident during the examination process. For example, the child may have generally poor health and be deconditioned. Deconditioning frequently is present in the child with chronic health problems or after recovery from long illnesses or surgery. If necessary, a reconditioning program similar to that used for any deconditioned child should be implemented.

The child's emotional and arousal state should be considered. An active, alert state is best to participate in and benefit from intervention. The inability to perform a movement must be distinguished from refusal. The child who is fearful may be hesitant to participate in movement-based activities; therefore activities need to be presented in a nonthreatening, playful manner. Generally, it is best to start intervention with activities in which the child perceives he or she is "safe" and will have some success. Activities gradually can be increased in complexity relative to various requirements of postural control.

Principles of motor learning should be incorporated in treatment sessions (see Chapter 1). The therapist needs to determine the target behavior, how frequently it will be practiced, and how frequently the child will be provided with knowledge of results. A systems approach suggests the therapist needs to consider the environments and materials used during treatment. Practice of specific daily functional tasks needed by the child in his or her normal environments should be a primary consideration in treatment. Practice should occur in each of the environments with different materials and different individuals, so generalization of the task can be achieved. Similarly, the percentage of time spent practicing postural responses to perturbations (eg, being tilted on a therapy ball) should be limited in comparison with the practice of postural adjustments and anticipatory postural control needed to maintain balance and perform active movements (eg, lifting the arm to reach for a toy while seated on a bench, or swinging a bat at a suspended ball).

Physical therapy intervention strategies will vary depending on the presenting level of postural control. For nonambulatory children, balance requirements in sitting, kneeling, and standing positions can be incorporated in therapy activities. Santamaria et al[90] suggested that providing external trunk support can assist children with CP with postural control and reaching proficiency. The level of trunk support should match the child's level of trunk control. Children with severe deficits will require a high level of support (eg, axillae), while moderately involved children may improve reaching performance with lower levels of support (eg, pelvis).

More challenging balance tasks can be stressed for ambulatory children. For example, Abdel-Aziem and El-Basatiny[91] studied the effect of additional backward walking training on postural control in 2 groups of children with hemiplegia CP between age 10 and 14 years. When compared with the children who did not practice backward walking, children in the intervention group demonstrated a significant improvement in overall antereoposterior and mediolateral stability indices.

Strength training is a major component of intervention for many children. Kordi et al[92] had 7- to 9-year-old children with DS participate in a strength training program. When compared with a control group of children with DS receiving routine exercises in physical education class, there was an improvement in static balance, but no effect on dynamic balance.

Nintendo Wii Fit video games have been used with children with varying diagnoses. Tarakci and colleagues[93] compared conventional balance training with Wii Fit balance-based video games in children (age 5 to 18 years) with CP. In this study, the Wii Fit balance-based video games improved balance parameters more than conventional exercises. Another study compared a 6-week period of nonintervention with a 6-week period of Wii Fit intervention in children with balance problems (probable DCD).[94] Following intervention, motor performance improved as assessed with the Movement Assessment Battery for Children, Second Edition; subtests of the Bruininks; and the Wii Fit Ski Slalom test (not practiced during intervention).

Taping often is suggested as an intervention strategy to improve postural stability.[95] In a review of databases through May 2015, 9 papers met the authors' inclusion criteria, but only 4 studies were considered high quality. Of these 4, only 2 were found to be effective in increasing activity in children with CP. Larger sample sizes and more specific taping procedures are needed to strengthen evidence for effectiveness with taping. Almeida et al[96] reviewed the effects of 13 interventions with therapeutic suits (clothing) on children's posture, balance, motor function, and gait. Of the 13 reviewed, 2 were a full-body suit, 2 were dynamic elastomeric fabric orthoses, 3 were TheraTogs, and 6 were Therasuit/Adeli Suit protocols. The conclusion was that low-quality evidence was present, and caution should be taken in recommending the use of any of these therapeutic suits.

There are many community-based activities that may positively affect postural control, including dance,[97,98] yoga, tai chi, karate, and adapted sports programs. Many of these interventions have not been subjected to research regarding effectiveness. One systematic review of exercise interventions that may improve postural control in children with CP included 45 studies with 13 exercise interventions.[99] Five interventions were supported by a moderate level of evidence: gross motor task training, hippotherapy, treadmill training with no body-weight support, trunk-targeted training, and reactive balance training.

An important therapeutic intervention is parent instruction. Parents are the primary caregivers of their children. They need to be instructed in reasonable therapeutic interventions that can be performed as part of the child's daily routines. Embedding these activities into daily routines will increase the likelihood that they will be performed and the child will have more opportunities to practice specific tasks. (See Chapter 4 on communication to establish rapport with children and their families.)

Examples of general intervention strategies for improving various aspects of postural control and specific treatment techniques are provided in the following case studies.

CASE STUDY #1: JASON

> *Medical Diagnosis:* Cerebral palsy, right hemiparesis
> *Gross Motor Function Classification System:* Level I
> *Age:* 24 months

Examination and Evaluation

Postural Responses to Perturbation

> *Righting Reactions:* Jason rights his head in all planes.
> *Protective Reactions:* In sitting, Jason has left anterior, lateral, and posterior protective reactions in response to tilt. The right arm initiates movement in response to tilt forward and sideward, but without full extension and weight bearing. The right arm does not respond effectively when Jason is tilted backward.
> *Equilibrium Reactions:* In sitting and standing when his balance is perturbed, left trunk musculature appears to respond appropriately, but trunk movement on the right is delayed or absent; he is more successful maintaining his balance during slow tilt. In standing, Jason tends to use a protective stepping reaction. This response is not consistent, and he often falls.

Postural Control During Active Movement

> *Mobility Skills:* Jason rolls easily on the floor and pushes up on all fours. He can creep on all fours, but does not bear weight fully on the right arm. He can assume standing independently from the middle of the floor and walks independently. He attempts to run, but is unsteady and falls frequently.
> *Transitions:* Jason transitions independently from sitting on the floor to quadruped or kneeling positions. He can assume a bear stance to move into standing. Some unsteadiness is noted in transitions, but Jason is generally successful and does not lose his balance.
> *Fine Motor Skills:* Jason has more difficulty maintaining his balance in sitting when lifting or manipulating objects and in standing when lifting or carrying objects. When attempting to lift heavy objects, he does not appear able to anticipate the load he needs to counteract, and he tends to fall forward.

Participation Restrictions

Jason has difficulty with mobility skills and cannot keep up with peers during some gross motor activities. He also has difficulty manipulating some objects for play. Both mobility and play limitations negatively affect the repertoire of toys he can access. Because he falls frequently, does not catch himself, and often bumps his head against the wall or environmental objects, his family limits his play environments for safety; therefore, opportunities for social interaction and cognitive and motor exploration are decreased.

Activity Limitations

Jason tends to move stiffly and cannot change directions quickly, especially to his right side. He has difficulty maintaining his balance in standing when lifting or carrying heavy objects. He cannot run as quickly as his peers, and stair climbing and descent are difficult. He has difficulty playing with toys that require bilateral hand use.

Impairments

Jason demonstrates weakness and poor motor control of his right extremities, especially the right upper extremity. He appears to have a mild disregard for the right side of his body and the right side of space, tending to use the left side of his body for motor tasks and to orient objects to the left side of space. He demonstrates tightness in the muscles of the right upper extremity and in the right hip muscles and lateral trunk flexors. His balance reactions in sitting and standing are adequate to slow tilt or mild perturbations, but are too slow to be effective during rapid tilt or large perturbations. Postural adjustments appear adequate during slow active movements, but are less efficient during rapid active movement or when lifting, carrying, or manipulating objects.

Functional/Participation Goals

After 3 months of intervention, Jason will be able to accomplish the following:
1. Walk up and down 5 steps, holding on to a railing, using a reciprocal pattern with standby supervision.
2. Extend the right upper extremity when losing his balance or falling toward his right side, 3 of 5 occurrences.
3. Decrease number of falls from 10 times to 3 times daily.
4. Spontaneously position toys at midline or slightly to the right side of the body during play, 2 of 5 trials.
5. Run 20 feet (6 m) without falling.
6. Change direction in playing tag without losing balance.
7. Throw a tennis ball with his right arm while standing without losing balance.

Interventions

1. Parent education and instruction.
2. Right upper and lower extremities strengthening activities.
3. Standing balance activities.
4. Orienting to the right side of space.
5. Active ROM of right extremities and trunk.
6. Opportunities to exhibit protective reactions of the right upper extremity.
7. Bimanual movement activities.

Therapeutic Activities

Jason's parents can be instructed to place toys on his right side so he has to reach with his right arm (Intervention #1) and to place toys slightly outside his BOS so he has to use an equilibrium reaction to reach the toy. These may seem simple tasks to the parents, but they need to know the importance of allowing Jason to use his body and not just making activities easy for him.

Strengthening activities (Intervention #2) can include practicing "wheelbarrowing" with adult assist. Using both arms to push open doors or to push against resistance offered by an adult or object (eg, pushing over a bench, pushing a chair across the kitchen floor) may improve elbow extension, shoulder protraction, and general upper extremity strength. In quadruped, Jason can be encouraged to bear weight equally on both extended arms. He can be encouraged to shift his weight onto the right arm and attempt to bat a suspended balloon or reach for a toy with the left arm.

Supporting the body by leaning with both arms on a bench or holding an adult's hands while trying to do one-leg knee bends is an example of a lower extremity strengthening activity. Reciprocal stair climbing and descent with assistance for balance also will improve strength and weight shift onto the right leg (Interventions #2 and #3). Small Velcro weight cuffs (eg, 1 pound [0.5 kg]) around the wrists or ankles during "weight-lifting" games can be used to improve strength and increase proprioceptive input.

Walking and attempting to run on uneven terrain outside, as well as up and down slight inclines, will improve upright balance control. Jason also can try walking a few steps backward (Intervention #3). Walking straddling a 4-inch- (10-cm-) wide elastic band laid flat on the floor or a 2- × 4-inch (5- × 10 cm) board placed on the ground will facilitate a weight shift to the right side (Interventions #3 and #4). Placing paper footsteps on the carpet or making footsteps with chalk on the sidewalk can be used to promote a weight shift to the right leg. Placing toys, the television, or a computer screen at midline and eventually to the right side of his body will help Jason orient to that side of space (Interventions #1 and #4).

Since Jason has tight right hip and lateral trunk flexors, activities to increase ROM in active right hip extension and lateral trunk flexion to the left should be encouraged (Intervention #5).

Playing games in sitting (eg, "rocking boat" on sofa cushion) and standing (eg, "dancing" to music) that require increased weight shifts will provide practice with losing his balance and catching himself (Intervention #6). Activities specific to improving equilibrium on an unstable base might include prone on a scooter board or ball, and use of a small trampoline or seesaw. The therapist will have to structure activities to emphasize falling to the right to promote active participation of the right upper extremity.

Constraint-induced movement therapy and bimanual intensive movement activities have been found to be effective for children with hemiplegia CP[100,101] (Intervention #7; see Chapter 13). Although a complete program might not be possible with Jason, his parents could be instructed in ways to encourage use of his right arm and not allow consistent use of the left arm (Intervention #1). Batting at bubbles with his right hand while he holds the bubble bottle in the left hand would be an example of bilateral hand use. Bilateral arm use in sitting and standing also would encourage postural control

CASE STUDY #2: JILL

> *Medical Diagnosis:* Cerebral palsy, spastic quadriparesis, microcephaly, intellectual deficits, seizure disorder
> *Gross Motor Function Classification System:* Level V
> *Age:* 7 years

Examination and Evaluation

Postural Responses to Perturbation

> *Righting Reactions:* Jill can maintain her head in neutral when held vertically. However, she cannot right her head when tilted more than 30 degrees from upright. She raises her head momentarily in prone, but not in supine.

> *Protective Reactions:* Protective reactions of the extremities are not present in response to imposed movement in any position.
> *Equilibrium Reactions:* These reactions are not present in response to imposed movement in any position.

Postural Control During Active Movement

> *Mobility Skills:* Jill can shift her position when lying on the floor and rolls from supine to side-lying. She is unable to maintain her balance in any position (ie, sitting, all fours, kneeling, standing).
> *Transitions:* Jill does not make any independent transitions of movement between positions. She can assist in standing pivot transfers by momentarily bearing weight on her legs.
> *Fine Motor Skills:* Jill attempts to grasp, but her hand often closes involuntarily prior to obtaining an object. She cannot manipulate objects with her fingers.

Participation Restrictions

Limitations in head control and position options negatively affect educational and social opportunities. Jill cannot maintain head control to consistently and effectively visually explore her environment. She usually is seated in her wheelchair and not at eye level with peers, which limits eye contact and communication. Jill has severe intellectual deficits that often limit her ability to understand and cooperate during motor activities.

Activity Limitations

Jill has not developed functional balance or postural control in any position (eg, sitting, kneeling, quadruped, and standing). She has poor head control and needs maximal support in all positions, either through adult assistance or the use of adapted equipment (eg, wheelchair, stander).

Impairments

Jill has a seizure disorder, intellectual deficits, and a severely compromised motor control system as a result of pathology involving her CNS. She does not demonstrate balance or protective reactions to passive tilt or actively during attempts to move. She has generalized stiffness in her extremities and trunk with associated tightness, especially in the end excursions of joint ROM. Jill's endurance is limited, and she is often lethargic. Periods of decreased arousal may be associated with her antiseizure medications.

Functional/Participation Goals

After 3 months of intervention, Jill will be able to accomplish the following:
1. Maintain current ROM (less than 10-degree limitation in hip and knee extension) to be comfortable in her prone stander and while positioned prone on the floor.
2. Maintain standing balance for 3 to 5 seconds with partial body support from an adult during standing pivot transfers.
3. Right and maintain her head in vertical when being lifted or carried as part of her daily care at home and school.
4. Maintain upright head control for 3 minutes in supported sitting in her adapted chair during a classroom activity.
5. Lift her head 3 to 5 times in a 1-minute interaction to achieve eye contact with a classmate while positioned in a prone stander.

Interventions

1. Parent instruction.
2. Active and assistive ROM.
3. Weight bearing in standing.
4. Trunk support for stability in sitting and standing through proper positioning and adapted equipment.
5. Head control activities in supported sitting, in her stander, and during caregiver handling.

Therapeutic Activities

Jill's parents and caregivers will be instructed (Intervention #1) in the intervention program, making certain the activities are embedded throughout her normal daily routine. Jill has a school and home schedule of positioning designed to maintain her ROM (Intervention #2). This includes being in her prone stander and lying prone on the floor to maintain hip and knee extension. When in prone she is assisted in bringing her arms up over her head to maintain forward flexion and external rotation of her shoulders as well as elbow extension. When on the floor she is encouraged to roll to maintain muscle function and ROM. During some classroom activities she long sits on the floor with support from a classroom aide (eg, leaning back against the adult). At home her family places her in her wheelchair for 15 minutes each evening with her legs in extension and propped on a footstool. Periodically, when knee joint tightness increases, night splints are used. These activities assist in maintaining elongation of the hamstrings and extension of the knee joint.

Part of Jill's daily routine at home and school is to assist in standing pivot transfers (Intervention #3). She currently has a molded seat insert for her wheelchair and a lap tray, which place her in an optimal position for classroom activities (Intervention #4).

Because Jill has some head control in an upright position, she is provided opportunities throughout the day to actively control her head position (Intervention #5). For example, Jill is placed astride the adult's lap, and while proper support is given to the trunk, a vertical head position and active contraction of the cervical muscles are encouraged. Jill is most successful when working from a neutral head position in sitting, where gravity offers the least resistance. Slowly moving in a small arc of motion in supported sitting encourages both concentric and eccentric muscle contractions. In supported sitting, either in a chair, rocking chair, or on an adult's lap, Jill is tilted from side to side and forward and back. The adult usually starts with 5 to 10 degrees of slow tilt, giving adequate time for a response. If no response occurs, Jill's head is positioned and a holding contraction requested. Progression to larger degrees of tilt and more rapid movement can occur. It is helpful to make this activity fun and meaningful by having her look out a window or in a mirror. At home Jill's family can use cartoons on a laptop computer to engage and maintain her interest (Intervention #1).

CASE STUDY #3: TAYLOR

▸ *Medical Diagnosis:* Myelomeningocele, repaired L1-2
▸ *Age:* 4 years

Examination and Evaluation

Postural Responses to Perturbations

▸ *Righting Reactions:* Taylor rights his head in all directions when tilted in sitting and in a supported upright position (held by an adult).

- *Protective Reactions:* All upper extremity protective reactions in sitting are present to passive tilt. Standing reactions are not testable.
- *Equilibrium Reactions:* In prone and supine, on a stable and unstable BOS, the upper trunk response to tilt is present. In sitting, the upper trunk response also is present; however, the quality of the response is poor. Taylor responds slowly to tilt and frequently has insufficient muscle strength or endurance to maintain an upright posture without reverting to a protective response. Equilibrium reactions were not tested in standing.

Postural Control During Active Movement

- *Mobility Skills:* Taylor rolls consecutively, sits with good balance, and attempts to pull to kneeling. He has difficulty using active muscle contractions to maintain his posture. He uses his arms to pull and belly crawl or to "scoot" on his bottom.
- *Transitions:* Taylor is able to get in and out of sitting and into an all fours position independently. He is working on transitions from his wheelchair, such as on and off a classroom chair and on and off the toilet. In these transitions, he demonstrates trunk instability and frequent loss of balance.
- *Fine Motor Skills:* Taylor has normal grasp, manipulation, and release. He has difficulty manipulating large or heavy objects because of difficulty in stabilizing his trunk.

Participation Restrictions

In his preschool classroom, Taylor is unable to maintain floor sitting during some academic, play, and social activities. During free play when he is using his long leg braces and walker, he cannot keep up with classmates as they move around the play area. He also tires quickly and chooses to "rest." These balance and mobility limitations negatively affect his educational and social opportunities and peer interactions. He also has difficulty with transitions to and from his wheelchair, which limits his independence in choosing alternative positions within the classroom.

Activity Limitations

Taylor cannot walk independently, but uses an anterior walker and a reciprocating gait orthosis (RGO). He has begun practicing standing wearing long leg braces and using forearm crutches. Poor endurance and balance limit his standing time. He has good independent sitting balance. However, when reaching for objects outside his BOS, he tends to fall. If he falls to the side in sitting, he usually catches himself with his arms and returns to sitting. When he loses his balance with crutches, he does not use his arms effectively to catch himself. His balance during transitions in and out of his wheelchair and on and off classroom chairs or toilet are precarious and he needs manual assistance of an adult for safety.

Impairments

Taylor has loss of motor and sensory function in his lower extremities secondary to his myelomeningocele. He has poor active trunk extension and demonstrates generalized weakness in his arms and trunk. Balance reactions to passive tilt in sitting and supported standing are slow. Taylor has visual-perceptual problems, particularly figure-ground discrimination. In addition, when he bends his head to look at the floor his balance often is disturbed.

Functional/Participation Goals

After 3 months of intervention, Taylor will be able to accomplish the following:

1. Lean laterally 20 to 30 degrees to either side with his walker and long leg braces and correct his balance without assistance.
2. Reach laterally in sitting to the limits of his base of stability for an object without using a protective reaction.
3. Actively fall forward from a standing position onto a 3-inch (7.5-cm) thickness mat and catch himself with his arms without hitting his head on the mat.
4. Walk across the classroom using long leg braces and crutches and follow a visual pattern (trail) on the floor without losing his balance with standby guarding from an adult.
5. Independently lift his body weight with his arms during transfers so he clears his buttocks off the surface.
6. Transfer in and out of his wheelchair to a classroom chair with standby guarding from an adult.
7. Walk around the classroom area intermittently with his walker and RGO for 10 minutes without fatiguing.

Interventions

1. Parent and school staff instruction.
2. Activities to strengthen trunk and upper extremities.
3. Practice of sitting transfers.
4. Balance activities in standing with walker and forearm crutches.
5. Balance activities in sitting.
6. Practice head bending in standing and walking with walker or crutches.
7. Endurance training during ambulation with his walker.
8. Facilitation of protective reactions in standing.

Therapeutic Activities

Coordination and communication are critical; therefore, the parents and school personnel need to be instructed in how to encourage Taylor's participation in his classroom and community (Intervention #1).

General upper extremity strengthening activities, such as modified prone push-ups and wheelchair push-ups can be included in Taylor's program (Intervention #2). Using small weights, pulleys, or elastic bands for upper extremity strengthening would add variety. Active trunk extension in prone, upper trunk flexion in supine, and lateral flexion in side-lying should be incorporated for trunk strengthening. These antigravity movements will help increase muscular endurance in those muscles necessary for equilibrium movements. Once Taylor can perform these antigravity movements, resistance can be added and diagonal patterns encouraged.

Taylor should practice a variety of transfers at home and at school (Interventions #1 and #3) to improve his efficiency and independence. Manual assistance should be gradually lessened to standby assistance.

In standing with his RGO, Taylor could practice reaching outside his BOS as far as possible for objects (Intervention #4). Swaying in standing or "dancing" also would improve his balance. When in sitting, he should be encouraged to reach for toys placed on the floor or suspended at ear level in an area around his body (Intervention #5). When he reaches for toys, resistance can be provided either by using elastic bands attached to the hanging toys or using heavy toys on the floor.

Interventions #4 and #5 can be addressed by having Taylor respond to tilt on an unstable BOS, such as a ball. Tilting could be performed in prone and supine to strengthen trunk muscles as well as in sitting. In addition to anterior, posterior, and lateral tilting, diagonal tilting should be provided.

Repetitive head bending in standing should be performed to tolerance to habituate Taylor to visual and vestibular inputs (Intervention #6). Activities that require him to look down while walking, such as following a pattern on the floor, should help him accommodate to the sensory input. As part of his classroom routine, Taylor should be encouraged to use his walker for longer periods of time (Intervention #7). In addition to using the walker in his classroom, moving to other areas in the school (eg, to the cafeteria or music room) should be gradually added to his routine. Taylor would benefit from specific activities to help him develop the ability to catch himself when he falls (Intervention #8). Controlled (by an adult) falls from standing will give him experience with these movements and the upper extremity responses that he needs to produce for protection. Eventually, he should be able to rock, fall forward on his own, and catch himself.

Case Study #4: Ashley

> *Medical Diagnosis:* Down syndrome
> *Age:* 15 months

Examination and Evaluation

Postural Responses to Perturbation

> *Righting Reactions:* All vertical and rotational reactions are present.
> *Protective Reactions:* In sitting, Ashley has anterior and lateral responses, but inconsistent responses to tilt in a posterior direction. All protective reactions are slow.
> *Equilibrium Reactions:* Equilibrium responses are present in prone and supine on a stable BOS. In sitting, anterior and posterior responses are present, but lateral equilibrium responses are delayed. Ashley was too fearful to permit testing in all fours or standing on an unstable BOS.

Postural Control During Active Movement

> *Mobility Skills:* Ashley can roll, sit independently, creep on hands and knees, pull to kneeling, and pull to stand. She does not cruise at furniture and does not walk independently. In standing she has a wide BOS with lumbar lordosis, knee hyperextension, and foot pronation. She does not use active muscle contraction to maintain her posture.
> *Transitions:* Ashley transitions in and out of sitting and in and out of a hands-and-knees position. She uses straight plane movements without trunk rotation. She is unsteady, particularly when trying to move quickly.
> *Fine Motor Skills:* Ashley grasps objects but does not have controlled release. She has difficulty manipulating small objects and will not attempt to lift or manipulate heavy objects.

Participation Restrictions

Ashley demonstrates "postural insecurity" (ie, fear of movement) and avoids exploring many environments. She moves away from other children, especially if they are moving quickly or engaged in gross motor play. If she loses her balance in crawling or sitting, she becomes upset and refuses to participate in the current activity. When seated at a small table, she does not maintain an erect posture for more than 1 to 2 minutes and leans on the table, limiting the use of both hands for exploration of toys or other objects.

Activity Limitations

Ashley has achieved some basic motor skills, such as sitting, creeping on hands and knees, and pulling to stand. However, she is unsteady in all positions and easily loses her balance when perturbed or when she moves quickly or becomes distracted. When she loses her balance, she tries to correct her position using her head, trunk, and extremities. Her attempts to right herself often are too slow to be effective. Protective reactions of the arms and legs are noted with loss of balance, but she tends to rigidly lock her extremities and her reactions are inefficient.

Impairments

Ashley has low muscle tone and joint hypermobility. She appears to have difficulty stabilizing her joints when in weight-bearing positions. She tends to move slowly and is fearful about participating in movement activities. She has slow protective and balance reactions. Ashley is a passive child and is not physically active unless encouraged or assisted by an adult. She appears to have generalized weakness and poor endurance for gross motor activities. Ashley has a general developmental delay, including intellectual and language deficits, associated with her diagnosis of DS.

Functional/Participation Goals

After 3 months of intervention, Ashley will be able to accomplish the following:
1. Maintain her balance in sitting when passively tipped or tilted 30 degrees to the left or right.
2. Maintain her balance in all fours when slightly perturbed at the hip or shoulder.
3. Reach laterally for a toy while on all fours without loss of balance.
4. Cruise 4 steps to the left and right.
5. Move from the stuffed animal area of her parent-infant classroom (any method) to the toy area independently.
6. Respond positively (ie, no crying) to being swung in a playground swing.
7. Creep on hands and knees within 12 inches (30.5 cm) of other children.
8. Sit at a table for 5 minutes playing with a toy without leaning on the table.
9. Take 3 independent steps before falling.

Interventions

1. Parent instruction.
2. Strengthening activities of trunk and extremities.
3. Balance activities in all positions (ie, sitting, all fours, kneeling, standing).
4. Activities to promote protective responses.
5. Endurance activities.
6. Playful movement activities to decrease fear of movement and falling.
7. Treadmill training.

Therapeutic Activities

The therapist works with the preschool teacher and parent to determine what movement activities Ashley will tolerate (Intervention #1). Examples may be repetitive tilting while sitting on an adult's lap, slowly progressing to using a therapy ball or bolster to encourage trunk activity and strengthening (eg, abdominal muscles, back extensors; Intervention #2). Playing tug-of-war with elastic bands and batting and kicking at a suspended balloon will help increase extremity strength.

Ashley's classroom has a small waterbed mattress in the play area. This is a safe environment to have Ashley work on her balance skills (Intervention #3) by having her sit, creep on all fours, and attempt to kneel on the waterbed. If she falls she will not be injured and may begin to enjoy movement and learn to use her extremities and trunk more effectively for controlling her balance and using protective responses. Her parents can have Ashley practice the same movements at home using the mattress on the bed (Interventions #1, #3, and #4). Favorite toys or rewards could be used to motivate her to move independently (Intervention #5). Games, such as "chasing" her on hands and knees, might motivate her to move more and faster.

The play area also has a small playground set, which includes a swing and slide. Ashley should be assisted in swinging and sliding to her tolerance (Intervention #6). Her family should be encouraged to assist Ashley in participating in movement-based activities at home, such as being held by an adult while the adult "dances," "sways," "bounces," and "turns in circles" (Interventions #1 and #6). A small rocking chair can be used to encourage Ashley to move herself in a controlled, nonthreatening activity and can be used both in the home and school environments.

Research suggests that treadmill training in children with DS can have a positive effect on the timely achievement of upright balance skills and ambulation.[102,103] There is a small treadmill in the preschool gym, and Ashley can be supervised and encouraged to use it for 2 minutes each day (Intervention # 7; see Chapter 12).

Case Study #5: John

> *Medical Diagnosis:* Developmental coordination disorder/attention-deficit hyperactivity disorder
> *Age:* 5 years

Examination and Evaluation

Postural Responses to Perturbation

> *Righting Reactions:* John rights his head in all directions in all positions tested (ie, sitting on ball, tilting in hands and knees, kneeling, and standing on a vestibular board).
> *Protective Reactions:* John demonstrates protective reactions in all positions tested.
> *Equilibrium Reactions:* John demonstrates equilibrium reactions in all positions tested.

Postural Control During Active Movement

> *Mobility Skills:* John ambulates independently, but is described as being "clumsy." He has difficulty with age-appropriate motor skills, such as running, hopping, skipping, and riding a bicycle. John appears to have difficulty performing 2 tasks at once, such as participating in a motor activity while talking.
> *Transitions:* John is independent in transitions of movement, although he demonstrates some slowness and incoordination with higher-level transition skills, such as moving on and off playground equipment.
> *Fine Motor Skills:* John has difficulty with "tool use" (eg, pencil, knife and fork). He is independent in dressing, but has difficulty with buttons, snaps, and zippers. When carrying large or heavy objects, he frequently bumps into furniture or walls.

Participation Restrictions

John is "clumsy" compared with same-age peers. He is self-conscious about his motor abilities and avoids participation in many age-appropriate gross motor activities. He bumps into objects frequently so he avoids crowded environments. His poor motor planning skills limit his social opportunities and negatively affect his overall physical fitness.

Activity Limitations

John has difficulty with motor skills, such as bike riding (eg, must use training wheels). He demonstrates incoordination and poor endurance for play activities such as hopping, jumping, and ball games.

Impairments

John easily becomes frustrated when trying to learn new motor skills. He has a poor attention span and is very distractible. He tends not to stick with a task long enough to perform enough repetitions to improve his performance, and he fatigues quickly when participating in gross motor activities. Upper extremity strength is decreased compared with other children his age.

Functional/Participation Goals

After 3 months of intervention, John will be able to accomplish the following:
1. Perform 5 prone push-ups within 1 minute.
2. Ride his bike (with training wheels) for 5 miles during family bike trips.
3. Perform 3 successive 2-foot (0.5-m) jumps, one of 3 attempts.
4. Walk in a crowded environment (eg, mall, grocery store, hallway in school) without bumping into objects or people.
5. Catch and throw a tennis ball from a standing position, 7 of 10 trials.

Interventions

1. Parent, teacher, and child education.
2. Strengthening activities.
3. Endurance activities.
4. Balance and coordination activities during gross motor games and walking.
5. Eye-hand coordination activities in conjunction with balance activities.

Therapeutic Activities

John's family will carry out a home program designed to improve his overall strength, endurance, and coordination (Intervention #1), which is embedded into family activities (eg, bike riding, playing tag). School and community activities (eg, soccer and T-ball) also will be encouraged (Interventions #1, #2, and #3). The physical therapist should suggest appropriate community activities for John. For example, the family could investigate having John participate in a "karate for kids" class to improve his strength, endurance, and motor control. In addition, John can accompany his father to the local health club and work with small weights as his father performs strength training.

Cognitive strategies can be used to assist John in remembering to walk slower and pay attention to his environment (Interventions #1 and #4). He can practice walking around the local playground on various terrains (eg, sand, gravel, grass) with environmental objects (eg, swings, slide, climbing structures) to navigate. This activity can be increased in complexity by having John carry objects of various sizes and weights and by having him talk while walking. John's father can work with him on throwing and catching balls of different sizes and weights, as John usually is motivated to do activities when his father participates (Interventions #1 and #5). The physical therapist will monitor John's motor program and progress, adapting or adding activities as John improves his motor skills.

Communication and coordination of services should occur between school and private therapists. If John does not qualify for school physical therapy services, the private physical therapist should try to coordinate services with his physical education and classroom teachers.

References

1. Hadders-Algra M. Typical and atypical development of reaching and postural control in infancy. *Dev Med Child Neurol.* 2013;55(suppl 4):5-8. doi:10.1111/dmcn.12298.
2. Karasik LB, Adolph KE, Tamis-Lemonda CS, Bornstein MH. WEIRD walking: cross-cultural research on motor development. *Behav Brain Sci.* 2010;33(2-3):95-96. doi:10.1017/S0140525X10000117.
3. Merzenich MM, Van Vleet TM, Nahum M. Brain plasticity-based therapeutics. *Front Hum Neurosci.* 2014;8:385. doi:10.3389/frhum. 2014.00385.
4. Houghton KM, Guzman J. Evaluation of static and dynamic postural balance in children with juvenile idiopathic arthritis. *Pediatr Phys Ther.* 2013;25(2):150-157; discussion 157. doi:10.1097/PEP.0b013e31828a2978.
5. Herskind A, Ritterband-Rosenbaum A, Willerslev-Olsen M, et al. Muscle growth is reduced in 15-month-old children with cerebral palsy. *Dev Med Child Neurol.* 2016;58(5):485-491. doi: 10.1111/dmcn.12950.
6. Willerslev-Olsen M, Lorentzen J, Sinkjaer T, Nielsen JB. Passive muscle properties are altered in children with cerebral palsy before the age of 3 years and are difficult to distinguish clinically from spasticity. *Dev Med Child Neurol.* 2013;55(7):617-623. doi:10.1111/dmcn.12124.
7. Mockford M, Caulton JM. The pathophysiological basis of weakness in children with cerebral palsy. *Pediatr Phys Ther.* 2010;22(2):222-233. doi:10.1097/PEP.0b013e3181dbaf96.
8. Begnoche DM, Chiarello LA, Palisano RJ, Gracely EJ, McCoy SW, Orlin MN. Predictors of independent walking in young children with cerebral palsy. *Phys Ther.* 2016;196(2):183-192. doi:10.2522/ptj.20140315.
9. Dusing SC. Postural variability and sensorimotor development in infancy. *Dev Med Child Neurol.* 2016;58(suppl 4):17-21. doi:10.1111/dmcn.13045.
10. Rine RM, Rubish K, Feeney C. Measurement of sensory system effectiveness and maturational changes in postural control in young children. *Pediatr Phys Ther.* 1998;10(1):16-22. doi:10.1097/00001577-199801010-00004.
11. Lui WY, Ya-TingHsu, Lien HY, et al. Deficits in sensory organization for postural stability in children with Tourette syndrome. *Clin Neurol Neurosurg.* 2015;129(suppl 1):S36-540. doi:10.1016/S0303-8467(15)30010-X.
12. Mazaheryazdi M, Moossavi A, Sarrafzadah J, Talebian S, Jalaie S. Study of the effects of hearing on static and dynamic postural function in children using cochlear implants. *Int J Pediatr Otorhinolaryngol.* 2017;100(9):18-22. doi:10.1016/j.ijporl.2017.06.002.
13. Hatzitaki V, Zisi V, Kollias I, Kioumourtzoglou E. Perceptual-motor contributions to static and dynamic balance control in children. *J Mot Behav.* 2002;34(2):161-170. doi:10.1080/00222890209601938.
14. Huang HJ, Mercer VS. Dual-task methodology: application in studies of cognitive and motor performance in adults and children. *Pediatr Phys Ther.* 2001;13(3):133-140. doi:10.1097/00001577-200110000-00005.
15. Huang HJ, Mercer VS, Thorpe DE. Effects of different concurrent cognitive tasks on temporal-distance gait variables in children. *Pediatr Phys Ther.* 2003;15(2):105-113. doi:10.1097/01.PEP.0000067886.96352.6B.
16. Blanchard Y, Carey S, Coffey J, et al. The influence of concurrent cognitive tasks on postural sway in children. *Pediatr Phys Ther.* 2005;17(3):189-193. doi:10.1097/01.PEP.0000176578.57147.5d.
17. Boonyong S, Siu KC, van Donkelaar P, Chou LS, Woollacott MH. Development of postural control during gait in typically developing children: the effects of dual-task conditions. *Gait Posture.* 2012;35(3):428-434. doi:10.1016/j.gaitpost.2011.11.002.
18. Prechtl HFR. *The Neurological Examination of the Full Term Newborn Infant.* 2nd ed. Philadelphia, PA: JB Lippincott; 1977:39-56.
19. Katz PS. Evolution of central pattern generators and rhythmic behaviours. *Philos Trans R Soc Lond B Biol Sci.* 2016; (1): 371. doi:10.1098/rstb.2015.0057.

20. Danner SM, Hofstoetter US, Freundl B, et al. Human spinal locomotor control is based on flexibly organized burst generators. *Brain*. 2015;138(pt 3):577-588. doi:10.1093/brain/awu372.

21. Danner SM, Wilshin SD, Shevtsova NA, Rybak IA. Central control of interlimb coordination and speed-dependent gait expression in quadrupeds. *J Physiol*. 2016;594(23):6947-6967. doi:10.1113/JP272787.

22. DeVries JIP, Visser GHA, Prechtl HFR. Fetal motility in the first half of pregnancy. In: Prechtl HFR, ed. *Continuity of Neural Functions from Prenatal to Postnatal Life*. Oxford, England: Spastics International Medical Publications; 1984:46-64.

23. Forssberg H. Ontogeny of human locomotor control. I. Infant stepping, supported locomotion and transitions to independent locomotion. *Exp Brain Res*. 1985;57(3):480-493. doi:10.1007/BF00237835.

24. Thomas A, Autgaerden S. *Locomotion From Pre- to Post-Natal Life: How the Newborn Begins to Acquire Psycho-Sensory Functions*. Clinics in Developmental Medicine. No. 24. London, England: Medical Books Ltd; 1966:1-88.

25. Lamb T, Yang JF. Could different directions of infant stepping be controlled by the same locomotor central pattern generator? *J Neurophysiol*. 2000;83(5):2814-2824. doi:10.1152/jn.2000.83.5.2814

26. Meyns P, Desloovere K, Molenaers G, Swinnen SP, Duysens J. Interlimb coordination during forward and backward walking in primary school-aged children. *PloS One*. 2013;8(4):e62747. doi:10.1371/journal.pone.0062747.

27. Ivanenko YP, Dominici N, Cappellini G, et al. Changes in the spinal segmental motor output for stepping during development from infant to adult. *J Neurosci*. 2013;33(7):3025-3036a. doi:10.1523/JNEUROSCI.2722-12.2013.

28. Cappellini G, Ivanenko YP, Martino G, et al. Immature spinal locomotor output in children with cerebral palsy. *Front Physiol*. 2016;7:478. doi:10.3389/fphys.2016.00478.

29. Kornhuber HH. The vestibular system and the general motor system. In: Kornhuber HH, ed. *Handbook of Sensory Physiology. Vestibular System Part 2: Psychophysics, Applied Aspects, and General Interpretation*. Vol VI/2. New York, NY: Springer-Verlag; 1974:581-586.

30. Magnus R (abstracted by Brunnstrom S). Haltung. *Phys Ther Rev*. 1953;33:281-290. Reprinted in Payton OD, Hirt S, Newton RA, eds. *Neurophysiologic Approaches to Therapeutic Exercise*. Philadelphia, PA: FA Davis Company; 1977:64-66.

31. Aiello I, Rosati G, Sau GF, et al. Interaction of tonic labyrinth and neck reflexes in man. *Ital J Neurol Sci*. 1992;13(3):195-201. doi:10.1007/BF02224389.

32. Georgopoulos AP, Grillner S. Visuomotor coordination in reaching and locomotion. *Science*. 1989;245(9):1209-1210. doi:10.1126/science.2675307.

33. Dubowitz LM, Dubowitz V. *The Neurological Assessment of the Preterm and Full-Term Newborn Infant*. Clinics in Developmental Medicine No. 79. Philadelphia, PA: JB Lippincott; 1981:334-338.

34. Dubowitz LM, Dubowitz V, Goldberg C. Clinical assessment of gestational age in the newborn infant. *J Pediatr*. 1970;77(1):1-10. doi:10.1016/S0022-3476(70)80038-5.

35. Hamer EG, Hadders-Algra M. Prognostic significance of neurological signs in high-risk infants—a systematic review. *Dev Med Child Neurol*. 2016;58 (suppl 4):53-60. doi:10.1111/dmcn.13051.

36. Øberg GK, Jacobson BK, Jørgenson L. Predictive value of general movement assessment for cerebral palsy in routine clinical practice. *Phys Ther*. 2015;95(11):1489-1495. doi:10.2522/ptj.20140429.

37. Datta AN, Furrer MA, Bernhardt I, et al. Fidgety movements in infants born very preterm: predictive value for cerebral palsy in a clinical multicentre setting. *Dev Med Child Neurol*. 2017;59(6):618-624. doi:10.1111/dmcn.13386.

38. Doidge N. *The Brain's Way of Healing*. New York, NY: Penguin Books; 2015.

39. Sporns O, Edelman GM. Solving Bernstein's problem: a proposal for the development of coordinated movement by selection. *Child Dev*. 1993;64(4):960-981. doi:10.1111/j.1467-8624.1993.tb04182.x.

40. Forssberg H, Hirschfeld H. Postural adjustments in sitting humans following external perturbations: muscle activity and kinematics. *Exp Brain Res*. 1994;97(3):515-527. doi:10.1007/BF00241545.

41. Hedberg A, Forssberg H, Hadders-Algra M. Postural adjustments due to external perturbations during sitting in 1-month-old infants: evidence for the innate origin of direction specificity. *Exp Brain Res*. 2004;157 (1):10-17. doi:10.1007/s00221-003-1811-z.

42. Hadders-Algra M, Brogren E, Forssberg H. Development of postural control—differences between ventral and dorsal muscles? *Neurosci Biobehavi Rev*. 1998;22(4):501-506. doi:10.1016/S0149-7634(97)00036-5.

43. Dietz V, Horstmann GA, Berger W. Interlimb coordination of leg-muscle activation during perturbation of stance in humans. *J Neurophysiol*. 1989;62 (3):680-693. doi:10.1152/jn.1989.62.3.680.

44. Thelen E, Cooke DW. Relationship between newborn stepping and later walking: a new interpretation. *Dev Med Child Neurol*. 1987;29(3):380-393. doi:10.1111/j.1469-8749.1987.tb02492.x

45. Thelen E, Spencer JP. Postural control during reaching in young infants: a dynamic systems approach. *Neurosci Biobehav Rev*. 1998; 22 (4):507-514. doi:10.1016/S0149-7634(97)00037-7.

46. Hadders-Algra M, Brogren E, Forssberg H. Training affects the development of postural adjustments in sitting infants. *J Physiol*. 1996;493(pt 1):289-298. doi:10.1113/jphysiol.1996.sp021383.

47. Sveistrup H, Woollacott MH. Practice modifies the developing automatic postural response. *Exp Brain Res.* 1997;114(1):33-43. doi:10.1007/PL00005621.
48. Roncesvalles MN, Woollacott MH, Jensen JL. Development of lower extremity kinetics for balance control in infants and young children. *J Mot Behav.* 2001;33(2):180-192.
49. Rachwani J, Soska KC, Adolph KE. Behavioral flexibility in learning to sit. *Dev Psychobiol.* 2017;59(8):937-948. doi:10.002/dev 21571.
50. Pavão SL, dos Santos AN, Woollacott MH, Rocha NA. Assessment of postural control in children with cerebral palsy: a review. *Res Dev Disabil.* 2013;34(5):1367-1375. doi:10.1016/j.ridd.2013.01.034.
51. Hadders-Algra M, Brogren E, Forssberg H. Postural adjustments during sitting at preschool age: presence of a transient toddling phase. *Dev Med Child Neurol.* 1998;40(7):436-447. doi:10.1111/j.1469-8749.1998.tb15393.x.
52. Hadders-Algra M, Brogren E, Katz-Salamon M, Forssberg H. Periventricular leukomalacia and preterm birth have different detrimental effects on postural adjustments. *Brain.* 1999;122 (pt 4):727-740. doi:10.1093/brain/122.4.727.
53. Brogren E, Forssberg H, Hadders-Algra M. Influence of two different sitting positions on postural adjustments in children with spastic diplegia. *Dev Med Child Neurol.* 2001;43(8):534-546.
54. Roncesvalles MN, Woollacott MW, Burtner PA. Neural factors underlying reduced postural adaptability in children with cerebral palsy. *Neuroreport.* 2002;13(18):2407-2410. doi:10.1097/01.wnr.0000048024.40536.9d.
55. Kenis-Coskun O, Giray E, Eren B, Ozkok O, Karadag-Saygi E. Evaluation of postural stability in children with hemiplegic cerebral palsy. *J Phys Ther Sci.* 2016;28(5):1398-1402. doi:10.1589/jpts.28.1398.
56. Harbourne RT, Willett S, Kyvelidou A, Deffeyes J, Stergiou N. A comparison of interventions for children with cerebral palsy to improve sitting postural control: a clinical trial. *Phys Ther.* 2010;90(12):1881-1898. doi:10.2522/ptj.2010132.
57. Goetz M, Schwabova JP, Hlavka Z, Ptacek R, Surman CB. Dynamic balance in children with attention-deficit hyperactivity disorder and its relationship with cognitive functions and cerebellum. *Neuropsychiatr Dis Treat.* 2017;13(3):873-880. doi:10.2147/NDT.S125169.
58. Fournier KA, Hass CJ, Naik SK, Lodha N, Caurauh JH. Motor coordination in autism spectrum disorders: a synthesis and meta-analysis. *J Autism Dev Disord.* 2010;40(10):1227-1240. doi:10.1007/s10803-010-0981-3.
59. Van der Fits IBM, Hadders-Algra M. The development of postural response patterns during reaching in healthy infants. *Neurosci Biobehav Rev.* 1998;22(4):521-526. doi:10.1016/S0149-7634(97)00039-0.
60. Van der Fits IB, Otten E, Klip AWJ, Van Eykern LA, Hadders-Algra M. The development of postural adjustments during reaching in 6- to 18-month-old infants. Evidence for two transitions. *Exp Brain Res.* 1999;126(4):517-528. doi:10.1007/s002210050760.
61. Van Balen LC, Dijkstra LJ, Bos AF, Van Den Heuvel ER, Hadders-Algra M. Development of postural adjustments during reaching infants at risk for cerebral palsy from 4 to 18 months. *Dev Med Child Neurol.* 2015;57(7):668-676. doi:10.1111/dmcn.12699.
62. Dinkel D, Snyder K, Molfese V, Kyvelidou A. Postural control strategies differ in normal weight and overweight infants. *Gait Posture.* 2017;55(6):167-171. doi:10.1016/j.gaitpost.2017.04.017.
63. Hedberg A, Schmitz C, Forssberg H, Hadders-Algra M. Early development of postural adjustments in standing with and without support. *Exp Brain Res.* 2007;178(4):439-449. doi:10.1007/s00221-006-0754-6.
64. Schmitz C, Martin N, Assaiante C. Building anticipatory postural adjustment during childhood: a kinematic and electromyographic analysis of unloading in children from 4 to 8 years of age. *Exp Brain Res.* 2002;142(3):354-364. doi:10.1007/s00221-001-0910-y.
65. Shiratori T, Girolami GL, Aruin AS. Anticipatory postural adjustments associated with a loading perturbation in children with hemiplegic and diplegic cerebral palsy. *Exp Brain Res.* 2016;234(10):2967-2978. doi:10.1007/s00221-016-4699-0.
66. Grasso R, Assaiante C, Prévost P, Berthoz A. Development of anticipatory orienting strategies during locomotor tasks in children. *Neurosci Biobehav Rev.* 1998;22(4):533-539. doi:10.1016/S0149-7634(97)00041-9.
67. Girolami GL, Shiratori T, Aruin AS. Anticipatory postural adjustments in children with typical motor development. *Exp Brain Res.* 2010;205(2):153-165. doi:10.1007/s00221-010-2347-7.
68. Liu WY, Zaino CA, McCoy SW. Anticipatory postural adjustments in children with cerebral palsy and children with typical development. *Pediatr Phys Ther.* 2008;19(3):188-195. doi:10.1097/PEP.0b013e31812574a9.
69. Chen HL, Yeh CF, Howe TH. Postural control during standing reach in children with Down syndrome. *Res Dev Disabil.* 2015;38(3):345-351. doi:10.1016/j.ridd.2014.12.024.
70. Tomita H, Fukaya Y, Ueda T, et al. Deficits in task-specific modulation of anticipatory postural adjustments in individuals with spastic diplegic cerebral palsy. *J Neurophysiol.* 2011;105(5):2157-2168. doi:10.1152/jn.00569.2010.
71. Johnston LM, Burns YR, Brauer SG, Richardson CA. Differences in postural control and movement performance during goal directed reaching in children with developmental coordination disorder. *Hum Mov Sci.* 2002;21(5-6):583-601. doi:10.1016/S0167-9457(02)00153-7.

72. Kane K, Barden J. Frequency of anticipatory trunk muscle onsets in children with and without developmental coordination disorder. *Phys Occup Ther Pediatr.* 2014;34(1):75-89. doi:10.3109/01942638.2012.757574.

73. Forssberg H, Nashner LM. Ontogenetic development of postural control in man: adaptation to altered support and visual conditions during stance. *J Neurosci.* 1982;2(5):545-552. doi:10.1523/JNEUROSCI.02-05-00545.1982.

74. Horak F, Nashner L. Central programming of posture movements: adaptation to altered support-surface configurations. *J Neurophysiol.* 1986;55(6):1369-1381. doi:10.1152/jn.1986.55.6.1369.

75. Roncesvalles MN, Woollacott MH, Jensen JL. The development of compensatory stepping skills in children. *J Mot Behav.* 2000;32(1):100-111. doi:10.1080/00222890009601363

76. Fiorentino MR. *Reflex Testing Methods for Evaluating CNS Development.* Springfield, IL: Charles C. Thomas; 1963.

77. Haley SM. Sequential analyses of postural reactions in nonhandicapped infants. *Phys Ther.* 1986;66(4):531-536. doi:10.1093/ptj/66.4.531.

78. Bayley N. *Bayley Scales of Infant Development.* New York, NY: Psychological Corporation; 1969.

79. Touwen B. *Neurological Development in Infancy.* Clinics in Developmental Medicine. No. 58, Philadelphia, PA: JB Lippincott; 1976.

80. Knobloch H. *Manual of Developmental Diagnosis.* New York, NY: Harper & Row Publishers; 1980.

81. Gilfoyle EM, Grady AP, Moore JC. *Children Adapt.* Thorofare, NJ: SLACK Incorporated; 1981:57-77.

82. Tower G. Selected developmental reflexes and reactions—a literature search. In: Hopkins HL, Smith HD, eds. *Willard and Spackman's Occupational Therapy.* 6th ed. Philadelphia, PA: Lippincott; 1983:175-187.

83. Peiper A. *Cerebral Function in Infancy.* New York, NY: Consultants Bureau; 1963:156-210.

84. Saint-Anne D'Argassies S. Neurodevelopmental symptoms during the first year of life. *Dev Med Child Neurol.* 1972;14(2):235-246. doi:10.1111/j.1469-8749.1972.tb02583.x.

85. Fisher AG. Objective assessment of the quality of response during two equilibrium tasks. *Phys Occup Ther Pediatr.* 1989;9(3):57-78. doi:10.1080/J006v09n03_04.

86. Rachwani J, Santamaria V, Saavredra SL, Woollacott MH. The development of trunk control and its relation to reaching in infancy: a longitudinal study. *Front Hum Neurosci.* 2015;24(2):9-94. doi:10.3389/fnhum.2015.00094.

87. Butler PB, Saavedra S, Sofranac M, Jaravis SE, Woollacott JH. Refinement, reliability, and validity of the segmental assessment of trunk control. *Pediatr Phys Ther.* 2010;22(3):246-257. doi:10.1097/PEP.0b013e3181e69490.

88. Saavedra SL, Woollacott MH. Segmental contributions to trunk control in children with moderate-to-severe cerebral palsy. *Arch Phys Med Rehabil.* 2015;96(6):1088-1097. doi:10.1016/j.apmr.2015.01.016.

89. Richter EW, Montgomery PC. *The Sensorimotor Performance Analysis.* Stillwater, MN: PDP Press; 1989.

90. Santamaria V, Rachwani J, Saavedra S, Woollacott M. Effect of segmental trunk support on posture and reaching in children with cerebral palsy. *Pediatr Phys Ther.* 2016;28(3):285-293. doi:10.1097/PEP.0000000000000273.

91. Abdel-Aziem AA, El-Basatiny HM. Effect of backward walking training on walking ability in children with hemiparetic cerebral palsy: a randomized controlled study. *Clin Rehabil.* 2017;3(6):790-797. doi:10.1177/0269215516656468.

92. Kordi H, Sohrabi M, Saberi Kakhki A, Attanzadeh Hossini SR. The effect of strength training based on process approach intervention on balance of children with developmental coordination disorder. *Arch Argent Pediatr.* 2016;114(6):526-533. doi:10.5546/aap.2016.eng.526.

93. Tarakci D, Ersoz Huseyinsinoglu B, Tarakci E, Razak Ozdincler A. Effects of Nintendo Wii-Fit video games on balance in children with mild cerebral palsy. *Pediatr Int.* 2016;58(10):1042-1050. doi:10.1111/ped.12942.

94. Jelsma D, Geuze RH, Mombarq R, Smits-Engelsman BC. The impact of Wii Fit Intervention on dynamic balance control in children with probable Developmental Coordination Disorder and balance problems. *Hum Move Sci.* 2014;33(2):404-418. doi:10.1016/j.humov.2013.12.007.

95. Güçhan Z, Mutlu A. The effectiveness of taping on children with cerebral palsy: a systematic review. *Dev Med Child Neurol.* 2017;59(1):26-30. doi:10.1111/dmcn.13213.

96. Almeida KM, Fonseca ST, Figueiredo PRP, Aquino AA, Mancini MC. Effects of interventions with therapeutic suits (clothing) on impairments and functional limitations of children with cerebral palsy: a systematic review. *Braz J Phys Ther.* 2017;21(5):307-320. doi:10.1016/j.bjpt.2017.06.009.

97. Strebling K, Christy J. Creative dance practice improves postural control in a child with cerebral palsy. *Pediatr Phys Ther.* 2017;29(4):365-369. doi:10.1097/PEP.0000000000000450.

98. Teixeira-Machado L, Azevedo-Santos I, DeSantana JM. Dance improves functionality and psychosocial adjustment in cerebral palsy: a randomized controlled clinical trial. *Am J Phys Med Rehabil.* 2017;96(6):424-429. doi:10/1097/PHM0000000000000646.

99. Dewar R, Love S, Johnston LM. Exercise interventions to improve postural control on children with cerebral palsy: a systematic review. *Dev Med Child Neurol.* 2015;57(6):504-520. doi:10.1111/dmcn.12660.

100. Bleyenheufat Y, Ebner-Karestinos D, Surana B, et al. Intensive upper- and lower-extremity training for children with bilateral cerebral palsy: a quasi-randomized trial. *Dev Med Child Neurol.* 2017;59(6):625-633. doi:10.1111/dmcn.13379.

101. Gelkop N, Burshein DG, Lahav A, et al. Efficacy of constraint-induced movement therapy and bimanual training in children with hemiplegic cerebral palsy in an educational setting. *Phys Occup Ther Pediatr.* 2015;35(1):24-39. doi:10.3109/01942638.2014.925027.

102. Ulrich DA, Ulrich BD, Angulo-Kinzler RM, Yun J. Treadmill training of infants with Down syndrome: evidence-based developmental outcomes. *Pediatrics.* 2001;108(5):E84. doi: 10.1542/peds.108.5.e84.

103. Ulrich DA, Lloyd MC, Tiernan CW, Looper JE, Angulo-Barroso RM. Effects of intensity of treadmill training on developmental outcomes and stepping in infants with Down syndrome: a randomized trial. *Phys Ther.* 2008;88(1):114-122. doi:10.2522/ptj.20070139.

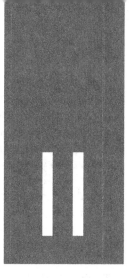

Facilitating Early Mobility

Lisa K. Kenyon, PT, DPT, PhD, PCS
Maria Jones, PT, PhD

Early mobility patterns, such as crawling and walking, broaden the world for typically developing (TD) infants and toddlers and start a cascade of developmental and social changes on the path to independence. But how can we, as therapists, provide similar early mobility experiences to young children who have mobility limitations? And perhaps more importantly, how might children with mobility limitations benefit from early mobility? This chapter explores the developmental impact of mobility and outlines various methods that therapists can use to provide early mobility experiences for young children with a wide range of abilities and limitations.

The Impact of Early Mobility in Typical Development

The onset of self-generated mobility patterns (eg, crawling, walking) radically changes the relationship between a developing infant or toddler and the environment.[1-4] For the very first time, the child is no longer dependent on others to move from one place to another. Self-generated mobility is, however, more than just a way to get from point A to point B. According to Piaget,[5] self-generated mobility, and the sensory information gained through such mobility, is the basis for intelligence in the young child. Gibson[3] proposed that a child's (and indeed an adult's) cognitive foundation is laid by the information and knowledge acquired as a result of the early exploratory activities afforded by self-generated mobility. From the perspective of brain development, Pallas[6] suggested that the impact of early postnatal experiences, such as those provided by moving and exploring the environment, are vital in shaping and molding cortical connectivity and function.

Self-generated mobility also provides a plethora of novel experiences and opportunities that contribute to learning, problem solving, spatial awareness, visual skills, memory, social and emotional processes, and overall development.[1-4] When you were a baby and you crawled under a low table and tried to stand up, you might have hit your head, but you also learned about maneuvering through space and concepts such as under, over, and through. Your ability to crawl gave you autonomy and encouraged persistence as you decided where you wanted to go and what

Connolly BH, Montgomery PC, eds. *Therapeutic Exercise for
Children With Developmental Disabilities, Fourth Edition* (pp 305-329).
© 2020 Taylor & Francis Group.

you wanted to do.[2] No matter how many times an adult may have tried to steer you away from something you wanted (eg, stairs, delicate objects, television remote), you were developing a sense of freedom while exploring. You also were learning that you could interact with your environment rather than passively waiting for adults to bring desired objects to you.[2] As you crawled, you were discovering spatial concepts and learning about spatial properties of objects, both of which contributed to your developing spatial cognition and your sense of self.[7,8] As your self-generated mobility skills improved, the ways in which you located and learned about objects evolved from using only visual information to being able to manipulate the spatial relationship between objects and your body. As your mobility patterns matured, you were able to remember where objects were located and started to understand the interrelationships between yourself and the objects within your ever-expanding world.[7,9]

As you moved and explored, you were developing the foundational skills necessary for *social cognition,* the ability to process, store, and use information about others and social situations.[10] Social cognition specifically relates to the interpretation of social signals and enables us to learn about the world through social interactions.[10] For example, when you were a baby and crawled toward something new or unusual in your environment, you learned to look at your mother or other trusted caregiver to determine whether it was OK to approach this novel object based on your interpretation of your caregiver's facial expressions.[10] In this way, you learned about what your caregivers perceived as "good" and "bad." Unbeknownst to you, the onset of crawling and the experiences you gained through crawling were accompanied by changes in cortical organization as connections likely were created between the frontal/occipital and parietal/occipital areas of the brain.[11] Given that the parietal lobe is associated with processing sensory information, spatial behavior, and motor planning,[12] these experience-related changes in your brain may have been directly related to the inherent requirements and sensory aspects of crawling.[11]

TD older infants and toddlers often are highly mobile. Adolph et al[13] explored spontaneous locomotion during free play in children age 12-19 months and found that walking infants averaged 2367.6 steps per hour, traveled 701.2 meters per hour, and fell 17.4 times per hour. To put this in perspective, walking 701.2 meters (767 yards) in an hour is roughly equivalent to moving the length of 7.7 American football fields.[13] With these practice rates over the span of only one hour, imagine how much walking practice these young children garnered throughout the course of their day. Assuming that these children were free to move about for just 6 hours a day, their daily practice "dose" would be approximately 14,000 steps over the length of 46 football fields.[13] This amount of motor practice alone is incredible, but the learning opportunities and sensory experiences that likely accompany this motor practice makes it is easy to see how TD children benefit from early mobility experiences.

THE IMPACT OF MOBILITY LIMITATIONS

Children with mobility limitations often are unable to reap the inherent developmental and functional benefits of independent mobility,[14,15] putting them at risk for secondary impairments in spatial cognition, communication, social development, and other developmental domains.[1,9,16,17] Passive mobility, such as being pushed in a wheelchair, does not provide the same experience as self-generated mobility and therefore does not promote the development of the spatial-cognitive skills necessary to understand the relationship between oneself and the environment.[4] Children who are unable to actively move and interact with their environment also may exhibit passive, dependent behaviors.[15,17] This lack of control and inability to interact with the environment may lead to the development of learned helplessness wherein children may believe they have no control over themselves or the social and physical events in their world.[18,19] These ongoing feelings may result in a negative affect, difficulties with problem solving, poor task mastery (especially with more challenging tasks), and limitations in executive function.[19,20] In addition, prolonged lack of control may result in decreased development of skills related to self-regulation, which ultimately may further perpetuate and amplify perceptions of helplessness.[19,20] Mobility devices, manual or power, provide children who have mobility limitations opportunities for self-generated mobility, allowing them a degree of independence that may discourage the development of learned helplessness.[15,17,18]

PROVIDING EARLY MOBILITY EXPERIENCES

Mobility devices enable people who have mobility limitations the opportunity to achieve mobility, benefit from human rights, and live with dignity.[21] The 2006 United Nations Convention on the Rights of Persons with Disabilities[22] asserted that nations have a responsibility to ensure access to mobility devices that provide the greatest possible level of independence for people with mobility limitations. Although there are likely limitless ways to provide early mobility experiences, this chapter focuses on providing early mobility through the use of power mobility devices and other assistive devices, such as gait trainers and a variety of self-propelled wheeled mobility options. Supplemental information illustrating the use of power mobility devices and other assistive devices to provide early mobility experiences is provided in Video 11-1, which accompanies this chapter.

The *International Classification of Functioning, Disability and Health* (ICF)[23] considers mobility devices both as an environmental and personal factors that may have a profound impact on a child's participation and independence. As outlined in Chapter 3, therapists can apply Gibson's model[24] for understanding human behavior as a way to construct "affordances" (objects in the environment) and elicit functional mobility.[25] In this way, mobility devices can be viewed as affordances[24,25] that may enhance and encourage self-generated mobility in young children who have mobility limitations. As stated in Chapter 3, when provided opportunities and encouragement, children often will explore movement and mobility options, which may in turn help to ameliorate the impact of mobility limitations.

PRACTICE CONSIDERATIONS WHEN PROVIDING EARLY MOBILITY EXPERIENCES

Benefits of Early Power Mobility

To provide children with mobility limitations movement experiences similar to their TD peers, therapists must consider providing such experiences at younger ages than previously reported in the literature.[26,27] In fact, according to the Rehabilitation Engineering Society of North America (RESNA),[28] age should not be a factor when considering power mobility use for children who have mobility limitations. Evidence supporting power mobility use in young children rapidly is increasing. A systematic review of power mobility outcomes in children from infancy to age 18 years found support for power mobility use across the ICF[23] domains.[14] In Body Functions and Structures,[14] power mobility positively affected areas such as developmental change,[29-34] intelligence quotient,[35] affect,[36] engagement,[37] sleep/wake pattern,[38] and psychological growth.[39] Improvements within the Activities domain[14] included power wheelchair and power mobility skills,[29,32,33,35,38] self-generated mobility,[30,37,39-42] communication,[37,42] interaction with objects,[37,42] and independence.[31,39,43] Participation enhancements within the ICF[23] model included social skills and interaction,[36,38,43] play,[37,40,41] and peer interaction and participation.[31,39-41,43] Although the majority of studies included in this review provided Level IV or V evidence,[44] studies by Jones et al[29] and Butler[42] provided Level II and III evidence,[44] respectively.

The Level II study by Jones and colleagues[29] provides the strongest evidence to date supporting early power mobility use in children with mobility limitations. This randomized controlled trial explored the effects of power mobility use in young children (age 14 to 30 months) who had severe motor impairments. Statistically significant improvements were found in the intervention group on the Battelle Developmental Inventory[45] in the area of receptive communication and on the Pediatric Evaluation of Disability Inventory[46] in the Mobility domain and the Mobility and Self-Care Caregiver Assistance scales. In addition, 4 of the 14 children in the intervention group achieved 100% of the skills on the Wheelchair Skills Checklist[47] in 12 to 42 weeks, whereas 7 children mastered between 2 and 6 skills, and all but 2 children learned to move forward 10 feet (3 m) in wide areas within 2 to 34 weeks.[29]

A Delphi study by Livingstone and Paleg[15] explored practice considerations related to power mobility introduction and use in children and achieved consensus among international pediatric power mobility researchers on 9 transferable practice messages. These messages detail factors pertinent to early power mobility use, including the age at which children should be introduced to power mobility and the potential benefits of power mobility.[15] Specifically, using specialized power mobility devices, infants with mobility limitations can participate in power mobility experiences as young as age 8 months.[15,30] Furthermore, infants and toddlers can learn to maneuver a power mobility device by about age 14 months, and those who have the physical ability to use a joystick can demonstrate competent control as young as 18 months.[14,29] Other messages in this Delphi study are that power mobility use promotes functional mobility, enhances overall development, provides independence, and increases participation in children who have mobility limitations or diagnoses that limit early functional mobility.[15,30,48] In addition, with sufficient practice and support, power mobility may augment self-initiated behavior and learning not only in children who have mobility limitations, but also in children who have severe intellectual or sensory impairments.[15,49-51] Although not every child will become a competent driver, all children with mobility limitations can benefit from power mobility use.[15] Despite evidence supporting these transferable messages, little is known about therapists' agreement with or implementation of the concepts outlined in these messages. A survey study exploring the views and practices of pediatric occupational therapists and physical therapists in Canada and the United States regarding power mobility use in children found that a majority (>80%) of respondents agreed or strongly agreed with many of these messages.[27] However, respondents reported performing various tasks related to the provision of power mobility (eg, ordering power wheelchairs, providing power mobility experiences, creating power mobility training programs) at a very low frequency (1 to 2 times per year or never).[27] Whether therapists are applying these messages related to the introduction and use of power mobility for children to practice is unclear, but because of the apparent discrepancy between research and practice, a more concerted effort to promote knowledge translation in this area is warranted.

Despite the abundance of evidence supporting early power mobility use, therapists and families may be concerned that early use of power mobility may negatively affect gross motor skill acquisition in young children. One transferable message in the Delphi study[15] clearly indicated that this concern is unfounded and that evidence does not support the myth that using power mobility at a young age hinders or blocks development of ambulation or other motor skills. The concept that power mobility use does not obstruct the development of ambulation is supported by multiple studies.[29,35,52]

Early Power Mobility Devices

Power mobility devices (Figure 11-1) used to provide early mobility experiences include modified battery-operated toy cars,[48,53,54] modified scooter boards and standers,[28] pediatric power wheelchairs,[29] and alternative power mobility devices involving custom-built mobile platforms[49-51] or robotic mobility devices.[55] The specific power mobility device used to provide early mobility experiences often depends on the availability of a specific device. However, factors such as positioning and postural support, as well as the goals for power mobility use, also must

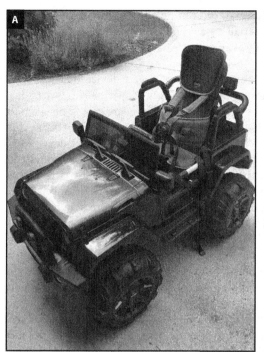
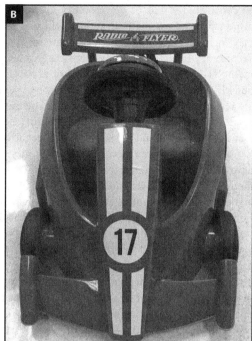
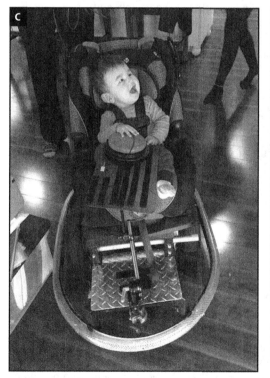
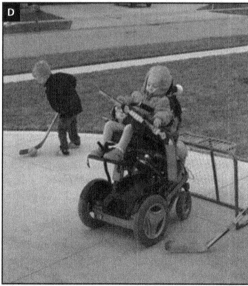

Figure 11-1. Select power mobility devices that can be used to provide early mobility experiences. (A) and (B) Modified battery-operated toy cars. (C) An alternative power mobility device involving a custom-built mobile platform. (D) A pediatric power wheelchair.

be considered.[28] For power mobility use to be optimal, or even possible, therapists must determine which access method a child will use to operate a power mobility device. Access options may include a type of joystick or some form of a switch. Tools such as the Wisconsin Assistive Technology Initiative[56] Assessment Package may be helpful in making decisions regarding access methods. When learning how to use a power mobility device, having a device that responds quickly when the child activates the access method is important. This allows the child to associate activation of the access method with the movement of the device.[28,57] Care should be taken to ensure that movement of the power mobility device is not too forceful or excessively jerky as this may startle a child and possibly create a negative perception of the movement and the device.[28,57]

Although children as young as age 18 months, who have the physical ability to use a joystick, have demonstrated competent joystick use,[15,29] many studies use a switch or switches as the access method for early power mobility.[48,49,51,54] Two main types of switches are available: mechanical and electrical. Mechanical switches (such as plate switches) require physical depression for activation and a release of depression to stop.[57] The amount of force needed to activate a mechanical switch varies depending on the specific switch. The auditory or tactile feedback associated with activating mechanical switches may be helpful for those beginning to learn to use a power mobility device.[57,58] Electrical switches (such a proximity switch) require a power source but do not rely on physical depression or release of force.[57] Mechanical and electrical switches come in many sizes, can be put in a variety of locations (eg, on a tray, head rest, foot plate), and should be positioned to allow children to activate the switch using whatever body part is most effective and efficient (eg, hand, finger, knee, foot, head).[57] Starting with a single, large switch that provides one direction of movement may allow young children the opportunity to experience initial success. As children progress and use more purposeful movement to activate the switch, additional switches can be added. Smaller switches can replace larger switches or the access method can be changed to a joystick. Sample mechanical and electrical switches are provided in Table 11-1. Additional details related to access methods are provided in Chapter 14 related to the selection and use of assistive technology devices.

Early Power Mobility Training Methods

Simply providing a power mobility device as a means to move often is not enough to allow most young children with mobility limitations the ability to independently move and explore. Article 20 of the 2006 United Nations Convention on the Rights of Persons with Disabilities[22] stated not only that nations must provide mobility devices to people who need them, but that nations also must provide training in the use of these devices as a way to ensure independence for persons with disabilities. The 2008 World Health Organization Guidelines on the Provision of Wheelchairs in Less-Resourced Settings[59] further emphasized the need for training in the safe and appropriate use of wheeled mobility devices. Despite these directives to ensure adequate training related to the use of mobility devices (including power mobility), few studies have explored the effectiveness of power mobility training methods for children of any age, and no study has compared specific power mobility training methods for use with children.[60,61] Very little evidence is available to support the dosage (ie, frequency and duration) of power mobility training interventions.[61]

A systematic review of power mobility training methods used in peer-reviewed, published research studies identified 26 publications encompassing 27 studies involving children age 21 years or younger.[61] The ages of the 216 children included in these 27 studies ranged from 5 months to 21 years. Twenty-one of the 27 studies involved children with mobility limitations who had diagnoses such as cerebral palsy, spinal muscular atrophy, arthrogryposis multiplex congenita, and Down syndrome. Although most of the included studies were case reports, case series, or mixed methods case studies providing Level IV[62] evidence, 2 single-subject research designs were identified as Level V,[63] 1 study provided Level III[62] evidence, and 5 studies were randomized controlled trials (Level II[62] evidence). The duration of training varied from one single day of training to a

TABLE 11-1. SAMPLE MECHANICAL AND ELECTRICAL SWITCHES

SWITCH	SWITCH TYPE	DESCRIPTION
AbleNet Candy Corn Proximity Switch	Electrical	Movement of a hand or other body part near the switch activates the switch. Does not require physical touch to activate. Auditory beep and visual feedback can be turned on and off. Size: 2 sizes, small (1.9-inch/5-cm wide activation area) and large (3.5-inch-/ 9-cm-wide activation area).
Adaptive Tech Solutions, LLC Honeybee Proximity Switch	Electrical	Movement of a hand or other body part near the switch activates the switch. Does not require physical touch to activate. Auditory feedback accompanies switch activation. Size: 3 × 1.5 × 0.5 inches (8 × 4 × 1.5 cm). Activation area of the switch adjusts to 1 of 4 distances: 6 inches/ 14 cm, 3 inches/7 cm, 1 inch/3 cm, or touch.
AbleNet Jelly Bean Twist	Mechanical	Requires 2.5 ounces/71 g of force to activate. Provides an auditory click and tactile feedback. Size: 2.5-inch/6.4-cm activation area.
AbleNet Possum Chin Switch	Mechanical	Positioned around neck with plastic tubing (like a necklace). Activated by movement of the head onto the switch. Requires 1.6 to 3.8 ounces/46 to 107 g of force to activate switch. Provides auditory click and tactile feedback. Size: 0.8 × 2.8 inches/2 × 7 cm.

Adapted from Kenyon LK, Hostnik L, PT, McElroy R, Peterson C, Farris JP. Power mobility training methods for children: a systematic review. *Pediatr Phys Ther*. 2018;30(1):2-8.

TABLE 11-2. POWER MOBILITY TRAINING APPROACHES	
APPROACH	**DEFINITION OF THE APPROACH**
Incorporating play	Using play to intentionally engage a child during power mobility use. Includes providing opportunities to use the power mobility device to enable and support a child's ability to play.
Natural environments	Providing opportunities for a child to functionally use a power mobility device in familiar locations where the child would typically be spending time during the day (eg, home, school, day care).
Goal-directed mobility	Using intentional placement of a toy, object, or person to entice the child to use the power mobility device in a meaningful and purposeful manner.
Self-exploration	Intentionally allowing a child to use the power mobility device to learn about the environment.
Adapted from Kenyon LK, Hostnik L, PT, McElroy R, Peterson C, Farris JP. Power mobility training methods for children: a systematic review. *Pediatr Phys Ther.* 2018;30(1):2-8.	

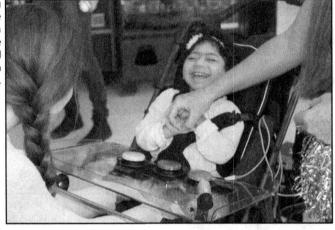

Figure 11-2. Power mobility training approaches incorporating play can be helpful for young children. The child in the photograph is participating in a tickle game with her sibling. Her hands are held during the tickle to prevent her from accidently activating one of the switches.

12-month period. Frequency of training ranged from daily opportunities for power mobility training to training one time per week. Individual training sessions ranged from 10 to 60 minutes. All included studies explicitly or implicitly stated the need for age-appropriate supervision during power mobility training and use, and even suggested increased supervision for some children. None of the included studies reported any adverse events. The specific power mobility training methods used in each study varied; however, approaches involving goal-directed mobility, incorporating play, natural environments, and self-exploration may be most pertinent when providing early power mobility experiences and are outlined in Table 11-2.

Given that TD infants and toddlers are not taught to move, self-exploration, incorporating play (Figure 11-2), and goal-directed mobility carried out within natural environments may allow power mobility training to more closely mimic the emergence of mobility in TD children.[61] Supplemental information related to power mobility training methods for young children is provided in Video 11-2.

Several studies suggest that power mobility training methods should be process based rather than skills based and must be individualized to meet the needs of a specific child.[64-66] Durkin[64] further suggested that rather than teaching a child specific power mobility skills, therapists should act as "responsive partners" who engage the child in individualized, motivating play activities to promote the emergence of power mobility use. Nilsson and Durkin[65] provided specific learning strategies to facilitate power mobility skill acquisition based on where a child is positioned along a continuum of learning. A qualitative study exploring the experiences related to learning to use a power mobility device found that "there isn't a cookbook."[67] This suggests that a generalizable recipe to teach a child how to use a power mobility device does not exist, but rather the recipe includes strategies that work for each individual child.[67] Additional research is needed to more fully explore power mobility training methods and to determine when the use of process-based or skills-based training methods might be beneficial for a specific child or during different phases of learning.

Assessing Outcomes of Early Power Mobility Use

The Evidence Alert Traffic Light Grading System (EATLS)[68] provides a global appraisal of the available evidence using the colors of traffic lights to denote the overall level of evidence related to a particular intervention. Within the EATLS,[68] Green—Go indicates high-level, quality evidence to support the intervention; Yellow—Caution Needed—Measure signifies limited or low-level evidence; and Red—Stop means high-level, quality evidence exists that the intervention is ineffective or harmful and should not be used. Owing to the dearth of high-level research dedicated to power mobility training methods for children, the lack of studies comparing specific training methods, and the limited evidence related to dosing of training, the aforementioned systematic review found the EATLS[68] rating for use of power mobility training methods in children age 21 years or younger was Yellow—Caution Needed—Measure.[61] Given this Yellow EATLS[68] rating, therapists are strongly encouraged to determine and measure outcomes of early power mobility use. Tests and measures used to evaluate outcomes should align with the specific desired outcomes. For example, if early power mobility outcomes are related to enhancing overall development, the Battelle Developmental Inventory,[45] used by Jones et al,[29] or the Bayley Scales of Infant and Toddler Development, Third Edition,[69] used by Lynch and colleagues,[30] may be appropriate. If the outcomes relate to improving functional skills, the Pediatric Evaluation of Disability Inventory—Computer Adaptive Test[70] could be used to document children's progress. Outcomes related to attaining power mobility skills are best measured using different tools that reflect the specific stage of a child's power mobility use.[71] A systematic review by Field and Livingstone[71] identified and explored measures of power mobility skills in children. Of the identified measures, the Wheelchair Skills Checklist,[47] the Power Mobility Training Tool,[72] and the Assessment of Learning Powered mobility use[65] were recognized as appropriate for use with children who are at the beginning stages of learning to use a powered mobility device.[71] As children's power mobility skills progress and desired outcomes evolve to include integration of power mobility devices into daily routines, the Assessment of Learning Powered[65] and the Powered Mobility Program[73] may be more helpful in assessing outcomes. Field and Livingstone[71] further noted that all of these measures are in the initial stages of development and that additional research is needed regarding the validity, reliability, and use of these measures. Sullivan[74] also reminded therapists that evidence-based practice involves the integration of research with family values and suggested that a family's desired outcomes may differ from the outcomes that have been explored in research studies (see Chapter 4).

Expectations for Children Learning to Use Power Mobility

When you were a teenager and drove a car for the very first time, it is highly unlikely that you drove the car perfectly. You likely drove under the supervision of an experienced, licensed driver for many hours before you took and passed your driver's test. Even after you earned a driver's license, the state in which you lived may have restricted when and with whom you could drive as you further developed your driving skills. Just as it takes time to learn how to drive a car, TD infants and toddlers do not just suddenly start crawling or walking with precision—such skills are obtained through a developmental process involving intensive practice as well as frequent failures and falls.[13,28] Although learning to drive a power mobility device is not the same as learning to drive a car or learning to walk, remember that learning complex skills is a process that develops over time. This may help families understand that learning to use a power mobility device is a complex skill that occurs in a developmental process.

Developmental Process

Many studies support learning to use a power mobility device as a developmental process.[64,67,71,75] Durkin[64] identified 3 developmental stages in learning to use a power mobility device: (1) learning the idea of movement, (2) learning how to operate the device, and (3) learning how to use the device in everyday life. Nilsson et al[75] described 8 phases in the developmental process of conscious use of a joystick. Another study suggested that learning to use a power mobility device is an individualized, cyclical process that often unfolds over time.[67] In their systematic review, Field and Livingstone[71] defined 3 groups of power mobility learners: exploratory, operational, and functional. Most young children begin as exploratory learners and need assistance and close adult supervision. Supplemental information related to introducing power mobility to young children is provided in the Video 11-2. Operational learners are focused on learning basic power mobility skills, whereas functional learners concentrate on using a power mobility device for a variety of activities within multiple environments.[71] Functional learners often meet criteria for purchase of an individually prescribed power wheelchair.[71] Some children may quickly progress from one group to another, whereas other children may remain at exploratory or operational levels and may not be considered for purchase of an individually prescribed power wheelchair.[71] Therapists can gauge their expectations for power mobility use based on where a child falls within the continuum of these 3 learner groups. Identifying a child's learner group also may provide insights into the power mobility device and training methods used. For example, an exploratory learner may benefit from ongoing training in familiar, predictable environments using modified battery-operated toy cars or shared/loaned power mobility devices. An exploratory learner may benefit further from engaging in activities that promote self-generated mobility.[15,71] An operational learner may benefit from continuing training, but be ready to drive in less restrictive environments and participate in specific activities to advance understanding of the power mobility device.[71]

Dosing to Achieve Competence

If the desired outcomes of early power mobility use relate to becoming what Butler et al[76] referred to as a "competent driver," how long does it take for a young child to learn how to proficiently use a power mobility device? Butler et al[47,76] conducted the seminal studies in this area more than 3 decades ago. In the first study,[76] 9 children age 20 to 39 months who had mobility and other physical limitations, but age-appropriate cognition, were provided power wheelchairs for use in their homes. Competence was defined as being able to consistently perform 7 skills using the power wheelchair: starting and stopping, moving straight forward in open areas, moving straight forward in narrow hallways, turning around in a circle, turning corners, backing up, and driving near people and furniture without hitting things.[76] Seven of these 9 children became competent drivers in less than 3 weeks and an eighth child, who was age 24 months, achieved competence in the seventh week.[76] The ninth child reportedly experienced repeated illness and hospitalizations during the 4-month period in which she had access to the power wheelchair.[76] These factors may have limited her opportunities to practice and use the power wheelchair. She was the only 1 of the 9 children who did not achieve competence.[76] The second study[47] involved 13 children age 20 to 37 months with mobility and other physical limitations and age-appropriate cognitive skills. Competence was defined as the ability to perform the 7 wheelchair skills comprising the

Wheelchair Skills Checklist.[47] Twelve of the 13 children achieved competency within an average of 16.3 days of driving (range, 3 to 50 days) and a mean cumulative practice time of 34.4 hours (range, 6.6 to 168 hours).[47] All the children in these 2 early studies were physically able to use a joystick.[47,76] More recent work by Huhn and colleagues[77] and Mockler et al[78] suggests children who are unable to use a joystick and require alternate access methods may require longer periods of time to learn to drive a power wheelchair.

Special Considerations for Young Children With Visual or Intellectual Impairments

Visual Impairments

Some therapists and parents may be concerned about providing power mobility experiences to young children who have visual impairments and question whether it is safe for these children to use power mobility devices. RESNA[28] advocates that limited vision in and of itself should not be a factor when considering power mobility for children. Although each case is unique and adequate supervision must be provided to ensure safety, children with visual impairments may benefit from the self-generated mobility provided through power mobility use.[49-51,79]

Cerebral visual impairment (CVI, also known as *cortical visual impairment*) is the most common cause of visual impairment in children living in industrialized nations.[80] CVI does not involve problems with the structures of the eyes, but rather is a result of damaged or malformed visual pathways or visual processing centers in the brain. In fact, children who have CVI often may present with a normal eye exam and yet functionally may not be able to process and use visual information.[80,81] Because of these difficulties with processing visual information, children with CVI may have a mild to moderate vision impairment, and in rare instances, may even have profound blindness.[80,81] Children who have periventricular leukomalacia or hypoxic ischemic encephalopathy are especially at risk for CVI.[81]

When working with the young child with CVI, subtle modifications in the environment may positively affect a child's ability to use a power mobility device.[79] An uncluttered, visually simplified environment may help the child who has CVI to focus attention on a particular visual stimulus (such as the switch or joystick being used to operate the power mobility device).[79,82,83] Intentional use of color (such as a brightly colored switch), use of high-contrast materials (such as placing the colored switch on a tray that has a plain black background), and allowing additional time to process visual information may help the child to better "see" the access method for the power mobility device.[79,82,83] Some children with CVI like shiny objects. In these cases, the switch can be covered with aluminum foil or foil wrapping paper.[79,82] Graded use of tactile or auditory stimulation to draw the child's attention to particular objects or environmental factors also may be helpful. For example, simply covering the switch with a brightly colored, textured fabric may draw the child's attention to the switch.[79,82,83] This can be accomplished easily by gluing fabric to a piece of cardboard and using Velcro to attach the cardboard to the switch. When the environment necessitates the child turn the power mobility device, placing an audio device playing the child's favorite song or talking to the child when on the left or right side may help the child orient to the direction of the turn. When working with the child, it is helpful for the therapist to wear nonpatterned or even solid black clothing as a way to further decrease the visual complexity of the environment.[79] A consistent and predictable environment may be particularly helpful especially in the early stages of learning to use a power mobility device.[79,82,83] Specific resources related to orientation and mobility for people who use wheelchairs may provide additional insights and suggestions.[84]

Intellectual Impairments

Therapists and parents may have concerns about providing power mobility experiences to young children who have intellectual impairments. Each case is unique, and adequate supervision

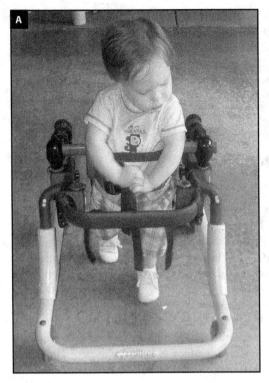

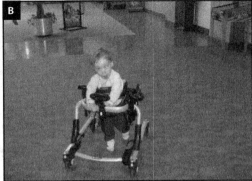

Figure 11-3. A gait trainer can provide early mobility experiences for the young child and may be used indoors or outdoors in (A) home or (B) community settings.

must be provided to ensure children's safety; however, children who have mobility limitations as well as intellectual impairments may benefit from power mobility use.[15,71] RESNA[28] asserts that intellectual limitations should not be a factor when considering power mobility for children. Children with intellectual impairments often fall into the group of exploratory learners outlined by Field and Livingstone[71] and may gain skills such as cause and effect, improved alertness, and basic power mobility skills through ongoing power mobility training.[49-51,58,75] Supplemental information related to power mobility training for children with intellectual impairments is provided in Video 11-3, which accompanies this chapter. Occasionally, children who have severe physical limitations may be unable to express their intellectual abilities. When provided with the opportunity to practice using a power mobility device, these children may quickly progress into the operational or functional groups of learners.[71]

When children have mobility limitations and a visual or intellectual impairment (or both), longer periods of time may be required to learn power mobility skills.[29,35,58,75] Studies by Nilsson et al[58,75] involved providing power mobility training for such children over extended periods of time (several years); however, other studies have found improved, although not competent, power mobility use following training periods of 8 to 15 weeks.[49-51]

USING GAIT TRAINERS TO PROVIDE EARLY MOBILITY EXPERIENCES

Gait trainers (Figure 11-3) can provide early mobility experiences for the young child.[85] Gait trainers, also known as support walkers,[86] are mobility devices that support a child's weight through a solid or fabric "seat" and may provide additional external support to stabilize the trunk and pelvis.[85] Gait trainers primarily incorporate either a U-shaped frame or a straddle frame.[85]

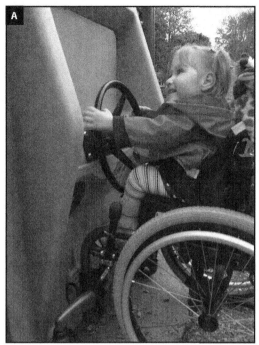
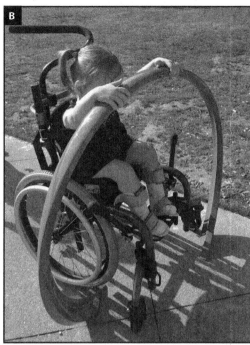

Figure 11-4. A manual wheelchair can offer mobility experiences and opportunities for (A) play and (B) exploration.

A U-shaped frame typically is open either in front or behind the child, making transfers in and out of the device easier, and allowing greater freedom of leg movements.[85] A straddle frame has a solid seat, and part of the frame goes between the legs at ankle level.[85] This design may be especially helpful for children who have a strong "scissor-gait" (ie, excessive adduction) that results in the feet frequently crossing and often getting stuck together.[85] Although many gait trainers can be used either anteriorly or posteriorly, evidence does not support one over the other.[85] The drive style and wheel size of a gait trainer can significantly influence the amount of force required to initiate movement of the gait trainer on different surfaces and should be considered when choosing a gait trainer.[85] Paleg and Livingstone,[87] in a systematic review of the outcomes of gait trainer use in children age 18 years or younger, found Level II[44] evidence related to an increased number of steps and a trend toward increased walking distance when using gait trainers. Two Level III[44] studies included in the review reported a significant impact on mobility, with one of these studies reporting a significant impact on bowel function and a positive association between the amount of time spent in a gait trainer and bone mineral density. The remaining 13 studies included in the review provided Level IV and V[44] evidence supporting the positive impact of gait trainer use on areas such as affect, motivation, and participation. The ages of children who participated in the studies ranged from 2 to 18 years with age 10 years being most prevalent.[87]

USING SELF-PROPELLED WHEELED MOBILITY TO PROVIDE EARLY MOBILITY EXPERIENCES

For children who have sufficient upper extremity function, early mobility experiences may be provided through various self-propelled wheeled mobility devices. Manual wheelchairs (Figure 11-4) and mobile standers (Figure 11-5) can offer mobility experiences for children who have the ability to adequately self-propel. Children can use scooter boards either in prone or sitting as a way to move and explore their environment. Modifications may be needed to these scooter boards to

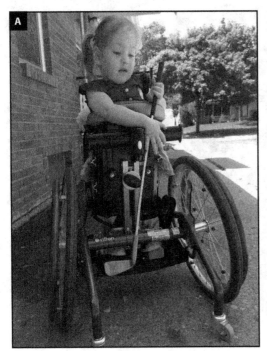
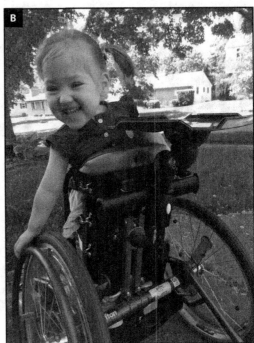

Figure 11-5. A mobile stander can offer mobility experiences and opportunities for (A) play and (B) exploration.

provide additional support (such as a seat back) and increased safety (seat belts or lap straps). Small adapted tricycles or hand cycles can provide young children an age-appropriate means of mobility and exploration. Specialized adapted trikes such as the DCP Mini by Freedom Concepts may allow children as young as age 18 months the opportunity to ride and explore. Optional components may allow caregivers to assist with steering or braking. Various types of caster carts are another option. Designed primarily for use indoors on smooth surfaces or outdoors on concrete or other similar even surfaces, caster carts are particularly helpful for young children with spina bifida who have thoracic or upper lumbar lesions.[88] The Star Car, a common type of caster cart, is no longer available commercially but can be built using instructions available online.[89] In a similar manner, a Bumbo seat can be modified into a "manual wheelchair" using instructions provided online.[90] Therapists must address the safety and appropriateness of any device but should be especially careful with devices that are not commercially made.

CREATING AN EARLY MOBILITY PLAN

Therapists may feel overwhelmed by the many options for providing early mobility experiences and wonder which option might be "best" for a specific child. Although therapists should consider providing energy efficient functional mobility, a child who has mobility limitations ideally should have different mobility options, depending on the goal and demands of the environment. As adults, we use different forms of mobility every day for different purposes: we walk the dog, we drive or take a bus to work, we take a bike ride, or we run on the treadmill for exercise. The child should have similar mobility options and not be limited to a single form of mobility (Figure 11-6). For example, perhaps a child uses a power mobility device to freely explore and keep up with his or her peers. Maybe this child also uses a gait trainer to run around on the driveway with his or her siblings and an adapted tricycle that includes a push handle to "walk" down the street with the family to get ice cream. When out in the community, where he or she might not

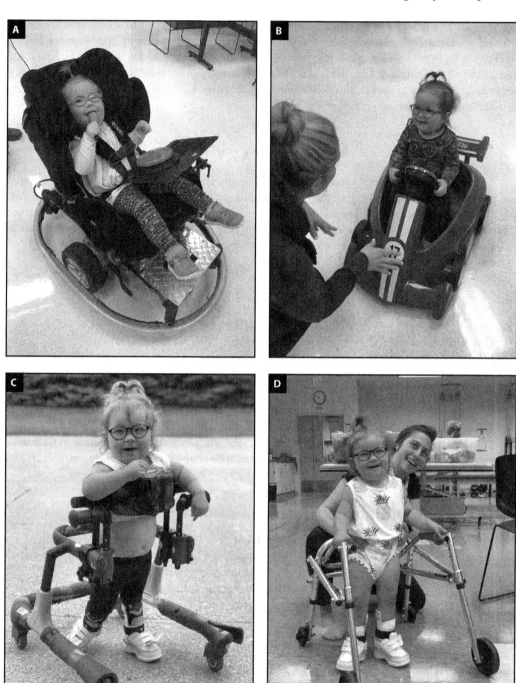

Figure 11-6. An early mobility plan can provide a young child mobility options that vary based on the goal and demands of the environment. (A) When this child was still learning to sit, she used an alternative power mobility device involving a custom-built mobile platform as a way to introduce her to power mobility. (B) As she started to sit independently, a modified battery-operated toy car was provided. (C) At the same time, she continued to focus on her assisted ambulation skills with a gait trainer. (D) Later, she progressed to using a walker.

yet be ready to use a power mobility device, maybe he or she is pushed in an adapted stroller or manual wheelchair. Think about how you feel after a hard exercise workout. Now imagine having to keep up this level of physical activity as you move throughout your day. Imagine having to do cartwheels all day long to get from one place to another. You would be exhausted. Mobility practice sessions and exercise opportunities should never be confused with functional mobility.[28] Mobility is functional only when it is efficient.

SUMMARY

This chapter has presented an overview of the many types of early mobility experiences that can be provided for young children who have mobility limitations. Create a mobility plan consisting of a variety of options to provide young children opportunities to move, explore, and learn through early mobility experiences. Children in the case studies will be addressed at age 6 to 18 months to illustrate the application of early mobility principles.

CASE STUDY #1: JASON

- ▸ *Medical Diagnosis:* Cerebral palsy, right hemiparesis
- ▸ *Gross Motor Function Classification System:* Level I
- ▸ *Age:* 15 months

Participation Restrictions

Jason is starting to belly crawl and has limited floor mobility. He has difficulties accessing toys and physically exploring all aspects of his environment. His limited mobility results in decreased opportunities for social interaction with other children or adults. Limited mobility also decreases opportunities for sensory exploration and perceptual learning experiences during play.

Activity/Functional Limitations

Jason is able to sit independently when placed, but does not make transitions of movement. He belly crawls 3 feet (1 m) and attempts to get on his hands and knees. He has difficulty with crawling and maintaining a quadruped position, as he is unable to support his weight well on his right arm. He supports his weight in standing when assisted and leans against furniture.

Impairments

Jason presents with general neglect of the right side of his body and space. He has decreased use and coordination of his right upper and lower extremities. Weakness in the right upper extremity is noted.

Early Mobility Intervention

Jason would benefit from use of a modified battery-operated toy car to help him to keep up during play activities with his brother out in the yard (Figure 11-7). Given his postural asymmetries, Jason may require use of a postural insert to promote symmetrical postural control in sitting. Turning to the right during play activities may help to improve his awareness of the right visuospatial field.[91] Modifying the toy car to require depression of a switch with his right hand while he steers the toy car with his left hand may encourage him to use his right hand. As he ages,

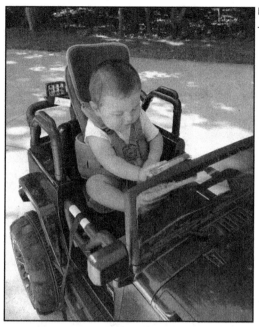

Figure 11-7. A modified battery-operated toy car will help Jason to keep up with his brother out in the yard.

he may benefit from use of an adaptive tricycle to increase his participation in family activities. Given his inefficient crawling pattern and delay in walking, he may benefit from use of a power mobility device as an infant.

Participation/Functional Goals

After 3 months of intervention, Jason will be able to accomplish the following:
1. Turn/steer to the right when using a power mobility device.
2. Use his right upper extremity to activate a switch.
3. Play with his twin while using a battery-operated car out in the yard.

CASE STUDY #2: JILL

> *Medical Diagnosis:* Cerebral palsy, spastic quadriparesis, microcephaly, intellectual deficits, seizure disorder
> *Gross Motor Function Classification System:* Level V
> *Age:* 18 months

Participation Restrictions

Jill has limited mobility in all positions and is unable to use her upper extremities to access toys. Her significant physical limitations reduce her ability to use vision and other sensory systems for learning experiences. All social interactions must be initiated by adults, which limits her opportunities for developing social skills and independence.

Figure 11-8. Power mobility training using an alternative power mobility device involving a custom-built mobile platform will provide Jill with early mobility experiences.

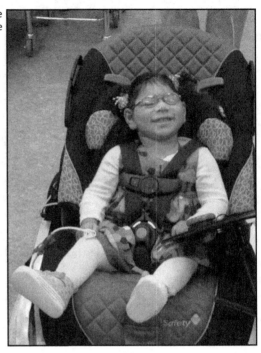

Activity/Functional Limitations

Jill is dependent for all mobility activities, transfers, and activities of daily living. She is unable to maintain a sitting position without external support. She does not have good head control in any position. Her manual skills are limited. Her parents and therapists are uncertain if Jill understands the concept of cause and effect.

Impairments

Jill has increased stiffness and limited active and passive movement in all 4 extremities. Her motor control is very limited. She appears lethargic and is hypersensitive to vestibular stimulation. She has a seizure disorder, and antiseizure medication may relate to her difficulties with maintaining alertness. Jill has microcephaly and associated intellectual impairments.

Early Mobility Intervention

Jill would benefit from power mobility training using either a shared/loaner power wheelchair or an alternative power mobility device involving a custom-built mobile platform (Figure 11-8).[49-51] The Power Mobility Training Tool,[72] developed to guide therapists in creating power mobility training programs for children who have multiple severe disabilities, may be helpful in identifying basic power mobility skills to target in her power mobility training program. Starting with a single, large switch positioned to allow Jill to activate the switch using whichever body part is most effective and efficient (eg, hand, finger, knee, foot, head) may help her to experience success. Given that Jill is hypersensitive to vestibular input, starting at a low speed with only forward movement may be helpful. Jill would also likely benefit from use of a gait trainer. As she grows, Jill may benefit from use of an adaptive tricycle that allows her to partake in physical activity.[92]

Participation/Functional Goals

After 3 to 6 months of intervention, Jill will be able to accomplish the following:

1. Increase her activation of a switch during use of a power mobility device by 50% over baseline levels.

2. Move forward 5 feet (1.5 m) to obtain a desired object while using a power mobility device.

3. Use more than one switch to drive a power mobility device.

4. Demonstrate understanding of cause and effect.

CASE STUDY #3: TAYLOR

> *Medical Diagnosis:* Myelomeningocele, repaired L1-2
> *Age:* 9 months

Participation Restrictions

Taylor's preferred method of mobility is rolling, but he occasionally attempts to belly crawl. Both methods of mobility are fatiguing, so he tends to remain stationary. Limitations in physical mobility result in decreased opportunities for accessing objects in his environment for play and cognitive learning. He is unable to keep up with peers and has few social interactions.

Activity/Functional Limitations

Taylor is able to roll repeatedly. He is unable to sit independently without assistance. Taylor is able to belly crawl 6 inches (15.24 cm) forward by pulling with his upper extremities, but he is unable to crawl on hands and knees or walk.

Impairments

Taylor has poor sensation in his lower body, and active motion is limited in his lower extremities. He has generalized trunk and extremity weakness. Taylor has visual-perceptual problems.

Early Mobility Intervention

Taylor would benefit from using a caster cart[89] or a Bumbo wheelchair[90] (Figure 11-9) to provide early mobility experiences. Additionally, using a power mobility device (such as a modified battery-operated toy car with a postural insert) may provide him the opportunity to explore and learn from his environment. As he ages, Taylor may benefit from using a power wheelchair to allow him to keep up with his peers and to more fully participate in age-appropriate activities. A hand-crank–adapted tricycle may provide an age-appropriate, fun mobility option that allows him to partake in physical activity and increase his upper extremity strength as he grows.

Participation/Functional Goals

After 3 months of intervention, Taylor will be able to accomplish the following:

1. Keep up with his friends during play activities indoors and outdoors using a power wheelchair or battery-operated riding toy.

2. Initiate exploration of his environment a minimum of 3 times in 15 minutes while seated in a Bumbo wheelchair.

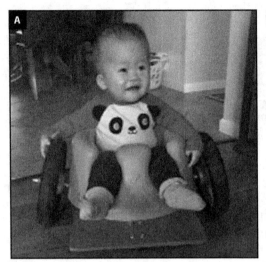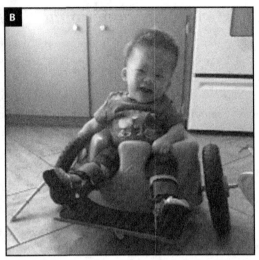

Figure 11-9. A Bumbo wheelchair, created using instructions found online, can be used to provide Taylor with early mobility experiences.

CASE STUDY #4: ASHLEY

> *Medical Diagnosis:* Down syndrome
> *Age:* 15 months

Participation Restrictions

Ashley has limited mobility skills and does not interact often with peers, decreasing social contacts. She avoids many age-appropriate play activities, which limits opportunities for spatial and cognitive learning.

Activity/Functional Limitations

Ashley is able to pull to stand and take steps with 2 hands held when provided maximal assistance. She observes other children but does not play with them. She has difficulties with fine motor control.

Impairments

Ashley presents with generalized hypotonia and hypermobility in her upper and lower extremities. She demonstrates hypersensitivity to sensory input and is fearful of movement-based activities. Intellectual skills are delayed (ie, 10- to 12-month level).

Early Mobility Intervention

Ashley would benefit from mobility experiences using a power mobility device. A modified battery-operated toy car with a postural insert (Figure 11-10), such as the one used by Logan et al,[48] may help promote her social skills and provide her with a means for functional mobility. Despite her fine motor difficulties, Ashley should be able to use a single, large switch to operate the power mobility device. Depending on how the toy car is modified and configured, the single switch may be able to either move the device forward or to spin the device. As she progresses in her use of a

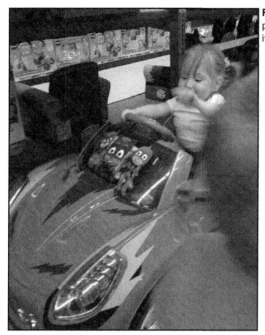

Figure 11-10. A modified battery-operated toy car with a postural insert will allow Ashley to benefit from early mobility experiences.

switch, adding additional switches or advancement to use of a joystick may be appropriate. Given Ashley's apprehension about movement activities, ensuring that the power mobility device moves smoothly without any excessive jerkiness and at a very slow speed is important.

Participation/Functional Goals

After 3 months of intervention, Ashley will be able to accomplish the following:

1. Increase the frequency of her social interactions with other children her age by 50% over baseline levels during free play.
2. Use a power mobility device at home and in her early intervention program to explore both environments.

Case Study #5: John

> *Medical Diagnosis:* Developmental coordination disorder/attention-deficit hyperactivity disorder
> *Age:* 12 months

John is walking independently and has achieved age-appropriate gross motor skills. At this time, is does not appear that John has impairments or functional limitations that require power mobility or mobility experiences with a gait trainer or wheeled mobility device.

REFERENCES

1. Anderson DI, Campos JJ, Witherington DC, et al. The role of locomotion in psychological development. *Front Psychol.* 2013;4(7):1-17. doi:10.3389/fpsyg.2013.00440.

2. Campos JJ, Anderson DI, Barbu-Roth M, Hubbard EM, Hertenstein MJ, Witherington DC. Travel broadens the mind. *Infancy.* 2000;1(2):149-219. doi:10.1207/S15327078IN0102_1.

3. Gibson EJ. Exploratory behavior in the development of perceiving, acting, and the acquiring of knowledge. *Ann Rev Psychol.* 1988:39(2):1-41. doi:10.1146/annurev.ps.39.020188.000245.

4. Foreman N, Foreman D, Cummings A, Owens S. Locomotion, active choice, and spatial memory in children. *J Gen Psychol.* 1990;117(2):215-233. doi:10.1080/00221309.1990.9921139.

5. Piaget J. *The Origins of Intelligence in Children.* New York, NY: International Universities Press; 1952.

6. Pallas SL. Pre- and postnatal sensory experience shapes functional architecture in the brain. In: Hopkins B, Johnson SP, eds. *Prenatal Development of Postnatal Functions.* Westport, CT: Praeger Publishers Incorporated; 2005:1-30.

7. Bremner JG, Bryant PE. Place versus response as the basis of spatial errors made by young infants. *J Exp Child Psychol.* 1977;23(1):162-171. doi:10.1016/0022-0965(77)90082-0.

8. Proulx MJ, Todorov OS, Taylor Aiken A, de Sousa AA. Where am I? Who am I? The relation between spatial cognition, social cognition and individual differences in the built environment. *Front Psychol.* 2016;7(2):64. doi:10.3389/fpsyg.2016.00064.

9. Yan JH, Thomas JR, Downing JH. Locomotion improves children's spatial search: a meta-analytic review. *Percept Mot Skills.* 1998;87(1):67-82. doi:10.2466/pms.1998.87.1.67.

10. Frith CD. Social cognition. *Philos Trans R Soc London B Biol Sci.* 2008;363(1499)2033-2039. doi:10.1098/rstb.2008.0005.

11. Bell MA, Fox NA. Crawling experience is related to changes in cortical organization during infancy: evidence from EEG coherence. *Dev Psychobiol.* 1996;29(7):551-561. doi:10.1002/(SICI)1098-2302(199611)29:7<551::AID-DEV1>3.0.CO;2-T.

12. Andersen RA. The neurobiological basis of spatial cognition: role of the parietal lobe. In Stiles-Davis J, Kritchevsky M, Bellugi U, eds. *Spatial Cognition: Brain Bases and Development.* Hillsdale, NJ: Lawrence Erlbaum Associates; 1988:57-80.

13. Adolph KE, Cole WG, Komati M, et al. How do you learn to walk? Thousands of steps and dozens of falls per day. *Psychol Sci.* 2012;23(11):1387-1394. doi:10.1177/0956797612446346.

14. Livingstone R, Field D. Systematic review of power mobility outcomes for infants, children and adolescents with mobility limitations. *Clin Rehabil.* 2014;28(10):954-964. doi:10.1177/0269215514531262.

15. Livingstone R, Paleg G. Practice considerations for the introduction and use of power mobility for children. *Dev Med Child Neurol.* 2014;56(3):210-221. doi:10.1111/dmcn.12245.

16. Kermoian R, Campos JJ. Locomotor experience: a facilitator of spatial cognitive development. *Child Dev.* 1988;59(4):908-917. doi:10.2307/1130258.

17. Butler C. Wheelchair toddlers. In: Furumasu J, ed. *Pediatric Powered Mobility: Developmental Perspectives, Technical Issues, Clinical Approaches.* Arlington, VA: Rehabilitation Engineering Society of North America Press; 1997:1-6.

18. Fernandes T. Independent mobility for children with disabilities. *Int J Ther Rehabil.* 2006;13(7):329-333. doi:10.12968/ijtr.2006.13.7.21410.

19. Ylvisaker M, Feeney T. Executive functions, self-regulation, and learned optimism in paediatric rehabilitation: a review and implications for intervention. *Pediatr Rehabil.* 2002;5(2):51-70. doi:10.1080/1363849021000041891.

20. Maier SF, Peterson C, Schwartz B. From helplessness to hope: the seminal career of Martin Seligman. In: Gillham JE, ed. *The Science of Optimism and Hope.* West Conshohocken, PA: Templeton Press; 2000:11-37.

21. United Nations. Standard Rules on the Equalization of Opportunities for Persons with Disabilities. https://www.un.org/development/desa/disabilities/standard-rules-on-the-equalization-of-opportunities-for-persons-with-disabilities.html. Published 1993. Accessed June 23, 2018.

22. United Nations. United Nations convention on the rights of persons with disabilities. https://www.un.org/development/desa/disabilities/convention-on-the-rights-of-persons-with-disabilities.html. Published 2006. Accessed June 23, 2018.

23. *International Classification of Functioning, Disability and Health (ICF).* Geneva, Switzerland: World Health Organization. http://www.who.int/classifications/icf/en/. Published 2001. Accessed June 23, 2018.

24. Gibson JJ. The theory of affordance. In: Shaw RE, Bransford J, eds. *Perceiving, Acting, and Knowing: Toward an Ecological Psychology.* Hillsdale, NJ: Lawrence Erlbaum Associates; 1997:67-82.

25. Osiurak F, Rossetti Y, Badets A. What is an affordance? 40 years later. *Neurosci Biobehav Rev.* 2017;77(16):403-417. doi:10.1016/j.neubiorev.2017.04.014.

26. Guerette P, Tefft D, Furumasu J. Pediatric powered wheelchairs: results of a national survey of providers. *Assist Technol.* 2005;17(2):144-158. doi:10.1080/10400435.2005.10132104.

27. Kenyon LK, Jones M, Livingstone R, Breaux B, Tsotsoros J, Williams K. Power mobility for children: a survey study of American and Canadian therapists' perspectives and practices. *Dev Med Child Neurol.* 2018;60(10): 1018-1025. doi:10.1111/dmcn.13960.

28. Rosen L, Plummer T, Sabet A, Lange ML, Livingstone RL. RESNA position on the application of power mobility devices for pediatric users [published online ahead of print March 26, 2018]. *Assist Technol.* doi:10.1080/10400 435.2017.1415575.

29. Jones M, McEwen I, Neas B. Effects of power wheelchairs on the development and function of young children with severe motor impairments. *Pediatr Phys Ther.* 2012;24(2):131-140; discussion 140. doi:10.1097/ PEP.0b013e31824c5fdc.

30. Lynch A, Ryu JC, Agrawal S, Galloway J. Power mobility training for a 7-month-old infant with spina bifida. *Pediatr Phys Ther.* 2009;21(4):362-368. doi:10.1097/PEP.0b013e3181bfae4c.

31. Nisbet P. Assessment and training of children for powered mobility in the UK. *Technol Disabil.* 2002;14(4):173-182.

32. Douglas J, Ryan M. A preschool severely disabled boy and his powered wheelchair: a case study. *Child Care Health Dev.* 1987;13(5):303-309. doi:10.1111/j.1365-2214.1987.tb00547.x.

33. Jones M, McEwen I, Hansen L. Use of power mobility for a young child with spinal muscular atrophy. *Phys Ther.* 2003;83(3):253-262. doi:10.1093/ptj/83.3.253.

34. Nisbet P, Craig J, Odor P, Aitken S. 'Smart' wheelchairs for mobility training. *Technol Disabil.* 1996;5(1):49-62. doi:10.1016/1055-4181(96)00147-1.

35. Bottos M, Bolcati C, Sciuto L, Ruggeri C, Feliciangeli A. Powered wheelchairs and independence in young children with tetraplegia. *Dev Med Child Neurol.* 2001;43(11):769-777. doi:10.1111/j.1469-8749.2001.tb00159.x.

36. Deitz J, Swinth Y, White O. Powered mobility and preschoolers with complex developmental delays. *Am J Occup Ther.* 2002;56(1):86-96. doi:10.5014/ajot.56.1.86.

37. Guerette P, Furumasu J, Tefft D. The positive effects of early powered mobility on children's psychosocial and play skills. *Assist Technol.* 2013;25(1):39-48; quiz 49-50. doi:10.1080/10400435.2012.685824.

38. Tefft D, Guerette P, Furumasu J. The impact of early powered mobility on parental stress, negative emotions, and family social interactions. *Phys Occup Ther Pediatr.* 2011;31(1):4-15. doi:10.3109/01942638.2010.529005.

39. Wiart L, Darrah J, Cook A, Hollis V, May L. Evaluation of powered mobility use in home and community environments. *Phys Occup Ther Pediatr.* 2003;23(2):59-75. doi:10.1080/J006v23n02_05.

40. Ragonesi CB, Chen X, Agrawal S, Galloway JC. Power mobility and socialization in preschool: a case study of a child with cerebral palsy. *Pediatr Phys Ther.* 2010;22(3):322-329. doi:10.1097/PEP.0b013e3181eab240.

41. Ragonesi CB, Chen X, Agrawal S, Galloway JC. Power mobility and socialization in preschool: follow-up case study of a child with cerebral palsy. *Pediatr Phys Ther.* 2011;23(4):399-406. doi:10.1097/PEP.0b013e318235266a.

42. Butler C. Effects of powered mobility on self-initiated behaviors of very young children with locomotor disability. *Dev Med Child Neurol.* 1986;28(3):325-332. doi:10.1111/j.1469-8749.1986.tb03881.x.

43. Home A, Ham R. Provision of powered mobility equipment to young children: the Whizz-Kidz experience. *Int J Ther Rehabil.* 2003;10(11):511-517. doi:10.12968/bjtr.2003.10.11.13462.

44. American Academy for Cerebral Palsy and Developmental Medicine methodology to develop systematic reviews of treatment interventions (Revision 1.2). https://www.aacpdm.org/UserFiles/file/systematic-review-methodology.pdf. Published 2008. Accessed June 23, 2018.

45. Newborg J, Stock JR, Wnek L, Guidubaldi J, Svinicki J. *Battelle Developmental Inventory.* Chicago, IL: Riverside Publishing; 1984.

46. Haley SM, Coster WJ, Ludlow LH, Haltiwanger JT. *Pediatric Evaluation of Disability Inventory: Development, Standardization and Administration Manual.* Boston, MA: New England Medical Center Publications; 1992.

47. Butler C, Okamoto GA, McKay TM. Motorized wheelchair driving by disabled children. *Arch Phys Med Rehabil.* 1984;65(2):95-97.

48. Logan S, Huang H, K S, Galloway JC. Modified ride-on car for mobility and socialization: single-case study of an infant with Down syndrome. *Pediatr Phys Ther.* 2014;26(4):418-426. doi:10.1097/PEP.0000000000000070.

49. Kenyon LK, Farris JF, Brockway K, Hannum N, Proctor K. Promoting self-exploration and function through an individualized power mobility training program: a case report. *Pediatr Phys Ther.* 2015;27(2):200-206. doi:10.1097/PEP.0000000000000129.

50. Kenyon LK, Farris JP, Gallagher C, Hammond L, Webster LM, Aldrich NJ. Power mobility training for young children with multiple, severe impairments: a case series. *Phys Occup Ther Pediatr.* 2017;37(1):19-34. doi:10.310 9/01942638.2015.1108380.

51. Kenyon LK, Farris J, Aldrich N, Rhodes S. Does power mobility training impact a child's mastery motivation and spectrum of EEG activity? An exploratory project. *Disabil Rehabil: Assist Technol.* In Press. doi: 10.1080/17483107.2017.1369587

52. Paulsson K, Christofferson M. Psychosocial aspects on technical aids—how does independent mobility affect the psychosocial and intellectual development of children with physical disabilities? In: Rehabilitation Engineering Society of North America, ed. *Second International Conference on Rehabilitation Engineering, Ottawa, Canada.* Arlington, VA: Rehabilitation Engineering Society of North America Press; 1984:282-286.

53. Huang H, Galloway JC. Modified ride-on toy cars for early power mobility: a technical report. *Pediatr Phys Ther.* 2012;24(2):149-154. doi:10.1097/PEP.0b013e31824d73f9.

54. Logan SW, Feldner HA, Galloway JC, Huang HH. Modified ride-on car use by children with complex medical needs. *Pediatr Phys Ther.* 2016;28(1):100-107. doi:10.1097/PEP.0000000000000210.

55. Larin HM, Dennis CW, Stansfield S. Development of robotic mobility for infants: rationale and outcomes. *Physiother.* 2012;98(3):230-237. doi:10.1016/j.physio.2012.06.005.

56. Wisconsin Assistive Technology Initiative (WATI) Assessment Package. Madison, WI: Wisconsin Department of Public Instruction. https://dpi.wi.gov/sites/default/files/imce/sped/pdf/at-wati-assessment.pdf. Published 2004. Accessed June 23, 2018.

57. Lange M. Switch assessment: determining type and location. Canadian Seating & Mobility Conference Proceedings. http://www.csmc.ca/docs/archives/2006_archive/ws/w29.pdf. Published 2006. Accessed June 23, 2018.

58. Nilsson L, Eklund M. Driving to learn: powered wheelchair training for those with cognitive disabilities. *Inter J Ther Rehabil.* 2006;13(11):517-527. doi:10.12968/ijtr.2006.13.11.22466.

59. Armstrong W, Borg J, Krizack M, et al. Guidelines on the provision of manual wheelchairs in less resourced settings. Geneva, Switzerland: World Health Organization. 2008. Accessed June 23, 2018.

60. Livingstone R. A critical review of powered mobility assessment and training for children. *Disabil Rehabil Assist Technol.* 2010;5(6):392-400. doi:10.3109/17483107.2010.496097.

61. Kenyon LK, Hostnik L, PT, McElroy R, Peterson C, Farris JP. Power mobility training methods for children: a systematic review. *Pediatr Phys Ther.* 2018;30(1):2-8. doi:10.1097/PEP.0000000000000458.

62. Oxford Centre for Evidence-Based Medicine Levels of Evidence. http://www.cebm.net/wp-content/uploads/2014/06/CEBM-Levels-of-Evidence-2.1.pdf. Published 2011. Accessed June 23, 2018.

63. Romeiser Logan L, Hickman RR, Harris SR, Heriza CB. Single-subject research design: recommendations for levels of evidence and quality rating. *Dev Med Child Neurol.* 2008;50(2):99-103. doi:10.1111/j.1469-8749.2007.02005.x.

64. Durkin J. Discovering powered mobility skills with children: 'responsive partners' in learning. *Int J Ther Rehabil.* 2009;16(6):331-341. doi:10.12968/ijtr.2009.16.6.42436.

65. Nilsson L, Durkin J. Assessment of learning powered mobility use—applying grounded theory to occupational performance. *J Rehabil Res Dev.* 2014;51(6):963-974. doi:10.1682/JRRD.2013.11.0237.

66. Nilsson L, Durkin J. Powered mobility intervention: understanding the position of tool use learning as part of implementing the ALP tool. *Assist Technol.* 2017;129 (7):730-739. doi:10.1080/17483107.2016.1253119.

67. Kenyon LK, Mortenson WB, Miller WC. "Power in mobility": parent and therapist perspectives of the experiences of children learning to use powered mobility. *Dev Med Child Neurol.* 2018;60(10):1012-1017. doi:10.1111/dmcn.13906.

68. Novak I, McIntyre S. The effect of education with workplace supports on practitioners' evidence-based practice knowledge and implementation behaviours. *Aust Occup Ther J.* 2010;57(6):386-393. doi:10.1111/j.1440-1630.2010.00861.x.

69. Bayley N. *Bayley Scales of Infant and Toddler Development.* 3rd ed. San Antonio, TX: PsychCorp; 2006.

70. Haley SM, Coster WJ, Dumas HM, Fragala-Pinkham MA, Moed R. Pediatric Evaluation of Disability Inventory—Computer Adaptive Test Manual. https://s3.amazonaws.com/pedicat/PEDI–CAT-Manual-1-3-6.pdf. Published 2012. Accessed June 23, 2018.

71. Field DA, Livingstone RW. Power mobility skill progression for children and adolescents: a systematic review of measures and their clinical application. *Dev Med Child Neurol.* 2018;60(10):997-1011. doi:10.1111/dmcn.13709.

72. Kenyon LK, Farris JP, Cain B, King E, VandenBerg A. Development and content validation of the power mobility training tool. *Disabil Rehabil Assist Technol.* 2018;13(1):10-24. doi:10.1080/17483107.2016.1278468.

73. Furumasu J, Guerette P, Tefft D. The development of a powered wheelchair mobility program for young children. *Technol Disabil.* 1996;5(1):41-48.

74. Sullivan KJ. President's perspective. Evidence for physical therapist practice: how can we reconcile clinical guidelines and patient-centered care? *J Neurol Phys Ther.* 2010;34(1):52-53. doi:10.1097/NPT.0b013e3181d055c2.

75. Nilsson L, Eklund M, Nyberg P, Thulesius H. Driving to learn in a powered wheelchair: the process of learning joystick use in people with profound cognitive disabilities. *Am J Occup Ther.* 2011;65(6):652-660. doi:10.5014/ajot.2011.001750.

76. Butler C, Okamoto GA, McKay TM. Powered mobility for very young disabled children. *Dev Med Child Neurol.* 1983;25(4):472-474. doi:10.1111/j.1469-8749.1983.tb13792.x.

77. Huhn K, Guarrera-Bowlby P, Deutsch J. The clinical decision-making process of prescribing power mobility for a child with cerebral palsy. *Pediatr Phys Ther.* 2007;19(3):254-260. doi:10.1097/PEP.0b013e31812c65cc.

78. Mockler S, McEwen IR, Jones M. Predictors of power mobility proficiency in young children with severe motor impairments. *Arch Phys Med Rehabil.* 2017;98(10):2034-2041. doi:10.1016/j.apmr.2017.05.028.

79. Kiger A. Cortical visual impairment: ideas for seating & mobility success. Proceedings from the 2018 International Seating Symposium. http://www.seatingsymposium.com/images/pdf/ISS2018_Syllabus_eVersion.pdf. 176-178. Published 2018. Accessed June 23, 2018.

80. Good WV, Jan JE, Burden SK, Skoczenski A, Candy R. Recent advances in cortical visual impairment. *Dev Med Child Neurol.* 2001;43(1):56-60. doi:10.1017/S0012162201000093.

81. Merabet LB, Mayer DL, Bauer CM, Wright D, Kran BS. Disentangling how the brain is "wired" in cortical (cerebral) visual impairment. *Semin Pediatr Neurol.* 2017;24(2):83-91. doi:10.1016/j.spen.2017.04.005.

82. Roman-Lantzy C. *Cortical Visual Impairment: An Approach to Assessment and Intervention.* New York, NY: AFB Press; 2007.

83. Groenveld M, Jan JE, Leader P. Observations on the habilitation of children with cortical visual impairment. *J Vis Impair Blind.* 1990;84(1):11-15.

84. Crawford JS. O&M for visually impaired wheelchair users. Affiliated Blind Of Louisiana. Lafayette, LA. http://www.affiliatedblind.org/Images/Interior/documents/wheelchair_om.pdf. Accessed June 23, 2018.

85. Paleg G, Livingstone R. Evidence-informed clinical perspectives on selecting gait trainer features for children with cerebral palsy. *Int J Ther Rehabil.* 2016;23(8):386-396. doi:10.12968/ijtr.2016.23.9.444.

86. Low SA, McCoy SW, Beling J, Adams J. Pediatric physical therapists' use of support walkers for children with disabilities: a nationwide survey. *Pediatr Phys Ther.* 2011;23(4):381-389. doi:10.1097/PEP.0b013e318235257c.

87. Paleg G, Livingstone R. Outcomes of gait trainer use in home and school settings for children with motor impairments: a systematic review. *Clin Rehabil.* 2015;29(11):1077-1091. doi:10.1177/0269215514565947.

88. Carroll NC. The orthotic management of spina bifida children present status—future goals. *Prosthet Orthot Int.* 1977;1(1):39-42. doi:10.3109/03093647709164604.

89. Jasinski R. Do-it-Yourself Star Car. http://www2.waisman.wisc.edu/~rowley/sb-kids/dme-dyi-star-car.html. Accessed June 23, 2018.

90. Build your own Bumbo wheelchair. http://www.whatdoyoudodear.com/wp-content/uploads/2014/08/Build-a-BUMBO-Wheelchair1.pdf. Accessed June 23, 2018.

91. Mountain AD, Kirby RL, Eskes GA, et al. Ability of people with stroke to learn powered wheelchair skills: a pilot study. *Arch Phys Med Rehabil.* 2010;91(4):596-601. doi:10.1016/j.apmr.2009.12.011.

92. Daly C, Haneline C, Johannes S, Middleton J, Kenyon LK. A school-based intervention to improve fitness and function in severe cerebral palsy: a pilot study. *Pediatr Phys Ther.* 2016;28(4):E1.

Assessment and Development of Gait Skills

12

Dora J. Gosselin, PT, DPT, PCS, C/NDT

Participation is an individual's ability to function within society: one's involvement in a real-life situation.[1] A number of studies have confirmed the relationship between higher levels of mobility and gross motor functioning and increased participation.[2-6] Walking is the most common form of human locomotion and is often an emphasis of therapeutic intervention.

This chapter will use the domains of the *International Classification of Functioning, Disability and Health* (ICF)[1] to discuss the basic concepts related to walking in common diagnostic groups. Guidelines for examination, treatment planning, and therapeutic interventions for the development of gait skills will be proposed. Finally, the 5 case studies used throughout this text will be used to demonstrate the processes described.

BASIC CONCEPTS

The terms *locomotion, walking, gait,* and *ambulation* frequently are used in the literature, and to prevent confusion the definition of each of these terms must be clear. Locomotion is the ability to move from one place to another[7] by any means, including rolling scooting, creeping, and propelling a wheelchair. Walking is to move along on foot, taking steps[7] and requires that a person have the ability to control his or her posture upright against gravity. Gait and ambulation can be used interchangeably and are defined as the manner or style of walking[7] or the posture and movement that one demonstrates when walking from place to place.

Applying these terms within the context of the ICF is helpful to contextualize the terms for a therapeutic setting. The ICF describes 3 main domains: Body Functions and Structures, Activities, and Participation. The Body Functions and Structures domain addresses the physiological processes and anatomical parts of human functioning. Activities is defined as a task or action executed by an individual, and, as described previously, Participation is related to the individual's involvement in a real-life situation. Locomotion is a functional activity and represents the summation of many components within the Body Functions and Structures domain. To apply this framework to walking and gait, the example of taking 10 steps can be used. The steps themselves represent an Activity;

Connolly BH, Montgomery PC, eds. *Therapeutic Exercise for Children With Developmental Disabilities, Fourth Edition* (pp 331-366).
© 2020 Taylor & Francis Group.

however, if those steps were being used in a meaningful, real-life environment, for example, on a playground, that would be classified within the Participation domain of the ICF. Gait is complex, and the ICF model is helpful to systematically describe functioning in each domain; in determining what is or what is not working; and in providing a structure for examination, evaluation, and development of a plan of care.

Locomotion

Although developmental sequences vary, a child often begins the process of moving in space by the fourth month of age with rolling activities. This typically is followed at age 5 to 6 months by pivoting as well as pushing backward through space when prone. Belly crawling usually is the first form of forward mobility and emerges at about age 7 months. Creeping on hands and knees follows at age 8 to 9 months. The ability to locomote around an environment greatly increases an infant's experiences by allowing exploration of novel surfaces, objects, and spaces. Looper et al[8] did not find a relationship between the ability to sit when placed and the onset of locomotion either by crawling, cruising, or walking. However, these researchers suggested that the transitional skills that require modulation of forces through the trunk and pelvis (eg, rotating into sitting, getting down to the floor by squatting, pulling to stand at furniture, and moving from squat to stand), allow an infant to develop the trunk and pelvic control necessary for locomotion via crawling, cruising, or walking.

Walking

When infants begin holding their posture vertically against gravity, there is a progression that involves transferring the base of support (BOS) from the upper extremities (either on a horizontal surface or held by a caregiver) to the lower extremities. Typically developing children begin to take assisted steps in the eighth or ninth month. Independent walking is defined as taking a minimum of 5 unaided steps[9] with the mean age for the onset of independent walking between 11.5 and 14.5 months.[10,11] Størvold and colleagues[11] investigated prewalking strategies and the onset of walking and found that infants who crawled on their hands and knees walked significantly earlier than those that shuffled on their bottoms.

To capitalize on the newly discovered form of upright mobility, the child must learn to ambulate in different directions; go up and down stairs; avoid obstacles in the pathway; stop, start, and change directions; carry items while walking; and walk and talk at the same time while coping with distractions in the environment. The emergence of these skills is well-documented in developmental charts and tests.[12-15]

Gait

Perry[16] defined gait as a repetitive sequence of stable upright postures in which the body weight is advanced over a constantly changing BOS. When gait is observed in typically functioning individuals, it is seen as rhythmical, stable, predictable, and yet individualized. Gait varies within each individual as changes in the neural and body systems occur both in real time and developmental time. Functional, healthy gait is the ability to cope with a wide breadth of environmental complexity, both predictable and unpredictable. For example, a student who is able to walk in an empty school hallway also must be able to walk in that hallway when it is bustling with students during a class period transition. In this example, when the requirements of the environment exceed the gait capacity of the student, the rhythm and efficiency of the gait will be altered, or, worse, safety will be compromised and the risk of falling increased.

Gait is complex and, for the sake of analysis, often is broken down into a variety of elements: cycles, periods, and phases. A gait cycle is defined as the time from initial contact to the next ipsilateral contact and is divided into 2 periods: (1) stance, about 60% of the gait cycle, and (2) swing,

TABLE 12-1. PARAMETERS OF GAIT	
SPATIOTEMPORAL VARIABLE	DEFINITION
Cadence	Step rate, reported in steps per minute.
Foot progression angle	The angle between the line bisecting the calcaneus and the second metatarsal and line of progression.
Stride length	The distance of one entire cycle in the gait process beginning when one foot contacts the ground and continuing until the same foot once again contacts the ground.
Step length	The distance between the initial contact point of the 2 opposite feet.
Step width	The perpendicular distance between the bisection of each calcaneus, perpendicular to the plane of motion.

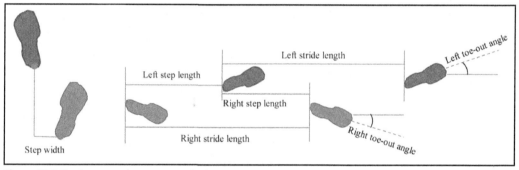

Figure 12-1. Spatiotemporal parameters of gait.

which compromises the other 40% of the cycle. Phases include more specific spatiotemporal, kinematic, and kinetic components of gait. The intent of this chapter is not to provide an in-depth review of gait biomechanics, but a general understanding of these elements, which is critical for proper examination and evaluation.

Symmetry is a hallmark of a healthy and efficient gait. Cadence, foot progression angle, step length, step width, and stride length are spatiotemporal parameters that are easily and frequently measured. (See Table 12-1 and Figure 12-1.) Whereas breaking down the components of gait may be essential for an accurate assessment, it is critical to realize that just as a symphony cannot be understood or appreciated by studying each note in isolation, gait cannot be understood by studying only the individual aspects.

GROWTH AND DEVELOPMENT

Gait parameters change across the lifespan. In general, younger children show greater variability in gait parameters than older children. Across childhood, step and stride lengths increase with age and cadence decreases, as step and stride lengths increase. The BOS decreases with age.[17] The changes in these parameters reflect changes in many of the body systems and continual refinements of global neuronal maps. Gait is thought to be mature by age 7 years.[17] (See Table 12-2 and Figure 12-2.)

TABLE 12-2. AGE-RELATED CHANGES IN GAIT			
AGE (YEARS)	SPEED (METERS/MINUTE)	MEAN CADENCE (STEPS/MINUTE)	STEP LENGTH (CENTIMETERS)
1	38	176	22
2	43	156	28
3	52	154	33
4	60	152	39
5	65	154	42
6	65	146	44
Adult	82	113	65 to 80

Adapted from Sutherland DH, Olshen RA, Biden EN, Wyatt MP. *The Development of Mature Walking*. London, England: Mac Keith Press; 1988.

Figure 12-2. Increased variability, especially during the first 3 months of walking.

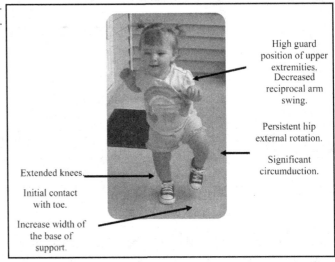

High guard position of upper extremities. Decreased reciprocal arm swing.

Persistent hip external rotation.

Significant circumduction.

Extended knees.

Initial contact with toe.

Increase width of the base of support.

Changes in the Musculoskeletal System

For walking to develop, remarkable shifts in physical skeletal growth must occur. The relative size of the head compared with the trunk and limbs in early infancy makes independent walking impossible. After age 12 months, trunk growth and the relative growth of the lower extremities provide a biomechanical advantage for walking. At the same time, there are changes in the shape of the bones that change the efficiency of gait. Specific examples include the decrease in the angle of inclination of the femur with the coexisting shift in the amount of femoral antetorsion, which contribute to a resultant decrease in the BOS. The knees demonstrate a gradual increase in genu valgum until age 2.5 years and then a decrease until age 6 years. In addition, the growth of the long bones in the lower extremities can account for increased step and stride lengths.[18]

The growth of the long bones is associated with growth of and increased length of the muscles and soft tissue. In muscle, the increase in length is an adaptive response by adding sarcomeres. In addition to increasing length, strength also increases dramatically in the early years. Increased strength of extensor muscles provides power for push-off, increasing step length. This increase in strength is also critical in developing skills such as stair climbing, jumping, and running.[19]

Changes in the Neuromuscular System

The neuromuscular system demonstrates changes both in control and coordination of muscle activity that are reflected in changes of gait parameters. During early walking, the child demonstrates increased cocontraction or "fixing."[20] This pattern of cocontraction diminishes with experience. There is a gradual increase in the recruitment of patterns of axial rotation with a period of hyperrotation. The changes in control of trunk rotation occur simultaneously, with increased isolated control between as well as within the extremities.[21]

Changes in Sensory Systems

There is evidence of changes in sensory systems that are reflected in changes in gait. Children younger than 3 years rely heavily on vision for postural alignment during stance. Between ages 4 to 6 years, the sensory systems reorganize with vestibular, somatosensory, and visual integration, resulting in more mature movement.[21]

Because growth in many body systems continues through adolescence and beyond, children are constantly making subtle adaptations to accommodate for changes. Of additional consideration are the nonbiomechanical contributions to locomotion including motivation and cognition.

IMPLICATIONS OF PATHOLOGY

In addition to the impact of growth and systems maturation discussed earlier, the impact of pathology on the parameters of gait must be considered. Certainly not all children with developmental disabilities have the potential to walk independently, but many do and intervention focused on gait is common in pediatric physical therapy.[22] There are clearer indicators for eventual ambulation in children within some diagnostic groups (eg, myelodysplasia) than there are others (eg, cerebral palsy [CP]).

Myelodysplasia

Children with myelodysplasia with lesions above L4-L5 will ambulate only with orthoses, crutches, or walkers.[23-25] In a study of 68 children with myelodysplasia, DeSouza and Carroll[24] were able to define criteria for ambulation (Table 12-3). Although the eventual ambulatory status seemed to depend primarily on the neurosegmental level, the extent and degree of orthopedic deformities also were significant factors.

Similarly, Hoffer and colleagues[23] followed more than 50 children with myelodysplasia and found that none of the children with thoracic level lesions walked, whereas all with sacral-level lesions became community ambulators. In children with lesions at the lumbar level, 45% were functional ambulators. In addition, those who achieved functional ambulation did so prior to age 9 years.

Intellectual Disability

Individuals with intellectual disabilities (IDs) may have abnormalities in gait.[26] However, a mental age for walking has never been determined.[25] Shapiro and colleagues reported that 92% of children with a profound ID (intelligence quotient less than 25) walked if the ID was not accompanied by another neurological dysfunction, although the median age of walking was delayed.[27] When ID was present with CP, the median age of walking was 63.5 months. A greater risk of falls in individuals with ID has been reported;[28] however, balance and gait are potentially trainable in people with ID.[29]

TABLE 12-3. AMBULATION STATUS BY NEUROSEGMENTAL LEVEL	
NEUROSEGMENTAL LEVEL	FUNCTIONAL ABILITY
Thoracic lesion with no power distal to the hip joint	Not community ambulators
High lumbar lesion with power in hip adductors or flexors or extensors of the knee	10% community ambulators
Low lumbar lesion with power in the knee flexors, dorsiflexors, or hip abductors	33% community ambulators
Sacral lesion with power in plantar flexors	50% community ambulators

Adapted from Hoffer MM, Feiwell E, Perry R, Perry J, Bonnett C. Functional ambulation in patients with myelomeningocele. *J Bone Joint Surg Am*. 1973;55(1):137-148.

Cerebral Palsy

Nearly all pediatric physical therapists treat children with CP. This group represents a very heterogeneous collection of individuals with varying pathophysiology, degrees of severity of primary and secondary impairments, and courses of intervention and recovery. This heterogeneity creates a challenge when attempting to determine the predictors of walking. Montgomery[30] reviewed 7 studies across 25 years that attempted to identify predictors of ambulation in children with CP and found that almost all children with hemiplegia walk before age 3 years. Most children with diplegia walk with or without assistive devices, whereas the majority of children with quadriplegia remain nonambulatory, and those who became ambulatory typically require an assistive device.

Begnoche and colleagues[31] used a number of items on the Gross Motor Function Measure (GMFM)[15] to investigate the predictors of independent walking in young children with CP. The researchers found that functional strength (tested as a sit to stand and stand to sit) was a predictor for independent ambulation. Additionally, children with CP take significantly fewer steps and have lower levels of physical activity compared with age-matched peers.[32,33]

Regardless of the diagnostic group, it is important to identify those children with the potential to ambulate to develop the most efficient interventions to reach that outcome. It also is important to identify those children who may not be ambulators so alternative interventions, such as acquiring needed assistive devices and making environmental modifications, can be implemented (see Chapters 11 and 14).

EXAMINATION

General Considerations

A useful assessment of a child's gait includes gathering a wide variety of information and performing specific examinations that are assimilated into a comprehensive evaluation, and, subsequently, the development of a plan of care. Gait can be examined in a number of ways, from a highly technical instrumented gait analysis, which generally requires expensive equipment and specific training, to clinical observational gait analysis, which takes place in a typical clinical setting and requires only tools that are customary in a clinical environment. Instrumented gait analysis will not be discussed in this chapter.

Generally, therapists follow a similar sequence and flow during patient examination; however, therapeutic style is unique and individualized and the following are suggestions for components to include in an examination. After obtaining a thorough history with a directed and comprehensive discussion of gait, particularly the child's motivation to walk and the details of the specific environment(s) in which the child desires to walk, the focus turns to examination.

Big Picture

The therapist can be most effective when beginning the process by obtaining a "big picture" of the child's life with observations of the child in various settings. It is important to understand how the child's ambulation supports or interferes with full participation at home, at school, or in the community. Observations made during the "big picture" examination could include the following:

- What is the general temperament of the child?
- Does the child seem to enjoy movement and walking in particular?
- Does the child's current form of locomotion appear safe?
- Does the child require assistance to walk?

Functional Abilities and Limitations

Specific functional limitations or abilities directly related to the ability to walk should be identified. To simply state that a child can walk a set distance is **not** a report of function. The examination must focus on the functional implications of walking that distance:

- Does the child need support to move from a sitting position to initiation of the first step?
- Are the child's ambulation skills sufficient for walking in the desired environments?
- Is the child able to navigate common environmental obstacles?
- Is the child able to readily change directions while walking?
- Is the child able to communicate while walking?
- Is the child able to carry an object while walking?
- Does the child require assistance to navigate while walking?
- Is the child's gait speed adequate?
- Where does the child seem to look while walking?
- Does fatigue affect the child's ability to walk?

It is through the integration of multiple functional skills that the individual demonstrates the ability to participate in typical experiences and roles associated with childhood. Once again, functioning must be explored in multiple environments. A child may walk independently in the home, but, once in school, be unable to demonstrate that same ability. Following intervention, a child may demonstrate progress by either acquiring a new functional ability or by generalizing a previously acquired skill in a new, more complex environment.

Therapy goals must be more than measurable, they must be child and family centered. Goal development should include the family, and, when able, the child. Once goals are established, the therapist may begin to educate and counsel the family as to the feasibility of the child reaching desired outcomes. For example, the family may indicate that it is most important to focus on ambulation in the home to increase independence in the bathroom and bedroom now that the family has a second child. In another circumstance, it may be more important that the adolescent walk longer distances (even if it is with an assistive device) in the school now that he or she must change classes every hour.

Gait Analysis

In an attempt to more accurately describe the environment in which an activity or participation is being executed, the ICF proposes the qualifiers of *capacity* and *performance*. Capacity defines the ability of a person in a standardized environment, whereas performance defines what a person does in a natural environment. Observational gait analysis should be conducted with consideration of what the desired level of measurement is—capacity or performance. Regardless, the analysis should be systematic and inclusive of a variety of gait skills, and, when possible, different environments.

Only a few basic tools are needed for clinical observational gait analysis: a stopwatch, a reliable method for measuring distance or premarked distances, open and closed environments, and elements to increase the challenge of the environment (ie, objects to carry and obstacles). With increased access to recording methods, whenever possible recordings should be taken in both planes with the camera positioned at a 90-degree angle to the walker. Recording allows multiple opportunities for analysis and can be reviewed in slow motion, thus allowing the examiner to make observations one joint or body segment at a time. Advancements in technology have resulted in more accessible and affordable options of motion analysis, many of which can be used with a standard smartphone and can offer even more accurate measurement.

When performing observational gait analysis, it is critical that the examiner views gait both in the sagittal and frontal planes and either proximal to distal or distal to proximal. Spatiotemporal parameters of gait (see Table 12-1) also should be analyzed. Determining the symmetry of gait is critical and defining whether and where asymmetry exists is an efficient way to focus the gait analysis. If asymmetry is observed, the examiner must determine the contributor(s) to the asymmetry. Doing this will require further investigation with other clinical measures, for example, range of motion (ROM), muscle strength, the presence of spasticity, and sensory integrity.

An additional framework for considering the posture and movement during gait, or any other movement, is the "ABCs" of examination:

> **Alignment:** Examine the alignment of the body in the upright posture. Is the alignment adequate for efficient antigravity control? Look at the entire body as well as specific joint relationships. At this point it may be more effective to begin looking from the BOS upward rather than the head-to-toe approach. Analyze the alignment of the foot, ankle, knee, hip, and spine, including the neck and head. What is the impact of each joint on the body above and below? Look at the impact of the ground forces on alignment and movement. Frequently, an examination in both non–weight-bearing and weight-bearing positions is needed to determine whether the observed deviation in alignment is a structural problem or a dynamic substitution.

> **Base of support:** Consider the size of the BOS and what portions of the body need to be included in establishing that BOS. For example, does the child rely on the upper extremities within the BOS by using an assistive device to increase his or her BOS? The larger the BOS, the more difficult it is to shift the center of mass (COM) over the base. For example, a child who walks with a scissoring-style gait with the feet close together while in a posture walker still is demonstrating a large BOS. Even though the feet are close together, the size of the BOS is large. It also incorporates the upper extremity contacts with the walker and subsequently the BOS includes the entire area within the walker base.

> **Center of mass:** In assessing posture and alignment, the therapist considers the relationship of the child's COM to the BOS. Is the child increasing stability by lowering the COM in a crouched gait pattern? How is weight shifting of the COM achieved? Does the child shift weight only by shifting upper body weight over a more stable base and shortening on the weight-bearing side or does the child control the weight shifting efficiently through the recruitment of patterns of rotation?

Perry[16] describes 5 prerequisites for normal gait: (1) stability in stance, (2) sufficient foot clearance during swing, (3) appropriate swing-phase prepositioning of the foot, (4) adequate step length, and (5) energy conservation. Considering the integrity of these components is an additional way to structure gait analysis.

Pediatric Clinical Gait Analysis Tools

Two systematic reviews[34,35] identified, evaluated, and reported on variables and psychometric properties of pediatric gait assessment tools. The majority of pediatric gait assessment tools included in these reviews measured the Body Functions and Structures (6/24) or Activities (24/24) components of the ICF, and only one tool included a component that assessed the Participation domain. For example, the commonly administered 6-Minute Walk Test measures heart rate, blood pressure and oxygen saturation (Body Functions and Structures), and total distance walked (Activities).[36] Assessment of the Body Functions and Structures and Activities domains of the ICF is important for monitoring progress as well as for choosing interventions. However, limiting assessment to these 2 domains may fail to accurately assess the way that a child walks in a participatory environment, arguably the most important from the child/parent point of view. Participatory environments are inherently more demanding than laboratory settings because they take into account other people, changes or shifts in environmental requirements, and higher-level tasks. Existing pediatric gait assessment tools are limited in their ability to capture these more complex environmental considerations related to gait.

EVALUATION

Once a thorough examination of the body systems and gait has been completed, the physical therapist engages in the evaluation process and hypothesizes the role of impaired body systems, postures, and movements in the abilities or limitations the child has in gait. The strengths of the child, family, and environment are compared with areas of concern. Barriers the child potentially may meet that can impair or prevent functional walking will be considered and the posture and movement problems interfering with walking will be prioritized so the plan of care can be developed.

PLAN OF CARE

Based on the evaluation, a plan of care is established that includes the following: (1) the frequency and duration of treatment, (2) the necessary equipment, (3) the adjuncts to therapy that may speed progress, (4) the therapeutic goals, (5) a plan to educate the client and family, and (6) the specific strategies and interventions that will be used to meet the goals.

INTERVENTION

The therapist will make decisions on specifics of intervention based on the *Guide to Physical Therapist Practice 3.0*[37] and anticipated outcomes from the Gross Motor Function Classification System (GMFCS).[38] The therapist selects direct intervention strategies based on the examination, evaluation, and anticipated outcomes. Forms of direct intervention that are included when focusing on changes in walking or gait are therapeutic exercise, functional training in self-care, communication and work integration, manual therapy, and the prescription of orthotic and assistive devices.

Palisano and colleagues[38,39] provided an additional framework for problem solving with the GMFCS. Five levels of severity of gross motor functioning in children with CP based on age-specific gross motor activities were described. Levels I to V demonstrate increasingly compromised functional locomotive abilities. Each level reflects the highest level of mobility anticipated for a child between ages 6 to 12 years. Descriptions of locomotion abilities at earlier age ranges (birth to 2 years, age 2 to 4 years, and age 4 to 6 years) also are provided. In this classification system, Level I includes children who walk without restrictions and with limitations being evident only in more advanced gross motor skills (Figures 12-3 through 12-5).

Figure 12-3. Level I, Emma walks well independently. Her difficulties in functional ambulation include walking while carrying items that require careful orientation, such as her cafeteria tray and ascending and descending stairs without a rail. Her personal goal is to be able to jump rope with friends at school. Here she is seen descending stairs.

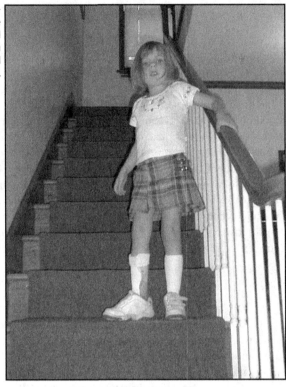

Figure 12-4. During ambulation on flat surfaces, asymmetry in the upper extremity is evident. She wears ankle-foot orthoses during ambulation and receives periodic injections of Botox (onabotulinumtoxinA).

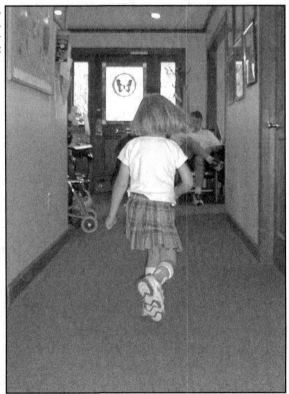

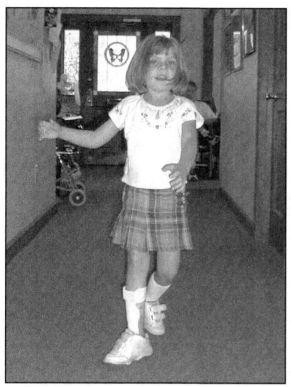

Figure 12-5. During running, posture- and movement-related impairments become more evident.

Level II includes children who walk without assistive devices but who demonstrate limitations in walking outdoors and in the community. The child in Level II might initially require an assistive device when very young and has more limitations in the ability to run and jump than children in Level I (Figures 12-6 and 12-7).

Level III includes children who walk with assistive mobility devices and who have limitations in walking outdoors and in the community. These children typically will always require an assistive device and perhaps the use of orthotics (Figures 12-8 through 12-18).

Level IV includes children who have self-mobility with limitations and who are usually transported or use power mobility outdoors and in the community. Children at this level typically function in sitting, usually with support, with very limited independent mobility (Figures 12-19 and 12-20).

Level V includes children whose self-mobility is severely limited even with the use of assistive technology. At this level the children have no means of independent mobility and are transported unless control of a powered wheelchair is mastered with extensive adaptations (Figures 12-21 through 12-23).

Descriptions of interventions will begin by addressing children who are in the most severely functionally limited groups (Levels IV and V) and proceed to those with less significant limitations. Although these functional levels describe children with CP, this chapter will focus on questions or general principles of practice for children with varying diagnoses but similar functional levels, with the goal of guiding clinicians toward the establishment of specific intervention plans.

Regardless of the child's functional level, prior to establishing any intervention plan it is critical to analyze the following:

> Is the cost, time, and effort worth the desired outcome?

> Are there secondary impairments that might emerge if no intervention is provided?

> What are the implications for the child's self-esteem or sense of well-being?

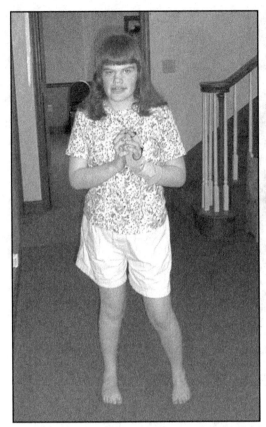 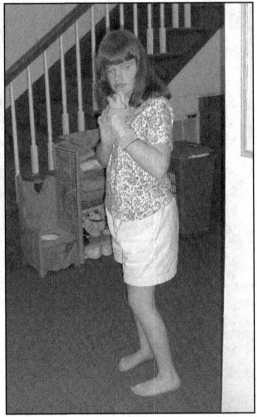

Figure 12-6. Level II. This 19-year-old girl has walked independently since age 4 years. However, because of significant visual impairments, decreased neuromuscular control and coordination, decreased range of motion at the ankles, and a scoliosis, her functional abilities in novel situations in the community are restricted.

Figure 12-7. She now wears ankle-foot orthoses bilaterally and periodically has Botox and taping to her back and legs. She participates in a therapeutic horseback riding program and gymnastics.

Intervention for Children at Level IV or V

Several appropriate, but possibly difficult, questions must be asked in regard to therapeutic intervention for a child who will probably never be able to walk in a functional manner:

> Is there any reason to work toward goals of ambulation?
> Is there any value to this child or family in ambulation assisted by another person or by extensive assistive devices?

For example, mobility in a powered chair may increase participation at school and in the community as well as at home; however, the child and caregivers may have particular reasons that a goal related to gait is feasible. For example, the child may be able to participate more in community activities if he or she is able to take steps with physical assistance into a restaurant or building that is not wheelchair accessible, or if the child is able to take assisted steps to move in and out of the family bathroom or bedroom. The family and child may believe that the functional outcome of being able to take assisted steps is worth the energy and financial cost of intervention.

These questions are very difficult to answer and require the careful consideration of the entire team. There is no one correct answer. Once the decision has been reached and specific outcome measures have been established, the clinician then develops specific strategies to address the impairments and motor component problems that interfere with successful performance of the desired outcomes.

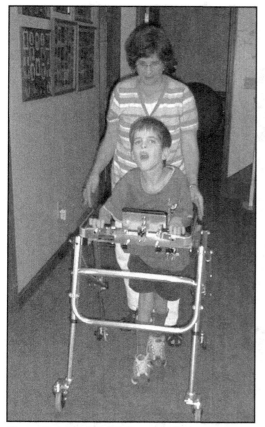

Figure 12-8. Level III. This 11-year-old boy moves independently by self-propelling a wheelchair and walking supported in a Pony (R82). He walks with standby guarding at household levels and is developing basic skills at community distances.

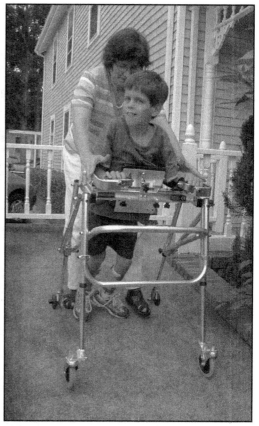

Figure 12-9. This boy requires physical assistance to descend a ramp.

Next, the team must consider the potential risks of not providing the intervention:

> Are there secondary impairments that might emerge if no intervention is provided?
> What is the potential of developing complications secondary to a more sedentary lifestyle?
> Are there risks of increased cardiopulmonary impairments?
> Are there risks to the musculoskeletal system, such as increased contractures, weakness, or osteoporosis?
> What are the implications for the child's self-esteem or sense of well-being?
> What will be the cost to the child or family if these complications occur?

If the answer to these questions lead the team to decide intervention is warranted, the intervention will include the use of extensive assistive technology as well as direct intervention. Activities in therapy will continue to focus on sitting function and on developing maximal skills for locomotion in the wheelchair. Additional equipment to aid the family in transport (eg, lifts or ramps for a van) may be indicated. The intervention may include the following:

> Using partial body weight-bearing (PBWB) training over a treadmill to establish basic patterns of ambulation[40,41]
> Instructing caregivers in supported ambulation
> Training the child to control a powered wheelchair
> Focusing on cardiopulmonary fitness

Figure 12-10. This 3-year-old girl moves around the floor by "bunny hopping."

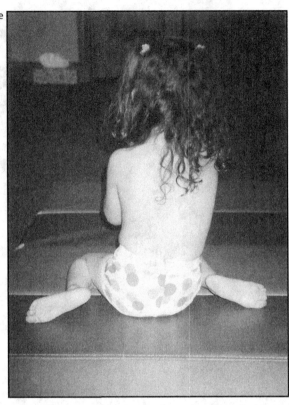

Figure 12-11. She pulls to stand and walks community distances with a posture walker.

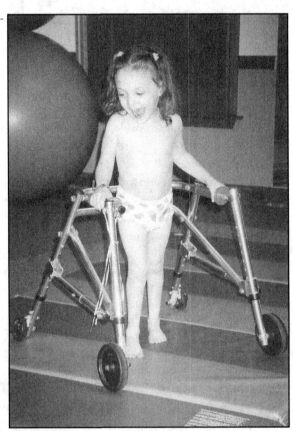

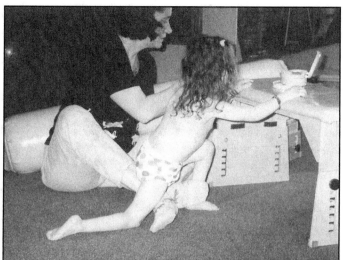

Figure 12-12. Transitions to and from the floor encourage lower extremity isolated control (one leg flexed and one extended).

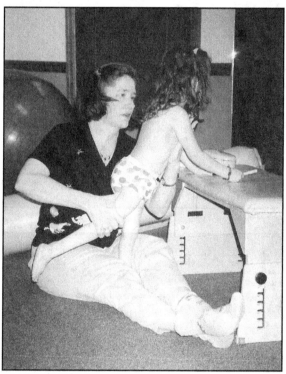

Figure 12-13. Transitions to and from the floor encourage lower extremity isolated control (one leg flexed and one extended).

Figure 12-14. Gait is facilitated to increase hip and knee extension in terminal ranges to increase her step length.

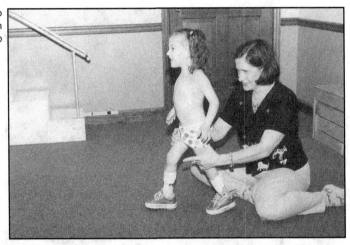

Figure 12-15. The muscles in the lower extremity are strengthened and ankle range of motion increased dynamically via a stair-climbing activity.

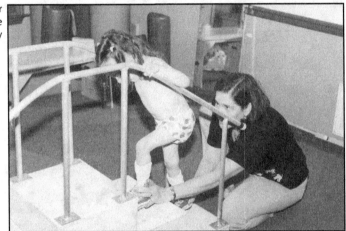

Figure 12-16. The child works in squatting activities to gain control of her center of mass over her base of support. Assistance is provided to minimize her tendency to adduct and internally rotate the lower extremities and to have a toe-only contact.

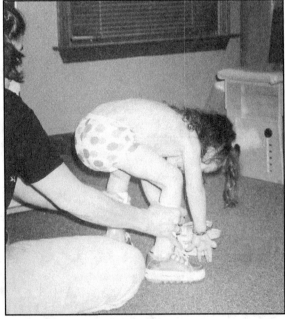

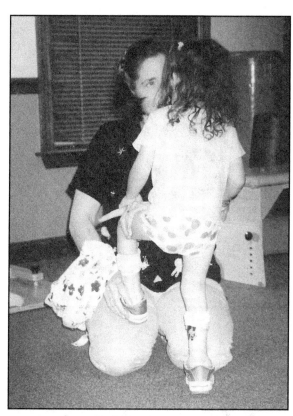

Figure 12-17. Another activity to promote motor learning is to teach family members about how she can assist in dressing in standing.

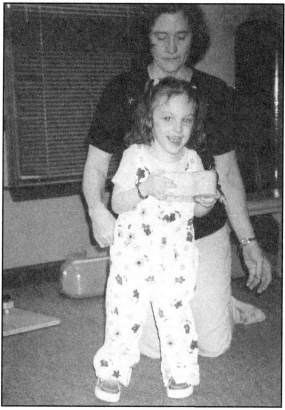

Figure 12-18. She is now able to stand and walk independently across the floor to give an object to a family member. This goal is important to the family as the child attends preschool and needs to walk from one area to another carrying objects.

Figure 12-19. Level IV. This teenager was involved in a motor vehicle accident 3 years ago. He has a power wheelchair.

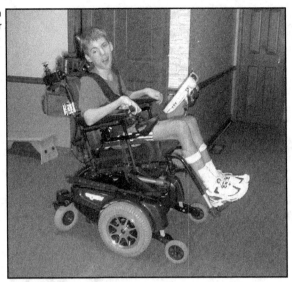

Figure 12-20. In recent months, he has demonstrated an increased ability to ambulate short distances with an assistive device. This makes it possible for him to walk from his bedroom to the bathroom or to walk into a restroom in the community that is not wheelchair accessible.

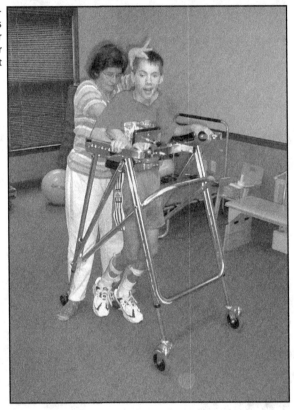

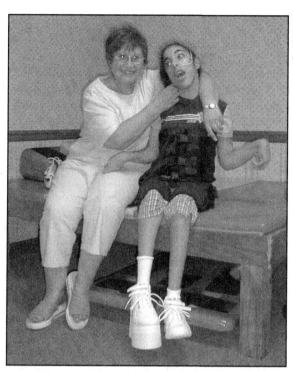

Figure 12-21. Level V. Michelle, age 16 years, sits with her mom. She has no independent mobility and is dependent on caregivers for all transfers. She has a dislocated hip and scoliosis.

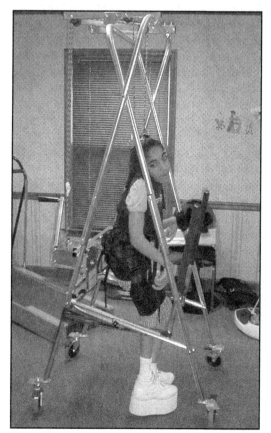

Figure 12-22. Michelle loves standing in a partial body weight-bearing device and can safely be positioned upright.

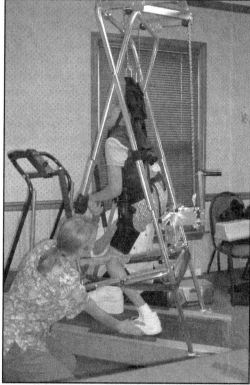

Figure 12-23. She enjoys ambulating on the treadmill with approximately 50% weight bearing. Her cardiopulmonary endurance has improved to 10-minute episodes of walking.

> Monitoring and addressing musculoskeletal issues (eg, ROM, strength)
> Addressing skeletal changes in bone mineral density
> Addressing issues related to self-esteem

The frequency and duration of intervention are established to match proposed functional outcomes, address the prevention of secondary impairments or greater functional limitations, address new issues related to growth or changes in body systems, address changes in environmental demands, and meet the needs of the individual family. Frank discussions with the family are important to ensure that the therapist and family all anticipate the same outcomes. For example, the family should not hope for an outcome of independent ambulation because intervention is addressing supported walking.

Basic Treatment Principles for Children at Level IV or V

1. Explore all options of locomotion or mobility, including independent wheelchair use, powered mobility, or modified battery-operated riding toys. Intervention strategies during direct services may include emphasis on sitting control, with upper extremities free for use to control the mobility device.

2. For upright posture and stability and forward propulsive-force generation, the therapist can provide equipment to compensate for postural and movement control limitations. These options might include the use of PBWB device, a gait trainer, or a Pony-type device. It may be possible to use an assistive device such as an anterior support walker for assisted household-level ambulation. These devices can be important to aid the caregivers and prevent injury to their backs, even when the child cannot use the device independent of standby assistance. During therapy sessions, intervention addresses increased postural control to hold the head and trunk upright with less assistance. Activities should be performed in the upright posture as the impact of gravity is reduced as compared with work in lower positions against gravity, and the postural synergies require less isolated control. Trunk extension is coupled with hip and knee extension. Ambulation over a treadmill may be useful to initially develop the sense of forward progression with a forward-propulsive force. It is important to work to obtain the correct alignment of the trunk over the extremities. The use of prone, supine, or vertical standers can be used to ensure this alignment. This is an important component of intervention if the child spends most of the day sitting. Orthotics are used to maintain biomechanical alignment and soft tissue mobility during other parts of the day when the child is not walking; however, he or she may be more successful during ambulation if the orthotics are removed.

3. Shock absorption concerns are addressed by supporting more appropriate alignment of the extremities and by limiting the amount of weight the child is expected to bear. A PBWB device can limit the amount of weight on an extremity, and the use of orthotics may reduce the valgus or varus stress to a limb. Orthotics are monitored for indications of excessive weight bearing and then modified to better distribute weight during ambulation.

4. The therapist is not expecting energy conservation to be a goal in this limited, assisted ambulation. The purpose of the assisted ambulation can be to challenge the child's cardiac and respiratory systems. The child may be participating in the activity as a form of aerobic exercise to increase cardiopulmonary fitness. The therapist first may need to address these issues with careful supervision in the therapy setting, but later the activity might occur in a classroom or physical education (PE) program without direct supervision by the therapist. It is important, however, to use caution during the decision-making process. Supported ambulation for these children involves risk both of immediate injury and the development of secondary impairments with additional functional limitations. Whereas almost every child needs a standing program to address issues of bone mineral density, alignment, and soft tissue length, not every child needs to participate in a walking program.

Intervention for Children at Level III

The therapist faces different questions with children at Level III. Most therapists and parents see the need for gait-focused therapeutic interventions for these children. The therapist begins by addressing participation of the children at home and in the community. The family identifies specific participation restrictions and desired outcomes. The therapist then selects potential strategies for intervention. In addition, the therapist and family must review the potential devices and orthotics that might be used by children within the key environments and then select and obtain the most appropriate ones. As these children typically use different forms of ambulation in different environments, a less cumbersome assistive device may be used at home than in the community. The therapist must train the child with those specific devices and then allow practice with the device in the critical environments to ensure functional use.

The therapist, with the family, identifies specific functional outcomes to be achieved in therapy. Once these outcomes are established, the therapist identifies and plans strategies to address the impairments as well as posture and movement problems that are hypothesized to interfere with the desired functional outcomes. The therapist must search for efficient strategies to address each of the impairments or posture and movement problems. The therapist plans activities to nurture motor learning. In addition, the therapist treats with the goal of minimizing anticipated future impairments. The balance between striving to improve function immediately and the need to anticipate and manage impairments that might influence future functional abilities and participation is critical for these children.

Intervention frequently includes coordination of services from a wide variety of professionals, including the possibility of orthopedic surgery, injections of Botox or phenol, use of medications, and considerations of neurosurgical or orthopedic interventions. The therapist is a resource for the family members, who are confronted with a wide array of possibilities for interventions from television, magazines, the internet, friends, and families.

Basic Treatment Principles for Children at Level III

1. For upright posture and stability, the therapist can begin with the ABCs of posture described in the Examination section. The therapist must treat to develop alignment for efficient upright posture. The ability to keep the head stable while scanning the environment during ambulation is critical. Activities to address alignment can include promoting soft tissue length throughout the body. Providing a BOS that is large enough for stability, but not so large as to limit mobility, will require both the careful selection of an assistive device as well as the selection of orthotics. It is critical for the child to develop strategies to control weight shifting of the COM. These strategies will lead to increased balance. Strengthening of the postural muscles should include isometric work in shortened ranges. Emphasis on strengthening the extensors of the trunk and lower extremities is needed. Extended practice or experience in locomotion on the floor (eg, creeping, "bunny hopping," or knee walking), may not carry over to the development of synergies required for upright postures. A child may use these methods of locomotion at home for increased independence. However, the relative cost and benefit of promoting these patterns of mobility for a child who is anticipated to have the potential for upright locomotion are part of the educational program for the family and the child alike. The team will need to discuss the selection and use of assistive devices in different environments to allow the child immediate independent mobility without jeopardizing greater independence in the future.

2. The development of smooth forward progression with forward-propulsive forces is a complex motor control problem for the child and the therapist to address. Focus in therapy is on developing efficient forward progression of the COM with less lateral and/or up and down movement. This is promoted by facilitating increased proximal cocontraction or coactivation with axial rotation to decrease the excursion of the COM during the gait cycle. A prerequisite

to this control is spinal and rib cage mobility in all planes. The forward-propulsive forces include both phasic-burst activity from the plantar flexors as well as hip extensors. These forces may be limited if the child wears orthotics to limit movement into plantarflexion. The therapist, therefore, should have the child work both in and out of the orthotics during direct services. Concentric burst work through the lower extremities is included as well as eccentric work to control the advancement of the COM. In addition, the child must develop isolated control both between and within the lower extremities. It is more effective to stress work in stride positions for mobility rather than in a static position as synergies, including isolated or fractionated control, are used. The use of supported ambulation over a treadmill can increase the speed of the child's gait through increased isolated control and reciprocity without compromising proximal control.

3. A child at Level III frequently demonstrates difficulties related to shock absorption. These problems can decrease the efficiency of gait. There also are implications for long-term independent ambulation due to injury to the joints or soft tissues or an increased likelihood of the development of arthritic changes. The most critical factor for the therapist is to be diligent in the observation and modification of alignment. Modifications with orthotics, taping, shoes, and assistive devices can alter alignment significantly. Particular attention should be given to knee alignment as the knees are at the greatest jeopardy from forces from both above and below. This problem is complicated by the use of orthotics that may improve alignment, but can simultaneously decrease the inherent ability of the child to absorb shock because interactions within the foot or between the foot, ankle, knee, and hip are limited.

4. Energy conservation is a key issue for the child at Level III. A child in this group may ambulate well in early childhood, but then rely more and more on wheelchair transport during adolescence or adult life because of the high-energy demands experienced during ambulation. The therapist needs to monitor and appropriately treat or manage the respiratory and cardiovascular impacts of ambulation. Treatment can include addressing the patterns of respiration as well as issues of endurance, particularly as the child matures into adolescence. Posture and movement problems also change the overall efficiency of gait. The therapist should address these problems to increase energy efficiency.

Intervention for Children at Level I or II

Children who are classified as a Level I or II can ambulate independently. The therapeutic focus is generally on the child's inability to adapt walking to meet a wide variety of functional demands in different settings. Most of these children are functioning in classrooms in community schools. The expectation that, because they can walk, they will be able to participate in all areas of family and school life may create unrealistic demands on their walking abilities. Many of these children still have significant functional limitations and restrictions in participation. For example, children may be able to walk independently by using weight shifting from the upper body with lateral trunk flexion, but need assistance at school because of an inability to carry a lunchroom tray independently.

For children who demonstrate marked asymmetries both in posture and movement, the risk of secondary impairment is high, and intervention may focus on strategies to improve symmetry of gait by addressing system impairments, and, possibly, incorporating orthotic intervention.

Although the child at Level I or II is able to walk, intervention may be needed to modify the quality of his or her gait that limits function. The therapist now is responsible for gait training. The therapist may develop a plan to address parameters related to step length or line of progression to increase overall efficiency. It is very important for the therapist to address ambulation in varying environmental contexts as well as focus on functional outcomes. The therapist must plan ahead for the anticipated functional and environmental challenges for the child. To meet these outcomes the therapist will need to address the specific impairments and atypical motor components that decrease the efficiency and effectiveness of gait.

An additional question or issue that can arise is the time at which to most effectively introduce independent ambulation as a therapy outcome or goal. For example, it can be assumed that the child with a hemiplegia will ambulate independently. However, if the child begins to ambulate very early, the gait often demonstrates marked asymmetries both in posture and movement that can have long-lasting impact. Would this child's gait be more functional and efficient in the long term if the onset of ambulation is delayed until greater postural control is developed? Although it is not advisable to actively restrict a child's attempts to ambulate, it may be appropriate to focus initially on increasing control and coordination in creeping on the floor rather than encouraging upright independent ambulation. This is an unresolved issue, however, as it is not clear how much transfer there will be of postural control in one position to postural control in another position (see Chapter 1).

Therapy for children in Level I or II may include more involvement in community-based activities in addition to or in place of traditional direct services. Therapy may be more effective if performed in water, on horseback, or in a karate gym.[42] Group activities may reflect more accurately the functional demands encountered by the child.

Basic Treatment Principles for Children at Level I or II

PRINCIPLE 1

For upright posture and stability, the therapist performs an ongoing analysis and evaluation of the child's postural control while ambulating in different functional activities and environments. It is common for children functioning at this level to recruit the 2-joint long muscles for postural stability even though these muscles are more typically used for movement. The implications are a reduction in the multifunctional tasks that require both postural stability and free use of the extremities during ambulation and a reduction of overall balance. For example, the child who uses the latissimus to increase stability in the trunk by stabilizing the upper extremity to the pelvis may be unable to walk and carry large items (eg, a large box or a tray) in front of the body with 2 upper extremities for support. In addition, the child may be unable to anticipate and respond to unexpected perturbations, such as remaining standing on a bus when it departs or walking across the uneven surface of the playground. The child often will return to less refined movement patterns for stability when postural control is challenged. Postural challenges can include complex tasks, the introduction of more complicated environments, or growth. A child may walk at home with good balance and be able to efficiently anticipate changes in floor surfaces, but when in the midst of the new kindergarten classroom, trip and fall over the edge of the carpet when moving to "circle time."

Therefore, the therapist facilitates and strengthens appropriate recruitment of the postural muscles and then adds the simultaneous recruitment of the movement muscles for tasks during ambulation. It is important to work in a variety of settings and with different associated functional demands. The therapist must provide the "just right" challenge both with tasks and environments. The parents and therapist also must be prepared for skills accomplished at one age to disappear after a major growth spurt. It may be necessary to return for an episode of more intense therapy. The therapist also carefully considers the use of orthotics and/or taping to simultaneously improve alignment but reduce the degrees of freedom available for postural adjustments.

Efficient and effective forward progression also can be a problem for the child. Key factors may contribute to this difficulty:

> Inability to develop axial rotation for the management of weight shifting to aid in step length

> Inefficient use of eccentric control to manage the speed of progression

> Lack of precise timing and sequencing of muscles that adapt quickly to changes in the environment on a moment-to-moment basis

PRINCIPLE 2

The therapist focuses on the smooth forward progression of the child's COM in which the child controls the speed and direction of gait to match environmental constraints as well as functional demands. The child must be able to manage all typical environmental barriers encountered in daily life. The posture and movement impairments relating to balance and function, and the individual system impairments that impede functional progress, are addressed within functional activities. Specific attention is directed to increasing the child's ability to isolate movement both between and within the lower extremities. More complex activities such as running, jumping, stair climbing, bicycling, and roller-skating challenge the child and aid in developing greater control and coordination. Orthotics must be reviewed on a regular basis for fit and function. The orthotic that worked well for the elementary-aged child may become ineffective in the middle school–aged child because of growth and social issues. Shifts in the style of the orthotic and the wearing schedule can alter the impact of orthotic use for the child. In addition to focusing on proximal issues discussed earlier, the therapist also focuses on details of the 3-rocker action (ie, heel strike, mid-stance, push-off) of the foot as it promotes the smooth forward progression of the body mass over the alternating feet.

The therapist must address difficulties related to the child's ability to absorb shock. The child's decreased ability to isolate movement, particularly in the foot, and to time foot movement with movement throughout the rest of the body, can lead to limited functional abilities related to decreased balance. The therapist also works on issues in the musculoskeletal system, such as ROM and strengthening, as well as neuromotor control and coordination. As the child grows and the biomechanics of upright posture change, revisions in the plans for orthotics, taping, or even the provision of direct services must be reconsidered.

PRINCIPLE 3

Many typically developing children in the United States demonstrate limited physical fitness and increased risk of obesity. Children with disabilities are at an even greater risk for a sedentary lifestyle and therefore changes in energy conservation during gait should be monitored. Inefficient gait patterns gradually may lead to functional limitations. The therapist should monitor heart and respiratory rates during gait-training activities and during the introduction of new functional activities, such as stair climbing or running. A regular fitness program for the child including aspects of flexibility, conditioning, and strength can be conducted through a community program or within the school program. The therapist may need to introduce the program, monitor it for initial safety, develop parameters or boundaries of the program, and then transfer responsibility for ongoing programming to the child and/or family.

SUMMARY

Children with developmental disabilities have multiple issues that can limit their ability to functionally ambulate and, therefore, to participate fully in home, school, and community life. The therapist needs an understanding of the basics of gait and of the changes that occur across development. An evaluation that includes examination of participation restrictions, activity/functional abilities and limitations, posture and movement strengths and problems, as well as individual system integrities and impairments, provides a basis for formulating hypotheses for intervention planning. The intervention plan needs to account for children's medical diagnoses and potential for ambulation as well as current status. The therapist then selects specific strategies for intervention to reach the anticipated outcomes. In the following case studies, examination, evaluation, and interventions focused on upright posture, standing balance, and ambulation will be illustrated.

Case Study #1: Jason

> *Medical Diagnosis:* Cerebral palsy, right hemiparesis
> *Gross Motor Function Classification System:* Level I
> *Age:* 24 months

Examination/Tests and Measures

> *Anthropometric Characteristics:* Jason is noted to have a slightly smaller right upper extremity compared with the left. His lower extremities currently measure the same in length and girth. He is scheduled for evaluation by an orthopedist for a baseline study of limb length and hip stability.

> *Posture/Gait/Balance:* Jason began walking at age 15 months. His most recent test scores revealed gross motor skills between age 12 and 15 months. In standing, Jason demonstrates an asymmetrical posture with anterior tilt of the pelvis and pelvic retraction on the right. He has an observable asymmetry in his rib cage. The right upper extremity usually is held in a posture of shoulder elevation, scapular adduction with humeral hyperextension and medial rotation, and elbow, wrist, and finger flexion. Weight is shifted to his left, and the left lower extremity is in slight genu recurvatum with the right lower extremity in a posture of hip and knee flexion with the ankle in slight plantar flexion.

> Jason can maintain an upright posture against gravity. In doing so he recruits and overuses muscles of movement for stability. This limits the freedom of movement of his trunk and upper extremity. He achieves forward propulsion through space but has difficulty with grading his speed. He does not manage the absorption of shock on the right side and is therefore at risk for injury to that side. He relies heavily on momentum to advance his body in space. His gait demonstrates a short swing phase on the right, short step length, with minimal right knee and ankle flexion at mid-swing. There is short stance on the right with genu recurvatum and a valgus position of the right foot at mid-stance. He always initiates steps with his left leg.

> *Muscle Performance:* Jason demonstrates tightness to passive stretch in the hip muscles and lateral trunk flexors on the right with limitation in trunk rotation. He has weakness in the right extremities.

> *Neuromotor and Sensory Processing:* Jason can initiate, sustain, and terminate motor unit activity throughout the body. He relies most heavily on concentric and isometric contractions, particularly on the right. He has difficulty in isolating muscle activation within both the upper and lower extremities. Jason demonstrates neglect of the right side of his body, upper extremity greater than lower extremity.

> *Reflex Integrity:* He demonstrates increased clonus at the right ankle when tested.

> *Ventilation and Respiration:* Breath holding is noted during stressful activity, such as during attempted running or transitioning from the floor to standing.

Evaluation

Jason is developing gross motor skills as anticipated for a child with a hemiplegia. He is at Level I of the GMFCS. It is anticipated that he will be a community ambulator without an assistive device. He may have functional limitations related to complex environments or tasks that require precise balance and symmetrical use of the upper extremities. The slower acquisition of functional skills of ambulation is related to the complex interaction of posture and movement asymmetries; the interaction of neuromotor, sensory, and musculoskeletal impairments; and his growth. He already is demonstrating asymmetries and is at risk for developing secondary impairments, such as a scoliosis or a subluxing or dislocating hip on the right from increased femoral ante torsion.

Although at this time his leg lengths measure the same, it is anticipated that with decreased weight bearing the bone growth on the right side might slow. It is assumed that intervention can minimize the appearance of these secondary impairments. Intervention will be most necessary during growth spurts and when there are new environmental or functional demands.

> *Participation Restrictions:* Jason is not able to walk as well as his brother at home while playing and is unable to play outdoors on the playground without falling.

> *Activity/Functional Limitations:* Jason falls frequently during the day. He attempts to run, but is "clumsy" and usually falls. When he falls, he is unable to catch himself with his right hand. He is unable to keep up with peers or sibling on the playground or when playing outside on uneven terrain.

> *Impairments:* Based on the examination, several impairments that relate directly to ambulation were identified: (1) tightness in the hip muscles and lateral trunk flexors on the right side, (2) difficulty in isolating muscle activation in the right lower extremity, and (3) neglect of the right side. Jason has an asymmetrical posture in standing and during ambulation. Specific gait deviations are a short swing phase on the right and short step length. Short stance on the right with genu recurvatum and a valgus position of the right foot at mid-stance also are observed.

Goals

Treatment goals are for Jason to demonstrate the following:

1. Increased symmetry in his standing posture.
2. Increased strength in the right extremities.
3. Increased isolated control within the right upper and lower extremities.
4. Longer and more equal step lengths.

Participation/Activity Outcomes

After 6 to 9 months of intervention, Jason will be able to accomplish the following:

1. Ambulate on a community playground, mounting and dismounting from at least 4 pieces of equipment without falling.
2. Walk in his playroom at home, pick up and carry items requiring 2 hands for support, and then place the items on a shelf at shoulder height.
3. In standing, be able to quickly turn to either his left or right without loss of balance.

Intervention

Jason will continue to receive direct services from the physical therapist. A knee immobilizer and an orthosis for the right lower extremity to wear occasionally at night will be recommended. A shoe insert to aid in the alignment of the right foot during ambulation can be considered depending on foot position during gait and whether leg length discrepancy is noted. An orthopedist will follow Jason both for hip integrity and spinal alignment.

Intervention activities will focus on increasing Jason's skill in ambulation in a wider variety of environments with increasing demands for the upper body. Sessions may occur in the home, at community playgrounds, or at an outpatient facility. Soft tissue elongation using myofascial and mobilization strategies, strengthening activities, and activities to increase control and coordination of the right side will be emphasized along with increasing meaningful sensory input to the right.

As Jason matures, tightness in the plantar flexor muscles of the lower extremity should be monitored. Studies with children[43] and adults[44] with CP have suggested that impaired gait function is associated with increased passive muscle stiffness and altered central drive to the ankle muscles rather than reflex-mediated stiffness (ie, spasticity). Treadmill interventions have been shown to decrease passive stiffness with toe lift and increase heel impact both during the treadmill training and overground walking and could be considered as a future intervention.[45,46]

The parents will be instructed in activities to perform at home to generalize functional use of upright balance activities and to provide greater opportunities for motor learning. Coordination of services among the physical, occupational, and speech therapists will be achieved via telephone conversations and written communication.

CASE STUDY #2: JILL

> *Medical Diagnosis:* Cerebral palsy, spastic quadriparesis, microcephaly, intellectual deficits, seizure disorder
> *Gross Motor Function Classification System:* Level V
> *Age:* 7 years

Examination/Tests and Measures

> *Posture/Gait/Balance:* Jill demonstrates a fixed kyphosis with an emerging scoliosis. These postural deviations are noted in all postures but are most evident in sitting and supported standing. Jill will assist briefly with standing pivot transfers, but she does not maintain standing unless supported in a stander. She has limited self-generated movement, preferring to keep her COM well within the BOS. Movement that occurs remains in the sagittal plane. Her upright stability against gravity is severely limited. She does not achieve any forward propulsion. She makes no attempts to manage shock absorption. All attempts to move independently through space are very costly in terms of energy conservation.
> *Neuromotor and Sensory Processing:* Jill is able to initiate and sustain motor unit activity, but at times has difficulty with termination of the activity. Muscle contractions are limited to either concentric or isometric contractions. She therefore frequently demonstrates excessive cocontraction with resulting stiffness throughout the extremities. She has a very limited repertoire of movements available to her. She also has very little ability to isolate muscle activation and therefore recruits total patterns of flexion or extension. Her upper extremities demonstrate patterns of full flexion, whereas the lower extremities can flex or extend briefly when coupled with full-body extension. She responds to vestibular input with autonomic distress.
> *Range of Motion:* Jill demonstrates limited ROM in the neck spine, hips, and shoulders.
> *Muscle Performance:* Her strength is reduced throughout and the size of her muscles is small compared with her peers.
> *Ventilation/Respiration:* Jill demonstrates shallow respiration that is frequently asynchronous in nature. She does not always coordinate respiration with other functional activities. The shape of her rib cage makes it difficult for her to achieve chest expansion when positioned in prone or when in her prone stander. She does not always breathe regularly during transitions. She also demonstrates difficulties in the cardiovascular system with decreased distal blood supply. Her limbs become purplish when in dependent positions for long periods.

Evaluation

Jill is a young child with multiple, severe impairments that result in significant functional limitations. She functions at Level V in the GMFCS. It is anticipated that Jill will remain dependent on others for her locomotion. She may be able to learn to take assisted steps to aid in transfers and to move very short distances in the home when supported by an adult. She may have a wider range of living possibilities as an adult if she is able to transfer with the assist of one and able to take assisted steps. It is not anticipated that she will be able to ambulate, but it is important that she achieve the ability to assist more with transfers. It may be possible for her to eventually be able to take a few assisted steps to assist during activities of daily living, such as bathing. It is important that she be positioned in standing on a regular basis to improve bone density, position the soft tissues for elongation, and to improve circulation and respiration. Jill will require ongoing monitoring. If programming to address her positional changes is not integrated into her daily routines, it is anticipated that she may develop significant secondary impairments with severe medical implications. These problems could relate to her respiratory, digestive, or orthopedic status.

- ▸ *Participation Restrictions:* Jill is unable to move independently to interact with peers or the physical environment.
- ▸ *Activity/Functional Limitations:* Jill has limited floor mobility and is unable to ambulate. She is dependent on others for mobility and self-cares.
- ▸ *Impairments:* Based on the examination, several impairments were identified. The primary impairments related to her ambulatory status are her limited repertoire of movements and restricted ROM in the trunk and lower extremities. She also has generally diminished strength, endurance, and respiratory function.

Goals

Treatment goals are for Jill to demonstrate the following:
1. Improved soft tissue mobility and bone mineral density.
2. Improved respiratory and cardiovascular endurance.
3. Increased strength.
4. Increased postural control.
5. Improved isolated control in the lower extremities to allow reciprocity for assisted stepping.

Participation/Activity Outcomes

After 6 to 9 months of intervention in her school program, Jill will be able to accomplish the following:
1. Stand and transfer, with the assist of one adult supporting her around the upper chest area, from her wheelchair to a classroom chair of equal height, requiring her to take 2 steps.
2. Tolerate without signs of autonomic distress being transitioned from sit to stand when positioned in an EasyStand at least twice daily with the assist of the classroom aide.
3. Stand for a classroom activity for a minimum of 30 minutes while positioned in a standing device and while wearing her orthotics, at least 3 times per week.
4. Participate in 20 minutes of aerobic exercise with her peers while positioned either in a gait trainer or a mobile stander and assisted by a classroom aide.

Intervention

Physical therapy services for Jill will continue in the school setting for 30 minutes per week. Most sessions will be indirect, but it is anticipated that occasional periods of more intensive direct services will be necessary to introduce new skills to Jill and her classroom attendant. Instruction will be provided to the teacher as well as to the adaptive PE instructor. The current stander will be exchanged for an EasyStand to allow introduction of more dynamic transfers. This stander will decrease weight bearing through her anterior chest, and therefore improve her depth of respiration and allow more frequent changes in her posture for circulatory stimulation. The correct positioning of Jill in her adaptive equipment, signs and symptoms of distress to be observed carefully, and the timing or scheduling of positional changes will be reviewed with the staff. This plan will be reviewed with her parents annually. It is suggested that the family arrange home-based services to assist in problem-solving issues related to transferring Jill to and from the bathtub as well as in and out of the family car. This could be arranged over a summer break.

Although independent physical activities are difficult for Jill to perform, Bryant and colleagues demonstrated that a 6-week exercise intervention can have a positive effect on gross motor function in nonambulant children with CP.[47] They randomly assigned 35 children (age 8 to 17 years, GMFCS Levels IV and V) to a static bike group, a treadmill group, or a control group. Blinded assessments performed at baseline and at 6 weeks and again at 12 and 18 weeks postintervention demonstrated significant differences in GMFM–88D scores between bike and control group and treadmill and control group. A modified stationary bicycle and/or body-weight–supported treadmill may offer exercise opportunities for Jill.

Case Study #3: Taylor

> *Medical Diagnosis:* Myelomeningocele, repaired L1-2
> *Age:* 4 years

Examination/Tests and Measures

> *Posture/Gait/Balance:* Taylor can scoot around on the floor in sitting. He can walk using a reciprocation-gait orthosis and a walker. In sitting and standing, Taylor demonstrates a marked lordosis related to his surgical repair. He compensates with increased kyphosis and slumps and hangs on the ligaments throughout his spine. He prefers a very large BOS and keeps his COM low and well within the BOS. Gait analysis reveals that Taylor uses his upper extremities effectively both for support and forward propulsion. He has difficulty adapting to changes in the floor surface. He demonstrates diminished control of lateral weight shifting as well as rotation. The activity is not yet energy efficient.

> *Anthropometric Characteristics:* Taylor has small lower extremities as compared with the rest of his body. In addition his head is slightly larger in proportion because of the hydrocephalus.

> *Range of Motion:* ROM is within normal limits in the upper body. He is somewhat tight at the hip in the hip flexors and adductors and can only bring the ankles to neutral (90 degrees of dorsiflexion). The plantar fascia is extremely tight.

> *Muscle Performance:* He has generalized weakness in the upper extremities and trunk, particularly in the abdominals. The lower extremities demonstrate 0 strength on a manual muscle test.

> *Sensory Integrity:* Taylor has good vision and hearing. He has no somatosensory awareness below L1-2. He demonstrates visual perceptual problems.

> *Integumentary Integrity:* Taylor has frequent skin breakdowns at the sacral area and in his feet and ankles.

> *Ventilation and Respiration:* Taylor tends to hold his breath to increase proximal stability. He has inadequate abdominal strength for sustained exhalation. Overall pulmonary endurance is decreased as compared with his peers.

Evaluation

Taylor is a cooperative, engaging young man with many strengths and resources that make him an excellent candidate for habilitation. He will, however, always require an assistive device and use of orthotics to walk. He demonstrates the musculoskeletal impairments of decreased ROM and strength in the lower extremities, along with decreased somatosensory awareness. He has limited respiratory support for gross motor activity. These impairments prevent him from locomotion at the speed of his peers, even in his wheelchair, and ambulation in his classroom and home, even with the use of assistive devices. He is, however, intrinsically motivated to ambulate with assistive devices and has the support of his family and teachers to reach these goals. Without ongoing intervention, Taylor may be unable to achieve these reasonable goals. Developing an active lifestyle is important at this age to avoid the health risks associated with the more sedentary lifestyle of children who remain in wheelchairs for locomotion.

> *Participation Restrictions:* Taylor is unable to self-propel manual wheelchair for long distances to keep up with peers or to use assistive devices effectively to maneuver within his classroom.

> *Functional Limitations:* Taylor is unable to assume or maintain an upright position without assistance and the use of orthotics and a walker or crutches. His endurance for ambulation is limited, and he moves slowly. He cannot propel his wheelchair fast enough to keep up with his peers, especially when playing outdoors.

> *Impairments:* Based on the examination, the most significant impairments that affect Taylor's ability to ambulate are the loss of muscle function and sensation in his lower extremities. Muscle tightness and limited ROM in the lower extremities may interfere with optimal use of orthotics. Taylor also has generalized weakness in the upper extremities and trunk, as well as poor respiratory function, all of which will adversely affect his use of ambulation aids and wheelchair.

Goals

Treatment goals are for Taylor to demonstrate the following:
1. Increased upper body and trunk strength.
2. Improved respiratory support for gross motor activity.
3. Improved control of lateral and diagonal weight shifting in the standing position.
4. Increased ROM in the lower extremities for proper alignment in standing.

Participation/Activity Outcomes

After 6 to 9 months of intervention, Taylor will be able to accomplish the following:
1. Walk 25 feet (7.5 m) to move from his bedroom to the living room or down the hall of his school to his classroom while wearing his hip-knee-ankle-foot orthoses with a walker and with supervision of an adult.
2. Propel his wheelchair from his classroom to the cafeteria at the same speed of his peers both while going to and returning from lunch.
3. Move from bench sit to standing at his walker, lock his braces, and begin ambulating independently. He also will unlock his braces and lower himself from standing at the walker to sitting on a bench safely.

Intervention

Taylor will continue to be seen twice weekly for physical therapy in his preschool program. Services will be coordinated with his parents, occupational therapist, and educators. An orthopedist will continue to follow Taylor annually. Gait training with bilateral long leg braces initially using a walker, but transitioning to crutches when possible, will be initiated to increase his functional use of walking. In addition, therapy will include activities to increase Taylor's skill in self-propelling the wheelchair at greater speeds and over more varied terrains. Strengthening for the upper body will be included as well as a positioning program to aid in soft tissue elongation.

Taylor's father will begin a modified weight-training program with Taylor at home. The adaptive PE program will stress aerobic conditioning while Taylor is in the chair and will work to increase abilities in the wheelchair in modified sports such as T-ball or soccer.

Case Study #4: Ashley

> - *Medical Diagnosis:* Down syndrome
> - *Age:* 15 months

Examination/Tests and Measures

> - *Posture/Gait/Balance:* Ashley is able to roll, assume and maintain sitting, move to all fours, kneel, and pull to stand at furniture. She can take steps with 2 hands held. Ashley can assume many antigravity positions and rise up to standing with support. In all positions she uses a wide BOS and keeps the COM low and well within the middle of the base. She relies on ligamentous integrity for alignment rather than dynamic activation of her postural system. She moves more with phasic bursts of activity and then rests on ligaments for mechanical stability. She, therefore, has least stability in weight-bearing postures such as all fours or standing with support. She does not demonstrate consistent balance in any antigravity posture. Movement is slow and tends to be in the sagittal plane with little to no spontaneous recruitment of patterns that include axial rotation.
> - *Mental Functions:* Ashley is a passive child who requires a great deal of stimulation to attend to either motor or cognitive tasks.
> - *Joint Integrity and Mobility:* Ashley demonstrates hypermobility and instability at all the joints in the body. She continues to overly stretch joint ligaments in her daily postures.
> - *Muscle Performance:* She has decreased strength throughout the body with poor muscle definition.
> - *Neuromotor and Sensory Processing:* Ashley is able to initiate, sustain, and terminate motor unit activity throughout her body. She has greatest difficulty sustaining postures, demonstrating more phasic-burst activity. An assumption is made that she is using more of her fast-twitch motor units than the slow-twitch ones. She uses more concentric muscle contraction with almost no isometric or eccentric control being noted. She can set only the lower levels of dynamic stiffness and cannot control or coordinate the stiffness to meet the demands of functional tasks. She has difficulty in recruiting complex synergies that include abductor/adductor control or axial rotation. She does not demonstrate any extraneous movements. She has a mild hearing loss and signs of decreased somatosensory awareness throughout her body. She avoids movement-based activities, which suggests immaturity or deficits in vestibular function.
> - *Ventilation and Respiration:* Ashley demonstrates a decreased respiratory base for motor activity. The decreased control in her rib cage contributes to a decreased vital capacity. She has small nasal passages and is a mouth breather. She holds her breath during difficult movement transitions.

Evaluation

Ashley is a child who demonstrates many of the musculoskeletal, neuromotor, and sensory impairments associated with Down syndrome (DS). She is demonstrating functional limitations based on these impairments. She should, however, be able to walk independently in the home and, eventually, community distances. She will require regular services to establish these skills and may periodically require additional services to address changes based on her growth (ie, episodic care).

Although at this time indirect services are being provided, an episode of direct services could be considered to try to speed the development of ambulation. Without intervention it is anticipated that the onset of ambulation may be further delayed. Ashley is at high risk for injury to her joints. She also is at risk for an increasingly sedentary lifestyle with the associated cardiovascular risks.

- *Participation Restrictions:* Ashley lacks the mobility to interact effectively with peers or to explore her physical environments.
- *Activity/Functional Limitations:* Ashley does not cruise at furniture or walk without support. She does not shift her weight in standing to be able to reach for objects that are not close to her or to change her position.
- *Impairments:* Primary impairments related to Ashley's limited ambulation skills are generalized weakness, joint hyperflexibility, limited balance and postural control, and sensory hypersensitivity, especially to movement.

Goals

Treatment goals are for Ashley to demonstrate the following:
1. Improve postural stability with increased muscle coactivation/cocontraction.
2. Increase control of lateral and diagonal weight shifts in standing.
3. Maintain postures with good alignment (eg, sitting, all fours, standing).

Participation/Activity Outcomes

After 6 to 9 months of intervention, Ashley will be able to accomplish the following:
1. Cruise in both directions the length of a sofa to obtain desired toys placed at the opposite end.
2. Take steps to walk 5 feet (1.5 m) between her parents in play.
3. Push and walk behind a weighted cart across the length of her classroom.

Intervention

Ashley will continue in the infant-mother early intervention program. Additional direct services provided in the home can be considered at the parents' discretion. The use of a small bench or chair for her to sit in during daily activities should be suggested to help decrease the size of her BOS. A small but heavy baby carriage or push toy could be used at home to encourage ambulation. If possible, and if Ashley will tolerate it, stepping on a small treadmill may be beneficial. Several studies using treadmill intervention with infants with DS have demonstrated an increase in the age of achieving locomotor skills, as well as higher levels of physical activity.[48-50] Looper and Ulrich[51] compared 2 groups of children with DS receiving treadmill training. One group also wore supramalleolar orthoses (SMOs) 8 hours per day, 5 days per week, and the other group did not wear SMOs. Treadmill training ended when the children could take 3 independent steps. Because the control group (without SMOs) had higher GMFM scores, the authors concluded that orthoses may have a detrimental effect on overall gross motor skill development before ambulation is achieved and recommended that children with DS should be walking before SMOs are prescribed.

Additional therapy activities will include strengthening; facilitation to recruit the postural muscles in higher positions against gravity; guarding of the joints during weight-bearing activities; and introduction of increased weight shifting laterally and in diagonal planes while in all positions, but especially in standing. The parent will be instructed in activities to increase somatosensory and vestibular input, such as extra toweling after her bath and regular visits to a playground with play on a swing. Physical therapy services will be coordinated with the occupational therapist and special educator as well as with her pediatrician. Education concerning sequelae of common impairments associated with DS will be provided for the family.

CASE STUDY #5: JOHN

> - *Medical Diagnosis:* Developmental coordination disorder/attention-deficit hyperactivity disorder
> - *Age:* 5 years

Examination/Tests and Measures

> - *Posture/Gait/Balance:* John is able to walk and run. He can perform most basic gross motor skills and can gallop. John demonstrates decreased postural control with a tendency to recruit long 2-joint muscles in the limbs to substitute for proximal postural control. Therefore, his legs frequently stiffen and he walks on his toes. He achieves forward progression by leaning forward and relying on momentum. He does not demonstrate refined isolated or fractionated movements in the limbs. The coordination of muscles diminishes the higher up against gravity he moves, as well as the more stressful the task or environment becomes. He has difficulty modifying the movement to match the specific task or environment. He has the greatest difficulty with movements or tasks that require multisegmental coordination (eg, upper extremities with lower extremities or eyes with hands or feet). He also has difficulty in selection of movements that require axial rotation as a component. He walks with stiffened legs and with a decreased arm swing. Thus, he gallops instead of skips, throws without trunk rotation, and cannot walk a balance beam. He also has difficulty with tasks that require varying the speed of movement.
> - *Mental Functions:* John has difficulty with gradation of arousal and selectivity of attention for work. He easily becomes frustrated and throws temper tantrums frequently. His attention has improved since he began taking his medication.
> - *Neuromotor and Sensory Processing:* John can initiate, sustain, and terminate motor unit activity throughout his body. However, he has difficulty with the control and coordination of muscle activity to match functional tasks. He most commonly uses concentric or isometric muscle contraction with decreased eccentric control, especially in the lower body. He does not recruit patterns of coactivation or cocontraction proximally and instead uses sustained holding in the distal movement muscles for stability. He cannot, therefore, quickly and efficiently recruit these muscles for dynamic actions. He also demonstrates poor grading of movements. He cannot accurately recruit the appropriate level of stiffness for a task (eg, increased stiffness in the lower extremities during ambulation). He has poor coordination with increased stiffness in the upper extremities in addition to that in the lower extremities during ambulation activities. He does not demonstrate extraneous movements. Testing indicates impairments related to tactile discrimination, kinesthesia, and stereognosis. He has limitations in motor planning.
> - *Muscle Performance:* His strength is decreased both in the upper as well as lower extremities. The greatest deficits occur proximally. Endurance for physical activities is decreased compared with his peers.

Evaluation

John is a 5-year-old child with complex and interacting impairments that significantly limit his ability to function effectively in his environments. He ambulates independently; however, the combination of decreased somatosensory awareness, decreased kinesthetic awareness, and decreased control and coordination of the neuromuscular system has resulted in poor midrange control and decreased dexterity and coordination. He is an excellent candidate for intervention. If intervention is not provided, it is anticipated that he may demonstrate increasingly limited functional skills, greater frustration, and therefore avoidance of these activities. This would be detrimental for general cardiovascular functioning as well as emotional health and well-being.

▸ *Participation Restrictions:* John has difficulty walking in crowded environments at school and in the community, frequently bumping into other people or objects. He often avoids gross motor play with peers during recess at school or at the playground in the community.

▸ *Activity/Functional Limitations:* John has difficulty with age-appropriate gross motor skills, such as being able to skip. He has difficulty with ball skills while standing, such as catching, throwing, and dribbling. He is less skilled in gross motor skills as compared with his peers, and has difficulty participating in gross motor games.

▸ *Impairments:* Primary impairments related to ambulatory skills are difficulties with motor planning, motor control, strength, and selective attention.

Goals

Treatment goals are for John to demonstrate the following:

1. Increased strength.
2. Improved eccentric control.
3. Increased repertoire of synergies including those with control of lateral weight shift and rotation.
4. Increased agility during gross motor activities with more refined timing and sequencing of motor activities.

Participation/Activity Outcomes

After 6 to 9 months of intervention, John will be able to accomplish the following:

1. Participate in a group community sport such as soccer, T-ball, or a swim team on a regular basis and complete all of the basic skills required by the sport.
2. Play safely and appropriately on equipment in a local fast food restaurant playground with other children being present.
3. Walk through a neighborhood store with parent supervision for 10 minutes without bumping into any of the displays or individuals in the store.

Intervention

John's parents are encouraged to have him wear more spandex-type clothing to increase sensory organization. They also are encouraged to have him participate in either a therapeutic horseback riding program or swimming in the community. Therapy will focus on organizing sensory perceptual information during complex motor tasks as well as increasing motor control and coordination. Strengthening activities of postural muscles with increased somatosensory feedback will be included. Rapid alternating movement through full range, including both concentric and then eccentric work, in the limbs will follow. John and his family will select preferred activities for focus, such as bicycling, gymnastics, soccer, or karate, to increase John's participation. Sessions will be structured with repetitions to provide increased opportunities for motor learning. As performance improves, small group work with other boys with similar impairments and interests will be used to improve motor and social skills.

Acknowledgments

The author of this chapter wishes to acknowledge the work of Janet Wilson Howle, MACT, PT and Judi Bierman, PT, DPT, C/NDT, who authored the chapter on gait in the previous 3 editions. Much of the original material has been incorporated into this chapter for this edition, and their input and mentorship regarding the content of this chapter is much appreciated.

References

1. World Health Organization. *International Classification of Functioning, Disability and Health (ICF)*. Paper presented at: World Health Organization 2002; Geneva.
2. Engel-Yeger B, Jarus T, Anaby D, Law M. Differences in patterns of participation between youths with cerebral palsy and typically developing peers. *Am J Occup Ther.* 2009;63(1):96-104. doi:10.5014/ajot.63.1.96.
3. Alghamdi MS, Chiarello LA, Palisano RJ, McCoy SW. Understanding participation of children with cerebral palsy in family and recreational activities. *Res Dev Disabil.* 2017;69(10):96-104. doi:10.1016/j.ridd.2017.07.006.
4. Donkervoort M, Roebroeck M, Wiegerink D, et al. Determinants of functioning of adolescents and young adults with cerebral palsy. *Disabil Rehabil.* 2007;29(6):453-463. doi:10.1080/09638280600836018.
5. Livingston MH, Stewart D, Rosenbaum PL, Russell DJ. Exploring issues of participation among adolescents with cerebral palsy: what's important to them? *Phys Occup Ther Pediatr.* 2011;31(3): 275-287. doi:10.3109/01942638.2011.565866.
6. Palisano RJ, Kang LJ, Chiarello LA, Orlin M, Oeffinger D, Maggs J. Social and community participation of children and youth with cerebral palsy is associated with age and gross motor function classification. *Phys Ther.* 2009;89(12): 1304-1314. doi:10.2522/ptj.20090162.
7. Merriam-Webster. www.merriam-webster.com. Accessed August 13, 2018.
8. Looper J, Talbot S, Link A, Chandler L. The relationship between transitional motor skills and locomotion. *Infant Behav Dev.* 2015;38:37-40. doi:10.1016/j.infbeh.2014.12.003.
9. Frankenburg WK, Dodds JB. The Denver Developmental Screening Test. *J Pediatr.* 1967;71(2):181-191. doi:10.1016/S0022-3476(67)80070-2.
10. Piper MC, Darrah J. *Motor Assessment of the Developing Infant*. Philadelphia, PA: WB Saunders; 1994.
11. Størvold GV, Aarethun K, Bratberg GH. Age for onset of walking and prewalking strategies. *Early Hum Dev.* 2013;89(9):655-659. doi:10.1016/j.earlhumdev.2013.04.010.
12. Bly L. *Motor Skills Acquisition in the First Year: An Illustrated Guide to Normal Development*. Tucson, AZ: Therapy Skill Builders; 1994.
13. Alexander R. Boehme R., Cupps B. *Normal Development of Functional Motor Skills: The First Year of Life*. Tucson, AZ: Therapy Skill Builders; 1993.
14. Folio MR, Fewell RR. *Peabody Developmental Motor Scales*. Austin, TX: PRO-ED; 2000.
15. Russell DJ, Rosenbaum PL, Avery LM, Lane M. *Gross Motor Function Measure (GMFM–66 and GMFM–88) User's Manual*. London, England: Mac Keith Press; 2002.
16. Perry J. *Gait Analysis: Normal and Pathological Function*. Thorofare, NJ: SLACK Incorporated; 1992.
17. Sutherland DH, Olshen RA, Biden EN, Wyatt MP. *The Development of Mature Walking*. London, England: Mac Keith Press; 1988.
18. Bleck EE. *Orthopedic Management in Cerebral Palsy*. London, England: Mac Keith Press; 1987.
19. Stout JL. Gait: Development and analysis. In Campbell SK, ed. *Physical Therapy for Children*. Philadelphia, PA: WB Saunders Company; 1994: 127-157.
20. Bernstein N. *Co-ordination and Regulation of Movements*. New York, NY: Pergamon Press; 1967.
21. Woollacott MH, Shumway-Cook A. *Development of Posture and Gait Across the Life Span*. Columbia, SC: University of South Carolina; 1989.
22. Chiarello LA, O'Neil M, Dichter CG, et al. Exploring physical therapy clinical decision making for children with spastic diplegia: survey of pediatric practice. *Pediatr Phys Ther.* 2005;17(1):46-54. doi:10.1097/01.PEP.0000154105.19384.D3.
23. Hoffer MM, Feiwell E, Perry R, Perry J, Bonnett C. Functional ambulation in patients with myelomeningocele. *J Bone Joint Surg Am.*1973;55(1):137-148. doi:10.2106/00004623-197355010-00014.
24. DeSouza LJ, Carroll N. Ambulation of the braced myelomeningocele patient. *J Bone Joint Surg Am.* 1976;58(8):1112-1118. doi:10.2106/00004623-197658080-00013.
25. Capute AJ, Shapiro BK, Palmer FB. Spectrum of developmental disabilities: continuum of motor dysfunction. *Ortho Clin North Am.* 1981;12(1):3-22.
26. Almuhtaseb S, Oppewal A, Hilgenkamp TI. Gait characteristics in individuals with intellectual disabilities: a literature review. *Res Dev Disabil.* 2014;35(11):2858-2883. doi:10.1016/j.ridd.2014.07.017.

27. Shapiro BK, Accardo PJ, Capute AJ. Factors affecting walking in a profoundly retarded population. *Dev Med Child Neurol.* 1979;21(3):369-373. doi:10.1111/j.1469-8749.1979.tb01629.x.

28. Hsieh K, Heller T, Miller AB. Risk factors for injuries and falls among adults with developmental disabilities. *J Intellect Disabil Res.* 2001;45(pt 1):76-82. doi:10.1111/j.1365-2788.2001.00277.x.

29. Enkelaar L, Smudlers E, van Schrojenstein Lantman-de Valk H, Geurts A, Weerdesteyn V. A review of balance and gait capacities in relation to falls in persons with intellectual disabilities. *Res Dev Disabil.* 2012;33(1):291-306. doi:10.1016/j.ridd.2011.08.028.

30. Montgomery PC. Predicting potential for ambulation in children with cerebral palsy. *Pediatr Phys Ther.* 1998;10(4):148-155. doi:10.1097/00001577-199801040-00003.

31. Begnoche DM, Chiarello LA, Palisano RJ, Gracely EJ, McCoy SW, Orlin MN. Predictors of independent walking in young children with cerebral palsy. *Phys Ther.* 2016;96(2):183-192. doi:10.2522/ptj.20140315.

32. Bjornson K, Belza B, Kartin D, Logsdon R, McLaughlin J. Ambulatory physical activity performance in youth with cerebral palsy and youth who are developing typically. *Phys Ther.* 2007;87(3):248-260. doi:10.2522/ptj.20060157.

33. Fiss AL, Jefferies L, Bjornson K, Avery L, Hanna S, Westcott McCoy S. Developmental trajectories and reference percentiles for the 6-Minute Walk Test for children with cerebral palsy. *Ped Phys Ther.* 2019;31(1):51-59.

34. Ammann-Reiffer C, Bastiaenen CH, de Bie RA, van Hedel HJ. Measurement properties of gait-related outcomes in youth with neuromuscular diagnoses: a systematic review. *Phys Ther.* 2014;94(8);1067-1082. doi:10.2522/ptj.20130299.

35. Rathinam C, Bateman A, Peirson J, Skinner J. Observational gait assessment tools in paediatrics—a systematic review. *Gait Posture.* 2014;40(2):279-285 doi:10.1016/j.gaitpost.2014.04.187.

36. ATS Committee on Proficiency Standards for Clinical Pulmonary Function Laboratories. ATS statement: guidelines for the six-minute walk test. *Am J Respir Crit Care Med.* 2002;166(1):111-117. doi:10.1164/ajrccm.166.1.at1102.

37. Introduction to the Guide to Physical Therapist Practice. Guide to Physical Therapist Practice 3.0. Alexandria, VA: American Physical Therapy Association; 2014. http://guidetoptpractice.apta.org/. Accessed September 9, 2018.

38. Palisano R, Rosenbaum P, Walter S, Russell D, Wood E, Galuppi B. Development and reliability of a system to classify gross motor function in children with cerebral palsy. *Dev Med Child Neurol.* 1997;39(4):214-223. doi:10.1111/dmcn.1997.39.issue-4.

39. Palisano RJ, Hanna SE, Rosenbaum PL, et al. Validation of a model of gross motor function for children with cerebral palsy. *Phys Ther.* 2000;80(10):974-985. doi:0.1093/ptj/80.10.974.

40. Zwicker JG, Mayson TA. Effectiveness of treadmill training in children with motor impairments: an overview of systematic reviews. *Pediatri Phys Ther.* 2010;22(4);361-377. doi:10.1097/PEP.0b013e3181f92e54.

41. Chrysagis N, Skordilis EK, Stavrou N, Grammatopoulou E, Koutsouki D. The effect of treadmill training on gross motor function and walking speed in ambulatory adolescents with cerebral palsy: a randomized controlled trial. *Am J Phys Med Rehabil.* 2012;91(9):747-760. doi:10.1097/PHM.0b013e3182643eba.

42. Winchester P, Kendall K, Peters H, Winkley T. The effect of therapeutic horseback riding on gross motor function and gait speed in children who are developmentally delayed. *Phys & Occup Ther in Pediatrics.* 2002;22(3-4):37-50. doi:10.1080/J006v22n03_04.

43. Willerslev-Olsen M, Andersen JB, Sinkjaer T, Nielsen JB. Sensory feedback to ankle plantar flexors is not exaggerated during gait in spastic hemiplegic children with cerebral palsy. *J Neurophysiol.* 2014;111(4):746-754. doi:10.1152/jn.00372.2013.

44. Geertsen SS, Kirk H, Lorentzen J, Jorsal M, Johansson CB, Nielsen JB. Impaired gait function in adults with cerebral palsy is associated with reduced rapid force generation and increased passive stiffness. *Clin Neurophysiol.* 2015;126(12):2320-2329. doi:10.1016/j.clinph.2015.02.005.

45. Willerslev-Olsen M, Lorentzen J, Nielsen BJ. Gait training reduces ankle joint stiffness and facilitates heel strike in children with cerebral palsy. *NeuroRehabilitation.* 2014;35(4):643-655. doi:10.3233/NRE-141180.

46. Willerslev-Olsen M, Petersen TH, Farmer SF, Nielsen JB. Gait training facilitates central drive to ankle dorsiflexors in children with cerebral palsy. *Brain.* 2015;138(3):589-603. doi:10.1093/brain/awu399.

47. Bryant E, Pountney T, Williams H, Edelman N. Can a six-week exercise intervention improve gross motor function for non-ambulant children with cerebral palsy? A pilot randomized controlled trial. *Clin Rehabil.* 2013;27(2):150-159. doi:10.1177/0269215512453061.

48. Ulrich DA, Ulrich BD, Angulo-Kinzler RM, Yun J. Treadmill training of infants with Down syndrome: evidence-based developmental outcomes. *Pediatrics.* 2001;108(5):E84. doi:10.1542/peds.108.5.e84.

49. Ulrich DA, Lloyd MC, Tiernan CW, Looper JE, Angulo-Barroso RM. Effects of intensity of treadmill training on developmental outcomes and stepping in infants with Down syndrome: a randomized trial. *Phys Ther.* 2008;88(1):114-122. doi:10.2522/ptj.20070139.

50. Angulo-Barroso R, Burghardt AR, Lloyd M, Ulrich DA. Physical activity in infants with Down syndrome receiving treadmill intervention. *Infant Behav Dev.* 2008;31(2):255-269. doi:10.1016/j.infbeh.2007.10.003.

51. Looper J, Ulrich DA. Effect of treadmill training and supramalleolar orthosis use on motor skills development in infants with Down syndrome. *Phys Ther.* 2010;90(3):382-390. doi:10.2522/ptj.20090021.

Promoting
Upper Extremity Control

13

Anne H. Zachry, PhD, OTR/L
Anita Witt Mitchell, PhD, OTR, FAOTA

Infants and young children learn about the world around them through exploration, and the use of the hands is key. Reaching, touching, grasping, and exploring with the hands all contribute to the development of body functions, such as cognitive and sensory motor skills. Just as the hands play a role in development, they also are important tools for accomplishing activities and participating in daily life. Hand function facilitates participation in activities of daily living, such as self-feeding, dressing, and hygiene tasks; educational activities, such as handwriting and manipulating puzzle pieces; and social activities, such as using a telephone or texting a friend.

Children with disabilities may have difficulty using their hands to accomplish self-care tasks, such as manipulating fasteners on clothing or opening food containers independently; school tasks such as handwriting or creating art projects; or activities involving social participation, such as playing board games with friends. These participation restrictions can affect the children's feelings of self-worth and self-respect. Unfortunately, research indicates that children with disabilities are more likely to be isolated and even bullied in comparison with their nondisabled peers. This is concerning because social inclusion contributes to overall well-being.[1]

Overcoming challenges with functional hand use leads to increased independence for children with disabilities and may break down barriers to social inclusion. For these reasons, a primary goal of therapists is to support children's development of upper extremity control and hand function to the greatest extent possible. This chapter will describe a dynamic systems approach to understanding hand function and typical development of upper extremity functioning. Suggestions for evaluation and intervention strategies for children with limitations in hand skills are provided.

DYNAMIC SYSTEMS THEORY

Traditional neuromaturational theories of development are based on the assumption that motor skill development is dictated by the central nervous system. From this perspective, development is genetically predetermined, linear, and hierarchical.[2] In contrast, dynamic systems theory (DST) posits that development is driven by intricate bidirectional interactions between the task,

Connolly BH, Montgomery PC, eds. *Therapeutic Exercise for Children With Developmental Disabilities, Fourth Edition* (pp 367-396).
© 2020 Taylor & Francis Group.

individual, and environment.[3] The DST of motor development can be used to guide therapeutic interventions in children with developmental delays. (See Chapters 1 and 9 for additional discussions of DST.)

The assumptions of DST are that development is complex, nonlinear, emergent, and self-organizing,[4] and that a child's brain is not preprogrammed to drive development through a predictable sequence of motor milestones. Rather, a complex interaction between the individual, the environment, and the task leads to the emergence of new motor behaviors.[5] For example, when an infant learns to reach, the emergence of this skill is influenced by subsystems such as body composition, muscle strength, musculoskeletal integrity, motivation, context, and the physical characteristics of the item for which the child is reaching. During the early stages of reaching, there is instability and considerable variability; however, with repetition and practice, a new, more stable pattern emerges.[5] Instability in movement patterns, or transition states, are called *perturbations* and can be triggered by a growth spurt, a period of illness, and a number of other external or internal factors.[5,6] With transitions, motor patterns have a tendency to become preferred "attractor states," which generally are stable; however, attractor states are not always fixed and have the potential for transformation.[7] During times of instability, motor skill patterns are especially amenable to change. As infants experiment with novel motor patterns, new forms of movement emerge, thus offering an opportune time for therapeutic intervention to facilitate more functional movement strategies.[8,9] This is the premise behind early intervention. That is, owing to a child's ongoing growth and development during the first 3 years of life, unstable periods are common. These early periods of instability offer optimal opportunities for therapeutic intervention.

When novel motor behaviors emerge, constraints in various subsystems within the child, the context, or the particular task may facilitate or restrict the developmental process.[10,11] These constraints, or rate-limiting factors, guide motor actions in a certain way and may prevent a child from successfully performing a developmental activity or functional task.[8] During intervention, therapists often alter rate-limiting factors to increase independence and improve function.[8] For example, low muscle tone is a constraint that could prevent an infant from engaging in hand-to-mouth exploration, and a therapist might use handling or positioning techniques to facilitate midline exploration and mouthing of the hands.

Person

From a dynamic systems perspective, the distinct mental and physical characteristics of an individual interact with environmental factors and task requirements to influence development. For example, body structures such as the central nervous system, the sensory systems, anatomical structures, height, and weight interact and influence the production of body functions such as perception, cognition, and motor actions. Body functions such as motivation, attention span, anxiety, and cognitive capacity also interact with the environment and task to influence development.

Historically, motor skill and intellectual development were considered to be independent of each other; however, a recent systematic review supports the premise that cognitive and motor skill development are interrelated.[12] This relationship is logical in that intellectual impairments may limit curiosity, decrease motivation, and deter goal setting, resulting in decreased environmental exploration, thus negatively affecting the acquisition of motor skills.[13] Additional research by van der Fels et al[12] reveals that bilateral coordination is strongly related to abstract reasoning and problem solving, and fine motor coordination is associated with visual-processing abilities. Moreover, a number of studies confirm a direct relationship between early motor proficiency and future cognitive functioning and academic achievement.[14-16] These findings are supported by studies that reveal cognitive processing and the execution of motor actions involve the activation of common brain structures (ie, the prefrontal cortex and the cerebellum).[17]

Our senses help us perceive our world, and perceptual processing is linked with cognitive and motor skill development.[18] For example, one method children use to distinguish features

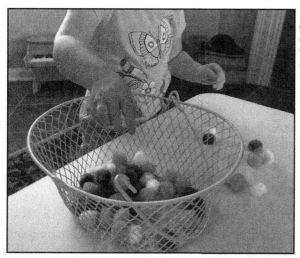

Figure 13-1. Task constraints that influence the dynamics of the reach include the size and shape of the object, the distance of the object from the child, and whether the object is stationary or moving.

of the environment is through processing of sensory input, such as visual, tactile, auditory, and proprioceptive information. Haptic perception, which involves using sensory feedback from the hands to take in and process discriminative information, is used to differentiate the sizes, shapes, and characteristics of objects. Sensory feedback also guides and directs movement, and conversely, motor actions, such as manipulating objects with the hands, influence how sensory information is processed[19,20] (see Chapter 9).

Musculoskeletal impairments in children can occur as a result of congenital anomalies, disease, or injury. These impairments may influence movement patterns and have the potential to lead to activity limitations. To understand how musculoskeletal impairments influence movement patterns, it is important for therapists to use their observation skills to identify any biomechanical constraints, and then analyze the complex interactions between the anatomical structures, the environment, and the task.[21] Frequently, biomechanical limitations lead to compensation or adaptation of the task.

Task

When a task is carried out, the movement pattern is influenced by the interaction between the individual, environmental factors, and the task at hand. Additionally, changes in task requirements can lead to variability in motor actions. For example, if a child is reaching for something, a variety of task constraints influences the dynamics of the reach, such as the size and shape of the object, the distance of the object from the child, and whether the object is stationary or moving[11] (Figure 13-1). This variability allows the individual to meet a wide range of task demands.

Environment

The environment is the third system in DST that influences motor skill development. Physical, social, and cultural aspects of the environment may constrain or promote development.[8,22] Cross-cultural research reveals that different parenting practices have the potential to influence motor skill development in a variety of ways[21] (see Chapters 1 and 2). For example, in cultures where babies have regular opportunities to practice standing and stepping, the babies have an accelerated onset of walking,[19,21] whereas children who are adopted from institutionalized settings often present with delayed motor skill development because of limited movement opportunities early in life.[22] Social deprivation has been found to negatively affect motor skills, specifically manual dexterity.[23] Conversely, increased exposure to manipulative activities in the home setting has a positive impact on fine motor skill development.[24] Considering this evidence, it is clear that the impact of environmental context on motor functioning is a key factor for therapists to consider during assessment and treatment planning and when recommending home programming.

Summary

When therapists use the DST perspective, all interactions among the individual, environment, and task carefully are considered. Therapy providers also need to have a thorough understanding of typical upper extremity development to guide the clinical reasoning process; therefore, an overview of hand skill development is presented.

OVERVIEW OF HAND SKILL DEVELOPMENT

At birth, infants have minimal control over their bodies, but soon purposeful movements begin to emerge. Motor skill development generally progresses directionally: cephalic to caudal, proximal to distal, and gross to fine. For example, neck and head control emerge first, followed by gains in trunk control, and eventually control of the arms and hands. The sequence of motor milestone achievement is relatively predictable, but the developmental rate varies from child to child,[25] likely because of differences in person, task, and environmental constraints.

Proximal to Distal Progression

The progression of proximal to distal control of the upper extremity can be observed in infant development. Examples include emergence of control of the proximal muscles and joints of the shoulder before fine control and skilled use of the hand are achieved, and the more proximal palmar grasp of objects appearing before development of a fine precision grasp with the fingers. Despite these examples of proximal to distal development, research suggests the relationship between proximal and distal control is not a causal one.[26-29] Instead, the relationship has been described as "interdependent"[26,30] and "functional."[26,27] Some authors suggest that neurological control systems for proximal and distal functions are separate,[31] and that only a small percentage of the variance in fine motor control is explained by postural stability in typically developing (TD) infants.[26,28,32]

The interdependent and functional relationship between proximal stability and upper extremity function is exemplified by the coordination between reach and postural control.[33,34] Anatomically and physiologically, the shoulder girdle is attached to the thorax, and reaching involves more than one joint. The shoulder girdle must have full flexibility to allow the arm to have full range of motion, thereby giving the hand access to a large range in space. At the same time, the shoulder girdle must have a variety of strong, stable, fixed points for actions specific to upper extremity function. Research has shown that the speed and accuracy of upper extremity movements increase with reduced postural demands.[29,35,36] Presitting infants demonstrate smoother coordination of reach with either external support for postural control in sitting or achievement of independent sitting.[35,36]

On the other hand, the act of reaching can challenge postural stability. Van Der Fits and Hadders-Algra[34] documented the complex postural adjustments that accompany reaching in 4-month-old TD infants. Use of the arms for reaching can destabilize the body, and the head and trunk must make compensatory movements to maintain the center of gravity and postural stability.[26,29,37] Thus, the infant practices postural responses during reaching, and postural stability is enhanced (see Chapter 10).

In preterm infants with delayed postural control, Wang and colleagues[30] found a significant relationship between postural control and fine motor skills. In these infants, up to 25% of the variance in fine motor scores on the Peabody Developmental Motor Scales, Second Edition was explained by postural control scores. This was particularly true for the younger (6 months' adjusted age) preterm infants with poor postural stability. Indeed, when flexibility and stability of the shoulder are missing and there is concomitant instability or immature postural control, compromised patterns of movement of the upper extremities often are observed. With poor joint alignment, the child may not be able to position the hips adequately to obtain a functional base of support for sitting. The child may lack postural control against gravity and be unable to maintain balance during the weight shift needed for a particular functional activity. The upper extremities may need to be used to assist the child to maintain a sitting position, preventing their use to explore and manipulate objects, thus thwarting the practice needed to develop hand skills.

When scapular instability on the rib cage is a problem, the child may compensate in a variety of ways. For example, in quadruped, the child may markedly internally or externally rotate the upper arms to achieve mechanical stability, or hip flexion may be used to keep most of the body weight on the legs instead of the arms. The child may move quickly between positions using momentum rather than postural control to shift weight. The child may coactivate muscles on one side of the body for stability and direct movements asymmetrically, always moving one favorite side. The child may not feel secure enough to attempt transitional movements, thereby limiting the ability to move and explore the world. Hence, poor proximal stability may inhibit interaction of the infant with the environment and hinder new actions such as reaching and manipulating objects. These new actions could contribute to the development of improved postural stability.

Sequential Development of Hand Skills

The following sections will describe the sequence of hand skill development. When assessing hand skills, therapists commonly use a development perspective as a framework for identifying delays, impairments, or absence of typical hand skills and determining the need for intervention. The typical developmental sequence also may be used as a guide for goal setting and treatment planning.

Reach

The upper arm plays a primary role in reaching. Specifically, its job is to project the hand appropriately in a wide and varied range of space with precise timing, allowing direction of the hand to an object, or placement of the hand on a surface for weight bearing. In the newborn, arm movements seem somewhat random, asymmetrical, and uncontrolled, but around age 2 months, as scapular–rib cage stability and integration of visual regard and proprioception improve, infants swipe and bat at objects.[38] Hand-to-mouth and self-touching behaviors also are observed. Self-touching is important as research suggests this behavior is a precursor that leads to the development of reach and grasp.[39] Scapulohumeral mobility develops between age 3 and 6 months, and successful reaching begins around age 3 months. Early on, reach is characterized by symmetrical, bilateral movements to midline, but little anticipatory control of distal joints or the hand in preparation for grasp. Poor planning and greater variability of movement contribute to clumsiness when reaching. At age 6 months, unilateral reaching emerges as internal stability of the scapula and shoulder improves. Although in sitting, infants up to age 8 or 9 months continue to use the rib cage to stabilize the humerus during manipulation. Active thoracic extension that occurs during prone play prevents excessive scapular winging and facilitates medial scapular stability. Humeral and trunk stability continue to increase through infancy, and once infants are able to sit independently and creep on all fours using alternating limb movements, a more mature unilateral pattern of reaching emerges.[40] Weight-bearing and weight-shifting experiences during creeping and crawling and transitions between positions (eg, all fours to sitting) contribute to further development of scapular and shoulder stability and controlled mobility. This allows for reaching, holding in space, and corrective movements during reach. The arm can be used to produce lateral protective responses, reach and grasp overhead objects, don and doff clothing, and perform personal hygiene. Specific movement patterns used vary with the constraints of the task, environmental factors, and the individual infant's body functions and structures.[37]

Dynamic elbow control also contributes to reach, allowing the elbow to move slowly through its range and hold in midrange. Thus, the arm can become shorter or longer, bringing the hand either closer to or farther away from the body for accurate reach and transitional movement patterns. These skills emerge around age 5 months, as the infant pushes up on extended elbows in prone and continues as the upper extremities are used to bear weight in transitions to sitting and all fours. Dynamic elbow control can then be integrated during self-care skills, such as holding a bottle at age 6 to 7 months or finger feeding at age 8 to 9 months.

The forearm and wrist orient the hand in space during reach and in preparation for weight bearing or weight shifting. Forearm rotation is critical for function and develops as a result of controlled humeral rotation, balanced elbow flexion and extension, and the prone weight-shifting experiences that begin around age 4 to 5 months. Prone weight-shifting on extended arms contributes to development of balance between long finger flexion and extension across the wrist joint, which is necessary for internal stability of the wrist. Prone-on-elbows play experiences allow the child to isolate forearm movements, while humeral movements are restricted by the weight-bearing posture. Bringing toys to the mouth while weight bearing in prone also allows isolated movement of the elbow with separation of forearm movements in space. The young child generalizes isolated wrist control by using it in self-feeding and play at age 8 to 9 months; however, in sitting, the infant initially stabilizes the humerus against the rib cage while experimenting with forearm rotation. Humeral and trunk stability continues to improve through infancy, and by age 12 months, the infant can control forearm supination and pronation in a variety of positions. As strength and control develop, the young child is able to turn doorknobs and eat with a spoon more efficiently.

Grasp

The newborn's hands follow the pattern of physiological flexion, with occasional opening observed. From the flexed posture, voluntary grasp emerges, first as a whole-hand or palmar grasp. As the infant uses this grasp in hand-to-hand, hand-to-knee, and hand-to-foot play, the hand experiences the potential for accommodation. Generally, the hand shapes itself around an object and accommodates its own shape to the shape to be held or the shape and contour of the weight-bearing surface. To do this, it must be expandable enough to flatten out for weight bearing. The hand also must be malleable enough to shape itself around large and small objects. Over time, tactile and visual input contribute to the development of anticipatory movements that assist the hand in shaping and accommodating to the size and shape of objects and surfaces, even before the hand contacts the object or surface.

The hand, at times, needs to be powerful and, at other times, delicate in its approach to grasp and manipulation. The ability of the hand to be functional in all these situations depends on a variety of arching systems in the palm. The capability for arch development in the hand relies on a balance of activity between the long finger flexors and extensors, the capability for neutral alignment between wrist and hand, mobility of the carpal and metacarpal bones, and activity of the intrinsic muscles of the hand. Ungraded pressure with the child's first attempts to grasp helps make the arches malleable. Early weight-shifting experiences on extended arms from around age 5 months and throughout the first year of life help to expand the hand and develop balance reactions from the arches. The web space of the thumb opens and allows for the development of thumb opposition.

Controlled grasp can begin once the hand is stable in a neutral position at the wrist. Weight-bearing and weight-shifting experiences contribute to stability of the wrist and metacarpophalangeal (MCP) joints, which in turn, allows differentiation of the ulnar and radial sides of the hand and more isolated movements of the hand and fingers. As the baby creeps while holding a toy in the hand, the muscles on the ulnar side of the hand are elongated, contributing to dissociation of the radial and ulnar sides of the hand. With the sides of the hand differentiated, the radial side can be used for a variety of fine grasp patterns, while the ulnar side provides power grip and stability during fine motor activities. The infant's interest in objects, along with sensory discrimination and feedback, encourages the use of the hands for exploration and further facilitates development of fine grasp patterns.

As the sides of the hand become differentiated around age 7 months, grasp transitions from a whole-hand or palmar grasp to a radial palmar or superior palmar grasp. In this grasp, the object is held by the radial side of the hand, while the ulnar side is used for stability. The infant also engages in scratching of surfaces and crude raking of small objects, providing additional sensory feedback. With improving finger isolation, the 8- to 9-month-old infant is able to grasp small objects using the radial fingers and thumb; however, poor intrinsic control precludes fine tip-to-tip precision grasp. Instead, scissors (thumb to lateral border of the index finger) and 3-point (thumb opposed to index and middle fingers) grasps are observed. Between age 9 to 12 months, the infant develops the ability to use MCP joint flexion with graded interphalangeal joint extension, allowing refinement of 2-point prehension. An inferior pincer, (ie, pad-to-pad) grasp emerges, followed by the more precise superior pincer (ie, tip-to-tip) grasp. Initially, external stability from the table surface is needed when these grasp patterns are used, but by age 12 months the infant is able to use a superior pincer grasp without external stabilization. Improved coordination, speed, and accuracy of grasp are observed. By age 15 months, the infant uses a variety of grasps and is able to shape and accommodate the hand to the size and shape of objects. However, force regulation is poor, and the infant may tend to crush paper cups or less sturdy objects. The ability to scale grip force and motor output to the size of objects continues to be refined through the first 7 years of life, and may not reach adult levels until age 8 to 10 years.[27,41]

Release

Through the first 5 months of life, release of objects occurs involuntarily and reflexively. A number of body functions must mature to allow the emergence of voluntary release, including tactile and proprioceptive discrimination, cognition, visual control, grip force regulation, timing of movement, and movement patterns characterized by inhibition of finger flexion and controlled contraction of the extensors. Purposeful release begins as the infant learns to transfer objects from hand to hand. At first, the infant may transfer objects by using one hand to pull a toy from the other or by bringing the toy to the mouth, placing both hands on the toy, and then removing one hand. Purposeful release using a surface or the mouth for assistance begins between age 7 and 10 months, at which time babies often begin flinging and casting objects. As graded finger extension improves, 12- to 24-month-old children start to stack blocks and other objects with more precision, at first externally stabilizing the arm on the surface (Figure 13-2).

Over the next several years, with improved internal stability of the upper extremity and increased control over the intrinsic muscles of the hand, graded release with precision, dexterity, and speed is observed. Young children learn to use release skills to throw a ball, using sequencing and timing of mobility and stability at joints throughout the upper extremity.

In-Hand Manipulation

Once grasp patterns have developed, the young child begins learning to use these skills to manipulate objects within the hand. This ability is called *in-hand manipulation*. In-hand manipulation allows the child to adjust the position of objects in the hand for efficient use, aiding in accomplishment of activities such as buttoning, snapping, tying, and using forks and pencils effectively. In-hand manipulation involves a complex set of skills that rely on many underlying body functions. These include stability of the upper extremity, particularly the forearm, wrist, arches, and thumb. Mobility and control of the hand and individual fingers, dissociation of the sides of the hand, sequencing and timing of movement, grading of grip force, motor planning, tactile and

Figure 13-2. A child stacking blocks with precision.

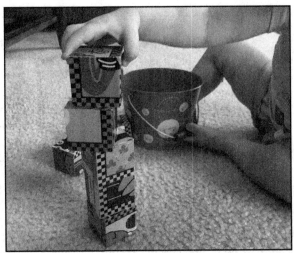

proprioceptive discrimination, visual acuity and perception, cognition, and motivation are all involved in in-hand manipulation. Three primary types of in-hand manipulation—translation, rotation, and shift—are described in the literature.[41]

Translational movements are linear movements of objects from the fingers to the palm or palm to fingers. For example, these movements are used to pick up coins and store them in the palm or to move a coin from the palm to the fingers for placement in a piggy bank or vending machine. Finger-to-palm translation is the first in-hand manipulation skill to emerge, as it involves more basic movements from finger extension to finger flexion. It occurs around age 12 to 15 months, whereas the isolated thumb control and controlled finger extension needed for palm-to-finger translation occur later, after age 2 years.[41]

Rotation is an in-hand manipulation skill that involves moving an object around its axis, for example, to open a small lid or turn a pencil over to erase. When objects are rotated more than 180 degrees, it is considered complex rotation, while rotating objects less than 180 degrees is considered simple rotation. Simple rotation is observed after age 2 years, but complex rotation does not emerge until age 3.5 to 5.5 years, as complex rotation requires thumb opposition and skilled isolation of the thumb and fingers.[41]

The third type of in-hand manipulation skill is called *shift*. Shift can occur horizontally or vertically. An example of horizontal shift is the movement used for aligning snaps. Vertical shift is used to position the fingers closer to the pencil lead for writing, to button a button, or to lace a bead on a string. Shift is observed in children age 3.5 to 5.5 years and requires isolated thumb movements with reciprocal finger movements.[41]

In-hand manipulation may occur with or without stabilization, that is, with or without holding other objects in the hand. In-hand manipulation with stabilization tends to be more difficult, as it requires manipulation by the radial side of the hand along with simultaneous use of the ulnar side of the hand for holding the additional objects. Combinations of in-hand manipulation skills, such as shift with stabilization and complex rotation with stabilization are accomplished around age 6 to 7 years. Continued refinement of the speed and skill of in-hand manipulation occurs up to age 12 years. Children with hand skill impairments may compensate for a lack of in-hand manipulation by using the alternate hand, body, or surface to assist with adjusting the position of the toy or object in the hand.[41]

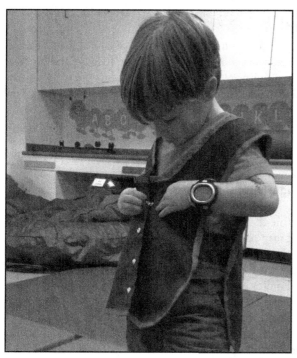

Figure 13-3. Bimanual skill practiced in self-care task of dressing.

Bimanual Skills

At age 4 to 5 months, infants begin to use both hands together in a more organized manner, for example, bringing both hands to a toy at midline. Seven-month-olds use bimanual skills for reaching and grasping large objects and will hold a toy with one hand while exploring it with the other. Bimanual skills also are practiced as the baby transfers toys from hand to hand. By age 9 months, the infant holds a toy in each hand and bangs them together, and around age 11 to 12 months, is able to use the 2 hands in complementary activities, during which one hand stabilizes the object while the other manipulates it.

Research has shown that the onset of upright locomotion influences bimanual skills.[40,42] That is, once infants begin to cruise around furniture, an increase in bimanual reaching often is observed. This apparent regression to a less mature bimanual reaching pattern has been attributed to a variety of factors, including motor reorganization, biomechanical influences related to the use of the upper extremities during cruising, new learning opportunities afforded by the upright position, and the need to shift attentional resources from reaching to the demands of upright locomotion.[40,42] Nevertheless, once infants have acquired the ability to walk unsupported, they return to the more mature unilateral pattern.[40]

By age 2 to 3 years, the young child is able to manipulate objects with both hands simultaneously and perform differentiated activities, such as cutting with scissors and stringing beads. Bimanual skills are practiced in many self-care tasks during the preschool and early school years (Figure 13-3).

By around age 6 years, children learn to coordinate the use of both hands in complex motor sequences such as tying shoes. Over time, with refinements in body functions such as visual-perceptual, cognitive, and motor skills, the ability to use bimanual skills with complexity, speed, accuracy, and precision increases.[27,41]

Tool Use

The use of tools is essential for everyday life, for children as well as adults. Children must learn to use forks and spoons to feed themselves, hairbrushes and toothbrushes for hygiene and grooming, and pencils for written communication. Tool use involves the integration of multiple body functions in the context of a particular task, considering the environment and its constraints. For example, a child's ability to use a writing utensil to successfully complete a handwritten assignment in the classroom may be limited by impairments in the motor skills needed to manipulate a pencil, visual-perceptual skills needed for letter formation, or cognitive skills needed to remember shapes of letters. Task constraints, such as the type of writing utensil and paper used, or time limits imposed are also considerations. Environmental constraints, such as distracting visual or auditory input, also may pose challenges for the child who is learning to use a pencil to produce written work in the classroom.

Between age 2 and 5 years, children refine the motor skills needed for tool use. Early motor patterns for tool use often involve a fisted grasp pattern, which is altered over time as the child explores and practices using the tool.[43] As the child practices tool use, visual and tactile perception facilitates exploration and learning about the tool characteristics that constrain its functions. Research has shown that preschoolers adjust motor output, such as movement amplitude and grip force, based on the characteristics of the tool.[44,45]

To use tools effectively, one must simultaneously stabilize the tool and manipulate it with the fingers. Separation of the sides of the hand is required to accomplish this. A stable wrist assists with forceful grip and use of tools and affords greater precision than movements controlled by the elbow or shoulder.[43] Effective tool use also requires an active MCP arch and the ability to flex, extend, abduct, adduct, and rotate at the MCP joints of the 2 radial digits. Full thumb range of motion is needed for stability of the open thumb web space. Bimanual skills often are involved in tool use, as one hand stabilizes the object while the tool is used to act on it. Examples include stabilizing paper while writing, or stabilizing a block of wood while hammering a nail into it.[43] The development of hand preference also contributes to the effective, efficient use of tools. Between age 4 and 5 years, children tend to automatically use the more skilled hand to grasp and manipulate tools. From middle childhood and into adulthood, skilled use of tools continues to improve to proficiency and mastery, and the variety of tools used increases.[27,46]

Given the number of systems that interact to influence tool use, it is not surprising that motor patterns and grasps used for a tool may vary widely and may change in response to the task or the environment.[47-50] In fact, research has shown that a variety of pencil grips can be used with equivalent speed, legibility, and endurance.[51-54] From a DST perspective, children need to adopt grasps that allow smooth coordination and fine control of the tool—given a particular task and environment—rather than to develop a particular grasp.

Eating utensils are some of the earliest tools used by infants. Cultural conventions dictate the type of utensil used for self-feeding, and social learning contributes to developing children's use of tools. In Western cultures, learning to use utensils for self-feeding begins with a fisted grasp of the spoon at age 10 to 11 months, but mastery of spoon-feeding (ie, gripping the spoon using the fingers and forearm supination) does not occur until around age 3 years. Forks and knives require additional force for their use and often are held in a fisted grasp until around age 10 years, when most children are able to feed themselves independently, using utensils with dexterity and control, including in-hand manipulation for positioning utensils in the hand.[27,46]

Tools used for hygiene include toothbrushes and hairbrushes. Use of these tools requires skilled use of the wrist and hand and the ability to manipulate the tools without vision or by using a mirror to assist. Supervision often is needed for these tasks through the preschool years, with independence achieved during the elementary school years, depending on the specific tools used and preferred hairstyles.[27]

Practice is required for children to develop efficient use of tools, including scissors. Besides experience with scissors, stability of joints throughout the upper extremity and dissociation of the ulnar and radial sides of the hand are needed to accomplish smooth, coordinated use of scissors to cut lines and shapes. During cutting, the ulnar fingers of the hand remain fairly still, while the radial fingers open and close the scissors. Without practice, 3-year-old children may have difficulty positioning the scissors in their hands and coordinating the upper extremity stability and mobility needed to use scissors effectively. At age 3 years, children tend to snip with scissors, using alternating total flexion and extension of the fingers rather than continuous, smooth movements with the ulnar fingers motionless.

The definition of a mature scissors grasp depends on the type of scissors. Mitchell and colleagues[47] found that adults used different grasps for scissors with circular loops than for scissors with oval loops. In both cases, the loops were positioned between the proximal and distal interphalangeal joints of the fingers; however, with oval loops, it was common for adults to place their index, middle, and ring fingers through the loops. With circular loops, only the middle finger was placed in the bottom loop, with the index finger stabilizing outside the bottom loop. In both cases, the ulnar fingers were flexed and used for stability, with the wrist slightly extended during cutting. The forearm was stable in mid-position and the elbow was flexed.

Ratcliffe et al[48] found that less than 25% of 4- to 6-year-old children grasped scissors by placing only the middle finger in the bottom loop. Whereas a majority of the 4-year-olds demonstrated mature forearm positions, wrist stability in extension was uncommon. These researchers also found the children used a less mature cutting approach for more complex shapes such as circles. When cutting circles, they tended to pronate the forearm, with abduction of the humerus. Based these findings, maturation of scissor skills appears to occur beyond age 6 years.[48]

As with other tools, the earliest grasps of pencils and crayons tend to be whole-hand or fisted. With exploration and practice, these power grips transition to static grips with the pencil held in the fingers and then to grasps allowing skilled movement of the radial side of the hand with ulnar stabilization. A common grasp used by TD children is a dynamic tripod grasp, in which the pencil is held between the index finger and thumb, while resting on the lateral surface of the middle finger. The thumb is opposed, with an open web space, and the ulnar fingers are flexed for stability. Although many children use the dynamic tripod grasp by around age 6 years, a number of grasps that can be used for efficient, effective handwriting have been identified. Consistent with DST, evidence suggests grasps used for writing utensils are influenced by characteristics of the individual, the task, and the environment. For example, changes in grasp patterns can be observed with changes in the characteristics of the writing implement and with changes from writing to coloring tasks.

ACTIVITY LIMITATIONS AND PARTICIPATION RESTRICTIONS

Therapists share a common goal in treatment, which is to guide the child toward a life of participation and independent functioning. For this reason, it is important to identify all impairments, activity limitations, and participation restrictions when assessing a child. Impairments such as spasticity, decreased balance, muscle weakness, range of motion limitations, poor motor control, and challenges with executive functioning often lead to activity limitations and participation restrictions.[55] For example, if a child presents with muscle weakness in the hands, the weakness may lead to an activity limitation of self-feeding, which could result in decreased mealtime participation.

Research suggests impairments, activity limitations, and participation restrictions are correlated, but this is not always found.[8,56,57] Therefore, therapists must carefully analyze and understand relationships that are present to guide assessment and treatment.[55] Because participation is the ultimate goal of treatment, it is important to consider how environmental factors affect participation.[58-60]

Figure 13-4. Body functions such as spasticity, abnormal synergies, weakness, impaired proprioceptive sense, and poor tactile discrimination may all contribute to difficulties using the hands for play, self-care, and other activities.

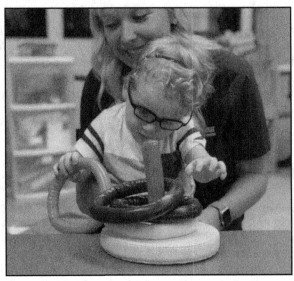

Children With Disabilities

Children with a wide variety of disabilities experience hand skill impairments, and specific impairments have been associated with certain disabilities. For example, children with attention-deficit hyperactivity disorder have been observed to reach more quickly than TD children, but these movements tend to be inaccurate and result in the need for additional movement to correct for endpoint errors. Children with developmental coordination disorder have difficulty anticipating where the hand will contact the object and preparing the hand for grasp. Visual perceptual impairments and poor motor learning can interfere with reach and grasp for children with spina bifida, and difficulty using feedback to control and monitor movements often affects reach and grasp skills of children with Down syndrome. A number of hand skill impairments have been identified in children diagnosed with cerebral palsy (CP). These include slower movement time, incoordination, disproportionate grip force, poor anticipatory shaping of the hand to match the shape and size of the object being grasped, poor timing of finger closure on an object, and mirror movements of the hands. Body functions such as spasticity, abnormal synergies, weakness, impaired proprioceptive sense, and poor tactile discrimination may all contribute to difficulties using the hands for play, self-care, and other activities (Figure 13-4).[27,29,61]

Examination and Assessment

The first step in assessment is to identify the child's strengths and needs in terms of the ability to accomplish activities and participate in necessary, expected, and desired aspects of life. Standardized tests such as the Pediatric Evaluation of Disability Inventory—Computer Adaptive Test,[62] the Roll Evaluation of Activities of Life,[63] or the School Function Assessment[64] can be used. Standardized tests such as the Melbourne Assessment, Second Edition[65]; the Functional Dexterity Test[66]; the Peabody Developmental Motor Scales, Second Edition[67]; and the Bruininks-Oseretsky Test of Motor Proficiency, Second Edition[68] can help define the role upper extremity dysfunction plays in activity limitations and participation restrictions. Chapter 2 provides in-depth discussion of factors used for selection of specific tests and measures. Standardized testing provides an objective, scientific basis for identifying developmental delays, determining the need for intervention, and monitoring the effects of intervention; however, standardized assessments may not provide the flexibility needed for assessment of young children or those who are severely involved. Using norm-referenced standardized tests to monitor progress may obscure improvements in children

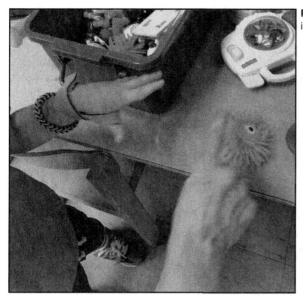

Figure 13-5. Lack of mobility and joint range that interferes with reach and grasp.

with permanent motor impairments, as the rate of progress may lag behind the rate of change in TD children. Further, Aslam et al[69] reviewed 19 commonly used pediatric upper extremity assessments and found that none of the instruments included items that comprehensively assessed body structures, body functions, activities, and participation. Interviews of family members and other professionals involved with the child and clinical observations in natural environments can provide the comprehensive information that is essential for intervention planning, regardless of the type or severity of the disability.

Basic questions can be used to guide clinical observations:

> Can the child use his or her upper extremities to help with movement in and out of positions?
> Can the child use one or both upper extremities to dress, use the toilet, and self-feed?
> Can the child use his or her hands for classroom learning?
> Can the child use his or her hands to explore and play with objects in the environment?
> Can the child use his or her arms and hands for mobility aids or transfers?

Questions should be asked about how the child uses the upper extremities during performance of activities. For example, does the child move his or her arms typically during activity? Is there an increase in muscle tone, atypical patterns, breath holding, or compensations? What consistent problems seem to interfere with activities that the child is unable to perform? What body functions and structures contribute to challenges using the upper extremities for activities and participation in physical, social, and cultural environments? For instance, activity limitations or participation restrictions may be due to a lack of mobility. The child may not have enough joint range to accomplish the activity or there could be poor joint alignment (Figure 13-5). Difficulties in sensory processing may also interfere with the child's motor abilities. Sensory organization contributes to the child's ability to plan movements and interact with the world. The inability to organize and process sensory information may make learning frustrating.

The child's use of each joint or segment of the upper extremity can be assessed and described. For example, the upper arm can be described in terms of the ability to move through the full range of reach, hold the reaching posture against gravity, correct the reach during movement, time the reach appropriately, reach with and without grasp, reach in a variety of directions, coordinate reach and postural control, accept weight on forearms, weight shift on forearms, move in and out of prone propping, demonstrate asymmetrical arm and hand use, use a bilateral approach, and demonstrate unilateral control. Assessment of the elbow may include the ability to bring the hand to the body, face, or foot; accept weight on extended arms; move in and out of extended-arm weight-bearing postures; orient the lower arm and hand appropriately in space in preparation for grasp; use a variety of forearm positions; or hold an object while moving the forearm and wrist. Evaluation of hand function may address the child's ability to bear weight on the hand; weight-shift over an open hand; use a variety of grasps with speed and precision or immobilize an object in the hand; orient and shape the hand and fingers based on the size and shape of the object; manipulate an object between 2 hands; perform various types of in-hand manipulation; regulate grip force appropriately; use tools efficiently; and release objects of varying sizes, shapes, and weights with precision and without having to fling the object or flex the wrist to let it drop.

INTERVENTION

Collaboration between the child, caregivers, and professionals involved in the child's care will result in goals that are meaningful and motivating for the child and the family. These goals then can be addressed in a variety of ways and may involve interventions that prepare the upper extremities for function, those that provide practice of upper extremity skills, and those that focus on the use of the upper extremities to participate in valued life activities.

Interventions Used to Prepare the Upper Extremity for Function

A splint or orthosis is a device worn by a patient that provides joint support and alignment and may improve upper extremity function.[70] There are 2 types of hand splints, nonfunctional and functional.[71] Nonfunctional hand splints are fabricated for the purpose of preventing or correcting contractures and often restrict active hand movements and hinder function. Alternately, functional hand splints position the hand for the purpose of improving hand function during tasks such as self-feeding or writing.[72] The evidence supporting the effectiveness of splinting in isolation is limited, but findings from several studies indicate functional hand splints may improve upper extremity function during tasks or activities.[70,71,73,74]

Strengthening is a frequently used approach during the preparation phase of intervention that involves the application of resistance during various activities or on a stand-alone basis to increase strength and endurance.[72] Therapists use a variety of strength training approaches, which is appropriate, as research suggests that upper extremity muscle weakness negatively affects a child's performance in daily activities.[75,76] Based on a critical review of the literature, Rameckers et al[72] suggested that strengthening programs should be carried out at least 3 times per week for a minimum of 8 weeks. For a child-centered focus, therapists should consider incorporating strengthening into purposeful activities or play.

Another preparatory technique often used by therapists is stretching, as it is important for flexibility. However, studies of passive stretching have not found stretching to have long-lasting benefits in patients with spasticity.[77] Increasing the duration and intensity of a stretching program and adding orthotics may be beneficial, and another option is to actively involve the patient in the stretching process while increasing ranges of movement.[78,79] Moreover, Wiart and colleagues[80] suggested that therapists emphasize active movement opportunities for children instead of focusing on stretching for maintenance of flexibility.

Voluntary movements used for functional activities require effort, and this may increase the atypical or less desirable muscle tone and poor postural control often observed in the child with CP. Preparing the child before practicing a skill will make the task less effortful and will help the child develop some of the motor components that may be missing. Achieving scapulohumeral mobility, for example, will give the child the potential for increased range of reach during functional movement. A TD infant acquires freedom of the humerus in the scapulohumeral joint while transitioning from supine to side-lying and rolling from supine to prone. As the weight of the trunk is loaded onto the upper arm in these transitional movement patterns, elongation of the musculature between the humerus and scapula and between the humerus and rib cage will give the child the freedom to initiate upper arm movements in a greater range. Reaching in prone then stimulates the child to use this new range. For the child with poor scapulohumeral mobility, activities incorporating rolling, transitional movements, and reaching in prone can provide experiences that help improve scapulohumeral mobility. For a young infant, these can be facilitated during developmental play, and for an older child, they can be integrated as part of an obstacle course or when playing a board game in the prone position.

Facilitating scapulothoracic activity will help develop the stability needed for controlling reach in mid-ranges. Active thoracic extension and scapular stability can be promoted through prone positioning and weight shifting during play. As body weight is transferred off the shoulders and onto the abdomen and thighs, the child can begin to push up on forearms and the spine extends. With volitional or accidental weight shifting, the scapula begins to hold onto the rib cage. As the child develops endurance in spinal extension, reach can be added.

Shoulder girdle and elbow strength allow use of the arms for transitional movements, for functional transfers, and as mobility aids. In typical development, infants develop strength and endurance in the shoulders and elbows by using slow, graded movements as the arms push the body from one position to another. This developmental play begins with the 5-month-old infant pushing up on extended arms in prone and continues as the child transitions from propping on his or her side up to sitting, sitting to quadruped, and creeping in quadruped. Incorporating these developmental skills in playful treatment activities can facilitate the development of shoulder girdle and elbow strength.

Developing isolated elbow movements is critical to self-care skills. Isolated elbow movements are used by young infants for hand-to-mouth play in supine and for prone weight-bearing and transitional movements. Dynamic elbow control developed in these positions can then be used for accurate, controlled reach when activating and exploring toys. Similar experiences can be used in treatment to assist the child in moving the elbow through the range of motion using slow, graded movements.

Isolated control of the forearm and wrist can be facilitated by prone play. The mobility needed for forearm rotation is enhanced by weight shifting prone on forearms as the child shifts weight back to the elbows and actively moves the forearm and wrist. Active weight shifting on extended arms in prone elongates the muscles around the wrist and facilitates internal stability of the wrist. These types of experiences can be used in therapy to help develop isolated control of the forearm and wrist for use during functional activities.

Facilitating hand function requires a combination of therapeutic activities. Weight shifting on extended arms in quadruped and in transitional movements helps to expand the hand so it will be malleable enough to actively arch during grasp and manipulation. The palm of the hand is the proximal point of control for the fingers. Ongoing hand-to-body play provides the hand a sensation of accommodation in which the hand shapes itself around objects. Helping the child grasp with the hand held in a neutral position at the wrist will facilitate an appropriate balance between flexion and extension over the wrist, through the palm, and over the metacarpal joints.

Simulating a skill through play helps the child use the movements and plan the sequence without the stress of the actual task. For example, pushing a large toy or therapy ball will give the child experience with elbow extension for crutch walking. Placing hoops on the feet will prepare the child for putting on socks, orthotic devices, and shoes.

Interventions Focusing on Practice

Children learn to develop skills through successive approximation with much repetition. Repetition brings the skill from a conscious to a more automatic level (ie, motor learning);

therefore, the skill must be practiced. For example, a study of TD children found that incorporating motor learning principles, such as randomly ordering and varying practice of tasks that allow exploration of different solutions, was effective not only for learning motor skills, but also had cognitive benefits.[81]

During practice, caregivers often need to help children with developmental delays cope with any problems that occur. Functional skills often are learned in small parts. If a child is not having success in the development of independence, the task may need to be broken down into smaller steps (refer to Chapter 1 regarding motor learning issues and Chapter 3 on short-term goals). Many verbal cues may be needed. Children can be coached while practicing in therapy, at home, or at school. They may not always know when they are being successful or recognize improved skill or efficiency of movement. Temporary adaptations also may be helpful during a training program. Seating devices, for example, help the child work on upper extremity movements required in a task without demanding control of his or her whole body at the same time. Temporary adaptations should be reevaluated frequently and removed when possible and when the child can function without them.

Occupational and physical therapists use a variety of therapeutic interventions that provide practice of upper extremity skills to improve function. Approaches that incorporate practice include constraint-induced movement therapy (CIMT), bimanual therapy, mirror therapy, neurodevelopmental treatment (NDT), and visual motor interventions. Some of these approaches are more evidence based than others.

Constraint-Induced Movement Therapy and Bimanual Therapy

CIMT was originally developed for adults recovering from stroke, and involves physical restraint of the nonaffected upper extremity to increase functional use of the affected arm and hand. A variety of restraints can be used with CIMT, such as casts, splints, mitts, and slings.[82] Classic CIMT involves physical restraint of the less affected limb for 90% of a child's waking hours for 2 weeks accompanied by intensive training for 6 hours each day. Early studies found that CIMT resulted in increased use and improved motor functioning of the affected arm in children with hemiplegic CP.[83,84] A meta-analysis by Sakzewski and colleagues[85] revealed CIMT is more effective in improving upper extremity function when compared with standard care. Chiu and Ada[86] conducted a systematic review and found CIMT to be more effective than no intervention, yet no more effective than a similar amount of upper extremity practice without restraint.

Modified CIMT is an approach in which variations in constraints are used, with a decreased intensity and duration of the repetitive unimanual task practice as compared with traditional CIMT. Modified CIMT is considered to be more child friendly than the traditional approach, and studies have found it to lead to improvements in the use of the affected upper extremity.[87,88]

Hand-arm bimanual intensive therapy (HABIT) is a child-friendly approach formalized by Charles and Gordon[89] that involves extensive bimanual practice that takes place during play and activities of daily living. Studies have shown intensive bimanual training leads to neurological changes, including increases in the motor map size of the affected hand, and improvements in functional bilateral upper extremity coordination.[90,91] CIMT and HABIT involve task-oriented practice, and both approaches have been found to be more effective than standard care in improving arm and hand function in children diagnosed with hemiplegic CP.[92] CIMT leads to greater improvements with unimanual performance of the affected upper extremity, whereas bimanual training leads to better bimanual coordination; therefore, when selecting a specific intervention, therapists should consider the particular outcomes desired by the child and family, as CIMT and HABIT are both useful approaches.

Mirror Therapy

Mirror therapy is an intervention in which a patient with hemiparesis observes the synchronous reflection of the unaffected arm in a mirror rather than directly viewing the movement of the affected limb. A number of studies have found that mirror therapy improves upper extremity motor functioning in adults. In children diagnosed with spastic hemiparetic CP, the research on mirror therapy is mixed but promising, with preliminary studies suggesting improvements in motor control, tactile perception, strength, and function.[93-96]

Neurodevelopmental Treatment

NDT is a hands-on intervention directed at improving the function of children who have difficulty controlling movement. With NDT, therapists use handling techniques to guide children's movements to improve motor function. The effectiveness of NDT has not been clearly established through research because of inconclusive and mixed findings.[97-99] However, in one study, short-term, intensive NDT was perceived to be beneficial by parents.[100]

Visual Motor Intervention

Children with developmental delays often have challenges with visual motor skills, and research has found visual-motor interventions to be effective.[101-106] For example, in a study by Ratzon et al,[103] after 12 weeks of intervention, the treatment group demonstrated improvements with fine motor skills, eye-hand coordination, and copying. Case-Smith[101] found improvements with scissor skills, motor accuracy, and writing in an intervention with preschool children who were receiving therapy services; and finally, another study revealed that a visual-motor intervention can be effective for children with and without disabilities.[104]

Interventions Focusing on Participation

Participation is a critical concept. Improving reach or in-hand manipulation in a clinical context, without carryover or transfer to daily-life activities, has little value for the child and caregivers. Using hand skills for successful and satisfying participation in everyday activities provides valuable sensory repetition, which contributes to hand-skill development as well as independence. A child with a disability may need even more repetition, especially if nonfunctional habits have developed. Thus, interventions that address preparation, practice, and participation may be complementary and overlapping.[87]

Motor-learning principles can provide a useful framework for interventions that focus on use of the upper extremities for participation in daily-life activities. Motor-learning principles incorporate a dynamic systems approach by considering the interaction of systems that may limit participation in desired activities, including those related to the child, the task, and the environment. Adaptations of the task itself or of the physical or social environment may be incorporated to support successful performance of the activity. Thus, goal-directed practice and feedback are provided within an environment that helps stimulate the child's exploration and development of motor patterns for successful accomplishment of the activity. For example, a child who has difficulty separating the skill and power sides of the hand to manipulate scissors effectively may benefit from modification of the physical environment by using adapted scissors that require simple whole-hand grasp and release for cutting sturdy construction paper rather than standard copy paper. Therapist feedback and guidance can supplement the intrinsic information the child receives from performing the task, focusing on the goal of staying on the lines to cut a shape. Physical and verbal guidance and demonstration may be helpful during early learning. The therapist can provide knowledge of performance or knowledge of results, assisting the child in assessing motor performance, detecting errors, and evaluating the outcome. This allows the child to problem solve and identify motor patterns and strategies that meet the demands of the task (ie, staying on the line to accurately cut the shape).[87,107]

For complex activities, interventions to address participation also may incorporate behavioral principles such as shaping, reinforcement, and scaffolding.[87,108,109] The desired activity may be broken into smaller steps, and reinforcement of approximations of each step can be provided as the child practices and learns the whole task or activity.[87,108] Research has shown that transferring the activity into natural physical and social environments by partnering with the family and incorporating play can be an important step in achieving effective outcomes.[108-111] Cognitive Orientation to Daily Performance (CO-OP) is a problem-solving approach that uses motor learning principles and cognitive strategies to improve performance of specific tasks. In the CO-OP approach, children are taught a Goal-Plan-Do-Check strategy to generate solutions to movement problems during chosen activities. Therapists use a guided discovery process to help the child determine the most effective solutions for improving task performance. CO-OP has been used effectively to assist children with CP in achieving goals related to donning and doffing clothing, using fasteners, eating with utensils, printing, throwing and catching, and tying shoes—all of which involve use of the upper extremities.[112] Similarly, a single case study demonstrated effectiveness for achieving handwriting and cutting goals, as well as improving motor performance, in children with attention-deficit hyperactivity disorder.[113] Children with developmental coordination disorder also have benefitted from the application of CO-OP for achieving writing, cutting, and utensil-use goals.[114] Research suggests children and families are satisfied with outcomes attained using CO-OP and that it may be effective for transfer and maintenance of skills.[112-114]

Home programs can be used to facilitate carryover of hand skills into daily activities and promote participation, as they provide repeated structured practice in natural environments.[115,116] Home programs should be based on reasonable expectations that consider individual and environmental factors. Expecting caregivers to work with their child on dressing in the morning before school may not be reasonable. It may be more feasible to work on dressing and undressing in the evening at bath time or in the family room after school when the child can practice in a leisurely manner. Home programs that address child and caregiver goals in a reasonable manner, use evidence-based interventions, and support and coach the caregiver in implementation are more likely to be effective.[115,116]

Morgan et al[117] conducted a systematic review of motor interventions for children with CP and found promising interventions were those incorporating principles consistent with a focus on participation, which included active movement by the child, task-specific training, and environmental modification. An earlier meta-analysis supported the use of goal-directed interventions targeting goals identified by the child and family and incorporating motor learning approaches.[85] Consultation and home programs can be effective means of service delivery when focusing on participation.[85,110]

Examples of intervention strategies for developing upper extremity function and addressing independence and participation are illustrated in the following case studies.

CASE STUDY #1: JASON

> *Medical Diagnosis:* Cerebral palsy, right hemiparesis
> *Gross Motor Function Classification System:* Level I
> *Age:* 24 months

Participation Restrictions

Jason experiences challenges with age-appropriate self-care tasks, school skills, and play. For example, he is unable to participate in games that require symmetrical weight bearing on his upper extremities, such as "frog jump."

Activity/Functional Limitations

Jason does not bear weight symmetrically on his upper extremities. He also does not use his right arm well for transitions such as moving from sitting on the floor to hands and knees, moving from supine into sitting, or moving from quadruped to right-side sitting. He demonstrates a gross grasp with poor control of release with his right upper extremity. He does not use his right hand and arm when undressing, nor does he use his right arm and hand effectively for manipulation of toys. Jason's lack of isolated forearm and wrist movements are reflected by the absence of symmetrical prone play experiences. He does not have the hand expansion that normally occurs during extended arm weight-bearing positions. He also does not participate in hand-to-body play that contributes to the ability to control and shape the hand for functional tasks.

Impairments

Jason presents with poor proximal control. Obvious instability is observed in scapular winging, but other subtle areas of instability also are found in the glenohumeral joint, clavicle, and right side of the rib cage. Poor scapulohumeral rhythm is noted with his attempts at movement. Because the scapula pulls away from the ribs, rather than upwardly rotating as he reaches, the humerus mechanically cannot move above 90 degrees. Atypical posturing of the right arm in humeral extension, adduction, internal rotation, and elbow flexion along with his associated reactions during effort may be Jason's attempt to control his posture and movements without the proximal control that should be present.

Jason presents with a lack of adequate protective responses with his right upper extremity when falling backward or to the right side in sitting or standing. He has poor motor control of the right upper extremity for fine motor tasks. Flexion dominates the posture of the involved arm with weakness in elbow extension, and stiffness in the hand that occurs with efforts at movement against gravity. Although a clinical description might indicate increased "tone," the underlying impairment may be more related to problems with motor control.

Jason demonstrates poor sensory awareness on the right side of his body, sensory disregard of the right upper extremity, and an inability to tolerate or interpret light touch. He also has a hypersensitive palmar grasp. Jason's feeding issues may be related to poor oral-motor control and oral sensory impairments.

Intervention

Intervention strategies to increase sensory input and awareness to the right side of the body can be incorporated into Jason's therapy sessions and home program (see Chapter 9). Weight bearing and weight shifting on the forearms and extended arms will increase sensory awareness as well as shoulder girdle stability, elbow extension strength (with arms extended), and endurance.

Obstacle courses and games such as "wheelbarrowing" and "frog jump" can be incorporated during therapy and his home program. Symmetrical flexion and extension upper extremity movements can be facilitated through assisted weight shifting in sitting or on hands and knees while on sofa cushions, bolsters, or balls. Playing in prone over a roll or wedge can facilitate increased range of reach of the right arm and facilitate a more extended and functional arm position. Playing with weight on the elbows, as in a prone-on-elbows position, can help free the forearm and wrist for functional activities such as manipulating toys.

A modified CIMT program can be implemented. For example, this program might involve Jason wearing a removable mitt on his left upper extremity during a therapy session or during prescribed home therapy activities once per day.

Sticker play will facilitate simultaneous use of 2 hands. Placing stickers on the left hand, forearm, and upper arm, for example, will require the stickers being removed with the right hand.

Finger feeding with the right hand will stimulate functional use, with the mouth serving as a point of stability. Using both hands to manipulate toys appropriate for his intellectual level (eg, toy accordion, pull-apart toys) will challenge him to develop improved fine motor control and bilateral hand use. These "prepare" and "practice" procedures may be used to prime the impaired systems for use during "participate" interventions. His play environment can be modified by using large balls, stackable blocks, and other large toys during play. Incorporating these types of toys can allow Jason to explore various movement solutions when playing with toys that typically require bimanual activity. Practice of these play activities would focus on the end goal (eg, successful stacking of large blocks) rather than the movement pattern, and varied practice would be incorporated by stacking blocks in various ways. During coloring activities using his left upper extremity, he should be prompted to stabilize the paper with his right arm. Age-appropriate feedback to assist with evaluating performance and detecting errors during goal-directed practice can facilitate Jason's identification of an optimal movement solution that promotes age-appropriate play with his sibling and peers (Video 13-1).

Jason occasionally assists with undressing using his left upper extremity and shows beginning interest in toilet training. Verbal and physical guidance can be used as necessary to shape and scaffold skills needed for successful age-appropriate donning and doffing of clothing. Modifying task and environmental constraints, such as the position for dressing, type of clothing (eg, elastic-waist pants), and size of clothing (eg, avoiding tight-fitting clothing), can support Jason's success at learning to undress and dress. Learning dressing skills through make-believe and dress-up games can vary the context for developing these skills and facilitate attention, motivation, and repetition. Shaping, chaining, and scaffolding, as well as physical and verbal guidance can be used as needed. A home program can be developed in collaboration with the caregivers to incorporate learned skills in natural environments. Caregivers can be coached to integrate motor learning principles during practice at home.

Participation/Functional Goals

After 3 months of intervention, Jason will be able to accomplish the following:

1. Demonstrate awareness of temperature differences in environmental objects with both hands (eg, warm oven surface vs cold metal surface).
2. Play reaching, throwing, and catching games with his sibling using a 12-inch (30-cm) diameter ball, incorporating forward reach with elbows extended with minimal assistance, 2 of 5 trials.
3. Grasp a hat with both hands and reach overhead with both arms to place it on his head, 2 of 5 trials.
4. Use both hands to take off socks independently, 2 of 5 trials.
5. Walk with the right arm flexed less than 90 degrees during outdoor play, using the right arm to attempt to break his fall when he loses his balance, 1 of 4 occurrences.
6. Run with the right arm flexed less than 90 degrees during outdoor play, using the right arm to attempt to break his fall when he loses his balance, 1 of 4 occurrences.
7. Stabilize paper with the right hand while scribbling with a large marker with the left hand.

CASE STUDY #2: JILL

> *Medical Diagnosis:* Cerebral palsy, spastic quadriparesis, microcephaly, intellectual deficits, seizure disorder
> *Gross Motor Function Classification System:* Level V
> *Age:* 7 years

Participation Restrictions

Jill is unable to feed herself, assist with dressing, or manipulate toys during play.

Activity/Functional Limitations

Jill lacks enough upper extremity control to propel her wheelchair or use other mobility devices. Her ability to assist with dressing is limited, such as consistently pushing her arm through a coat sleeve. Impaired upper extremity range and control prevent free and varied reach for play and environmental interactions. Her lack of upper extremity control also presents challenges with using a communication board. Jill's eye-head coordination is limited. She attempts to grasp, but her hand closes involuntarily prior to obtaining objects. Without a basic palmar grasp pattern, the development of release and manipulation is inhibited.

Impairments

Jill presents with impaired upper extremity range and control. Her use of head and neck hyperextension with tongue retraction virtually "locks" the neck and upper body together. She responds to head and neck hyperextension by pulling the shoulders forward. The shoulder elevation she maintains helps to support her head but limits attempts at head movement, contributing to her poor head control.

Jill's eye tracking is inadequate because she cannot visually scan her environment efficiently. Her lack of downward gaze is consistent with neck hyperextension. Her eyes and head may attempt to move together but her head control is too poor to allow coordinated eye-head coordination.

Shoulder girdle immobility limits her reach to 60 degrees of humeral abduction. Limited spine and rib cage mobility result in a poor base of support for dynamic shoulder girdle function. Scapulohumeral and humeral-rib cage immobility limit her arm movements to humeral extension, adduction, and internal rotation, indicating she has not yet developed voluntary control of her hands. In summary, Jill has generally decreased range of motion of the spine, rib cage, and shoulder girdle. She has poor motor control over her head, trunk, and upper extremities. Poor ocular control contributes to lack of eye-hand coordination. Additionally, Jill has intellectual and attentional deficits.

Intervention

Activities should be incorporated into Jill's daily routine to facilitate relaxation and increased range of motion of her trunk and upper extremities. Slow, passive trunk rotation in supine or sitting will increase spinal and rib cage mobility. This will facilitate general relaxation and decreased stiffness. Slow oscillating movements of each glenohumeral joint will facilitate relaxation and increase her potential range and variety of reach. Assisted movement in and out of side-lying will improve mobility between the scapula and humerus. Assisted expansion of her hand in weight bearing or onto body parts (such as the pressure of her hand onto her knee) may assist her in developing body awareness and control of grasp and release.

Strategies that prepare and practice should be implemented followed by opportunities to reach actively to accomplish functional or recreational tasks (eg, touch a communication board, bat at a joystick, activate a switch toy, bat a balloon). Practicing these skills in the natural environment will allow Jill to problem solve in the context of typical constraints she may encounter. Varying her position or the position of the target objects can facilitate adaptive problem solving and assist with generalizing skills to the ever-changing natural environment. Physical guidance can be provided as needed. Owing to attention and intellectual impairments, Jill may require longer processing time when practicing goal-directed activities. The tasks and environment can be modified to support Jill's successful participation, but errors and mistakes during practice may provide learning opportunities.

Participation/Functional Goals

After 3 to 6 months of intervention, Jill will be able to accomplish the following:

1. Reach above 60 degrees in 3 of 5 trials while in supported sitting to accurately touch a communication (eg, picture) board.
2. In supported sitting, visually follow moving objects to 30 degrees left and right from midline or scan nonmoving stimuli to find appropriate pictures on a communication board.
3. Grasp an object placed in her hand to activate a switch during a play activity, 5 out of 10 attempts while in supported sitting.
4. Release a beanbag that is stabilized by an adult into a target container during play, 1 of 5 attempts while in supported sitting.
5. Use one upper extremity to bat at a joystick in preparation for a trial with a power mobility device.
6. Maintain elbow extension while pushing her arm through a coat sleeve with no more than 2 physical prompts.
7. Use a switch to activate the television and videos.

CASE STUDY #3: TAYLOR

> *Medical Diagnosis:* Myelomeningocele, repaired L1-2
> *Age:* 4 years

Participation Restrictions

Taylor presents with participation restrictions during play, preschool academic activities, and self-care. He is unable to keep up with peers when propelling his wheelchair long distances in the community.

Activity/Functional Limitations

When playing with toys in unsupported sitting, Taylor fatigues more quickly than his peers. He also has difficulty with tracing circles and squares and connecting dot-to-dot patterns with crayons (preschool academic activities). Taylor has a limited ability to assist with lower extremity dressing and undressing tasks, needing adult assistance and supervision.

Impairments

Taylor demonstrates generalized weakness and poor endurance in his upper extremities. He also has visual-motor and visual-perceptual impairments. He presents with a loss of sensory integrity and motor control in his lower extremities related to the level of his myelomeningocele.

Intervention

Negotiation of scooter board obstacle courses will provide practice with visual-motor integration, spatial perception, and coordinated use of the arms for planned movements. This activity also will contribute to increased strength and endurance of the upper extremities. General strengthening activities such as prone push-ups, wheelchair push-ups, and "tug-of-war" games would be appropriate. Hand strength can be improved by completing arts and crafts or other activities using pinch-type clothespins or a paper punch. Balloon "tennis" using a lightweight badminton or ping-pong racket will require eye-hand coordination.

Direct practice of adapted dressing techniques on the floor, bench, toilet, or mat table should be incorporated into his daily routines. Arts and crafts activities will provide practice with visual-spatial tasks. Varying practice will promote development of different strategies that can be used for participation in daily activities. Verbal cueing can be used to help Taylor attend to relevant features of the varied tasks and the environment. Task and environmental modifications may include positioning for stability or clothing modifications such as Velcro closures on shoes. Demonstration and physical guidance can be used as necessary. Assistance with performance evaluation and error detection can be provided after the task is completed.

Participation/Functional Goals

After 3 months of intervention, Taylor will be able to accomplish the following:

1. Maneuver through an obstacle course for 3 minutes while using his arms to push a scooter board (supported prone on the scooter board).
2. Put on and remove sweatpants with minimal assistance while sitting on the floor, leaning against furniture or a wall, 3 of 5 trials.
3. Trace a circle and square with 1/8-inch (3 mm) lines using a large colored marker, deviating from the line 2 times or less, 3 of 5 trials.
4. Self-propel his wheelchair for 10 to 15 minutes during community outings with 3 brief rest breaks.

CASE STUDY #4: ASHLEY

› *Medical Diagnosis:* Down syndrome
› *Age:* 15 months

Participation Restrictions

Ashley is limited in her play repertoire as compared with her preschool classmates, and she is unable to keep up with her peers.

Activity/Functional Limitations

Ashley is slow during anterior and posterior movement transitions. She uses her upper extremities to assist but locks her elbows into extension and externally rotates her humerus during the transitions. Ashley has not yet developed goal-directed play. Rather than manipulate toys, she prefers to bang all objects on surfaces. She "flings" objects to dispose of them, and she is unable to feed herself.

Impairments

Ashley has generalized hypotonia, poor scapulothoracic stability, weakness, and limited endurance for motor activities. She also has poor balance (ie, impaired postural control). Ashley is unable to control movement patterns that require rotation of body weight over either arm, and she cannot pick up small pellet-sized items or release objects with control. Ashley demonstrates sensitivity to movement-based activities and has a mild hearing loss. Intellectual deficits are present.

Intervention

Assisted bouncing on extended arms in a hands and knees position on a small trampoline or therapy ball will help increase muscle coactivation around joints and provide increased proprioceptive and vestibular input. Activities with assisted transitions in and out of side-sitting and hands and knees will provide Ashley movement experiences requiring trunk rotation. The therapist should assist Ashley during these transitions and manually prevent her from locking her elbows. Playing in a quadruped position (eg, "horsey" or "doggie") with diagonal movements also requires improved motor control involving the shoulder girdle. Ashley should be provided weighted, resistive toys to improve hand strength, increase sensory input, and upgrade prehension patterns. Sticker play and finger feeding, with facilitation of palmar arches, will help develop pinch. Tearing paper of different thickness will require bilateral hand use and facilitate increased hand strength. These activities can help Ashley prepare and practice underlying skills needed for participation in daily activities.

Goal-directed play should be emphasized during Ashley's preschool sessions. Encouraging reaching and grasping of toys in different positions during the activities described above will help challenge postural control and assist Ashley in developing strategies for functional reaching in a variety of positions. The objects themselves may be presented at varying distances. Sitting on different surfaces (eg, the floor, a firm mattress, a foam mat) can provide variability and promote problem solving for motor solutions to the problem of maintaining postural control during reaching. Physical cues and guidance can be used to assist as needed. Presenting objects such as rings and a ring stack or shapes and a shape sorter in a vertical plane may assist with grasp and release as well as purposeful play, and again, provide variability in the task. Sizes and textures of objects also should be considered when choosing toys to challenge but promote success. Ashley can practice finger-feeding various types of "meltables" at snack time to facilitate practice of self-feeding skills.

Participation/Functional Goals

After 3 months of intervention, Ashley will be able to accomplish the following:
1. Release simple shapes into a shape sorter on verbal request (without flinging) while playing with her caregiver, 5 of 10 trials.
2. Pick up and feed herself a "meltable" textured food (eg, a small piece of graham cracker), without "raking," 3 of 10 times.
3. Participate successfully in 2 goal-directed activities with adult encouragement during each preschool session.

CASE STUDY #5: JOHN

> • *Medical Diagnosis:* Developmental coordination disorder/attention-deficit hyperactivity disorder

> • *Age:* 5 years

Participation Restrictions

John does not like to participate in age-appropriate games, such as catch, as he is uncoordinated in relation to his peers.

Activity/Functional Limitations

John is clumsy with utensils, such as silverware, and demonstrates poor coordination with paper and pencil tasks in his academic setting. He also has difficulty with buttons, snaps, and zippers on clothing.

Impairments

John has a decreased attention span. He has upper extremity weakness and poor endurance for gross and fine motor activities. John has poorly coordinated movements for fine motor tasks associated with academic skills and self-cares. Right-/left-hand dominance is not consistent, and he has sensory processing problems in the areas of tactile discrimination, kinesthesia, and stereognosis.

Intervention

Because tactile discrimination problems often are associated with fine motor and motor-planning problems, emphasis on tactile activities (eg, using water, play dough, sand) and games requiring stereognosis and other aspects of tactile perception should be included in John's therapy and home programs (see Chapter 9). Activities providing proprioceptive input to his hands (eg, navigating through obstacle courses on all fours, scooter board games, and resistive activities such as molding with clay) can help prepare John for participation in activities requiring fine motor coordination. John can be supervised at the local playground with emphasis on climbing skills to develop upper extremity strength and provide proprioceptive input. An individualized exercise video ("starring John") using elastic tubing and small hand weights can be developed to exercise along with 2 to 3 times each week. His karate class also will provide opportunities to develop upper extremity strength.

Repeated structured practice will help promote John's participation in everyday activities. He should be encouraged to use a knife, fork, and spoon during mealtime. He can help make simple snacks, for example, using a knife to put peanut butter and jelly on bread. Using different types of foods will provide varied practice. A slanted writing surface will help with wrist extension and grip positioning on pencils, crayons, and markers for academic activities. Multisensory prewriting activities will be beneficial, such as forming shapes and lines in shaving cream or textured finger paint.

John's parents can modify dressing tasks by purchasing clothing that is easier for him to manage independently (eg, shirts with large buttons, jackets with large zippers) until his skill with clothing closures improves. If he expresses interest and it is not frustrating for him, piano lessons would provide an opportunity for participation while facilitating fine motor control and planning. When practicing these activities, feedback to assist with error detection and exploration of various movement strategies can be provided, along with light physical guidance and verbal cues as needed during practice. The CO-OP approach would be appropriate, with John incorporating the Goal-Plan-Do-Check strategy.

Participation/Functional Goals

After 3 months of intervention, John will be able to accomplish the following:

1. Use a fork during mealtime to successfully stab food, 4 of 5 trials.
2. Use a butter knife during mealtime to spread butter on a slice of bread evenly, 4 of 5 trials.
3. Independently button and unbutton large buttons on a shirt, 4 of 5 trials.
4. Independently zip and unzip the zipper on his jacket after being assisted to engage the zipper, 4 of 5 trials.
5. Be able to identify a quarter, nickel, and penny in his pocket without using vision.
6. Cut out large, simple shapes (eg, circle, square) with 3/8-inch (10-mm) lines with scissors, deviating from the line fewer than 2 times.

REFERENCES

1. Murray C, Greenberg MT. Examining the importance of social relationships and social contexts in the lives of children with high-incidence disabilities. *J Spec Educ.* 2006;39(4):220-233. doi:10.1177/00224669060390040301.
2. Adolph K. Motor and physical development: locomotion. In: Haith MM, Benson JB, eds. *Encyclopedia of Infant and Early Childhood Development.* San Diego, CA: Academic Press; 2008.
3. Thelen E. The (re)discovery of motor development: learning new things from an old field. *Dev Psychol.* 1989;25(6):946-949. doi:10.1037/0012-1649.25.6.946.
4. Fischer KW, Bidell TR. Dynamic development of action, thought, and emotion. In: Damon W, Lerner RM, eds. *Theoretical Models of Human Development. Handbook of Child Psychology.* 2nd ed. New York, NY: Wiley; 2006.
5. Thelen E. Dynamic systems theory and the complexity of change. *Psychoanal Dialogues.* 2005;15(2):255-283. doi:10.1080/10481881509348831.
6. Royeen CB. Chaotic occupational therapy: Collective wisdom for a complex profession. *Am J Occup Ther.* 2003;57 (6):609-624. doi:10.5014/ajot.57.6.609.
7. Spencer JP, Perone S. Defending qualitative change: the view from dynamical systems theory. *Child Dev.* 2008;79(6):1639-1647. doi:10.1111/j.1467-8624.2008.01214.x.
8. Darrah J, Bartlett D. Dynamic systems theory and management of children with cerebral palsy: unresolved issues. *Infants Young Child.* 1995;8(1):52-59. doi:10.1097/00001163-199507000-00007.
9. Law M, Darrah J, Pollock N, et al. Family-centered functional therapy for children with cerebral palsy: an emerging practice model. *Phys Occup Ther Pediatr.* 1998;18(1):83-102. doi:10.1080/J006v18n01_06.
10. Newell KM. Constraints on the development of coordination. In: Wade MG, Whiting TA, eds. *Development in Children: Aspects of Coordination and Control.* Netherlands: Martinus Nijhoff Publishers; 1986.
11. Thelen E, Kelso S, Fogel A. Self-organizing systems and infant motor development. *Dev Rev.* 1987;7(1):39-65. doi:10.1016/0273-2297(87)90004-9.
12. van der Fels IM, Te Wierike SC, Hartman E, Elferink-Gemser MT, Smith J, Visscher C. The relationship between motor skills and cognitive skills in 4-16 year old typically developing children: a systematic review. *J Sci Med Sport.* 2015;18(6):697-703. doi:10.1016/j.jsams.2014.09.007.
13. Von Hofsten C. Action, the foundation for cognitive development. *Scand J Psychol.* 2009;50(6):617-623. doi:10.1111/j.1467-9450.2009.00780.x.
14. Cadoret G, Bigras N, Duval S, Lemay L, Tremblay T, Lemire J. The mediating role of cognitive ability on the relationship between motor proficiency and early academic achievement in children. *Hum Mov Sci.* 2018;57(2):149-157. doi:10.1016/j.humov.2017.12.002.
15. Piek JP, Dawson L, Smith LM, Gasson N. The role of early fine and gross motor development on later motor and cognitive ability. *Hum Mov Sci.* 2008;27(5):668-681. doi:10.1016/j.humov.2007.11.002.
16. Pitchford NJ, Papini C, Outhwait LA, Guilliford A. Fine motor skills predict math ability better than they predict reading ability in the early primary school years. *Front Psychol.* 2016;7:783. doi:10.3389/fpsyg.2016.00783.
17. Diamond A. Close interrelation of motor development and cognitive development and of the cerebellum and prefrontal cortex. *Child Dev.* 2000;71(1):44-56. doi:10.1111/1467-8624.00117.
18. Gibson EJ. Exploratory behavior in the development of perceiving, acting, and the acquiring of knowledges. *Annu Rev Psychol.* 1988;39:1-41. doi:10.1146/annurev.ps.39.020188.000245.
19. Adolph KE, Franchak JM. The development of motor behavior. *Interdiscip Rev Cogn Sci.* 2017;8:1-2. doi:10/1002/wcs.130.
20. Levac D, DeMatteo C. Bridging the gap between theory and practice: dynamic systems theory as a framework for understanding and promoting recovery of function in children and youth with acquired brain injuries. *Physiother Theory Pract.* 2009;25(8):544-554. doi:10.3109/09593980802667888.

21. Abbott A, Bartlett DJ. The relationship between the home environment and early motor development. *Phys Occup Ther Pediatr.* 1999;19(1):43-57. doi:10.1080/J006v19n01_04.

22. Roeber BJ, Tober CL, Bolt DM, Pollak SD. Gross motor development in children adopted from orphanage settings. *Dev Med Child Neurol.* 2012;54(6):527-531. doi:10.1111/j.1469-8749.2012.04257.x.

23. McPhillips M, Jordan-Black JA. The effect of social disadvantage on motor development in young children: a comparative study. *J Child Psychol Psychiatry.* 2007;48(12):1214-1222. doi:10.1111/j.1469-7610.2007.01814.x.

24. Suggate S, Stoeger H, Pufke E. Relations between playing activities and fine motor development. *Early Child Dev Care.* 2017;187(8):1297-1310. doi:10.1080/03004430.2016.1167047.

25. Johnson CP, Blasco PA. Infant growth and development. *Pediatr Rev.* 1997;18(7):224-242.

26. Flatters I, Mushtaq F, Hill LJ, Holt RJ, Wilkie RM, Mon-Williams M. The relationship between a child's postural stability and manual dexterity. *Exp Brain Res.* 2014;232(9):2907-2917. doi:10.1007/s00221-014-3947-4.

27. Henderson A, Pehoski C. *Hand Function in the Child: Foundations for Remediation.* 2nd ed. St. Louis, MO: Mosby; 2006.

28. Rosenblum S, Josman N. The relationship between postural control and fine manual dexterity. *Phys Occup Ther Pediatr.* 2003;23(4):47-60. doi:10.1080/J006v23n04_04.

29. Shumway-Cook A, Woollacott MH. *Motor Control: Translating Research Into Practice.* 5th ed. Philadelphia, PA: Wolters Kluver; 2017.

30. Wang TN, Howe TH, Hinojosa J, Weinberg SL. Relationship between postural control and fine motor skills in preterm infants at 6 and 12 months adjusted age. *Am J Occup Ther.* 2011;65(6):695-701. doi:10.5014/ajot.2011.001503.

31. Kuypers HG. The organization of the motor system. *Int J Neurol.* 1963;4(1):78-91.

32. Case-Smith J, Fisher AG, Bauer D. An analysis of the relationship between proximal and distal motor control. *Am J Occup Ther.* 1989;43(10):657-662. doi:10.5014/ajot.43.10.657.

33. Thelen E, Spencer JP. Postural control during reaching in young infants: a dynamic systems approach. *Neurosci Biobehav Rev.* 1998;22(4):507-514. doi:10.1016/S0149-7634(97)00037-7.

34. Van der Fits IBM, Hadders-Algra M. The development of postural response patterns during reaching in healthy infants. *Neurosci Biobehav Rev.* 1998;22(4):521-526. doi:10.1016/S0149-7634(97)00039-0.

35. Hopkins B, Rönnqvist L. Facilitating postural control: effects on the reaching behavior of 6-month-old infants. *Dev Psychobiol.* 2002;40(2):168-182. doi:10.1002/dev.10021.

36. Rachwani J, Santamaria V, Saavedra SL, Woollacott MH. The development of trunk control and its relation to reaching in infancy: a longitudinal study. *Front Hum Neurosci.* 2015;9:94. doi:10.3389/fnhum.2015.00094.

37. Harbourne R, Kamm K. Upper extremity function: what's posture got to do with it? *J Hand Ther.* 2015;28(2):106-112. doi:10.1016/j.jht.2015.01.008.

38. Campbell JM, Marcinowski EC, Babik I, Michel GF. The influence of a hand preference for acquiring objects on the development of a hand preference for unimanual manipulation from 6 to 14 months. *Infant Behav Dev.* 2015;39:107-117. doi:10.1016/j.infbeh.2015.02.013.

39. Thomas BL, Karl JM, Whishaw IQ. Independent development of the reach and the grasp in spontaneous self-touching by human infants in the first 6 months. *Front Psychol.* 2014;5:1526. doi:10.3389/fpsyg.2014.01526.

40. Atun-Einy O, Berger SE, Ducz J, Sher A. Strength of infants' bimanual reaching patterns is related to the onset of upright locomotion. *Infancy.* 2014;19(1):82-102. doi:10.1111/infa.12030.

41. Case-Smith J, O'Brien JC. *Occupational Therapy for Children and Adolescents.* 7th ed. St. Louis, MO: Mosby; 2015.

42. Dosso JA, Herrera SV, Boudreau JP. A study of reaching actions in walking infants. *Infant Behav Dev.* 2017;47:112-120. doi:10.1016/j.infbeh.2017.03.006.

43. Kahrs A, Jung WP, Lockman JJ. When does tool use become distinctively human? Hammering in young children. *Child Dev.* 2014;85(3):1050-1061. doi:10.1111/cdev.12179.

44. Fitzpatrick P, Wagman JB, Schmidt RC. Alterations in movement dynamics in a tool-use task: the role of action-relevant inertial tool properties. *Z Psychol.* 2012;220(1):23-28. doi:10.1027/2151-2604/a000087.

45. Klatzky RL, Lederman SJ, Mankinen JM. Visual and haptic exploratory procedures in children's judgments about tool function. *Infant Behav Dev.* 2005;28:240-249. doi:10.1016/j.intbeh.2005.05.002.

46. Deák G. Development of adaptive tool-use in early childhood: sensorimotor, social, and conceptual factors. In: Benson JB, ed. *Advances in Child Development and Behavior.* Waltham, MA: Elsevier Academic Press; 2014:149-181.

47. Mitchell AW, Hampton C, Hanks M, Miller C, Ray N. Influence of task and tool characteristics on scissor skills in typical adults. *Am J Occup Ther.* 2012;66(6):e89-e97. doi:10.5014/ajot.2012.004135.

48. Ratcliffe I, Concha M, Franssen D. Analysis of cutting skills in four to six year olds attending nursery schools in Johannesburg. *South African Journal of Occupational Therapy.* 2007;37(1):4-9.

49. Schneck CM, Henderson A. Descriptive analysis of the developmental progression of grip position for pencil and crayon control in nondysfunctional children. *Am J Occup Ther.* 1990;44(10):893-900. doi:10.5014/ajot.44.10.893.

50. Yakimishyn JE, Magill-Evans J. Comparisons among tools, surface orientation, and pencil grasp for children 23 months of age. *Am J Occup Ther.* 2002;56(5):564-572. doi:10.5014/ajot.56.5.564.

51. Dennis JL, Swinth Y. Pencil grasp and children's handwriting legibility during different-length writing tasks. *Am J Occup Ther.* 2001;55(2):175-183. doi:10.5014/ajot.55.2.175.

52. Koziatek SM, Powell NJ. Pencil grips, legibility, and speed of fourth-graders' writing in cursive. *Am J Occup Ther.* 2003;57 (3):284-288. doi:10.5014/ajot.57.3.284.

53. Schwellnus H, Carnahan H, Kushki A, Polatajko H, Missiuna C, Chau T. Effect of pencil grasp on the speed and legibility of handwriting after a 10-minute copy task in grade 4 children. *Aust Occup Ther J.* 2012;59(3):180-187. doi:10.1111/j.1440-1630.2012.01014.x.

54. Schwellnus H, Carnahan H, Kushki A, Polatajko H, Missiuna C, Chau T. Writing forces associated with four pencil grasp patterns in grade 4 children. *Am J Occup Ther.* 2013;67(2):218-227. doi:10.5014/ajot.2013.005538.

55. Park EY, Kim WH. Relationship between activity limitations and participation restriction in school-aged children with cerebral palsy. *J Phys Ther Sci.* 2015;27(8):2611-2614. doi:10.1589/jpts.27.2611.

56. Beckung E, Hagberg G. Neuroimpairments, activity limitations, and participation restrictions in children with cerebral palsy. *Dev Med Child Neurol.* 2002;44(5):309-316. doi:10.1017/S0012162201002134.

57. Mutlu A, Bügügan S, Kara ÖK. Impairments, activity limitations, and participation restrictions of the international classification of functioning, disability, and health model in children with ambulatory cerebral palsy. *Saudi Med J.* 2017;38(2):176-185. doi:10.15537/smj.2017.2.16079.

58. Goldstein DN, Cohn E, Coster W. Enhancing participation for children with disabilities: application of the ICF enablement framework to pediatric physical therapist practice. *Pediatr Phys Ther.* 2004;16 (2):114-120. doi:10.1097/01.PEP.0000127567.98619.62.

59. Hammal D, Jarvis SN, Colver AF. Participation of children with cerebral palsy is influenced by where they live. *Dev Med Child Neurol.* 2004;46(5):292-298. doi:10.1111/j.1469-8749.2004.tb00488.x.

60. Mihaylov SI, Jarvis SN, Colver AF, Beresford B. Identification and description of environmental factors that influence participation of children with cerebral palsy. *Dev Med Child Neurol.* 2004;46(5):299-304. doi:10.1017/S0012162204000490.

61. Li-Tsang CWP. The hand function of children with and without neurological motor disorders. *British Journal of Developmental Disabilities.* 2003;49(97):99-110. doi:10.1179/096979503799104093.

62. Haley S, Coster W, Dumas H, Fragala-Pinkham M, Moed R. *Pediatric Evaluation of Disability Inventory Computer Adaptive Test: Development, Standardization And Administration Manual.* Boston, MA: Health and Disability Research Institute; 2012.

63. Roll W, Roll K. *Roll Evaluation of Activities of Life.* New York, NY: Pearson; 2013.

64. Coster W, Deeney T, Haltiwanger J, Haley S. *School Function Assessment.* San Antonio, TX: Pearson; 1988.

65. Randall M, Johnson L, Reddihough D. *The Melbourne Assessment 2: A Test of Unilateral Upper Limb Function.* Melbourne, AU: The Royal Children's Hospital; 2012.

66. Aaron DH, Stenick-Jansen CW. Development of the functional dexterity test (FDT): construction, validity, reliability, and normative data. *J Hand Ther.* 2003;16(1):12-21.

67. Folio MR, Fewell RE. *Peabody Developmental Motor Scales.* 2nd ed. Austin, TX: PRO-ED; 2000.

68. Bruininks RH, Bruininks BD. *BOT-2: Bruininks-Oseretsky Test of Motor Proficiency Manual.* Minneapolis, MN: Pearson Assessments; 2005.

69. Aslam R, van Bommel A, Southwood TR, Hackett J, Jester A. An evaluation of paediatric hand and upper limb assessment tools within the framework of the World Health Organisation International Classification of Functioning, Disability and Health. *Hand Ther.* 2015;20(1):24-34. doi:10.1177/1758998315574431.

70. Shierk A, Lake A, Haas T. Review of therapeutic interventions for the upper limb classified by manual ability in children with cerebral palsy. *Semin Plast Surg.* 2016;30(1):14-23. doi:10.1055/s-0035-1571256.

71. Jackman M, Novak I, Lannin N. Effectiveness of hand splints in children with cerebral palsy: a systematic review with meta-analysis. *Dev Med Child Neurol.* 2014;56(2):138-147. doi:10.1111/dmcn.12205.

72. Rameckers EA, Janssen-Potten YJ, Essers IM, Smeets RJ. Efficacy of upper limb strengthening in children with cerebral palsy: a critical review. *Res Dev Disabil.* 2014;36(10):87-101. doi:10.1016/j.ridd.2014.09.024.

73. Elliott CM, Reid SL, Alderson JA, Elliott BC. Lycra arm splints in conjunction with goal-directed training can improve movement in children with cerebral palsy. *NeuroRehabilitation.* 2011;28(1):47-54. doi:10.3233/NRE-2011-0631.

74. Ten Berge SR, Boonstra AM, Dijkstra PU, Hadders-Algra M, Haga N, Maathuis CG. A systematic evaluation of the effect of thumb opponens splints on hand function in children with unilateral spastic cerebral palsy. *Clin Rehabil.* 2012;26(4):362-371. doi:10.1177/0269215511411936.

75. Brændvik SM, Elvrum AK, Vereijken B, Roeleveld K. Involuntary and voluntary muscle activation in children with unilateral cerebral palsy—relationship to upper limb activity. *Eur J Paediatr Neurol.* 2013;17(3):274-279. doi:10.1016/j.ejpn.2012.11.002.

76. Smits-Engelsman BC, Rameckers EA, Duysens J. Muscle force generation and force control of finger movements in children with spastic hemiplegia during isometric tasks. *Dev Med Child Neurol.* 2005;47(5):337-342.

77. Craig J, Hilderman C, Wilson G, Misovic R. Effectiveness of stretch interventions for children with neuromuscular disabilities: evidence-based recommendations. *Pediatr Phys Ther.* 2016;28(3):262-275. doi:10.1097/PEP.0000000000000269.

78. Damiano DL. Rehabilitative therapies in cerebral palsy: the good, the not as good, and the possible. *J Child Neurol.* 2009;24(9):1200-1204. doi:10.1177/0883073809337919.

79. Pin T, Dyke P, Chan M. The effectiveness of passive stretching in children with cerebral palsy. *Dev Med Child Neurol.* 2006;48(10):855-862. doi:10.1017/S0012162206001836.

80. Wiart L, Darrah J, Kembhavi G. Stretching with children with cerebral palsy: what do we know and where are we going? *Pediatr Phys Ther.* 2008;20(2):173-178. doi:10.1097/PEP.0b013e3181728a8c.

81. Pesce C, Masci I, Marchetti R, Vazou S, Sääkslahti A, Tomporowski PD. Deliberate play and preparation jointly benefit motor and cognitive development: mediated and moderated effects. *Front Psychol.* 2016;7(5):349. doi:10.3389/fpsyg.2016.00349.

82. Gordon AM, Hung YC, Brandao M, et al. Bimanual training and constraint-induced movement therapy in children with hemiplegic cerebral palsy: a randomized trial. *Neurorehabil Neural Repair.* 2011;25(6):692-702. doi:10.1177/1545968311402508.

83. Taub E, Griffin A, Nick J, Gammons K, Uswatte G, Law CR. Pediatric CI therapy for stroke-induced hemiparesis in young children. *Dev Neurorehabil.* 2007;10(1):3-18. doi:10.1080/13638490601151836.

84. Taub E, Ramey SL, DeLuca S, Echols K. Efficacy of constraint-induced movement therapy for children with cerebral palsy with asymmetric motor impairment. *Pediatrics.* 2004;113(2):305-312. doi:10.1542/peds.113.2.305.

85. Sakzewski L, Ziviani J, Boyd RN. Efficacy of upper limb therapies for unilateral cerebral palsy: a meta-analysis. *Pediatrics.* 2014;133(1):e175-e204. doi:10.1542/peds.2013-0675.

86. Chiu HC, Ada L. Constraint-induced movement therapy improves upper limb activity and participation in hemiplegic cerebral palsy: a systematic review. *J Physiother.* 2016;62(3):130-137. doi:10.1016/j.jphys.2016.05.013.

87. Eliasson AC, Krumlinde-Sundholm L, Shaw K, Wang C. Effects of constraint-induced movement therapy in young children with hemiplegic cerebral palsy: an adapted model. *Dev Med Child Neurol.* 2005;47(4):266-275.

88. Psychouli P, Kennedy CR. Modified constraint-induced movement therapy as a home-based intervention for children with cerebral palsy. *Pediatr Phys Ther.* 2016;28(2):154-160. doi:10.1097/PEP.0000000000000227.

89. Charles J, Gordon AM. Development of hand-arm bimanual intensive training (HABIT) for improving bimanual coordination in children with hemiplegic cerebral palsy. *Dev Med Child Neurol.* 2006;48(11):931-936. doi:10.1017/S0012162206002039.

90. Bleyenheuft Y, Dricot L, Gilis N, et al. Capturing neuroplastic changes after bimanual intensive rehabilitation in children with unilateral spastic cerebral palsy: a combined DTI, TMS and fMRI pilot study. *Res Dev Disabil.* 2015;43-44:136-149. doi:10.1016/j.ridd.2015.06.014.

91. Friel KM, Kuo HC, Fuller J, et al. Skilled bimanual training drives motor cortex plasticity in children with unilateral cerebral palsy. *Neurorehabil Neural Repair.* 2016;30(9):834-844. doi:10.1177/1545968315625838.

92. Tervahauta MH, Girolami GL, Øberg GK. Efficacy of constraint-induced movement therapy compared with bimanual intensive training in children with unilateral cerebral palsy: a systematic review. *Clin Rehabil.* 2017;31(11):1445-1456. doi:10.1177/0269215517698834.

93. Auld ML, Johnston LM, Russo RN, Moseley GL. A single session of mirror-based tactile and motor training improves tactile dysfunction in children with unilateral cerebral palsy: a replicated randomized controlled case series. *Physiother Res Int.* 2017;22(4). doi:10.1002/pri.1674.

94. Feltham MG, Ledebt A, Deconinck FJ, Savelsbergh GJ. Mirror visual feedback induces lower neuromuscular activity in children with spastic hemiparetic cerebral palsy. *Res Dev Disabil.* 2010;31(6):1525-1535. doi:10.1016/j.ridd.2010.06.004.

95. Gygax MJ, Schneider P, Newman CJ. Mirror therapy in children with hemiplegia: a pilot study. *Dev Med Child Neurol.* 2011;53(5):473-476. doi:10.1111/j.1469-8749.2011.03924.x.

96. Park E, Baek SH, Park S. Systematic review of the effects of mirror therapy in children with cerebral palsy. *J Phys Ther Sci.* 2016;28(11):3227-3231. doi:10.1589/jpts.28.3227.

97. Anttila H, Suoranta J, Malmivaara A, Mäkelä M, Autti-Rämö I. Effectiveness of physiotherapy and conductive education interventions in children with cerebral palsy: a focused review. *Am J Phys Med Rehabil.* 2008;87(6):478-501. doi:10.1097/PHM.0b013e318174ebed.

98. Brown GT, Burns SA. The efficacy of neurodevelopmental treatment in paediatrics: a systematic review. *Br J Occup Ther.* 2001;54(5):235-244. doi:10.1177/030802260106400505.

99. Lee KH, Park JW, Lee HJ, et al. Efficacy of intensive neurodevelopmental treatment for children with developmental delay, with or without cerebral palsy. *Ann Rehabil Med.* 2017;41(1):90-96. doi:10.5535/arm.2017.41.1.90.

100. Evans-Rogers DL, Sweeney JK, Holden-Huchton P, Mullens PA. Short-term, intensive neurodevelopmental treatment program experiences of parents and their children with disabilities. *Pediatr Phys Ther.* 2015;27(1):61-71. doi:10.1097/PEP.0000000000000110.

101. Case-Smith J. Fine motor outcomes in preschool children who receive occupational therapy services. *Am J Occup Ther.* 1996;50(1):52-61. doi:10.5014/ajot.50.1.52.

102. Dankert HL, Davies PL, Gavin WJ. Occupational therapy effects on visual-motor skills in preschool children. *Am J Occup Ther.* 2003;57(5):542-549. doi:10.5014/ajot.57.5.542.

103. Ratzon NZ, Efraim D, Bart O. A short-term graphomotor program for improving writing readiness skills of first-grade students. *Am J Occup Ther.* 2007;61(4):399-405. doi:10.5014/ajot.61.4.399.

104. Bazyk S, Mitchaud P, Goodman G, Papp P, Hawkins E, Welch MA. Integrating occupational therapy services in a kindergarten curriculum: A look at the outcomes. *Am J Occup Ther*. 2009;63(3):160-171. doi:10.5014/ajot.63.2.160.

105. DeGangi GA, Wietlisback S. Goodin M. Scheiner N. A comparison of structured sensorimotor therapy and child-centered activity in the treatment of preschool children with sensorimotor problems. *Am J Occup Ther*. 1993;47(9):777-786. doi:10.5014/ajot.47.9.777.

106. Ohl AM, Graze H, Weber K, Kenny S, Salvatore C, Wagreich S. Effectiveness of a 10-week Tier-1 Response to Intervention program in improving fine motor and visual-motor skills in general education kindergarten students. *Am J Occup Ther*. 2013;67(5):507-514. doi:10.5014/ajot.2013.008110.

107. Valvano J. Activity-focused motor interventions for children with neurological conditions. *Phys Occup Ther Pediatr*. 2004;24(1-2):79-107. doi:10.1300/J006v24n01_04.

108. Basu AP, Pearse J, Kelly S, Wisher V, Kisler J. Early intervention to improve hand function in hemiplegic cerebral palsy. *Front Neurol*. 2015;5:281. doi:10.3389/fneur.2014.00281.

109. Case-Smith J, Frolek Clark GJ, Schlabach TL. Systematic review of interventions used occupational therapy to promote motor performance for children ages birth-5 years. *Am J Occup Ther*. 2013;67(4):413-424. doi:10.5014/ajot.2013.005959.

110. Clark GF. Kingsley, K. *Occupational Therapy Practice Guidelines for Early Childhood: Birth Through 5 Years*. Bethesda, MD: American Occupational Therapy Association, Inc; 2013.

111. Lobo MA, Galloway JC, Heathcock JC. Characterization and intervention for upper extremity exploration and reaching behaviors in infancy. *J Hand Ther*. 2015;28(2):114-125; quiz 125. doi: 10.1016/j.jht.2014.12.003.

112. Cameron D, Craig T, Edwards B, Missiuna C, Schwellnus H, Polatajko HJ. Cognitive Orientation to daily Occupational Performance (CO-OP): a new approach for children with cerebral palsy. *Phys Occup Ther Pediatr*. 2017;37(2):183-198. doi:10.1080/01942638.2016.1185500.

113. Gharebaghy S, Rassafiani M, Cameron D. Effect of cognitive intervention on children with ADHD. *Phys Occup Ther Pediatr*. 2015;35(1):13-23. doi:10.3109/01942638.2014.957428.

114. Thornton A, Licari M, Reid S, Armstrong J, Fallows R, Elliott C. Cognitive Orientation to (Daily) Occupational Performance intervention leads to improvements in impairments, activity and participation in children with developmental coordination disorder. *Disabil Rehabil*. 2016;38(10):979-986. doi:10.3109/09638288.2015.1070298.

115. Novak I, Cusick A, Lannin N. Occupational therapy home programs for cerebral palsy: double-blind, randomized, controlled trial. *Pediatrics*. 2009;124(4):e606-e614. doi:10.1542/peds.2009-0288.

116. Novak I, Berry J. Home program intervention effectiveness evidence. *Phys Occup Ther Pediatr*. 2014;34(4):384-389. doi:10.3109/01942638.2014.964020.

117. Morgan C, Darrah J, Gordon AM, et al. Effectiveness of motor interventions in infants with cerebral palsy: a systematic review. *Dev Med Child Neurol*. 2016;58(9):900-909. doi:10.1111/dmcn.13105.

Selection and Use of Assistive Technology Devices

14

Patricia C. Montgomery, PT, PhD, FAPTA
Barbara H. Connolly, PT, DPT, EdD, C/NDT, FAPTA

Assistive technology (AT) devices refer to a wide range of appliances or tools with a goal of ameliorating problems faced by individuals with disabilities. Public Law 100-407[1] defined an AT device as, "any item, piece of equipment or product system whether acquired commercially off the shelf, modified, or customized that is used to increase, maintain, or improve functional capabilities of individuals with disabilities." The AT device can vary from low to high technology and can target a wide range of objectives. The primary focus of this chapter is on adaptive equipment (AE; ie, low-technology AT), which includes wheelchairs, ambulation aids, and positioning equipment. High-technology AT, which includes computerized communication systems, electronic environmental control devices, and educational aids, will be addressed briefly.

Over the past 25 years, several public laws have been passed that mandate children be included in the least-restrictive environments and include specific provisions regarding AT[2-4] (see Chapter 15). The Americans with Disabilities Act of 1990[5] prevents discrimination of individuals with disabilities in employment, state and local government agencies, public transportation, public accommodations, and telecommunications. Public laws emphasize the importance of including AT devices in the lives of individuals with disabilities to ensure their participation and increase their independent functional abilities in all meaningful environments.

The selection of AE and the integration of this equipment into the total plan of care are complicated and often time-consuming processes for therapists and families. Historically, families and professionals alike have included AE as an integral part of the treatment and management of the child with special needs. Parents often begin the process by selecting and using something as simple as a rolled up towel placed in a high chair to help position their infant during mealtime, or by using an infant-style walker for a period of time to allow a nonambulatory child the freedom of moving around the room more easily. Therapists frequently search for AE to increase functional abilities, improve posture and movement, or promote carryover of intervention strategies.

The process begins with a comprehensive examination, based on a thorough understanding of AE and the purposes for use. The team, including the family and professionals, navigates through the selection of the required item(s), seeks the approval for funding of the equipment, and then establishes a plan for the acquisition, use, modification, and monitoring of the equipment selected.

Connolly BH, Montgomery PC, eds. *Therapeutic Exercise for
Children With Developmental Disabilities, Fourth Edition* (pp 397-416).
© 2020 Taylor & Francis Group.

For the process to work smoothly, the child, family, therapists, physicians, educators, and durable medical equipment (DME) representative must work together with a shared purpose and clearly stated goals.

Purposes for Using Adaptive Equipment

The purpose of using AE must be clear to all members of the team. There are times when a single piece of equipment can meet several different purposes, whereas in other situations several different devices will be needed to meet a single or multiple objectives. For example, the parents of a young infant can find a single device to safely and appropriately position the baby in the car, act as a seat in public settings, and act as a stroller when placed in a frame for mobility through the mall or in the neighborhood. However, the family of an older child may need to obtain nighttime positional devices, a support for standing, and a specialized chair at school to address objectives of positioning the lower extremities to address musculoskeletal impairments, as well as to increase the child's participation in the classroom.

An "enablement" model provides a framework to relate various dimensions of disability with the objectives for using AT. This chapter uses an enablement model, which is based on the *International Classification of Functioning, Disability and Health* (ICF) model from the World Health Organization.[6]

AT for children includes the following general purposes:

> Facilitating participation of the child into a wider variety of environments
> Increasing independence or functional skill/activity level
> Improving the quality of postural control, alignment, and movement
> Minimizing, preventing, or managing system impairments
> Preventing the emergence of secondary impairments or additional pathophysiology

Facilitating Participation

AE often is used to increase a child's ability to participate in age-appropriate activities within the family or community. For example, AE may allow the child to direct his or her energies toward participation in educational or social programs rather than having to concentrate solely on maintaining posture or gaining mobility.

A specific device may address a specific system or motor impairment and reduce a participation restriction, but, if it is too complicated to use, or too large to fit in the physical setting, its use is diminished in encouraging participation. For example, a free-standing prone stander with a tray top may ideally position an adolescent child in full hip extension, provide weight bearing to lessen the development of osteoporosis, and place the child at the same level for social interaction with peers. However, if the prone stander consumes a large portion of a small classroom, breaks frequently, is not mobile, requires frequent readjusting, or requires 2 adults to safely transfer and position the child in the device, then the overall impact may be to decrease the teen's participation in the class. In another example, if a device is perceived as less than aesthetically pleasing to either the child or to the child's peers, it might result in decreasing rather than increasing participation. For example, the child may sit well positioned in a wheelchair inside the classroom, but choose not to join his or her classmates at recess because he or she is embarrassed to be seen outside by his or her able-bodied peers in the chair. A child may remove and discard parts of AE, such as an abductor wedge on the wheelchair, if it's considered unacceptable in a particular social or functional setting. Most therapy centers have at least one closet or room filled with "pieces and parts" of equipment that have been removed by either a family member or staff member for some reason. Likewise, when a therapist suggests that an accessory may improve the child's positioning, it is not infrequent for the family member to recall having

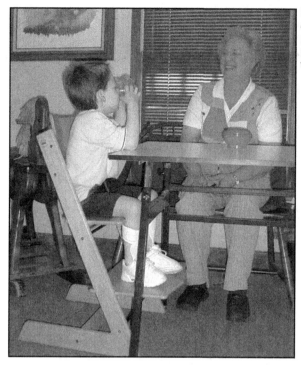

Figure 14-1. This young boy with Angelman syndrome enjoys a snack with his grandmother while positioned in his Tripp Trapp chair. He is well positioned and safe, and the chair fits well into the family home.

that particular piece "somewhere at home." The intervention team always must keep in mind what is acceptable to the child and family in order to expect AE to increase or, at least, not to limit participation by the child in appropriate settings.

Clinical Examples

An adapted stroller, even though it may not provide the best possible position, allows a parent to include the child on short excursions such as a quick stop at the grocery store, library, or drug store when time is short or the weather is bad. The parent, otherwise, might be inclined to leave the child at home if the only option is to unload and set up the child's wheelchair.

In the home setting, a Tripp Trapp seat (Stokke) permits the child to sit at the family dinner table for meals and participate in family conversation and social mealtime activities (Figure 14-1). A bath or toilet seat may increase the independence of a teenager who does not want adult supervision in daily hygiene activities. Positional devices (eg, corner chairs or small chairs and tables) and switches to activate toys or computer games can increase independence in play activities for the young preschool or school-aged child.

For example, Ríos-Rincón et al demonstrated an increase in playfulness in 4 children (Gross Motor Function Classification System [GMFCS] Levels IV and V) between the children and their mothers in free play sessions using a Lego robot.[7] At home or school the child may use a computer with specialized software, such as voice-activated programs, to play with or communicate with friends. An adapted chair may provide the postural support that allows the child to operate a computer mouse.

As the child moves outdoors, the use of walkers, crutches, adapted tricycles, or battery-operated riding toys increases participation in outdoor activities with the family as well as with peers (Figures 14-2 and 14-3; see Chapter 11).

Finally, for community activities or school-based activities, car seats, vans with lifts, powered chairs, walkers, crutches, sports equipment (eg, sport wheelchairs, modified ski equipment), augmentative communication devices, and specialized classroom seating can increase the participation of the child into a wider variety of settings and activities (Figures 14-4 through 14-6).

Figure 14-2. These siblings are able to fish together using the posture walker with a seat modification for extra support. Participation in recreational activities is enhanced.

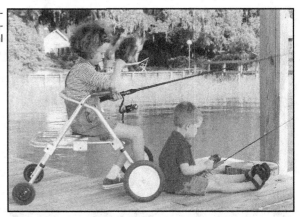

Figure 14-3. Bicycling on the beach with her sister is feasible with the modified 3-wheeled bike.

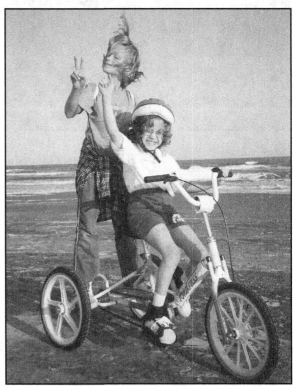

Addressing Activity/Functional Limitations

One of the major objectives in physical therapy intervention is to increase the child's ability to function in all critical environments. Functional gains may be observed in multiple domains related to a single item of AE. For example, the multiple benefits of early power mobility were reviewed in Chapter 11, and Haley and colleagues,[8] in the Pediatric Evaluation of Disability Inventory—Computer Adaptive Test, include additional items for children who use mobility devices to assess mobility. Increasing functional independence includes the following examples:

➤ A child may be able to demonstrate a functional ability that was not possible without AE. For example, a child might use the toilet purposefully when provided an adaptive toilet seat (Figure 14-7).

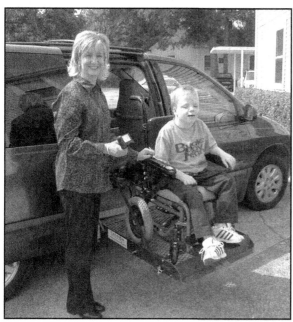

Figure 14-4. This youngster can be transferred into the family vehicle when transported to school, to medical appointments, to the mall, and to a friend's home alone by the mother, who also has 2 younger children. Although the child is still young, he is heavy and does not assist effectively with this difficult transfer into the family vehicle.

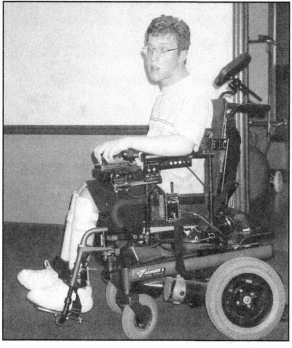

Figure 14-5. This teenager is now independent in his power wheelchair. He moves through his home and school well. He can now get home from school in the afternoons, let himself into the house, and start homework before his parents get home from work.

> ➤ A child may perform a task in broader contexts. The child who could sit on a bench at home while watching television or listening to audiotapes now can bench sit safely in the family vehicle when positioned with an EZ-ON Vest (EZ-ON Products; Figure 14-8).
>
> ➤ A child may be able to perform a familiar task with less assistance. A bath seat may allow bathing with assistance only for shampooing.

Figure 14-6. This young man uses a chair that has elements of a sports chair for participation in basketball and soccer. He uses a more supportive, higher-backed chair for postural support during the school day.

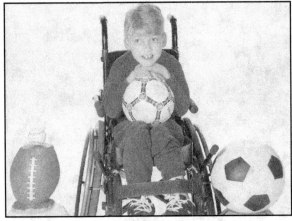

Figure 14-7. Increased independence in toileting will allow this young girl to participate in a school program more appropriately.

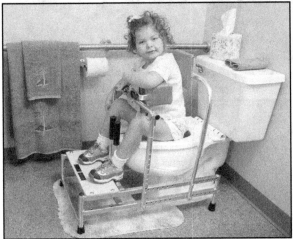

Figure 14-8. This 11-year-old is safely transported in the family car with his special car seat. He is well positioned with a 5-point seat belt, and the entire device is tethered to the car for safety.

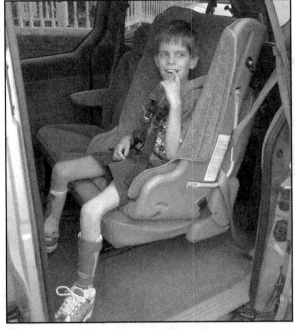

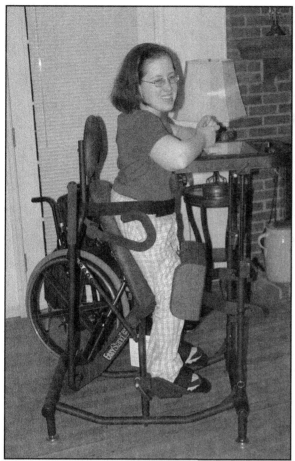

Figures 14-9. Joan can transfer from her wheelchair to the EasyStand independently. She is able to use the pump mechanism to raise herself to a standing posture without assistance.

> A child may be able to perform the same function with less assistive AE. A child may progress from ambulating with a walker to ambulating with forearm crutches and thus be able to move through a wider variety of environments with equipment that is easier to transport.

In the following section applications of AE in gross motor activities, fine motor activities, activities of daily living (ADLs), and intellectual functions are reviewed.

Gross Motor Activities

This domain includes activities such as the ability to move against gravity independently and through space. Gross motor functions include getting out of bed, rising from the classroom chair, crossing a room, and going down the hall to the cafeteria, or moving across town using public or private transportation.

> *Clinical Examples:* A wheelchair, push toy, or walker may increase mobility within the home. (See Video 14-1.) In school, a child may be able to move from sit to stand while positioned in an EasyStand with a hand-pump lift mechanism (Figure 14-9). Another child may be able to move from the classroom to the cafeteria with peers and obtain lunch independently by using a walker modified with a tray holder. Finally, a teenager may be able to drive him- or herself to school when the vehicle is modified with hand controls (Figure 14-10).

Figure 14-10. This 15-year-old adolescent has learned to load and unload his wheelchair and crutches to drive using specialized hand controls. His goal is to have his driver's license, as do his peers at school.

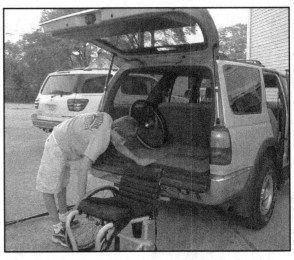

Fine Motor Activities

This domain includes activities such as managing tools or objects to solve environmental problems. Many investigators have explored the relationship between seating and upper extremity functioning. Angsupaisal and colleagues[9] studied the effect of 4 seated conditions in 19 children age 6 to 12 years with cerebral palsy (CP; GMFCS Levels I to III). Reaching was improved with a 15-degree forward inclination of the seat vs a horizontal position in children with hemiparesis, but performance of children with diplegia was negatively affected (independent of foot support). In contrast, Tsai et al[10] demonstrated that a 15-degree anterior inclined seat resulted in improved postural stability in 12 children with spastic diplegia (GMFCS Levels I to III). Physical therapists will need to evaluate the effect of seating position on postural control and upper extremity function for each individual child, as the results of current studies do not provide clear clinical guidelines.

> *Clinical Examples:* At home, the child may use switches to activate battery-operated toys, household appliances, or environmental controls (eg, remote control). Modified crayons may allow the child to color with a gross palmar grasp. Specialized clothing or shoes with Velcro fasteners may permit independent dressing for a child with poor bilateral hand use. At school, a laptop computer may substitute for note taking in a classroom when printing is too slow. Adapted scissors may permit the child to complete projects independently, rather than depending on an attendant's assistance.

Activities of Daily Living

This domain includes activities such as performing daily hygiene, preparing and consuming meals, and dressing and undressing. Typically these activities require the individual to participate in "multitasking" or performing a fine motor task while simultaneously completing a gross motor activity (Figure 14-11).

> *Clinical Examples:* At home, the family may use a mechanical lift to move the child from the bathtub or bed to a chair. The child may use devices such as bath seats or adapted toilet seats to increase independence in personal hygiene. Adapted spoons, forks, cups, or plates can increase independence during mealtimes. At school, a bathroom modified with grab bars can increase the child's independence and safety during toileting. An electronic feeder and cup holder may allow the child to eat independently, rather than relying on an adult to assist in feeding (Figure 14-12).

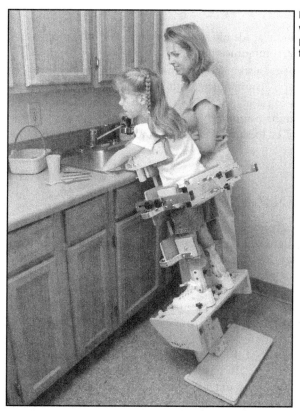

Figure 14-11. This mother and daughter work on washing dishes while the child is positioned in a prone stander. Both mother and daughter are free for the task while the child is well aligned.

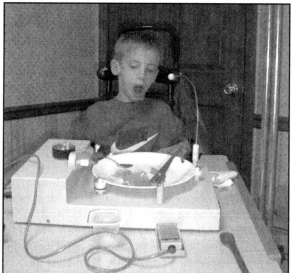

Figure 14-12. Justin can feed himself using this electronic feeder.

Intellectual Functions

This domain includes the ability to achieve academic skills, problem solve, and receive and express ideas, thoughts, wants, and needs (ie, communication).

> *Clinical Examples:* At home, a child may use a simple communication board to make choices during daily life. The mother may wear a "communication bib" during meals to allow the child to select whether he or she wants to eat another bite of food, have a swallow of his or her drink, or stop eating all together. In the community, a child can use a DynaVox to communicate meal selection in a restaurant or to share an answer in a timely fashion within a classroom.

IMPROVING ALIGNMENT AND MOTOR CONTROL

AE can be used to align single or multisegmental joints or the whole body. AE might be selected to support, assist, or require a specific alignment needed for a functional activity. Promoting appropriate alignment also can minimize or prevent secondary impairments from occurring. For example, Gibson and colleagues[11] found that incorporating a lumbar support, as well as lateral supports, in wheelchairs of children with Duchenne muscular dystrophy decreased the severity of their scoliosis. For those individuals with more significant postural or spinal deformities, the use of total-contact systems such as contoured foam systems can provide more complete support and therefore improve alignment.

Ryan et al[12] had parents complete a measure of the impact on performance before and after their child received a new adaptive seating system. The parents reported a large improvement in functioning for children younger than age 4 years, maintenance of skills in children age 4 to 12 years, and a moderate decline in children between ages 13 and 17 years. This inverse relationship with age suggests that adaptive seating systems need to be monitored as the child ages.

A systematic review of supported standing programs in children with CP suggested that effectiveness was related to duration and frequency.[13] This review documented that standing 5 days per week positively affected bone mineral density (60 to 90 minutes per day); hip stability (60 minutes per day in 30 to 60 degrees of total bilateral hip abduction); range of motion (ROM) of hip, knee, and ankle (45 to 60 minutes per day); and spasticity (30 to 45 minutes per day). In another study of children with CP, 10 children, ages 5 to 14 years (GMFCS Levels I to V), wore long leg orthoses for a minimum of 30 minutes/day, 5 days per week over 8 weeks.[14] Improved passive ROM for all 20 hamstring muscles and in 12 of 14 knee extension measurements was noted.

The most efficient relationship of the center of mass to the base of support (BOS) in standing is one that minimizes the amount of sway. This stable position is considered the "cone of economy."[15] A goal of AE is to support this efficiency while providing the fewest restraints to free, active, dynamic functional movements. The therapist also must consider the dichotomy of providing adequate stability while permitting necessary mobility. A walker might provide greater stability because it increases the size of the BOS and therefore immediately increases function for a child beginning to take assisted steps. Yet this same factor eliminates the need for the child to practice control of lateral weight shift of the center of mass over the BOS and reciprocity in the lower extremities. The walker, then, might slow the development of unsupported ambulation.

The design, placement, and use of AE also can modify movement patterns. The selection and use of AE can have an impact on symmetry, and increase or reduce activation of specific muscles for function. For example, poor placement of a head-control system for a powered wheelchair might increase the tendency for the child to push backward into cervical extension. This pattern of mass extensor muscle recruitment is a movement that is frequently discouraged during intervention because it may decrease the ability of the child to separate movements of the eyes from head movement, focus the eyes in midline, bring the hands together in midline, and achieve lip closure. Using a contoured head support system, or altering the place where the system contacts the occiput, can ensure that the time the child spends in the chair facilitates, rather than opposes, the posture and movement goals. In another example, a child who uses a partial weight-bearing device during early gait training may be able to practice task-specific movements, recruit the appropriate muscles, and reduce coactivation of the leg muscles to compensate for decreased strength.

Environmental Constraints

To fully address participation restrictions, functional/activity limitations, and impairments of a child, the key environments also must be considered. (Refer to discussions of dynamic systems theory in previous chapters.) Palisano et al[16] demonstrated that children use different amounts of adult support and assistance, as well as AT devices based on the environmental conditions. Children who were independent ambulators in the home environment and who used only walls or furniture for support frequently required adults, walkers, or crutches for support when outdoors or in community settings. Likewise, children communicate with familiar adults with fewer augmentative communication devices than when in different environments or with different listeners.

In addition, equipment that is functional in one setting may be dysfunctional or nonfunctional in another. A power wheelchair may appear to be a perfect solution for a child in a school with wide halls and doorways built on a single level with access to appropriate bus services. If, however, that child lives in a trilevel home with multiple staircases and with access to only a small family vehicle, this same solution will not be appropriate. The therapist must consider all the key environments. This analysis includes the immediate home as well as the homes of extended family members. If the child spends weekends at the grandparents' home or is in the home of an aunt each afternoon after school, the characteristics of those environments and the individuals in them must be considered. The therapist must review schools, day care centers, or community sites that the child frequently visits. The therapist must consider if the AE will stay at the family home or if it must be able to be regularly transported to a babysitter's, and if so, how it is going to be transported? Finally, a long-term view of the child and various environments is important. If the child is now in a preschool that is totally accessible, but the neighborhood elementary school is not, the therapist considers both environments when selecting equipment if it is expected to meet the needs of the child during this entire time frame.

Examination, Evaluation, and Intervention

Examination

A comprehensive examination includes data collection or history of the key information related to medical, social, and educational background as related to AT. An accurate medical diagnosis and an understanding of the implications of that diagnosis have a direct bearing on the decisions related to AT. Does the child have a progressive disorder with a limited life expectancy? Is the current condition temporary with spontaneous recovery anticipated within 6 months? Is this a chronic condition that is expected to affect, with little change, the child's functioning across the life span? Has an event, such as a surgery or a growth spurt, caused a temporary change in the child's health condition?

The therapist then examines the child's participation restrictions, functional activities and limitations, and impairments. The child's age and history of growth and development are recorded. It is critical to examine all the relevant body systems as well as typical postures and movements that will have an impact on the child's use of AT devices. In addition, it is important to consider other contextual factors such as the child's ability to adapt to change. For example, how easily is the child frustrated? Although physically capable, a child who is easily frustrated may not be willing to use a feeding device he or she must wait for an adult to set up, as it slows down the mealtime process. These contextual issues can dramatically affect the acceptance and use of AT.

In addition to determining the needs of the child, the therapist must determine caregivers' needs regarding their ability to understand and use AE. Caregivers must be able to understand the purpose of AE in the child's life and find it convenient to use. Caregivers might include parents, siblings, teachers, personal care attendants, babysitters, grandparents, or volunteers. The therapist evaluates the caregivers' understanding of the child's abilities and acceptance of AE to meet some of the child's needs. The therapist assesses the physical ability of the caregivers to handle the child and the equipment. A parent with a history of back pain may find it difficult to manage a large piece of equipment requiring transport in the family car. A grandparent may not be able to lift and position a child onto a prone stander. Whereas the parent or therapist may be able to independently transfer a child from the wheelchair to the toilet, the attendant at school may find that a 2-person transfer is needed.

Caregivers should be involved in the entire process of obtaining AT as the end result can have negative or positive effects on them. Mortenson and colleagues[17] interviewed 27 caregivers regarding their experience with AT, and 3 broad themes were identified:

1. "A partial piece of mind" (eg, decreasing stress and shift from physical tasks to a monitoring role)
2. "Working together" (eg, sense of collaboration)
3. "Overcoming barriers" (eg, addressing lack of funding and wait times for service providers)

The therapist also identifies key environmental constraints. Where does this child spend each day? Does the child go to school? How is the child transported? What are other settings in which the child regularly functions? Does the child attend a day care center, go to a babysitter's home, or stay at a relative's home? What changes in these environments will occur? Will the child change from home-based to school-based therapy? Is an upcoming surgery going to result in an inpatient rehabilitation stay? Will the child transition to a group home in the future? Equipment used in schools and day care centers frequently must meet different standards for safety and durability. Space available for use, as well as for storage of equipment, will be different based on the size and type of home or school. Will the equipment be shared with other children or be used around other children? Will there be other individuals, such as siblings, who might assist the child in the use of the equipment?

Evaluation

The team, including the child, family, DME representative, and therapist, establishes functional outcomes for the use of AT devices for long-term as well as for short-term timelines. For example, the long-term outcome for a 4-year-old child may be to become independently mobile in the home using a power wheelchair. The short-term objective is to drive the power chair the length of the hallway without scraping the walls. Because this is a growing child who will use the chair indoors, an appropriate choice for the team is a chair that is very maneuverable, rather than one that is durable on all terrains. A second chair, when the child has outgrown this one, may be one that can manage terrains around the home, school, and community. The specific choices are made based on these anticipated outcomes. Hypotheses are developed that relate the information in the examination to equipment options. For example, based on the examination, the team hypothesizes that a 4-year-old child who has limited upper extremity control will be able to operate a power wheelchair in the home and preschool environment. The team also hypothesizes that the child's visual-perceptual impairments and impulsive behaviors currently will prevent use of a wheelchair in outside environments without close adult supervision.

In addition to establishing these outcome measures, the therapist evaluates the caregivers' understanding of the use and potential abuse of equipment as the child grows and develops. AE needs may change across time. The equipment will need to be monitored for fit and for continued need. The equipment may need adjustment because of growth, changes in functional ability, different environments, or different tasks. For example, a child may require a head support system on the wheelchair and a trunk harness while being transported on the bus, but may need to have times during the day to work on developing head control without use of these optional supports.

Finally, it is important for the therapist to have a clear picture of the caregivers' lifestyle before selecting equipment. The therapist must understand that families come from a wide range of cultures, with varying priorities, values, interests, and ethics (see Chapter 4). With these differences come marked differences in the need, use, and acceptance of AE. Some families want to be able to include the child in as many outings as possible and, therefore, lightweight strollers are more convenient and appropriate. Other families tend to leave the child at home with an adult and the focus is more on positioning devices that do not need to be as portable. As much as possible the equipment should meet the needs of the caregivers' lifestyle and make care easier while still meeting the child's needs.

The evaluation also focuses on the specific objectives for each piece of recommended equipment, the costs of equipment, and available funding sources. The team must agree on the specific objectives that any piece of equipment is expected to meet. Options for renting, buying, constructing, or borrowing AE should be explored based on the needs and resources of the child and family. The funding may come from the family directly, from third-party payers, or from service organizations or groups. At this time the role of the DME representative becomes increasingly more important. This person often is knowledgeable about options in equipment, measurement of equipment, and the eligibility of equipment for payment under different systems. For example, in some states third-party payers may routinely pay for one type of stander and deny another one based on cost. The therapist should be well informed as to equipment options as well as to the DME representative's skills and biases.

Determining Specific Durable Medical Equipment

The first decision is to select the method of positioning or assistance. Ward[18] described 3 options to enhance a child's functional abilities. The first option is using an adult's body to hold or position the child. Parents, therapists, and teachers universally use this system. It has many advantages, including being dynamic and being the only system that includes sensory feedback and cognitive problem solving. The biggest disadvantage is that it requires the presence of an adult and limits the child's and the adult's independence.

The second option is the use of standard furniture. Many ideas for AE have originated from families modifying a standard piece of equipment. The advantage is that the device is more readily available from more sources and may fit into a wider variety of settings. The disadvantage is that the nonspecific nature of household items may not entirely meet the needs of the child.

A third option is to construct or purchase a specialized product. If there is a team member who is capable of constructing a device, the equipment may be specifically tailored to meet the needs of the child. While material costs may be less expensive, construction of a "one-of-a-kind" piece of AE generally involves intensive labor costs. Volunteers, such as family members, neighbors, and members of houses of worship and social organizations, often find constructing a chair or stander a rewarding experience. The end product, however, clearly is based on the skill of the individual(s) fabricating the device. The time taken to complete a project is subject to the fabricator's other commitments. It is not possible to pressure volunteers to hurry the construction. This type of construction may not be acceptable in various public settings because of fire or safety requirements. Another disadvantage is that the device may be less adaptable to the growth of the child and, therefore, may need to be reconstructed frequently.

If equipment is purchased, there are different advantages and disadvantages. One advantage is that purchased equipment often is more adaptable to growth and to use by a wider variety of children. Therefore, one chair may be ordered for a classroom and can be used with several different children throughout the day as well as across the years. The equipment tends to be more durable and carries with it the manufacturer's guarantees, such as being crash tested if the device is used in transportation. In addition, the equipment is more likely to be funded through third-party payers.

A disadvantage is the need to go through the approval process, which can be time consuming, labor intensive, and frustrating. Finally, although the equipment may be able to be used for several different children and accommodate to greater growth, it may be more difficult to get a specific fit to accommodate one child's needs or body.

A more recent role for therapists has been in selecting individuals who would benefit from service dogs and in finding reputable providers for service dogs.[19] Service dogs have been used for adults for many years and now are being used for children with autism and physical disabilities, for seizure alert and response, and for diabetic alert.

Intervention/Plan of Care

The plan of care includes an outline of the intervention provided, personnel involved, and timelines in terms of frequency and duration of the use of the AT device in direct services and home programs. In addition, specific strategies and equipment to be used as well as instruction to be provided to the family, caregivers, or child are determined. A specific plan for AE is included in the overall plan of care. A sample intervention would be that the child will use a corner chair during mealtimes to aid symmetry of trunk and head and facilitate head and oral posture for eating and drinking. The chair will be adjusted with the seat elevated so the knees are flexed at 90 degrees with the feet flat on the footrests. This will aid in achieving vertical pelvic position and normal spinal curves. The tray should be attached so the back of the chair inhibits scapular adduction as the child actively reaches forward and places the hands on the tray. The child then has the postural alignment and positioning of the upper extremities to pick up finger foods or to hold a cup in midline (functional outcomes). In addition to mealtimes, the child should use the corner chair for periods of 30 minutes several times during the day to use the same posture while playing with toys on the tray. The child should not be placed in the corner chair for more than a total of 4 hours during any given day and should always be supervised directly by an adult. The fit of the chair and its use will be evaluated in 6 months as part of the reexamination.

Acquisition

The team now must acquire the selected AE. If the family has a third-party payer involved, it is necessary to write a letter of medical necessity. The more specific the justification, the more effective the request will be. It is not adequate to write that the child requires a wheelchair because he or she has CP. It is necessary to write that the child needs an ultra-lightweight frame with removable armrests and footrests and a solid seat and back with a subanterior superior iliac spine bar to position the pelvis in a vertical symmetrical position. This position will help prevent further hip joint asymmetry and a possible scoliosis. The removable footrests and armrests will make it easier for the child to transfer into the chair from a walker and will make it feasible to be transported in the family vehicle. The lightweight frame will make it possible for the child with compromised cardiopulmonary support to propel the chair independently. This chair should meet the child's needs for the next 3 years or until substantial growth occurs. Remember, the equipment must be "medically necessary" for the child and not just make care easier for the caregivers. Typically, the therapist and the physician must sign the letter prior to submittal for approval. It is frequently very beneficial to contact the child's case manager with the third-party payer if one has been assigned. This person should know whether additional information is required or would be helpful. The appropriate information can be submitted with the original request rather than waiting for a denial and a subsequent resubmittal. In the case of requesting a power wheelchair for a young child, a video of the child demonstrating the ability to use the wheelchair can be provided as supplemental evidence of appropriateness.

The time to obtain approval for DME may be lengthy. If the therapist can inform the family prior to the process of expected timetables, it can be less frustrating to everyone involved. It is not unusual for the process to take many months and, therefore, it may be beneficial to develop a follow-up checklist with the DME representative to avoid unnecessary lapses.

Direct Use

Once the AE has been ordered, received, and assembled, the therapist or DME dealer fits the equipment to the child. At this time the therapist provides the caregivers detailed instructions in the use and care of the device. This includes specific use schedules. The therapist provides a schedule to monitor the fit and continued need for the equipment. A chair well adjusted for a child in January may need adjusting again in July if a major growth spurt has occurred. The therapist should include in annual reevaluations and quarterly summaries a report from the caregivers on equipment use, fit, and, whenever possible, how the child is using the equipment in the typical environments for which it was selected.

SUMMARY

When included in comprehensive examination, evaluation, and intervention, AT can play an important role in increasing functional independence and the ability of the child with a developmental disability to participate in age-appropriate environments.

In summary, the therapist evaluates the child, the caregivers, and the environments in which daily life occurs for the child and considers possible solutions that AE devices can offer. Based on familiarity with the strengths and limitations of many AE devices and the options for obtaining the devices, therapists can make decisions on whether to include AE as an intervention strategy.

A brief review of the participation restrictions, AT concerns, and AE interventions will be applied to the children in the 5 case studies.

CASE STUDY #1: JASON

› *Medical Diagnosis:* Cerebral palsy, right hemiparesis
› *Gross Motor Function Classification System:* Level I
› *Age:* 24 months

Participation Restrictions

Jason has difficulty keeping up with peers in gross motor play, especially outdoors or on playgrounds without falling. His family also wants him to be able to participate more in self-help skills, such as dressing, toileting, and self-feeding.

Adaptive Technology Concerns

Jason is demonstrating postural asymmetries and is at risk for developing secondary orthopedic impairments, such as a scoliosis, as well as asymmetrical limb lengths (upper and lower extremities). Limitations in bilateral upper extremity use and balance skills adversely affect his self-care skills, such as dressing and undressing.

Adaptive Equipment Interventions

An orthotic and a knee immobilizer to wear occasionally at night for the right lower extremity may be indicated to maintain ROM. Additionally, a shoe insert to aid in alignment of the right foot is an option. In addition, Jason may benefit from a small neoprene or other type of hand splint on the right hand to position the thumb in opposition for more effective grasp and release. Therapists often construct temporary lower extremity orthotics (using plastic of varying thickness) as well as upper extremity splints. If not constructed by the therapist, these items could be ordered through a vendor with the necessary prescriptions and letters of medical necessity. As Jason is interested in toileting, it is suggested that the family obtain a small potty seat with an attached tray to encourage him to stay on the toilet for an adequate length of time. He also could benefit from sitting at the table to encourage greater symmetry and stability at the hips. A Tripp Trapp chair could be used both for Jason and his brother. Finally, a small bench or chair for play, television time, and dressing activities could be obtained. These positioning alternatives would encourage increased symmetry by getting Jason up off the floor. These items could be acquired commercially, through yard sales, or from friends or relatives.

CASE STUDY #2: JILL

> *Medical Diagnosis:* Cerebral palsy, spastic quadriparesis, microcephaly, intellectual deficits, seizure disorder
> *Gross Motor Function Classification System:* Level V
> *Age:* 7 years

Participation Restrictions

Jill has limited gross and fine motor skills and needs adult assistance to participate in activities at home, at school, and in the community. She has limited communication skills for social interactions with adults or peers. Jill has poor eye-head control, which negatively affects her visual skills.

Adaptive Technology Concerns

The family reports increasing difficulty with transferring Jill. They have the most difficulty with transfers into the bathtub and into the family vehicle. Although the current wheelchair will go into the bathroom, there is little space to move once it is in the room. They anticipate that the next wheelchair will not go through the door. The mother is worried that Jill will have a seizure while she is in the bathtub or in midtransfer and that she may be hurt. The family also realizes it is time to order a new car seat as Jill has outgrown the one currently being used. The family would like additional options, other than her wheelchair, stander, or floor for safe positioning when Jill is at home in the afternoons and on weekends. Jill does not have any form of floor mobility and cannot sit without support. While she will assist briefly with standing pivot transfers, she does not maintain standing unless supported in a stander or by an adult.

Adaptive Equipment Interventions

At school, the current prone stander will be exchanged for an EasyStand to allow introduction of more dynamic transfers. This stander also will decrease the weight bearing through her anterior chest and therefore improve depth of respiration. Correct positioning of Jill in her AE and signs and symptoms of distress will need to be observed carefully. The therapist will recommend timing and scheduling of positional changes in conjunction with the school staff.

At home, the family will need to acquire a bath seat, a new car seat or EZ-ON Vest, a lift, and a small bench. The parents can purchase a lightweight plastic bench the height of Jill's wheelchair footrests to ease the transfer in and out of their vehicle (ie, using a standing pivot transfer). When she outgrows her current prone stander at home, a vertical-type stander will be recommended to capitalize on Jill's improved head control in the upright position. In addition, Jill could benefit from an additional activity chair for positioning for play activities. This chair should have a tray with the option to suspend toys for reach and activation. When seated in the chair, a trial of gaze-based AT could be attempted. This type of communication device has been shown to improve the repertoire of computer activities in children with severe physical impairments without speaking ability.[20]

The therapist can request the local equipment vendor to bring several different types of lifts into the home for a trial. A lift for the bathtub and other transfers would need to be tried in the home setting to make sure it will fit into all of the appropriate rooms (eg, bathroom). The car seat, bath seat, lift, and stander may be purchased with preapproval from the third-party payer. The intervention team, after trials with several items, will recommend the best options.

CASE STUDY #3: TAYLOR

> *Medical Diagnosis:* Myelomeningocele, repaired L1-2
> *Age:* 4 years

Participation Restrictions

Taylor has limited ability to self-propel his wheelchair long distances to keep up with his peers while outdoors and to be able to walk using long leg braces and crutches in the house and the classroom. He seldom plays with neighborhood friends.

Adaptive Technology Concerns

Taylor demonstrates the musculoskeletal impairments of decreased ROM and strength in the lower extremities, along with decreased sensory awareness in the lower body related to his L1-2 myelomeningocele. He has limited respiratory support for gross motor activities. He does not have the physical mobility necessary to interact with peers during gross motor play.

Adaptive Equipment Interventions

Taylor will continue to use his manual wheelchair. When a new wheelchair needs to be ordered, the family should consider one with a power assist to increase his ability to self-propel at higher speeds. The chair needs to be as light as possible, as the mother usually transports him and she is a small woman. Another option, if a heavier chair is required, is to purchase a portable ramp to be used for the family van and a tie-down system so the wheelchair and Taylor can be transported easily. Taylor recently received long leg braces. He is using an anterior support walker, but also has bilateral forearm crutches to use with his new braces. If funding is available, it would be beneficial for Taylor to obtain a mobile stander (ie, prone stander with wheels allowing for self-propulsion). This stander would place him at eye level with peers, help maintain lower extremity ROM, and increase his upper extremity strength as well as overall endurance. Most important, a mobile stander would promote independence in moving throughout his environment and facilitate social interactions.

A tricycle that is propelled with the upper extremities may be obtained for Taylor through a local philanthropic group. Another option would be the purchase of a battery-powered hand-controlled riding toy for him, so he could ride outside with neighborhood friends.

Case Study #4: Ashley

> *Medical Diagnosis:* Down syndrome
> *Age:* 15 months

Participation Restrictions

Ashley does not play independently with toys, usually throwing them. She does not interact often with other children, and avoids movement-based activities. Ashley does not assist in ADLs, except with feeding; however, she needs adult supervision.

Adaptive Technology Concerns

Ashley has poor floor mobility and does not ambulate independently. She does not have environmental structures to facilitate practice of fine motor skills and social interactions with peers. Her self-feeding skills are limited.

Adaptive Equipment Interventions

Although AE can be useful in aiding Ashley to reach her functional potential and minimizing the development of secondary impairments, her family is hesitant to incorporate dramatic changes in their home. Therefore, the therapist will provide recommendations for standard furniture or toys commercially available.

The therapist also can provide the parents an article describing how to convert riding toys to power mobility.[21] If Ashley's parents express interest in doing that for Ashley, they can be directed to websites and online videos that provide additional instructions.

A small bench or chair for Ashley to sit in during daily activities should be purchased to help decrease the size of her BOS. If a tray top is used, it would help limit the throwing of toys. A small but heavy baby carriage or push toy would be beneficial to encourage ambulation. Ashley also may benefit from a small swing to increase vestibular input. A swing could be obtained from a local toy store or the family could make frequent visits to a neighborhood park. Specific recommendations for a NUK toothbrush and adaptive spoon, plates, and cups to increase independence at snack and mealtimes also can be made. The therapists and school staff providing intervention will continue to assess the family's interest in using AE at home.

Case Study #5: John

> *Medical Diagnosis:* Developmental coordination disorder/attention-deficit hyperactivity disorder
> *Age:* 5 years

Participation Restrictions

John is unable to go with his family to the mall, into other homes, and to playgrounds without falling or knocking down other people or objects. He often is frustrated in the classroom and appears to have poor self-esteem. John avoids physical activity and group sports. He has difficulty with ball skills and cannot ride a bike without training wheels, which limits his interaction with peers. He demonstrates poor printing skills, has difficulty using utensils during meals, and is not totally independent in ADLs.

Assistive Technology Concerns

John walks independently and has basic gross motor skills. Although he does not need a mobility device, intervention to improve his gross and fine motor skills, as well as his performance of ADLs, is appropriate.

Adaptive Equipment Interventions

John can benefit from careful selection of equipment that is available in standard department stores. There are many games or toys that would promote improved motor planning. For example, during the examination process the therapist found that John avoided playing catch with a tennis ball, but seemed to enjoy playing badminton with the therapist. This is a low-cost activity that could be set up in his backyard and would improve eye-hand coordination and overall fitness. It would be helpful for the therapist to accompany John and his parents to a local store to select appropriate items.

In addition, the family may find that John's behavior will improve if more consistent sensory cues are provided in his environment. John could try more spandex-type clothing to increase sensory input. Eating utensils that are heavier and provide more tactile feedback might improve his fine motor control during mealtime. A standard, bright-colored placemat to indicate his place at the table, combined with a small patch of nonskid material in his seat cushion, may improve his participation during meals. An electric toothbrush may increase his proficiency and interest in toothbrushing, and a bath mitt could be used during bathing. Electric scissors, a squiggle or vibrating pencil, and printing with his paper positioned over a lined screen may be strategies that will improve his fine motor academic skills.

Children with developmental coordination disorder often have difficulty in a variety of sequencing tasks. François et al[22] reviewed research suggesting that positive neuroplastic changes in cortical and subcortical regions of motor, auditory, and speech processing networks occur with musical training. Whether playing a musical instrument (eg, piano, trumpet) or singing in a choir, music activities require sequencing (eg, reading musical notes in a series, motor sequencing for playing an instrument). Depending on family resources and John's level of interest, music-related activities may be beneficial and provide another opportunity not only to improve sequencing skills, but also to facilitate social interactions with peers.

ACKNOWLEDGMENTS

The editors wish to express appreciation to Judith C. Bierman, PT and Janet Wilson Howle, MACT, PT for their contributions to this chapter in previous editions.

REFERENCES

1. Technology-Related Assistance for Individuals with Disabilities Act: Public Law 100-407, 1988; reauthorized 1994.
2. Rehabilitation Act of 1973 and Amendments of 1998 PL 105-220, Sect.508, 29 USC Sec 794 d.
3. Individuals with Disabilities Education Act Amendments of 1997, Public Law (20 USC, SEC 1400 et.seq.) 1997; 105-117.
4. Assistive Technology Act of 1988: PL 105-394, codified at-Title 29 of United States Code at Section 3001 and following (29 USC Sec. 3001 et seq.), amending PL 103-218 (1994) and PL 100-407 (1998).
5. Americans with Disabilities Act of 1990: PL 101-336 Title 42 USC 12101 et seq.6.
6. World Health Organization. *International Classification of Functioning, Disability and Health (ICF)*. Geneva, Switzerland: World Health Organization; 2001.
7. Ríos-Rincón AM, Adams K, Magill-Evans J, Cook A. Playfulness in children with limited motor abilities when using a robot. *Phy Occup Ther Pediatr.* 2016;3(3):232-246. doi:10.3109/01942638.2015.1076559.

8. Haley S, Coster W, Dumas H, Fragala-Pinkham M, Moed R. *Evaluation of Disability Inventory Computer Adaptive Test: Development, Standardization and Administration Manual.* Boston, MA: Health and Disability Research Institute; 2012.

9. Angsupaisal M, Dijkstra LJ, la Bastide-van Gemert S, et al. Best seating condition in children with spastic cerebral palsy: one type does not fit all. *Res Dev Disabil.* 2017;71(12):42-52. doi:10.1016/j.ridd.2017.09.016.

10. Tsai YS, Yu YC, Huang PC, Cheng HY. Seat surface inclination may affect postural stability during Boccia ball throwing in children with cerebral palsy. *Res Dev Disabil.* 2014;35(12):3568-3573. doi:10.1016/j.ridd.2014.08.033.

11. Gibson DA, Koreska J, Robertson D, et al. The management of spinal deformities in Duchenne muscular dystrophy. *Orthop Clin North Am.* 1978;9:437-450.

12. Ryan SE, Sawatzky B, Campbell KA, et al. Functional outcomes associated with adaptive seating interventions in children and youth with wheeled mobility needs. *Arch Phys Med Rehabil.* 2014;95(5):825-831. doi:10.1016/j.apmr.2013.09.001.

13. Paleg GS, Smith BA, Glickman LB. Systematic review and evidence-based clinical recommendations for dosing of pediatric supported standing programs. *Pediatr Phys Ther.* 2013;25(3):232-247. doi:10.1097/PEP.0b013e318299d5e7.

14. Laessker-Alkema K, Eek MN. Effect of knee orthoses on hamstring contracture in children with cerebral palsy: multiple single-subject study. *Pediatr Phys Ther.* 2016;28(3):347-353. doi:10.1097/PEP.0000000000000267.

15. Haddas R, Lieberman IH. A method to quantify the "cone of economy." *Eur Spine J.* 2018;27(5):1178-1187. doi:10.1007/s00586-017-5321-2.

16. Palisano R, Tieman B, Walter S, et al. Effect of environmental setting on mobility methods of children with cerebral palsy. *Dev Med Child Neurol.* 2003;45(2):113-120. doi:10.1111/j.1469-8749.2003.tb00914.x.

17. Mortenson WB, Pysklywec A, Fuhrer MJ, Jutal JW, Plante M, Demers L. Caregivers' experience with the selection and use of assistive technology. *Disabil Rehabil Assist Technol.* 2018;13(6):562-567. doi:10.1080/17483107.2017.1353652.

18. Ward D. *Positioning the Handicapped Child for Function.* 2nd ed. Chicago, IL: Phoenix Press; 1984.

19. Stace LB. Welcoming Max: Increasing pediatric provider knowledge of service dogs. *Complement Ther Clin Pract.* 2016;24(8):57-66. doi:10.1016/j.ctcp.2016.05.005.

20. Borgestig M, Sandqvist J, Ahlsten G, Falkmer T, Hemmingsson H. Gaze-based assistive technology in daily activities in children with severe physical impairments—an intervention study. *Dev Neurorehabil.* 2017;20(3):129-141. doi:10.3109/17518423.2015.1132281.

21. Hsiang HH, Galloway JC. Modified ride-on toy cars for early power mobility: a technical report. *Pediatr Phys Ther.* 2012;24(2):149-154. doi:10.1097/PEP.0b013e31824d73f9.

22. François C, Grau-Sánchez J, Duarte E, Rodriguez-Fornells A. Musical training as an alternative and effective method for neuro-education and neuro-rehabilitation. *Front Psychol.* 2015;6:475. doi:10.3389/fpsyg.2015.00475.

Physical Therapy in the Educational Environment
Early Intervention and School-Based

Joanell A. Bohmert, PT, DPT, MS

The goal of education is to prepare children for adult life. The role of the physical therapist in the educational setting is to assist children with disabilities to attain this goal. Children fulfill many roles—that of son/daughter, sibling, friend, student, and worker. Their jobs are to play, learn, and work. Their work sites include home, day care, parks, stores, shopping centers, job sites, and school. The physical therapist working with these children is not only a pediatric therapist but also an industrial therapist. The physical therapist's primary purpose is to assist children with disabilities to function at their "work."

The purpose of public education is to provide a free and appropriate education for all children. Federal and state laws and regulations establish minimum standards for general education and special education. It is a challenge to provide an education that will prepare children and youth with disabilities for their adult life. This challenge is significant in that the percentage of youth with disabilities who graduate from high school (69% vs 84%),[1] percentage of youth with disabilities who complete a bachelor's degree or higher (16% vs 34%),[2] and the percentage of adults with disabilities who work (19% vs 67%)[3,4] is significantly less than that of youth and adults without disabilities. Many children with disabilities complete their high school program with a certificate of completion vs a diploma (11% vs 69%),[1] making it more difficult for them to pursue competitive employment.[1,4-7] Children with disabilities need to attain not only the ability to complete academic components of education, but also the functional skills necessary for postsecondary education, jobs and job training, independent living, and social competence for adult life.[5-12]

EDUCATION LAWS

Education laws are the bases for the provision of services for children with disabilities in public schools. To understand the role and function of the physical therapist in an educational setting, we must understand the contents and implications of the laws. We also must understand the history of educational law, interaction between federal and state laws, and the interaction between physical therapy practice laws and professional standards and educational laws.

Connolly BH, Montgomery PC, eds. *Therapeutic Exercise for Children With Developmental Disabilities, Fourth Edition* (pp 417-450).
© 2020 Taylor & Francis Group.

Historical Overview

In 1965, Congress passed the Elementary and Secondary Education Act (ESEA). This act established funding and minimum standards for public education for children. In 1975, Congress passed Public Law (PL) 94-142, the Education for All Handicapped Children Act (EHA). By mandating a free and appropriate public school education for all school-aged children with disabilities, PL 94-142 opened schools' doors to children with severe disabilities who had not been served previously. As stated by Congress, the purposes of PL 94-142 are[13]:

(1) To insure that all handicapped children have available to them a free and appropriate public education; (2) to assure that the rights of handicapped children and their parents are protected; (3) to assist states and localities to provide for the education of all handicapped children; and (4) to assess and insure the effectiveness of all efforts to educate such children.

In 1986, the EHA was amended again through enactment of PL 99-457, significantly changing services for infants and young children. Congress stated there was an urgent and substantial need to[14]:

(1) Enhance the development of handicapped infants and toddlers and to minimize their potential for developmental delay; (2) reduce the educational costs to our society, including our Nation's schools, by minimizing the need for special education and related services after handicapped infants and toddlers reach school age; (3) minimize the likelihood of institutionalization of handicapped individuals and maximize the potential for their independent living in society; and (4) enhance the capacity of families to meet the special needs of their infants and toddlers with handicaps.

Through PL 99-457 Congress established a policy to financially assist states to[14]:

(1) Develop and implement a statewide, comprehensive, coordinated, multi-disciplinary, interagency program of early intervention services for handicapped infants and toddlers and their families; (2) facilitate the coordination of payment for early intervention services from Federal, State, local, and private sources (including public and private insurance coverage); and (3) enhance its capacity to provide quality early intervention services and expand and improve existing early intervention services being provided to handicapped infants and toddlers and their families.

PL 99-457 did not mandate services for infants and toddlers, but provided financial support for states that chose to provide services for these children.

A major revision and reauthorization of EHA occurred in 1990 when the act was renamed the Individuals with Disabilities Education Act (IDEA).[15] IDEA was reauthorized and amended in 1997[16] with federal regulations finalized in 1999.[17] IDEA was reauthorized in 2004.

EHA, PL 94-142, and PL 99-457 established the foundation and framework for special education, and although amended several times, the essential components still remain a part of IDEA today.

From the initial enactment of the ESEA in 1965, it has been reauthorized and amended over the years. In 2001, Congress reauthorized and renamed the ESEA to the No Child Left Behind Act 2001 (NCLB).[18] The US Department of Education stated this law[18]:

Represents a sweeping overhaul of federal efforts to support elementary and secondary education in the United States. It is built on 4 common-sense pillars: (1) accountability for results; (2) an emphasis on doing what works based on scientific research; (3) expanded parental options; and (4) expanded local control and flexibility.

The major thrust of the act was to ensure that all children would read and demonstrate progress in reading, math, and science as measured by statewide assessments. This law had significant impact on students with disabilities as it required special education students to participate in testing and demonstrate progress in academic areas. The constructs of the 4 pillars also were carried over into the reauthorization of IDEA in 2004, especially as related to additions regarding "doing what works based on scientific research." There was also the expectation that students of minority background, who had traditionally been overrepresented in special education, would be supported through NCLB rather than IDEA.

NCLB was to be reauthorized in 2007, but because of difficulties with implementation of several of its requirements, input was sought from interested parties including educators, administrators, parents, agencies, organizations, and the public. The result was the Every Student Succeeds Act (ESSA), a bipartisan act signed into law December 10, 2015, reauthorizing ESEA and ending NCLB.

Laws and regulations are dynamic documents that can change through legislative processes. Readers are encouraged to check the US Department of Education and Office of Special Education for current information on ESSA and IDEA.

CURRENT EDUCATION LAWS

Every Student Succeeds Act

ESSA, as the reauthorization of the ESEA of 1965,[19] sets forth the standards and requirements for the education of students in public schools. The ESSA was enacted in December 2015 with the purpose to: "provide all children significant opportunity to receive a fair, equitable, and high quality education, and to close the educational achievement gap" (20 USC 6301).

To achieve this goal, ESSA revised the assessment process with the requirement that all children be assessed using standard testing. This includes students with significant cognitive impairments. The standardized testing must be of universal design as all children will be assessed.

Universal design means[20]:

A concept of philosophy for designing and delivering products and services that are usable by people with the widest possible range of functional capabilities, which include products and services that are directly accessible (without requiring assistive technologies) and products and services that are interoperable with assistive technologies (34 USC 3002).

Individuals with Disabilities Education Act

The last reauthorization of IDEA occurred in 2004 with the latest amendments in 2015 as a result of the passage of ESSA; technical amendments continue to be added as rules are finalized. The following is a description of IDEA as reauthorized in 2004 and amended through 2018.[21] The information is from the IDEA Statute and the Notice of Final Regulations for IDEA published in the Federal Register and compiled on the IDEA website by the Department of Education covering the period of 2006 to the present (August 2018).[21] The Department of Education has a separate website for IDEA, which has the most current information on IDEA law and regulations (https://sites.ed.gov/idea/).

Contents

The IDEA statute or law, contains 4 parts: (1) Part A—General provisions; (2) Part B—Assistance for education of all children with disabilities (addresses special education for children age 3 through 21 years); (3) Part C—Infants and toddlers with disabilities (addresses special education for children birth through age 2 years); and (4) Part D—National activities to improve education of children with disabilities (addresses grants, research, personnel preparation, technical assistance, and dissemination of information). Statutes or laws have specific coding, United States Code (USC), based on their topic. Chapter 20 of the USC is for education law. IDEA is coded as 20 USC 1400 (section number). Federal regulations are rules that are developed to further explain the law and are identified with a separate numbering system. Part B and Part C are the sections most often referred to for the provision of services. The Federal Regulations identify Part B as Part 300 Section 300.1 to 300.818 and Part C as Part 303 Section 303.1 to 303.734.

Purpose

Congress determined the need for IDEA based on the following finding:

Disability is a natural part of the human experience and in no way diminishes the right of individuals to participate in or contribute to society. Improving educational results for children with disabilities is an essential element of our national policy of ensuring equality of opportunity, full participation, independent living, and economic self-sufficiency for individuals with disabilities (20 USC 1400[c][1]).

Congress stated the purposes of the IDEA:

(1) (A) to ensure that all children with disabilities have available to them a free appropriate public education that emphasizes special education and related services designed to meet their unique needs and prepare them for further education, employment, and independent living; (B) to ensure that the rights of children with disabilities and parents of such children are protected; and (C) to assist States, localities, educational service agencies, and Federal agencies to provide for the education of all children with disabilities;
(2) to assist States in the implementation of a statewide, comprehensive, coordinated, multidisciplinary, interagency system of early intervention services for infants and toddlers with disabilities and their families;
(3) to ensure that educators and parents have the necessary tools to improve educational results of children with disabilities by supporting systemic improvement activities; coordinated research and personnel preparation; coordinated technical assistance, dissemination, and support; and technology development and media services; and
(4) to assess, and ensure the effectiveness of, efforts to educate children with disabilities (20 USC 1400[d]).

Constructs

To implement the purposes of IDEA, Congress embedded several constructs within the law. These included a whole child approach, a family-focused approach for infants and toddlers, use of the least restrictive environment (LRE), obligation to provide a free appropriate public education (FAPE), collaboration of services at all levels, and due process procedures.

WHOLE CHILD

IDEA requires that all aspects of the child be addressed in all aspects of education. The whole child approach means the evaluation and Individualized Education Program (IEP) must address all areas of development and the skills needed to learn, work, and live independently as an adult. This includes the ability to access general education curriculum, transition activities, and the preparation for further education, employment, and independent living. ESSA and IDEA stress the need to prepare all students for success in college and careers and to lead productive and independent adult lives to the maximum extent possible.[17-19]

FAMILY FOCUS

A significant difference in Part C (infants and toddlers) is the transition from child-focused service to family-focused service. Family-focused means the assessment and present level of development and needs must address not only the child, but also the family. The parents, while being part of the focus, also are a part of the team. Parents need, and want, to be involved in the entire process, especially before decisions are made.[22-24] The focus on the family is needed as the parents are the child's primary caregivers and as such the child's primary teachers.[25-27] To empower the parents, to recognize the knowledge they have regarding their child, and to acknowledge their ability to become the child's "teachers" are important aspects of intervention.[28-30]

LEAST RESTRICTIVE ENVIRONMENT

The law requires that children with disabilities be educated in the LRE with children without disabilities. The intent of LRE is that all children first should try to function in the regular classroom, first without support or modifications, and then with support or modifications. If this does not work, only then should other alternatives for instruction be attempted.

> ▸ Part B—"To the maximum extent appropriate, children with disabilities, including children in public or private institutions or other care facilities, are educated with children who are not disabled, and special classes, separate schooling, or other removal of children with disabilities from the regular educational environment occurs only when the nature or severity of the disability of a child is such that education in regular classes with the use of supplementary aids and services cannot be achieved satisfactorily" (U.S. 612[a][5][A]).

> ▸ Part C—"To the maximum extent appropriate, services are provided in natural environments, including the home and community settings in which children without disabilities participate" (USC 1432[4][G]). Services to meet the needs of infants and toddlers with disabilities and their families should be provided in natural environments as much as possible with children without disabilities. For most infants and toddlers this would be the home; however, it also may include day care or preschool settings.

FREE APPROPRIATE PUBLIC EDUCATION

When EHA was first enacted, states were required to provide students with disabilities the same resources as students without disabilities. To ensure equal treatment, Congress specifically stated that all children with disabilities are to receive a "free appropriate education, which includes special education and related services."[31] FAPE is currently available for all children with disabilities between ages 3 and 21 years in all states. FAPE for children younger than 3 years is not federally mandated but determined by individual states. IDEA Part C is the statute that states must follow if they decide to provide education for infants and toddlers.

Congress never intended that education assume all of the health costs incurred by children with disabilities but that other agencies would continue providing health or medical services. There has been confusion as to the extent the schools are responsible for providing health-related services. Congress amended the EHA and the IDEA to provide clarification so that states may use "whatever State, local, Federal, and private sources of support are available in the State"[17] and that funds for Part C may not be used to "satisfy a financial commitment for services that would have been paid for from another public or private source."[17] States also may not "reduce medical or other assistance available or to alter eligibility under Title V of the Social Security Act (relating to maternal and child health) or Title XIX of the Social Security Act (relating to Medicaid for infants and toddlers with disabilities) within the State."[17] The law further states that education is the payer of last resort if funding from private or public sources would have paid for the same service. However, educational services cannot be delayed or denied pending reimbursement from an agency. These provisions continue to be included in the current IDEA.

COLLABORATION OF SERVICES

The IDEA recognizes the complex and varied needs of families of children with disabilities. It also recognizes that one agency cannot meet all these needs. To meet the needs of families, collaboration of services is required from multiple agencies. The designated agency for services for children ages 3 through 21 years is education; however, each state must designate a lead agency (education or other) to manage the implementation of services for infants and toddlers. States also must establish collaborative relationships to aid in the transition from education to adult services.

The construct of collaboration also applies to the educational team. The physical therapist must perform coordination, communication, and documentation for each child. This activity in the educational setting is consistent with the *Guide to Physical Therapist Practice 3.0* framework of coordination, communication, and documentation that is a component of practice provided throughout the patient/client management process.[32] Therapists employed in educational settings are responsible for coordinating care and services with physicians and outside providers as well as other school personnel. Private physical therapists providing services in the community or in educational settings also need to coordinate and communicate their services with educational personnel.

DUE PROCESS

IDEA requires documentation of due process and the plan for special education. Due process consists of procedural safeguards to ensure that the rights of parents and children with disabilities are maintained in the educational setting. Due process includes the following:

> - Informed consent
> - Confidentiality
> - Timelines for assessment, placement, and service
> - Procedures for the development and implementation of individualized programs
> - Procedures for the resolution of conflicts

Part B and Part C include due process requirements but vary in the specific requirements and timelines.

Definitions

The following definitions form the basis for special education programs and services. As a result of public comments, court decisions, and amendments, IDEA has been refined to better address the needs of children with disabilities. For the most current definitions, please refer to current federal law (https://www.ed.gov/).

CHILD WITH A DISABILITY

The definition of "child with a disability" in the law is virtually unprecedented in its inclusiveness. The terms included in the definitions are different for Part B and Part C and are considered educational categories of disability based on specific eligibility criteria. To be defined as a child with a disability in the educational setting, a child must meet the eligibility criteria for one of the disability categories defined by the law:

> - Part B—A child with intellectual disabilities, hearing impairments (including deafness), speech or language impairments, visual impairments (including blindness), serious emotional disturbance (hereafter referred to as emotional disturbance), orthopedic impairments, autism, traumatic brain injury, other health impairments, specific learning disabilities—who by reason therefore, needs special education and related services (Sec. 300.8[a][1]). The term also includes "children age 3 through 9 years experiencing developmental delays" at the discretion of the state education agency (SEA) and the local education agency (LEA) (Sec. 300.8[b]).
> - Part C—Infant or toddler with a disability means an individual younger than 3 years who needs early intervention services because the individual is experiencing a developmental delay

in one or more of the following areas: cognitive development, physical development including vision and hearing, communication development, social or emotional development, adaptive development, or has a diagnosed physical or mental condition that has a high probability of resulting in developmental delay (Sec. 303.21[a][1,2]). The term also may include, at a state's discretion, an at-risk infant or toddler as defined in Section 303.5 (an individual younger than 3 years who would be at risk of experiencing a substantial developmental delay if early intervention services were not provided).

ELIGIBILITY

Eligibility identifies the 4 main requirements children must meet to receive special education services: (1) appropriate age, (2) complete an educational evaluation, (3) meet eligibility criteria, and (4) demonstrate a need for services. Part B and Part C have different age and disability categories with associated eligibility criteria. Children in either part must complete an evaluation and demonstrate a need for services. It is not enough to have a medical diagnosis, as this does not equate to an educational disability. For example, a child may have a diagnosis of cerebral palsy, but may not meet the eligibility criteria for an educational disability. By law, a child must meet the eligibility criteria for a disability category *and* demonstrate a need for special education. In addition, a child may have needs for physical therapy, but IDEA, Section 300.8(2)(i), specifically states that even though the child may meet the eligibility criteria for a disability category, "but only needs a related service and not special education, the child is not a *child with a disability* under this part" unless the related service being considered is a special education service.

> Part B—Children age 3 through 21 years must complete a full and individual initial evaluation, must meet the eligibility criteria for the above-listed disability categories, and also must demonstrate a need for special education and related services (Sec. 300.8).

> Part C—Children birth through age 2 years must complete an initial evaluation; must meet eligibility criteria for one of the areas of delay or have a diagnosed physical or mental condition that has a high probability of resulting in developmental delay; and also must demonstrate a need for early intervention services (Sec. 303.21).

SPECIAL EDUCATION/EARLY INTERVENTION SERVICES

Special education is the program available to children with disabilities in the educational setting. It includes primary program areas based on the disability categories, such as specific learning disability, intellectual disability, speech or language impairment, visual impairment, emotional disturbances, traumatic brain injury, physical impairment, and other health impairment. Individual states use the disability categories identified in IDEA and may define their own specific disability categories and change the terms as they see appropriate to provide services in their state.

Special education services are mandated for children eligible under Part B. Services for children eligible for Part C are permissive at the federal level, allowing individual states to determine whether they will provide services to this age group. Check your state's education laws to see whether and how children, birth through age 2 years, are provided services.

> Part B—Special education means specially designed instruction, at no cost to the parents, to meet the unique needs of a child with a disability, including instruction conducted in the classroom, in the home, in hospitals and institutions, and in other settings and instruction in physical education. The term also includes speech-language pathology services or any other related service if the service is considered special education rather than related services under state standards, travel training, and vocational education (Sec. 300.39[a]).

> Part C—Early intervention services means developmental services that are provided under public supervision; selected in collaboration with the parents; provided at no cost; and designed to meet the developmental needs of an infant or toddler with a disability and the needs of the family to assist appropriately in the infant's or toddler's development as identified by the Individualized Family Service Plan (IFSP) team in one or more of the following

developmental areas: physical, cognitive, communication, social or emotional, or adaptive (Sec. 303.13). These services are provided at no cost, in natural environments, and provide training for the family. Early intervention services are defined as developmental services and may include assistive technology, audiology, family training, counseling, home visits, special instruction, occupational therapy, physical therapy, and speech and language therapy. Additionally, psychological services, medical services for diagnostic or evaluation purposes, health services, nursing services, nutrition services, transportation and related costs for travel, social work services, and service coordination are included (Sec. 303.13).

RELATED SERVICES

Related services are those services required for the student to benefit from special education. Part B uses the term *related services* to specifically define the services available for a student to benefit from special education. Part C does not use the term related services, but includes the specific services available in the definition of early intervention services.

- ▶ Part B—Transportation and such developmental, corrective, and other supportive services (including speech-language pathology and audiology services, interpreting services, psychological services, physical and occupational therapy, recreation [including therapeutic recreation], social work services, school nurse services designed to enable a child with a disability to receive a free appropriate education as described in the IEP of the child, counseling services [including rehabilitation counseling], orientation and mobility services, and medical services, except that such medical services shall be for diagnostic or evaluation purposes only) as may be required to assist a child with a disability to benefit from special education, and includes the early identification and assessment of disabling conditions in children. Related services also include school health services and school nurse services, social work services in schools, and parent counseling and training (Sec. 300.24).
- ▶ Part C—Early intervention services definition lists the services available for infants and toddlers (Sec. 303.13). Federal law allows physical therapy to be a primary early intervention service; however, states may define this differently, requiring the infant or toddler also to receive services from an early intervention teacher.

PHYSICAL THERAPY

Physical therapy is defined differently in Part B and Part C. In addition to the stated definitions, physical therapists must meet the requirements of personnel qualifications that are "SEA-approved or SEA-recognized certification, licensing, registration, or other comparable requirements that apply to the professional discipline in which those personnel are providing special education or related services (Sec. 300.23) or conducting evaluations or assessments or providing early intervention services" (Sec. 303.31). This requires physical therapists to review their state education law, as most states require licensure only as a physical therapist. Some states, however, require additional certification of the physical therapist to work in a school district.

- ▶ Part B—"Physical therapy means services provided by a qualified physical therapist" (Sec. 300.34[c][9]).
- ▶ Part C—"Physical therapy includes services to address the promotion of sensorimotor function through enhancement of musculoskeletal status, neurobehavioral organization, perceptual and motor development, cardiopulmonary status, and effective environmental adaptation:
  - ∘ "Screening, evaluation, and assessment of infants and toddlers to identify movement dysfunction;
  - ∘ "Obtaining, interpreting, and integrating information appropriate to program planning to prevent, alleviate, or compensate for movement dysfunction and related functional problems; and

TABLE 15-1. INDIVIDUALIZED EDUCATION PROGRAM

Components of the Individualized Education Program must address how a child's disability affects involvement and progress in a general education curriculum; extracurricular and other nonacademic activities; and for preschool participation in activities:

- A statement of the child's present levels of academic achievement and functional performance
- A statement of measurable annual goals, including academic and functional goals
- A description of how the child's progress toward annual goals will be measured and when periodic reports will be provided (at least as often as reports for nondisabled students)
- A statement of specific special education and related services and supplementary aids and services to be provided to the child and a statement of the programs, modifications, or supports for school personnel
- An explanation of the extent, if any, to which the child will not participate with nondisabled children in the regular class and activities
- A statement of any individual modification in the administration of state- or district-wide assessments, or why the child cannot participate and alternative assessment selected
- The projected date for initiation of services and modifications and the anticipated frequency, location, and duration of those services
- At age 16 years, or earlier, a statement of transition needs
- Transfer of rights at age of majority (Sec. 300.320)

○ "Providing individual and group services or treatment to prevent, alleviate, or compensate for movement dysfunction and related functional problems" (Sec. 303.13[b][9]).

INDIVIDUALIZED PROGRAMS

A separate individualized program must be written for each child who qualifies for special education. The child's parent(s) and, when appropriate, the child, must be involved in the development of the program. Under Part B the program is the IEP, while under Part C it is the IFSP.

- ➤ Part B—IEP for all children age 3 through 21 years; for children age 3 to 5 years an IFSP can be used. An IEP is a written statement that describes the present levels of academic and functional performance of a child with the goals and objectives to address these identified needs. The IEP and IFSP are developed by the child's team, which includes the parent(s) and, when appropriate, the child. Table 15-1 lists the components of the IEP.
- ➤ Part C—IFSP for infants and toddlers, age birth through 2 years. The IFSP is a written statement of the child's present developmental levels, family's resources, priorities and concerns, and expected outcomes (Sec. 303.344). The IFSP is developed by the child's team, which includes the parent(s), and if requested, providers from outside agencies. Table 15-2 lists the components of the IFSP.

TRAVEL TRAINING

Travel training was added to IDEA as a special education service when IDEA was reauthorized in 1997. It is different from orientation and mobility training and applies to any student with a disability demonstrating a need for this type of training. Services may be an integral part of special education and are necessary for the student to prepare for transition to adult programs.[33]

TABLE 15-2. INDIVIDUALIZED FAMILY SERVICE PLAN

The Individualized Family Service Plan must contain the following information:

- Information about the child's status: A statement of the infant's or toddler's present levels of physical development, cognitive development, communication development, social or emotional development, and adaptive development
- Family information: A statement of the family's resources, priorities, and concerns
- Results or outcomes: A statement of the measurable results or outcomes expected to be achieved for the child and family
- Early intervention services: A statement of specific early intervention services including a statement of the natural environments in which early intervention services shall appropriately be provided, justification as to why services will not be provided in natural environments, and for a child at least age 3 years educational components that promote school readiness, preliteracy, language, and numeracy skills
- Other services: Identify medical or other services needed or receiving and, if not currently provided, steps to take to assist securing them
- Dates and duration of services: The projected dates for initiation of services and the anticipated duration of such services
- Service coordination: The name of the service coordinator
- Transition from Part C: The steps to be taken to support the transition of the infant and toddler to services provided under Part B (school-aged services) (Sec. 303.344)

The general definition of travel training means:

Providing instruction, as appropriate, to children with significant cognitive disabilities, and any other children with disabilities, who require this instruction, to enable them to— (i) develop an awareness of the environment in which they live; and (ii) learn the skills necessary to move effectively and safely from place to place within that environment (eg, in school, in the home, at work, and in the community) (Sec. 300.39[b][4]).

ASSISTIVE TECHNOLOGY

Assistive technology devices and services are included both in Part B and Part C. IDEA mandates that assistive technology be considered by the IEP/IFSP team as a method to meet the child's needs. Assistive technology devices and services must be provided at no cost to the child if the IEP/IFSP team determines they are necessary to ensure FAPE. Assistive technology can be considered a related service or a supplementary aid and service in Part B and an early intervention service in Part C.

- *Assistive technology device* means any item, piece of equipment, or product system, whether acquired commercially off the shelf, modified, or customized, that is used to increase, maintain, or improve the functional capabilities of a child with a disability (Sec. 300.5, 303.13[b] [1][i]).
- *Assistive technology service* means a service that directly assists a child with a disability in the selection, acquisition, or use of an assistive technology device (Sec. 300.6, 303.13[b][1][ii]).

TRANSITION SERVICES

Transition services are defined differently in Part B and Part C. Whereas both definitions address the need to plan for the transition of the child from one type of service or program to another, Part B specifically addresses areas of transition.

> Part B is a "coordinated set of activities" that "is designed within a results-oriented process, that is focused on improving the academic and functional achievement of the child with a disability to facilitate the child's movement from school to post school activities, including postsecondary education, vocational education, integrated employment (including supported employment), continuing and adult education, adult services, independent living, or community participation"; is based "on individual child's needs, taking into account the child's strengths, preferences, and interests"; and includes instruction, related services, community experiences, the development of employment and other postschool adult living objectives, and, if appropriate, acquisition of daily living skills and provision of a functional vocational evaluation (Sec. 300.43). Transition services are required for all students beginning at age 16 years, or earlier, if appropriate.

> Part C activities are used "to ensure a smooth transition for infants and toddlers with disabilities under the age of 3 years and their families receiving early intervention services under this part to preschool or other appropriate services or exiting the program for infants and toddlers with disabilities" (Sec. 303.209).

EXTENDED SCHOOL YEAR

Extended school year (ESY) services are available to children under Part B who may experience a loss of skills or regression and will not be able to recoup the skills in a reasonable amount of time.[18,22] Services are generally provided over the summer; however, they also could be provided over long breaks in the school calendar. ESY may be considered for children who turn age 3 years over the summer.

> Part B—ESY services are determined on an individual basis by the child's IEP team. A state or LEA may not limit the services to a specific disability category or limit the amount, type, or duration of services (Sec. 300.106[a]). ESY are defined as "special education and related services provided to a child with a disability, beyond the normal school year of the public agency, in accordance with the child's IEP, at no cost to the parents, and meet the standards of the State Education Agency (SEA)" (Sec. 300.106[b]).

> Part C—ESY services may be considered for a child who turns age 3 years during the summer if the child has been receiving Part C services.

OTHER LAWS THAT AFFECT EDUCATIONAL SETTINGS

In addition to understanding education laws, physical therapists need to be familiar with other laws that affect children with disabilities in the educational setting. All these acts are designed to protect the rights of individuals with disabilities in a variety of settings. These laws address civil rights not only in the educational setting, but also in community, health, and work settings in the real world. Table 15-3 provides an overview of federal laws that affect individuals with disabilities. See the Resources at the end of the chapter for websites that address disability.

Section 504 of the Rehabilitation Act[34] has the most impact in the educational setting. Section 504 can be used if a child does not qualify or demonstrate a need for special education service but has an identified disability. This law requires that schools provide reasonable accommodations for any individual that is defined by the act's definition as a person with a disability. The act defines a person with a disability as "any person who has a physical or mental impairment which substantially limits one or more of the major life activities, has a record of such impairment, or is regarded by others as having such impairment" (34 C.F.R. 104.3[j][1]). Schools or LEAs should have a process by which to identify and implement services for individuals, students, and staff who meet the criteria for a 504 plan. Physical therapists may be involved in the process to identify and implement a 504 plan; however, this would not be considered a special education or related service.

TABLE 15-3. LAWS THAT AFFECT INDIVIDUALS WITH DISABILITIES	
ACT	APPLICATION
Section 504 of the Rehabilitation Act of 1973	Protects rights in programs that receive federal financial assistance from the US Department of Education. Must provide reasonable accommodations.
Americans with Disabilities Act	Protects rights in public and private programs. Must provide reasonable accommodations.
Assistive Technology Act of 1998	Requires states to provide programs and training for assistive technology.
Family Educational Rights and Privacy Act	Protects rights regarding confidential health and education information.
Health Insurance Portability and Accountability Act	Protects rights for health insurance coverage and standards for privacy of individually identifiable health information. Rule does not apply to records covered by the Family Educational Rights and Privacy Act but may apply if information is used for outside billing or for research.

PHYSICAL THERAPIST PRACTICE ACTS

Physical therapists and administrators need to be knowledgeable of their state's physical thera-py practice act and its impact on educational services. Physical therapists are obligated to meet the requirements of their practice act, regardless of the setting in which they practice. Physical therapist assistants may or may not be regulated by their state. Additionally, state rules and regulations may or may not address the way a physical therapist should interact with the physical therapist assistant.

Physical therapist assistants may work in an educational setting, but must function under the direction and supervision of a physical therapist. Based on professional standards and education, physical therapist assistants cannot perform an evaluation or diagnosis but can assist the physical therapist in the implementation of selected interventions.[35] A physical therapist assistant can-not work independently of a physical therapist and should never be the only provider of physical therapy. It is important to review the regulations that apply to your state before providing service.

In addition to physical therapy practice regulations, states may have regulations that apply to all health care providers. It is important to review all the regulations that apply to health care providers, in addition to those that specifically apply to physical therapy.

ROLES AND FUNCTIONS OF PHYSICAL THERAPISTS IN THE SCHOOLS

The *Guide to Physical Therapist Practice 3.0* (the *Guide*) provides a description of physical therapist practice including an overview of roles, constructs, and the patient and client manage-ment process[32] (see Chapter 6). The focus of physical therapy is to address movement necessary for optimal function in the performance of activities and participation for positive quality of life. Physical therapists perform many roles, including primary, secondary, and tertiary care; preven-tion and promotion of health wellness, and fitness; consultation; education; critical inquiry; and administration. These are the physical therapist's role regardless of the setting or patient popula-tion. The role of the physical therapist in the educational setting, as defined by IDEA, is to assist the child with a disability to benefit from special education. The challenge for the physical thera-pist is (1) to determine the roles of the child in the educational setting, (2) then with the child's educational (IEP/IFSP) team determine if the identified needs affect the educational program, and (3) if the expertise of a physical therapist is necessary to assist the child to meet those needs. The emphasis of therapy will depend on the special education and general education program in which the child is participating, as well as the goals and objectives developed by the IEP or IFSP team. The primary focus for the physical therapist in the educational setting is to assist the child in the development of functional mobility, to assist the child to access the educational environment, and to assist the child to understand his or her disability and its impact on wellness and fitness.

Physical therapists play a unique role in addressing prevention, health, wellness, and fitness as they not only have expertise in these areas but also have knowledge and understanding of a child's condition, the natural course of that condition, and how the condition affects the health, wellness, and fitness of the child.[36-38] The physical therapist also has the unique role of understanding the impact of health, wellness, and fitness on learning[39-41] and, as such, is able to incorporate move-ment strategies into educational plans and while consulting and collaborating with schools and communities.[42-44]

The models of service in an educational setting are unlike those in the typical medical setting, in which direct one-to-one services are provided to each patient. Physical therapists in schools need to adjust and redefine their intervention programs and objectives to assist the child to ben-efit from special education.[25,30,45] Physical therapists are considered a member of the child's IEP or IFSP team whose members jointly identify needs, develop goals and objectives, and determine programs and services.

General Functions

Teaming

A critical aspect of working in an educational setting is the ability to function effectively on a team. The basic constructs of IDEA require that the child participate in the least restrictive envi-ronment and natural setting. The purpose of teaming is to bring a group of "experts" together to address the "whole child" and what that child needs to be successful throughout the educational day. For each child, the team needs to be familiar with the age-appropriate general education cur-riculum, the daily classroom routine, and the typical expectations for same-age peers so they may determine how that specific child's disability and identified needs interfere with his or her ability to participate and learn in general education. For any child with a disability to be successful in the educational environment, the team must be able to work together. Collaboration is essential throughout due process from the identification and prioritization of needs through the develop-ment and implementation of the IEP/IFSP.[22,46,47] Teaming is considered a dynamic process, and each member bringing a different perspective and expertise. Utley and Rapport[48] identified 4 ele-ments that special education teachers and related service providers identified as essential to effec-tive teaming: (1) problem solving, (2) willingness to share and combine intervention methods, (3) importance of assessment data, and (4) and decision making. The ability of the team to problem solve is reported to be the highest value of teaming.[46,48]

Basic components for an effective team include defined purpose for the team; clearly estab-lished team goals; high communication among team members; high commitment from team members; understanding of own and other professionals' roles; respect and value for each other's profession; equal participation, power, and influence; participation by all members; defined decision-making and conflict-resolution processes; and encouragement of differing opinions.[45-49] For effective teaming to occur, adequate time must be committed to and provided for on a regular basis by the administration and team members.[44,50]

INTERDISCIPLINARY VERSUS TRANSDISCIPLINARY

Teaming in the educational setting generally is viewed as interdisciplinary or transdisciplinary. Both models require regular communication and a team approach to the development and implementation of the IEP/IFSP. Transdisciplinary teaming requires members of the team to teach others aspects of their own discipline and to learn aspects of the other team members' disciplines.[51] Although this is defined as role release, many believe they are "giving away their profession" and are threatened by this process.[52] York and colleagues[52] attempted to clarify some of the misconceptions of transdisciplinary teamwork and integrated therapy. They stated that loss of direct student contact is not a result of released professional skills, but rather is cooperation among team members to enhance the child's ability to function in natural settings. Rainforth[53] addressed the legal and ethical concerns of role release by physical therapists and found that the activities can be both legal and ethical. An important aspect of working in an educational setting is teaching others how to set up the environment to facilitate the practice of specific skills when the child needs to use those skills. Teachers and paraprofessionals in the educational setting function as caregivers. This allows physical therapists to provide instruction and training of these individuals as part of patient/client-related instruction of the patient and client management process.[32]

Caution must be used so that the concept of the transdisciplinary approach is not used to limit the availability of or access to any discipline. It is critical in this discussion to remember that physical therapy can be performed only by a physical therapist or a physical therapist assistant under the direction and supervision of a physical therapist.[35] When activities or techniques are taught to other individuals, they are performing the activities, not physical therapy, and it should be documented as such on the child's IEP/IFSP.

Medical Versus Educational Services

For many years, administrators, legislators, parents, physicians, and even physical therapists have been trying to define the difference between medical and educational physical therapy services.[50] Many believe it is critical to define the difference since education is responsible for paying only for educational services, and many private and public insurers will pay only for medically necessary services. With the passage and amendments to educational laws and PL 100-360, Section 411(k)(13), educational agencies have been allowed to seek reimbursement for "medically necessary" health-related services provided as part of a child's special education program (IEP/IFSP). These changes have added to the confusion because "medical" services can now be provided and reimbursed in an "educational" setting.

Overlaps also exist in the provision of medical and educational services. Education now encompasses teaching children in a variety of settings that include the home, classroom, playground, lunchroom, bus, community, and work sites.[54] At the same time, the medical model has changed from the hospital setting to the home, community, and work site.[55-57] Another overlap is the philosophical basis for practice of the physical therapist. The *Guide,* as described in Chapter 6, describes the practice of the physical therapist, which is the same, regardless of setting. Based on this, the physical therapist in either the educational or medical setting needs to base practice on the 4 constructs and concepts of the *Guide 3.0:* (1) the disablement-enablement model of the *International Classification of Functioning, Disability and Health* (ICF) and biopsychosocial model, (2) evidence-based practice, (3) professional values, and (4) quality assessment.[32] This results in the physical therapist in both settings addressing the "whole child," the child's functional skills, and the roles of the child.

Perhaps one way to differentiate medical and educational services is to address the regulations and purpose of the service. Physical therapists in both settings are obligated to follow their state physical therapy practice act. In the medical setting, the additional regulations that oversee the service would be that of either federal and state health care laws, public or private insurers' policies, or, in cases of direct reimbursement, the desires of the patient/client. The purpose of physical therapy in the medical setting is to assist the patient/client to be as functionally independent as possible. This is accomplished by addressing the patient's/client's pathology or health condition, impairments in body functions and structures, activity limitations, participation restrictions, risk factors, and health, wellness, and fitness needs. In other words, medical necessity may be defined as services needed to impact the process of disablement or enablement.[55-57]

In the educational setting, the additional regulations that oversee the service are federal and state education laws. The purpose of physical therapy in the educational setting is to assist the identified special education student to be as functionally independent as possible to benefit from the educational program. Like the medical model, this is achieved by addressing the student's pathology or health condition, impairments in body functions and structures, activity limitations, participation restrictions, risk factors, and health, wellness, and fitness needs. However, it is only in relation to how these needs interfere with the student's ability to participate in the educational program. In other words, educational necessity may be defined as services needed to allow the student to benefit from education.[54]

One major difference between medical and educational services is the process for accessing the service. In the medical model, any child can receive physical therapy service. In the educational model, the child must meet a minimum of 2 conditions before physical therapy services can be considered. First, the child must be identified as having an educational disability, as defined by federal and state laws. Second, the child must demonstrate a need for special education and related services. For children ages 3 through 21 years, only when these first 2 conditions are met can physical therapy be considered to assist in meeting the child's identified special education needs. Infants and toddlers also must be identified with an educational disability and in need of early intervention services. However, federal law allows physical therapy to be the primary early intervention service for these children.

Deciding whether therapy services are medically or educationally necessary is up to the individual states, school districts, and individual IEP/IFSP teams. The law requires that physical therapy must be provided when it is necessary to "assist the child to benefit from special education."[21] IEP and IFSP teams that include the physical therapist must determine what is educationally necessary for that specific child and provide the appropriate services.

Role in Due Process

The physical therapist plays a vital role throughout educational due process. Figure 15-1 identifies Minnesota's model of the therapist's role and responsibilities at the various stages of due process.[50]

Therapists should check their state for specific guidelines.[54] Although the physical therapist participates in all the aspects of due process, it is not until the step involving the development of the IEP/IFSP, step 7 of 9, that the team discusses the need for the expertise of the physical therapist and services are determined.

Role in Identification

Identification is used to identify children birth through age 21 years who may have a need for special education and related services. Activities may include screening, interagency activities, and prereferral activities including consultation and education of staff. Districts need to have a plan for identifying children within the community, including children attending private schools. Therapists in educational settings may participate in any of the identification activities. Therapists in other settings need to be familiar with their state's identification process and the role of the LEA so children and families with suspected educational needs may be referred for evaluation.

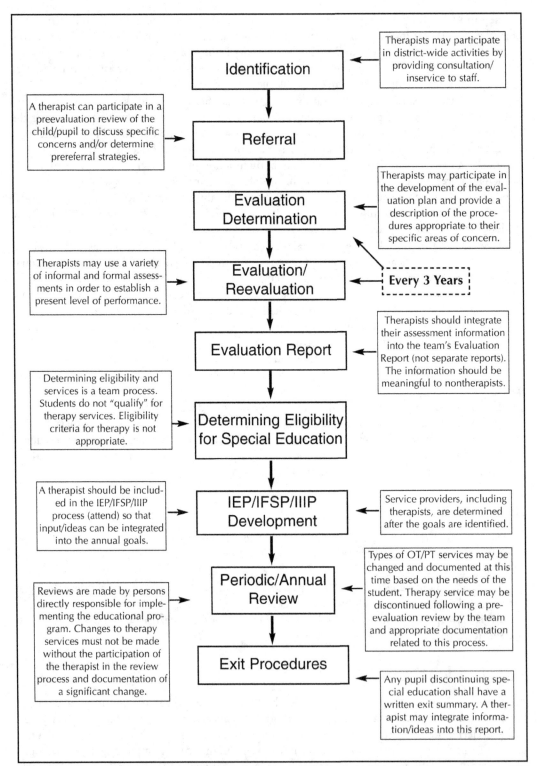

Figure 15-1. Therapist's role and responsibilities in due process. IEP indicates Individualized Education Program; IFSP, Individualized Family Service Plan; IIIP, Individual Interagency Intervention Plan; OT, occupational therapy; PT, physical therapy.

Role in Referral

Referral is the process of recommending children who are suspected of having a disability for review and possible evaluation by an educational team. There are many sources of referrals, including parents, teachers, physicians, physical therapists, and other professionals. Physical therapists may participate in the referral process by recommending a child for an educational evaluation and by consulting with educational staff regarding prereferral strategies to address motor concerns expressed by staff.

The process for referral is different for Part B and Part C. Therapists will need to review the requirements in law as well as SEA and LEA requirements.

Role in Evaluation

An evaluation is conducted "to determine whether a child is a child with a disability and the nature and extent of the special education and related services that the child needs"(Sec. 300.15). The information from the evaluation is used to determine whether the child is eligible for a disability category and whether the child qualifies for special education. This information also may be used in the development of the IEP/IFSP for the child. IDEA identifies a specific process for evaluation for Part B and Part C. Both parts require that all areas of a child, including functional development and academics, be reviewed and assessed even if the areas are not commonly associated with the disability category that is most appropriate for the child. The tools and materials selected must be culturally appropriate and valid for the purpose for which they are to be used. Information from the parents and general education staff must be included in the evaluation. Parents must give informed consent to perform an initial evaluation and also must provide consent to obtain or release information from other providers. Parents may refuse to have the evaluation performed and may refuse to release information. The LEA may choose to pursue due process to obtain the ability to have an evaluation performed.

Therapists need to work in collaboration with the entire team to determine the areas that need assessment and the tools and materials to be used. Procedures used by the physical therapist in performing an evaluation include administration of standardized tests, informal assessment, observation, interview, and review of records. As in the medical setting, the therapist must determine what is interfering with the student's ability to perform appropriate roles. Tests addressing functional skills, such as the School Function Assessment[58] and the Pediatric Evaluation of Disability Inventory,[59] are helpful in identifying needs and establishing a baseline of function (see Chapter 2). Impairments also are assessed, but evaluated in relation to how they affect the student's ability to function in the educational setting.

Determining Eligibility for Special Education

Following the evaluation, the team must determine whether the child qualifies for one or more disability categories. Generally, the disability categories require that the student fulfill the following:

- Performs at or below a specific level on a standardized test
- Demonstrates through observation difficulty managing academic activities, difficulty with organization, or difficulties as a result of an identified condition (eg, cerebral palsy, deaf or hard of hearing, attention deficit)
- Demonstrates a need for special education

The only criteria for receiving physical therapy are that the child qualify for special education **and** demonstrate a need for special education and related services. Individual states or school districts should not have additional criteria for physical therapy. The need for physical therapy is not determined at the time of evaluation or determination of eligibility but at the end of the development of the IEP or IFSP.

Children who qualify for special education must be reevaluated every 3 years to determine whether they still need special education. The physical therapist should participate in the reevaluation of children for whom they are a part of the IEP/IFSP team. They may also participate in the reevaluation for any child that that child's team determines needs the expertise of the physical therapist to determine the needs of the child.

An integrated team report must be written by the team summarizing the child's present level of performance and needs. This information then is the basis for the development of the child's IEP/IFSP.

INDIVIDUALIZED EDUCATION PROGRAM/ INDIVIDUALIZED FAMILY SERVICE PLAN DEVELOPMENT

The IEP and IFSP are legal contracts between the school district and the child and the child's family. They establish the framework for the child's special education program and any support or related services. Tables 15-1 and 15-2 list the components of the IEP and IFSP, respectively.

The process for development of the IEP/IFSP begins by identifying the "child's strengths, concerns of the parents for enhancing the education of their child, results of the initial or most recent evaluation of the child, and the academic, developmental, and functional needs of the child" (Sec. 300.324). Information from the child when appropriate, child's parent(s), staff, and other appropriate individuals including outside providers is used as the basis for identifying the child's strengths, abilities and needs, and the family's concerns and priorities. From the child's identified needs, the team prioritizes and develops goals and objectives that address these needs. Consideration is given to special factors such as behavioral needs, vision or hearing impairments, physical or health needs, and needs for assistive technology devices or services. It is important to address the identified needs as they relate to the educational program and recognize that not all identified needs have to be implemented in the IEP/IFSP. The team should prioritize which identified needs are important for the child for this IEP/IFSP and develop goals and objectives. In the development of the IFSP, the family's priorities and needs should be addressed before establishing expected outcomes or goals and objectives.[23,24,28,60] Once the goals and objectives are established they should not be considered static, but rather dynamic, changing and evolving.[50] For those identified needs that the team determines will not be included, a statement should be made regarding why they will not be addressed. Following the selection of goals and objectives, the team determines the services necessary for the child to achieve the identified goals and objectives. The team must determine whether the expertise of the physical therapist is needed for the child to benefit from the identified educational program.

The goals and objectives form the basis for measuring change in the child's abilities and determining effectiveness of the selected program and services. As in the medical setting, the goals and objectives should be child focused, measurable, and context specific.[60,61] In the educational setting, the physical therapist works with the team to develop the child's goals and objectives. Whereas the physical therapist may have more responsibility to develop and monitor a goal related to mobility, the entire team is responsible for implementing the goal. Just as the physical therapist incorporates the child's communication and cognitive goals into activities and interactions with the child, the teacher incorporates the child's mobility goals into the classroom activities. The goals need to reflect what the child can attain within 1 year, how the child's condition affects educational abilities, and have a direct link to the identified needs statements.[50]

Periodic Review

IDEA requires that the team review the child's progress at least as frequently as that done for the child's peers in general education. This means that the child's progress would be provided when reports are sent home for general education students, such as midterm reports and end-of-quarter reports. Data will need to be obtained throughout the year to determine progress and need for modification or development of new goals. ESSA legislation requires that **all** children make progress. It is important that teams establish reasonable, attainable goals and objectives so the child can demonstrate progress.

Periodic review is the time when the team can decide to change goals and services, including physical therapy services. A reevaluation is required to provide data to support the change in services. The physical therapist needs to be involved in the process to add, change, or discontinue physical therapy services.

Exit Procedures

Exit procedures generally apply to the discontinuation of special education. States define the procedures for determining whether a student continues to qualify and has need for special education. The procedures that allow for discontinuation of physical therapy are incorporated into the IEP/IFSP development and progress review as well as the reevaluation process. The physical therapist needs to be involved in the process to add, change, or discontinue physical therapy services.

Reimbursement of Therapy Services

Federal law requires states seek funding from public and private sources. Individual states determine how they will coordinate state agencies and reimbursement from public and private sources. Following passage of EHA some private and public payers changed their policies to reduce or deny coverage of covered services for children if they received covered services through their school system. To address this, Congress passed the Medicare Catastrophic Coverage Act, PL 100-360. Section 411(k)(13), which specifically says that states cannot deny payment for Medicaid services "because such services are included in the child's Individualized Education Program established pursuant to Part B of the Education of the Handicapped Act or furnished to a handicapped infant or toddler because such services are included in the child's Individualized Family Service Plan adopted pursuant to Part H of such Act."[26] Because this amendment was a technical amendment to Medicaid law, it has no impact on Medicare or private insurers unless they are involved in the state Medicaid program. To address private insurers, the IDEA was amended to allow states to seek reimbursement by having education be the payer of last resort; however, private payers are not required to participate and may deny payment. IDEA requires that when accessing a private payer, parents must provide informed consent and that parental refusal to access private insurance does not "relieve the responsibility to provide all required services at no cost to the parent" (Sec. 300.103).

Rogers[62] discussed "dangers to the family" that exist when schools access the family's private insurance. These include "depletion of available lifetime coverage; depletion of annual or service charge; loss of future insurability; premium increase; or discontinuation of coverage."[62] LEAs also have expressed concerns regarding the use of private insurance as they are obligated to provide a "free" and appropriate public education. Their concerns include payment of copays; request to pay increased premiums as a result of using the insurance; and potential litigation because, resulting from the depletion of lifetime caps, the child, now an adult, no longer has access to services.

The impact on school therapists may include additional documentation to meet the standards of the insurer, preauthorization, and denial with possible appeal. Each state determines the laws and rules and regulations that LEAs and therapists must follow. An important point is that the LEA cannot delay or deny any service that the child's IEP or IFSP team determines is necessary to meet the child's needs just because the service may or may not be reimbursed (Sec. 300.103).

Provision of Service

Intervention Options

IDEA does not specify the types of intervention options that must be available to children with disabilities, leaving it to states to define the types of services in their education laws. Generally, 2 types of service that apply to special education and related or support services are defined. These are *direct* and *indirect*. Direct service usually is defined as those services provided directly to the child. The focus of direct service is to instruct the child. Indirect service may be defined as those services provided to the child, staff, and parents when appropriate. The focus of indirect service is to train the student and those working with the student throughout the day to incorporate activities that address the student's needs into the daily routine. An assumption should not be made that one type of service is better or worse than the other.[45,53] The service the child receives will depend on the individual child's identified needs, goals, and objectives as well as the specific educational program and setting.

The role of the physical therapist in the educational setting is to examine and evaluate the child (health condition, impairments of body functions and structures, activity limitations, participation restrictions, and health, wellness, and fitness); the work environment (home, school, community, job); and the job (play, learn, work) expectations, then determine how the child's condition affects the ability to function and learn. Intervention should include the following: (1) adaptation or modification of the environment or task; (2) expectations for performance; (3) provision of assistive technology; (4) training and instruction of the child, staff, and family; (5) coordination and communication with appropriate providers; and (6) interaction with the child. The specific type of interaction with the child will vary based on a multitude of factors,[32,63,64] but the focus for the physical therapist always must be on improving function in the educational setting, not on fixing the impairments.[50]

When determining the type of service necessary to assist the child to benefit from special education, the physical therapist may wish to think in terms of what type of interaction is necessary, then apply the appropriate label. To assume that direct, one-to-one or "pull-out" service (ie, removing the child from the classroom to therapy room or other environment) is the only way to have the physical therapist involved is erroneous.[45] Indirect service allows and frequently requires the physical therapist to be actively involved with the child and the team. In many cases, it may be the preferred interaction as it embodies the principles of movement and the educational constructs of a whole child approach within the natural or least restrictive environment.

When making service delivery decisions, physical therapists must consider the following:

▸ Personal beliefs for how the brain learns, organizes, and uses information

▸ Role of environment in learning

▸ Role of family and social/emotional factors on learning

▸ Evidence-based practice that includes literature, self-experiences/knowledge, and patient/client preferences

▸ Purpose of education

▸ Impact of lifelong condition on learning

▸ Management of lifelong condition across the life span

▸ Continuum of service

▸ Models of service

▸ Timing and frequency of service that considers typical brain and body maturation, typical development for that specific condition, readiness of brain and child to learn the task, and level of expertise needed to assist the child to accomplish the goal

Evidence-based practice, which incorporates research, therapist experience, and desires of the child and family, forms the basis for making service-delivery decisions.[22,65-67] Therapists need to evaluate their own beliefs and how those beliefs relate to current evidence.[68,69] Should the normal motor developmental sequence be used as the basis for pediatric therapy? Although this may be a method to determine eligibility for special education, there is a need to address functional abilities and participation restrictions using a motor-learning approach emphasizing the interaction of the child with the task and the environment.[70-76] Understanding of brain-based research and motor learning theory is essential for the physical therapist (see Chapter 1). To affect learning, the child must be motivated to perform the task and must be able to repeatedly practice the task as it occurs within the natural setting.[73,77,78] Based on motor-learning theory, Byl[79] stated therapists would be unable to provide the amount of practice needed to affect learning and that our task should be to "mentor, guide, motivate, and teach our patients about the potential of their nervous system to adapt."[79p91] As we learn more about the brain and how it functions, we need to consider how these advancements affect how we provide interventions. We need to understand the movement system[80] and the importance of prevention, prediction, plasticity, and participation.[36,81,82]

Another important aspect to consider is that children who qualify for special education and related services generally have pathologies or conditions that are lifelong. One of the physical therapist's roles is to help the family and child understand the condition and how to manage it as the child ages. (See Chapter 18 for more information.) It is important for the child and his or her family to be aware of the implications of the condition, not only as they relate to the educational program, but also how they may affect the child's ability to be independent as an adult and obtain postsecondary education, employment, health insurance, and a positive quality of life.[5-12]

It should be expected that the involvement of the physical therapist will vary if the child's needs, priorities, and educational program change. It also is expected that the physical therapist will be involved as the child ages and environments and expectations increase. As the child and child's brain matures, body dimensions increase, attention improves, movement becomes quicker and more skilled, and the need for strength, endurance, and energy increases as environments enlarge. It generally has been thought that motor development is critical when children are young, plateauing in middle school and high school.[83] Whereas motor-developmental skill scales show motor skills being developed in early childhood or elementary age, motor learning continues throughout the life span and is dependent on the interaction of the child with the context of the task in a specific environment.[78] Physical fitness needs also increase as the child grows and environments expand.[83] Preparing students for life includes addressing needs to participate in the home, community, postsecondary education, and work.[9,10,11,36,83]

An "episode of care" in the educational setting should not be birth through 21 years, but rather there should be multiple episodes of care in which the therapist moves in and out of service meeting the changing needs of the child. The *Guide 3.0* provides information related to the patient and client management system including development of a plan of care and expected outcomes. Therapists also should consider factors that may modify the plan when considering the frequency and duration of service.[32,64] See Chapter 6 of this text for specifics on the *Guide 3.0*.

There are a number of questions to consider when determining whether the service to be provided is educationally necessary:

> What role(s) does the child perform?
> What are the expectations for typically developing peers?
> How is the child functioning in the educational environments (home, school/community/work)?
> What is interfering with the child's ability to perform his or her role?
> Is the environment facilitating or interfering with the child's ability to perform his or her role?
> Is there assistive technology, and how is it facilitating or interfering with the child's ability to perform his or her role?[84]

> Is this something that can be remediated, accommodated, or modified?
> Is this a priority to the child and/or family?
> Is this an educational priority as determined by the child's IEP/IFSP team?
> Is there a need to provide accommodations or modifications to the environment?
> Is there a need to provide assistive technology?
> Is the expertise of a physical therapist necessary to educate or train the child, family, or educational team?
> Is the expertise of a physical therapist necessary to address the identified needs, goals, and objectives?
> Is the expertise of a physical therapist necessary to assist the child to meet his or her educational goals?

Service Delivery Models

The models for delivery of service have changed with the understanding of motor learning and the acceptance of children with disabilities in all educational settings. Evidence-based practice is not only a standard for the practice of physical therapy but also a requirement for education under ESSA and IDEA. It is because of the evidence for learning in natural environments, performing real tasks and activities, and the legislative push to have all children benefit or be a part of general education that models for delivery of all educational services have changed.

Models can range from a more traditional "pull-out" service to a full inclusion model with teachers and therapists providing services in the classroom to a cooperative model with teachers and therapists providing consultation to classroom staff.[45,85] Sekerak et al[45] described an integrated model of service delivery in which there is a continuum of service delivery models from which the therapist can select based on the specific needs of the child. They noted that consultation, working with the child's team, is a critical component of each model. As a result of their study, Sekerak and colleagues[45] developed guidelines for integrating physical therapy services into preschool classrooms and identifying key components for successful integration. Although these guidelines were based on interviews with therapists in preschool settings, the components easily can be applied to children in all settings.

The key to the provision of physical therapy is not what it is called, but rather how well it is integrated into the child's educational program. In an integrated model, the physical therapist has the option of providing service in or out of the classroom; working with the classroom staff, caregivers, and families; and providing patient-/client-related instruction and coordination, communication, and documentation as needed to those in the educational program as well as to outside providers and agencies.

In the integrated model, the therapist does not have separate goals, but the goals are the child's goals and are developed and implemented by the team.[25] When developing goals that are child or family focused, it may be helpful to ask the child and family what is important to them now, what their lifestyle is, and what is important in the future.[10,11,23,24,49,61] When working with families, therapists need to recognize and acknowledge that each family is different. Each family has a different value system, which may be different from that of the therapist.[28] Cultural differences need to be addressed in the evaluation, identification of expected outcomes, and in materials and techniques used in intervention. The family's level of acceptance of the child and assistance from outsiders will affect their ability to participate in the IEP/IFSP process. The responsibility of the team is to determine which model and tools will address the individual family's needs appropriately (see Chapter 4).

ADDITIONAL ROLES OF THE PHYSICAL THERAPIST IN EDUCATIONAL SETTINGS

The *Guide 3.0* describes a number of roles of the physical therapist in addition to that of working with children with disabilities. These roles include consultation, education, critical inquiry, and administration. The physical therapist in the educational setting has the opportunity to participate in these roles in addition to their primary role of working with students, families, and staff. Listed below are the roles that may apply to the educational setting as adapted from the *Guide 3.0*[32] and the *Occupational Therapy and Physical Therapy in Educational Settings: A Manual for Minnesota Practitioners, Third Edition*, by Bathke et al.[50]

Consultation

The *Guide 3.0* defines consultation as "the rendering of professional or expert opinion or advice by a physical therapist."[86] In the educational setting this includes interaction with teachers, administrators, parents, physicians, outside providers, community members, and other professionals or agencies. This also can include prevention, health, wellness, and fitness activities such as classroom program development; special education continuous improvement plan; general educational programming and long-range planning for children with disabilities; review of architectural plans or specific sites for accessibility; development of forms for documentation; providing peer review; and serving as a resource to administration. Owing to educational and data privacy laws, child-specific consultation occurs only if the physical therapist is a part of that specific child's evaluation process or a member of that child's IEP/IFSP team.

Education

The *Guide 3.0* defines education as "the process of imparting information or skills and instructing by precept, example, and experience so that individuals acquire knowledge, master skills, or develop competence."[86] Activities include planning and conducting general educational in-service for staff, students, and parents about specific disabilities, body mechanics and lifting, evacuation and emergency plans for individuals with disabilities, general handling and positioning principles, and other topics that would complement the teacher-directed educational program. Physical therapists also can provide information regarding removal of architectural barriers; transportation needs; evacuation and emergency plans; special equipment needs; transition planning; prevocational and vocational planning; travel training; job site analysis health, wellness, and fitness plans; and long-range planning for students with disabilities. Again, owing to educational and data privacy laws, patient/client-related education/instruction occurs only if the physical therapist is a part of that specific student's evaluation process or a member of that student's IEP/IFSP team.

Critical Inquiry

Critical inquiry, as defined in the *Guide 3.0*, is the "process of applying the principles of scientific methods to: read and interpret professional literature; participate in, plan, and conduct research; evaluate outcomes data; and assess new concepts and technologies."[87] Activities include review of the literature, evidence-based practice, collaborative research with physical therapist educational programs, outcomes data collection and analysis, and participation in study groups.

Administration

The *Guide 3.0* defines administration as the "skilled process of planning, directing, organizing, and managing human, technical, environmental, and financial resources effectively and efficiently."[86] Activities include coordination and implementation of services in a manner consistent with district, state, and federal educational and physical therapy practice regulations; purchase of equipment and supplies; staffing considerations; employment options; work and office space considerations; direction and supervision of physical therapist assistants; performance reviews; and clinical education of physical therapy students.

EMPLOYMENT OPTIONS

Physical therapists generally have 2 employment options, direct hire or contracting. In the direct hire option, the physical therapist is hired directly by a LEA or by a cooperative agency that serves several LEAs. Through this system, the therapist is placed on a teacher's contract and receives the same benefits as a teacher. The advantages of being an employee of the LEA are more direct contact with other staff, availability, flexibility in scheduling, and inclusion in the LEA "system," which includes professional liability insurance and health and disability benefits. The disadvantages may include supervision by an educational administrator, requirement to perform educational-related duties such as bus supervision, and limited contact with other therapists.

Contracting may occur as an independent therapist or through an agency that employs therapists. The therapist does not receive any of the "system" benefits of the LEA and must show proof of professional liability insurance. The advantages of contacting for the therapist may be in having more independence in determining the amount of time spent in the LEA and in the number of children being provided services. Generally, contracting is advantageous to the LEA when there are few students who require physical therapy service. Disadvantages include limited availability for additional meetings and interaction with staff and a payment system that frequently results in the LEA requesting therapist involvement only for direct student contact time and essential meetings. The Minnesota State manual for occupational therapists and physical therapists in the educational environment advises therapists that a contract should include the following[50]:

> Purpose of the agreement, evidence of appropriate licensure of the therapist, professional liability insurance, availability of replacement therapists from agency, working conditions, documentation of expectations, identification of supervisory relationships and evaluation of staff performance, identification of how parties will resolve differences, payment schedule, cost of service and travel, effective dates, renewal conditions, and liability.

The contract also should address nonstudent contact activities, such as meetings, staff training, and preparation time. Therapists should investigate all alternatives before deciding which option is best. Additional information may be available to the therapist by checking with the state's education department regarding any guidelines for school-based therapists, each state's American Physical Therapy Association (APTA) chapter, and the APTA Academy of Pediatric Physical Therapy.

STAFFING CONSIDERATIONS

The need for physical therapy services for a specific student is determined on an individual basis during that student's IEP or IFSP meeting. The type of service, direct or indirect, and the amount of time and frequency are listed for the physical therapy service. The typical approach to staffing has been to look at the number of students on IEPs/IFSPs and set a case load for the therapist. This case load approach takes into consideration the service time for the students, but not the amount of work involved with providing service to the students or for training activities or other administrative tasks.

A different method of determining staffing is the work load approach. This approach looks at not only the number of students on IEPs/IFSPs, but also all the other responsibilities and work related to providing service. For example, consideration must be given not only for student-related IEP/IFSP time, but also for the time needed for administrative tasks, including program development and planning and documentation requirements (development and writing of evaluations, IEPs, and IFSPs); assistive technology services and devices; classroom programs; and third-party billing. In addition, student-related meetings, including evaluation determination planning meetings, IEPs/IFSPs reviews, staff training activities, and general training and specific student training may be required. The work load approach to staffing provides a more accurate picture of the actual time needed for each student, as well as the amount of time needed to perform other duties and responsibilities.

Each therapist needs to work with the administration to ensure that the needs of students as well as the therapist are being addressed. Federal laws do not address case load limits for physical therapy; however, therapists should check within their state to see whether the state has specific guidelines or recommendations. To assist therapists and school districts, 3 professional therapy organizations—the American Occupational Therapy Association, the APTA, and the American Speech-Language-Hearing Association—developed a joint document: *Workload Approach: A Paradigm Shift for Positive Impact on Student Outcomes*.[88] This document is available through the respective professional organizations.

PERFORMANCE REVIEW

As in all physical therapy settings, the performance review is an essential component to ensure quality services. However, unlike most physical therapy practice settings, in which the evaluating supervisor is a physical therapist, school physical therapists often are responsible to educational personnel, such as the school principal or the special education director. Performance standards such as professionalism, communication skills, organizational abilities, and adaptability and flexibility should be addressed in addition to the abilities of the therapist to perform specific examination or intervention techniques. If you are an employee of the school district, you may be required to participate in their performance-appraisal process.

Peer review is a "system by which peers with similar areas of expertise assess the quality of physical therapy provided, using accepted practice standards and guidelines,"[89] and may be used as a method of performance review. This process can include internal peer review, by which therapists within the same setting evaluate their services, and external peer review, by which therapists outside the setting evaluate the services. In either review, peers use recognized professional standards and guidelines to determine the quality of service provided. The APTA provides an overview of peer review and a self-assessment form that may be downloaded and used to assess the therapist's focus.[89]

SUMMARY

The purpose of education is to prepare children for adult life. The role of physical therapists is to assist children with disabilities with that preparation, and physical therapists play an important role in the educational environment. As integral members of an educational team, physical therapists work to ensure the most appropriate education for children with disabilities. Physical therapists have unique skills in the understanding and implementation of motor-learning principles and the impact of disease/conditions on function and health, wellness, and fitness. These skills are used to assist teachers, parents, administrators, and other educational staff in addressing needs of children with disabilities. Physical therapists also can assist families, schools, and communities to address the need for prevention, health, wellness, and fitness to promote a full, healthy lifestyle.

Physical therapists in the educational setting have an ideal job—they practice in the actual setting in which their clients need to perform. They have an excellent opportunity to implement strategies that facilitate motor learning and directly affect function. They can make a difference in the long-range life outcomes of a child by addressing the challenges of living with a disability. These challenges include employment, independence, relationships, and self-determination. To accomplish this, the goals of the child need to be established in terms of safe and efficient mobility, rather than "walking"; working on a task for 1 to 2 hours, rather than developing head control; and health and wellness to have the physical capacity to work and play, rather than improving range of motion. We need to focus on the functional components of life, not the impairments of the condition. We need to educate the child and family as to the lifelong implications of the condition and how to manage the condition so the child can as independent and self-reliant as possible. What an exciting challenge!

This chapter has provided an overview of the laws, roles, and functions of the physical therapist in the educational setting. Application of these topics will now be addressed in the case studies.

Case Study #1: Jason

> *Age:* 24 months: Practice Pattern 5C: Impaired Motor Function and Sensory Processing Associated With Nonprogressive Disorders of the Central Nervous System—Congenital Origin or Acquired in Infancy or Childhood
> *Medical Diagnosis:* Cerebral palsy, right hemiparesis
> *Gross Motor Function Classification System:* Level I
> *Current Age:* 16 years: Practice Pattern 4C: Impaired Muscle Performance

History

Initially, based on birth history and medical diagnosis, Jason was referred to the county inter-agency by his physician. Following an evaluation by the local school district, an interagency team meeting was held with the family to discuss the results of the evaluation and determine eligibility for special education. Based on the evaluation, Jason met the eligibility criteria for early intervention services, having a diagnosed physical condition that has a high probability of resulting in developmental delay, and demonstrating a need for services in the areas of communication, adaptive development, and motor development. Jason's team developed an IFSP with the school, addressing needs in the areas of communication, self-help skills, and the family, and through a private physical therapist, addressing the needs related to mobility. Through the school district, Jason received home-based services weekly, alternating visits from an early intervention teacher and an occupational therapist. He also received consultative services from the school physical therapist to coordinate services provided by his private physical therapist and to assist with transition to a school-based program when he was age 3 years. Jason also participated in a center-based family support and play group once every other week. Through a private provider, Jason received private physical therapy for 3 months, 1 time per week focusing on mobility in the home and community, as well as family education for his home program. Private physical therapy was to decrease to 1 time every 2 weeks, with the private therapist coordinating services with the school physical therapist.

At age 3 years, Jason was eligible to participate in a community-based preschool program with support from special education. Jason's IFSP team began the transition to a center-based program that offered a model of inclusion with typically developing peers and coordination of special education and related services.

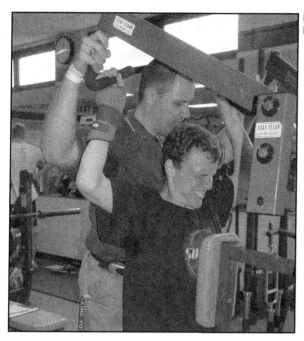

Figure 15-2. Strength training program for an adolescent with special needs.

Depending on how Jason's impairments affect his ability to participate in his educational program, he may or may not continue to demonstrate a need for special education. He may continue to demonstrate a need for special education in elementary school but may not need the expertise of a physical therapist. Some states provide additional services in the area of developmental/adapted physical education (D/APE), through which Jason's general motor skills and fitness needs may be addressed. It is appropriate for the physical therapist to be involved in Jason's 3-year reevaluation as a part of the evaluation team.

Current Status

Jason is now 16 and a sophomore in high school. As a part of his comprehensive 3-year reevaluation, the physical therapist and occupational therapist determine the impact of his disability on the transition areas. His parents have requested assistance in obtaining an evaluation to determine modifications or adaptations for driving. Jason states he would like to be able to drive as well as shoot baskets with both hands. As a result of growth and avoidance of use, Jason's right arm has become contracted so that he is unable to shake hands and has difficulty steering a car for driving. The team determines that Jason continues to meet the eligibility criteria for category (physically impaired), and demonstrates needs in the transition area for driving a car (travel training), ability to shake hands (jobs and job training, community participation), and fitness (overlies all transition areas) as related to flexibility, strength, and endurance of the right arm and hand. Jason's IEP is developed with goals for driving, appropriate interaction with individuals in the community or on the job, and development of an individualized fitness plan. Jason's program includes a driving evaluation at a center for individuals with disabilities (interagency agreement with agency allows school district to send students to facility for evaluation and training), and participation in strength training classes at school. To facilitate attainment of his goals in strength training, a paraprofessional with additional training in high-intensity strength training is assigned to work with Jason daily, and a physical therapist is placed on indirect service with a burst of service 3 to 4 times per week for the first 3 weeks then weekly for the remaining 7 weeks. The physical therapist's role is to work with the strength training teacher and paraprofessional to develop, implement, and modify a high-intensity strength training program for Jason that addresses his specific condition and needs[90,91] (Figure 15-2).

CASE STUDY #2: JILL

> ▸ *Age:* 7 years: Practice Pattern 5C: Impaired Motor Function and Sensory Processing Associated With Nonprogressive Disorders of the Central Nervous System—Congenital Origin or Acquired in Infancy or Childhood
> ▸ *Medical Diagnosis:* Cerebral palsy, spastic quadriparesis, microcephaly, intellectual deficits, seizure disorder
> ▸ *Gross Motor Function Classification System:* Level V
> ▸ *Current Age:* 17 years

Current Status

Jill is now a senior in high school. She participates in a functional curriculum in the moderate-severe cognitive impairment program, attends music class 4 times per week, and attends D/APE 3 times per week. As a part of her functional curriculum, Jill participates in a community outing once per week, prevocational training 2 times per week, and apartment living 1 day per week. Jill's IEP team has exempted her from the statewide academic testing, and she has completed the alternative assessment. Jill's needs are addressed as they relate to the state's 5 areas of transition: jobs and job training, postsecondary education, recreation-leisure, community participation, and home living.[92,93]

Jill has a tilt-in-space wheelchair with a custom seating system. She is not able to propel her wheelchair; however, she is able to assist with cares by relaxing and assisting with movement and can perform a standing pivot transfer with minimal to moderate assistance. Jill never developed maintained head control, but she is able to lift and control her head when motivated by the activity and is able to stay focused on a task for 5 to 10 minutes at a time. Her needs related to fitness include maintaining flexibility, functional strength, and endurance to participate in her educational program. She communicates through vocalizations and a simple augmentative device. She uses switches to interact with her environment. To participate in off-site community and work activities, Jill needs to tolerate sitting for 3 to 4 hours, and be on task for a 10- to 15-minute period of time. She also needs to be able to manage cares with one staff person to assist and requires a private area with a changing table.

Assistive Technology Needs

The focus of Jill's program is on providing her assistive technology that addresses her needs and facilitates her participation in her educational program. The physical therapist participates on Jill's IEP team to assist with problem solving for positions and equipment that will enhance her ability to participate in school and work activities. A hydraulic sit-to-stand upright stander is used at her work site to allow Jill to work while standing, take a break sitting, and resume standing to finish her work. Jill uses a supported-gait trainer as part of her fitness plan in D/APE class. The physical therapist also has trained staff to incorporate movements into her daily routine and cares to address her flexibility. The physical therapist is able to assist with evaluation of community and potential work sites for accessibility and need for evacuation plans.

Transition Plan

A major focus of Jill's program is on transition from high school. Jill's parents have decided that they would like Jill to continue in the district in the 18- to 21-year-old transition program. As a result, Jill is able to go through graduation ceremonies but will not accept her diploma. Jill's parents have been advised as to their need to address guardianship, as Jill will become her own guardian at age 18.[94] The physical therapist provides consultation regarding transition of medical providers from pediatric services to adult services and implications for future equipment needs.

Case Study #3: Taylor

> *Age:* 4 years: Practice Pattern 5C: Impaired Motor Function and Sensory Processing Associated With Nonprogressive Disorders of the Central Nervous System—Congenital Origin or Acquired in Infancy or Childhood
> *Medical Diagnosis:* Myelomeningocele, repaired L1-2
> *Current Age:* 12 years: Pattern 4C: Impaired Muscle Performance

Current Status

Taylor is now in seventh grade attending his neighborhood middle school. Taylor's middle school is a 2-story building serving grades 6 to 8 with an average of 250 students per grade level. There are 7 class periods, each 45 minutes, and a daily advisory period of 15 minutes, with a 5-minute passing time between classes and 30 minutes for lunch. He rides a regular bus route, using a regular bus equipped with a lift. Taylor has classes on the first and second floors, but his locker is located on first floor. Taylor decided in sixth grade to only use his manual wheelchair at school because of the amount of energy and time it took to walk between classes and because he was self-conscious of his body image (eg, less developed legs) when standing. He is independent in mobility within the building but has difficulty wheeling outside on the nature paths for science class and fields for physical education class. He is able to access all his learning stations in the classrooms either by transferring to a desk or wheeling under an adjustable height table. Taylor is independent in use of the elevator and opening inside and outside doors from his wheelchair. Taylor's evacuation plan, when on the second floor for fire situations, is to report to the fire rescue room. His method of evacuation is for the staff to lift and carry him in his solid-frame wheelchair down the stairs. Taylor has a Tuk-N-Kari sling that he carries on his wheelchair in case there is a situation in which staff members are unable to lift him and his wheelchair. Taylor reports he sometimes has difficulty transferring into his friends' parents' cars. His parents report that they have a family membership at the YMCA and would like to have a specific program for Taylor to use when there.

Taylor demonstrates needs in the area of fitness as related to outside mobility and transfers. Taylor and his family also need education on how his condition affects his ability to train and improve his fitness, as well as how Taylor can manage his condition as he ages. The physical therapist participates on Taylor's IEP team to assist with developing, implementing, and monitoring his evacuation plan, ability to access educational areas, and mobility. The physical therapist works with the physical education and D/APE teachers to address Taylor's fitness plan. The physical therapist also works with Taylor's family to develop a training program at the YMCA and provides education to Taylor and his family regarding how his condition changes with age and what Taylor needs to do to manage his condition.

Case Study #4: Ashley

> *Age:* 15 months: Practice Pattern 5B: Impaired Neuromotor Development
> *Medical Diagnosis:* Down syndrome
> *Current Age:* 8 years

Current Status

Ashley attends her neighborhood school in the third grade. Ashley's IEP team identified needs in preacademics (number and letter recognition, matching); social skills (turn taking, waiting in line, play, initiating interactions, independence); communication skills (conversation skills, written expression); motor skills (general endurance, ball skills, game skills, use of classroom tools); and functional skills (staying on task, following classroom routines, functional words, awareness of safety). Ashley's parents would like her to be able to play with children her age and be aware of what's going on around her, especially when they are out in the community. The team prioritized the needs and developed goals and objectives and determined that Ashley would benefit from a program that included participation in the general education second-grade classroom with a combination of in-class and out-of-class time to address her needs. The team prioritized safety areas and functional words that all staff would incorporate into their activities with Ashley. The general education and special education teacher agreed to collaborate on instruction of safety in the community, as the classroom works on bus safety and general traffic and stranger safety as part of the general curriculum. The physical education teacher and the D/APE teacher agreed to collaborate on instruction of game and motor skills as well as general fitness.

To address Ashley's needs for improving her general endurance, following directions and classroom routines, and the parents' desire for Ashley to be able to play with her peers, the physical therapist proposed that the classroom participate in the Courageous Pacers[95] program as it addresses general fitness for kids and is an activity that Ashley could participate in with the whole class. The team agreed and the physical therapist worked with the classroom teacher to understand and incorporate the program into the classroom routine. Physical therapy services on the IEP were indirect, weekly for the first 4 weeks, then monthly for the remainder of the IEP. The physical therapist put the following statement in the accommodations section of the IEP: "The physical therapist is available for consultation in the areas of fitness, mobility, and accessing educational activities and areas as needed by the team. The physical therapist will contact the IEP team a minimum of once per month to monitor Ashley's program."

CASE STUDY #5: JOHN

> *Practice Pattern 5B:* Impaired Neuromotor Development
> *Medical Diagnosis:* Developmental coordination disorder/attention-deficit hyperactivity disorder
> *Current Age:* 5 years

History

John's parents requested an educational evaluation following his medical work-up that resulted in the dual diagnoses of developmental coordination disorder and attention-deficit hyperactivity disorder. As a result of the parent request, the school referred John for an evaluation. An evaluation plan determination meeting was held at John's school and included the parent, kindergarten teacher, special education teacher, speech and language pathologist, school psychologist, principal, and a representative from the district's motor team (occupational therapist, physical therapist, and D/APE teacher). The team reviewed the medical reports and parent concerns. John's teacher provided information on how John was functioning in the classroom. An evaluation plan was developed in the motor area with the D/APE teacher assessing motor skills and the physical therapist and occupational therapist assessing motor abilities and functional skills.

Following the evaluation the team met with the parents to discuss the results and determine if John met any of the eligibility criteria for special education. Review of the evaluation results documented that John demonstrated difficulty with some tasks and activities; however, he did not meet the criteria for special education. The team discussed John's educational needs, and it was determined that he did not need special education but would benefit from a 504 plan that addressed simple modifications and strategies for motor activities and behavior. The physical therapist, occupational therapist, and special education teacher are available to assist with the development and training of strategies for the teacher.

REFERENCES

1. National Center for Education Statistics, Institute of National Sciences. Chapter 1. Children and Youth with Disabilities. *The Condition of Education 2018.* https://nces.ed.gov/programs/coe/indicator_cgg.asp. Accessed October 1, 2018.

2. Bureau of Labor Statistics, US Department of Labor, *The Economic Daily.* People with a disability less likely to have completed a bachelor's degree. https://www.bls.gov/opub/ted/2018/employment-of-workers-with-a-disability-in-2017.htm#bls-print. Accessed October 1, 2018.

3. Bureau of Labor Statistics. US Department of Labor. *The Economics Daily.* Employment of workers with a disability in 2017. https://www.bls.gov/opub/ted/2018/employment-of-workers-with-a-disability-in-2017.htm#bls-print. Accessed October 1, 2018.

4. The Kessler Foundation. The Kessler Foundation 2015 National Employment and Disability Survey: report of main findings. West Orange, NJ; 2015. http://kesslerfoundation.org/sites/default/files/filepicker/5/KFSurvey15_Results-secured.pdf. Accessed October 1, 2018.

5. Johnson DR, Stodden RA, Emanuel EJ, Luecking RG, Mack M. Current challenges facing secondary education and transition services: what research tells us. *Except Child.* 2002;68(4):519-531. doi:10.1177/001440290206800407.

6. Benz MR, Lindstrom L, Yovanoff P. Improving graduation and employment outcomes of students with disabilities: predictive factors and student perspectives. *Except Child.* 2000;66(4):509-529. doi:10.1177/001440290006600405.

7. Babbitt BC, White CM. "R U ready?" Helping students assess their readiness for postsecondary education. *Teach Except Child.* 2002;35(2):62-66. doi:10.1177/004005990203500209.

8. Test DW, Browder DM, Karvonen M, Wood WM, Algozzine B. Writing lesson plans for promoting self-determination. *Teach Except Child.* 2002;35(1):8-14. doi:10.1177/004005990203500102.

9. Haung IC, Holzbauer JJ, Lee EJ, Chronister J, Chan F, O'Neil J. Vocational rehabilitation services and employment outcomes for adults with cerebral palsy in the United States. *Dev Med Child Neurol.* 2013;55(1):1000-1008. doi:10.1111/dmcn.12224.

10. Johnson CC, Rose DS. School-based work capacity evaluation in young people with intellectual disability: 2 case reports. *Pediatr Phys Ther.* 2017;2(2):166-172. doi:10.1097/PEP.0000000000000367.

11. Liljenquist K, O'Neil ME, Bjornson KF. Utilization of physical therapy services during transition for young people with cerebral palsy: a call for improved care into adulthood. *Phys Ther.* 2018;98(9):796-803. doi:10.1093/ptj/pzy068.

12. Kang LJ, Palisano RJ, Orlin MN, Chiarello LA, King GA, Polansky M. Determinants of social participation—with friends and others who are not family members—for youths with cerebral palsy. *Phys Ther.* 2010;90(12):1743-1757. doi:10.2522/ptj.20100048.

13. Education for All Handicapped Children Act of 1975. 20 USC 1401.

14. Education of the Handicapped Act Amendments of 1986. 20 USC 1400.

15. Individuals with Disabilities Education Act of 1990. 20 USC 1400.

16. Individuals with Disabilities Education Act Amendments of 1997. 20 USC 1400.

17. Assistance to States for the Education of Children With Disabilities and the Early Intervention Program for Infants and Toddlers With Disabilities; Final Regulations, Appendix A to Part 300. *Fed Regist* 1999;64(suppl 48).

18. US Department of Education. No Child Left Behind Act of 2001. https://www2.ed.gov/nclb/landing.jhtml.

19. Every Student Succeeds Act of 2015 reauthorizing Elementary Secondary Education Act. 20 USC 6301. https://www.gpo.gov/fdsys/pkg/BILLS-114s1177enr/pdf/BILLS-114s1177enr.pdf. Accessed September 10, 2018.

20. Assistive Technology Act of 2005. 34 USC 3002. https://www2.ed.gov/legislation/FedRegister/announcements/2005-2/063005a.html. Accessed September 10, 2018.

21. Individuals with Disabilities Act of 2015. 20 USC 1400. https://sites.ed.gov/idea/. Accessed September 3, 2018.

22. Palisano RJ. A collaborative model of service delivery for children with movement disorders: a framework for evidence-based decision making. *Phys Ther.* 2006;86(9):1295-1305. doi:10.2522/ptj.20050348.

23. Almasri N, Palisano RJ, Dunst C, Chiarello LA, O'Neil ME, Polansky M. Profiles of family needs of children and youth with cerebral palsy. *Child Care Health Dev.* 2012;38(6):798-806. doi:10.1111/j.1365-2214.2011.01331.x.

24. Palisano RJ, Almarsi N, Chiarello LA, Orlin MN, Bagley A, Maggs J. Family needs of parents of children and youth with cerebral palsy. *Child Care Health Dev.* 2010;36(1):85-92. doi:10.1111/j.1365-2214.2009.01030.x.

25. McEwen I. *Providing Physical Therapy Services Under Parts B & C of the Individuals with Disabilities Education Act (IDEA).* 2nd ed. Alexandria, VA: Section on Pediatrics, American Physical Therapy Association; 2009.

26. Olmsted MG, Bailey DB Jr, Raspa M, et al. Outcomes reported by Spanish-speaking families in early intervention. *Topics Early Child Spec Educ.* 2010;30(1):46-55. doi:10.1177/0271121409360827.

27. Applequist KL, Bailey DB Jr. Navajo caregivers' perceptions of early intervention services. *J Early Interv.* 2000;23(1):47-61. doi:10.1177/10538151000230010901.

28. Byington TA, Whitby PJS. Empowering families during the early intervention process. *Young Exceptional Children.* 2011;14(4):44-56. doi:10.1177/1096250611428878.

29. Blackman JA. Early intervention: a global perspective. *Infants Young Child.* 2002;15(2):11-19.

30. O'Neil ME, Palisano RJ. Attitudes toward family-centered care and clinical decision making in early intervention among physical therapists. *Pediatr Phys Ther.* 2000;12(4):173-182. doi:10.1097/00001577-200001240-00005.

31. Code of Federal Regulations 300.550(b)(1-2), July 1988.

32. Guide to Physical Therapist Practice 3.0. Alexandria, VA: American Physical Therapy Association; 2014. http://guidetoptpractice.apta.org/. Accessed August 26, 2018.

33. Assistance to States for the Education of Children with Disabilities and the Early Intervention Program for Infants and Toddlers With Disabilities; Final Regulations, Analysis of Comments and Changes. *Federal Register* 1999;64(Suppl 48).

34. Rehabilitation Act of 1973 as Amended through PL 114-95 enacted December 10, 2015, Section 504, 29 USC 794.

35. APTA. *House of Delegates Standards, Policies, Positions and Guidelines.* Alexandria, VA: American Physical Therapy Association. 2018. http://www.apta.org/uploadedFiles/APTAorg/About_Us/Policies/Practice/DirectionSupervisionPTA.pdf#search=%22direction%20supervision%22. Accessed October 5, 2018.

36. Quinn L, Morgan E. From disease to health: physical therapy health promotion practices for secondary prevention in adult and pediatric neurologic populations. *J Neurol Phys Ther.* 2017;41(3):S46-S54. doi:10.1097/NPT.0000000000000166.

37. Rowland JL, Frangala-Pinkham M, Miles C, O'Neil ME. The scope of pediatric physical therapy practice in health promotion and fitness for youth with disabilities. *Pediatr Phys Ther.* 2015;27(1):2-15. doi:10.1097/PEP.0000000000000098.

38. Zhao M, Chen S. The effects of structured physical activity program on social interaction and communications with autism. *Biomed Res Int.* 2018;2018:1825046. doi:10.1155/2018/1825046.

39. Zeng H, Ayyub M, Sun H, Wen X, Xiang P, Gao Z. Effects of physical activity on motor skills and cognitive development in early childhood: a systematic review. *Biomed Res Int.* 2017;2017:2760716. doi:10.1155/2017/2760716.

40. Han GS. The relationship between physical fitness and academic achievement among adolescent in South Korea. *J Phys Ther Sci.* 2018;30(4):605-608. doi:10.1589/jpts.30.605.

41. Burns RD, Brusseau TA, Fu Y, Myrer RS, Hannon JC. Comprehensive school physical activity programming and classroom behavior. *Am J Health Behav.* 2016;40(1):100-107. doi:10.5993/AJHB.40.1.11.

42. Fuemmeler B, Behrman P, Taylor M, et al. Child and family health in the era of prevention: new opportunities and challenges. *J Behav Med.* 2017;40(1):159-174. doi:10.1007/s10865-016-9791-1.

43. Pope M. Preventing weight gain in children who are school age and African-American. *Ped Phys Ther.* 2016;28(2):207-216. doi:10.1097/PEP.0000000000000243.

44. Nunez-Gaunaurd A, Moore JG, Roach KE, Miller TL, Kirk-Sanchez NJ. Motor proficiency, strength, endurance, and physical activity among middle school children who are healthy, overweight, and obese. *Pediatr Phys Ther.* 2013;25(2):130-138; discussion 139. doi:10.1097/PEP.0b013e318287caa3.

45. Sekerak DM, Kirkpatrick DB, Nelson KC, Propes JH. Physical therapy in preschool classrooms: successful integration of therapy into classroom routines. *Pediatr Phys Ther.* 2003;15(2):93-104. doi:10.1097/01.PEP.0000067501.03241.28.

46. Snell ME, Janney RE. Teachers' problem-solving about children with moderate and severe disabilities in elementary classrooms. *Except Child.* 2000;66(4):472-490. doi:10.1177/001440290006600403.

47. Bartlett DJ, McCoy SW, Chiarello LA, Avery L, Galuppi B. A collaborative approach to decision making through developmental monitoring to provide individualized services for children with cerebral palsy. *Phys Ther.* 2018;98(10):865-875. doi:10.1093/ptj/pzy081.

48. Utley BL, Rapport MJK. Essential elements of effective teamwork: shared understanding and differences between special educators and related service providers. *Phys Disabil.* 2002;20(2):9-47.

49. Ovland Pilkington K, Malinowski M. The natural environment II: uncovering deeper responsibilities with relationship-based services. *Infants Young Child.* 2002;15(2):78-84.

50. Bathke L, Bohmert J, Lillie L. *Occupational Therapy and Physical Therapy in Educational Settings: A Manual for Minnesota Practitioners.* 3rd ed. Arden Hills, MN. Minnesota Department of Education, Special Education Division, Minnesota Low Incidence Projects, Metro ECSU; 2014.

51. Szabo J, Panikkar RK. Bridging the gap between physical therapy and orientation and mobility in schools: using a collaborative team approach for students with visual impairments. *J Vis Impair Blind.* 2017;111(6):491-510. doi:10.1177/0145482X1711100602.

52. York J, Rainforth B, Giangreco MF. Transdisciplinary teamwork and integrated therapy: clarifying the misconceptions. *Pediatr Phys Ther.* 1990;2(2):73-79. doi:10.1097/00001577-199002020-00003.

53. Rainforth B. Analysis of physical therapy practice acts: implications for role release in educational environments. *Pediatr Phys Ther.* 1997;9(2):54-61. doi:10.1097/00001577-199700920-00003.

54. Vialu C, Doyle M. Determining need for school-based physical therapy under IDEA: commonalities across practice guidelines. *Pediatr Phys Ther.* 2017;29(4):350-355. doi:10.1097/PEP.0000000000000448.

55. Friedman C, Feldner HA. Physical therapy services for people with intellectual and developmental disabilities: the role of Medicaid home- and community-based service waivers. *Phys Ther.* 2018;98(10):844-854. doi:10.1093/ptj/pzy082.

56. Hanson H, Harrington AT, Nixon-Cave K. Implementing treatment frequency and duration guidelines in hospital-based pediatric outpatient setting: administrative case report. *Phys Ther.* 2015;95(4):678-684. doi:10.2522/ptj.20130360.

57. Dumas HM, Fragala-Pinkham MA, Rosen EL, Folmar E. Physical therapy dosing: frequency and type of intervention in pediatric postacute hospital care. *Ped Phys Ther.* 2017;29(1):47-53. doi:10.1097/PEP.0000000000000339.

58. Coster W, Deeney T, Haltiwanger J, et al. School Function Assessment. Pearson Education; 1998. https://www.pearsonclinical.com/therapy/products/100000547/school-function-assessment-sfa.html. Accessed October 5, 2018.

59. Haley SM, Coster WJ, Dumas H, Fragala-Pinkham M, Moed R. *Evaluation of Disability Inventory Computer Adaptive Test: Development, Standardization and Administration Manual.* Boston, MA: Health and Disability Research Institute: 2012.

60. Dole RL, Arvidson K, Byrne E, Robbins J, Schasberger B. Consensus among experts in pediatric occupational and physical therapy on elements of individualized education programs. *Pediatr Phys Ther.* 2003;15(3):159-166. doi:10.1097/01.PEP.0000083046.14713.EF.

61. Randall KE, McEwen IR. Writing patient-centered functional goals. *Phys Ther.* 2000;80(12):1197-1203. doi:10.1093/ptj/80.12.1197.

62. Rogers JJ. Schools, insurance, and your family's financial security. *Exceptional Parent.* 1991;21(6)76-78.

63. Thomason HK, Wilmarth MA. Provision of school-based physical therapy services: a survey of current practice patterns. *Pediatr Phys Ther.* 2015;27(2):161-172. doi:10.1097/PEP.0000000000000127.

64. Effgen SK, Kaminker MK. Nationwide survey of school-based physical therapy practice. *Pediatr Phys Ther.* 2014;26(4):394-403. doi:10.1097/PEP.0000000000000075.

65. Sackett DL, Straus SE, Richardson WS, Rosenberg W, Haynes KB. *Evidence-Based Medicine.* New York, NY: Churchill Livingston; 2000.

66. Law M. Strategies for implementing evidence-based practice in early intervention. *Infants Young Child.* 2000;13(2):32-40. doi:10.1097/00001163-200013020-00008.

67. Dorling J, Salt A. Assessing developmental delay. *BMJ.* 2001;323(7305):148-149. doi:10.1136/bmj.323.7305.148.

68. Schreiber J, Stern P, Marchetti G, Provident I, Turocy PS. School-based pediatric physical therapists' perspectives on evidence-based practice. *Pediatr Phys Ther.* 2008;20(4):292-302. doi:10.1097/PEP.0b013e31818bc475.

69. Palisano RJ. Practice knowledge: the forgotten aspect of evidence-based practice. *Phys Occup Ther Pediatr.* 2010;30(4):261-263. doi:10.3109/01942638.2010.513221.

70. Atwater SW. Should the normal motor developmental sequence be used as a theoretical model in pediatric physical therapy? In: Lister MJ, ed. Contemporary Management of Motor Control Problems. Proceedings of the II Step Conference. Fairfax, VA: Foundation for Physical Therapy; 1991:89-93.

71. Van Sant AF. Motor control, motor learning, and motor development. In: Montgomery PC, Connolly BH, eds. *Clinical Applications for Motor Control.* Thorofare, NJ: SLACK Incorporated; 2003:79-106.

72. Attermeir S. Should the normal motor developmental sequence be used as theoretical model in patient treatment? In: Lister MJ, ed. Contemporary Management of Motor Control Problems. Proceedings of the II Step Conference. Fairfax, VA: Foundation for Physical Therapy; 1991:85-87.

73. Kamm K, Thelen E, Jensen JL. A dynamical systems approach to motor development. *Phys Ther.* 1990;70(4):763-775. doi:10.1093/ptj/70.12.763.

74. Van Sant AF. Life-span motor development. In: Lister MJ, ed. Contemporary Management of Motor Control Problems. Proceedings of the II Step Conference. Fairfax, VA: Foundation for Physical Therapy; 1991:77-83.

75. Heriza C. Motor development: traditional and contemporary theories. In: Lister MJ, ed. Contemporary Management of Motor Control Problems. Proceedings of the II Step Conference. Fairfax, VA: Foundation for Physical Therapy; 1991:99-126.

76. Higgins S. Motor skill acquisition. *Phys Ther.* 1991;71(2):123-129. doi:10.1093/ptj/71.2.123.

77. Hanft B, Pilkington KO. Therapy in natural environments: the means or end goal for early intervention? *Infant Young Child.* 2000;12(suppl 4):1-13. doi:10.1097/00001163-200012040-00006.

78. Lobo MA, Harbourne RT, Dusing SC, McCoy SW. Grounding early intervention: physical therapy cannot just be about motor skills anymore. *Phys Ther.* 2013;93(1):94-103. doi:10.2522/ptj.20120158.

79. Byl NN. Neuroplasticity: applications to motor control. In: Montgomery PC, Connolly BH, eds. *Clinical Applications for Motor Control.* Thorofare, NJ: SLACK Incorporated; 2003:79-106.

80. Van Sant AF. Movement system diagnosis. *J Neurol Phys Ther.* 2017;41(suppl 3):S10-S16. doi:10.1097/NPT.0000000000000152.

81. Harris SR, Winstein CJ. The past, present and future of neurorehabilitation: from NUSTEP through IV STEP and beyond. *J Neurol Phys Ther.* 2017;41 (suppl 3):S3-S9. doi:10.1097/NPT.0000000000000193.

82. Kimberley TJ, Novak I, Boyd L, Fowler E, Larsen D. Stepping up to rethink the future of rehabilitation: IV STEP considerations and inspirations. *J Neurol Phys Ther.* 2017;41(suppl 3):S63-S72. doi:10.1097/NPT.0000000000000182.

83. McCoy JO. Continued ambulation gains through high school in a student with cerebral palsy: a case study. *Pediatr Phys Ther.* 2011;23(4):391-398. doi:10.1097/PEP.0b013e31823525c6.

84. Morgan RL, Ellerd DA, Gerity BP, Blair RJ. That's the job I want! How technology helps young people in transition. *Teach Except Child.* 2000;32(4):44-49.

85. Rainforth B. The primary therapist model: addressing challenges to practice in special education. *Phys Occup Ther Pediatr.* 2002;22 (2):29-51. doi:10.1080/J006v22n02_03.

86. Glossary. *Guide to Physical Therapist Practice 3.0.* Alexandria, VA: American Physical Therapy Association; 2014. http://guidetoptpractice.apta.org/content/1/SEC42.body. Accessed August 26, 2018.

87. Introduction to the Guide to Physical Therapist Practice. *Guide to Physical Therapist Practice 3.0.* Alexandria, VA: American Physical Therapy Association; 2014. http://guidetoptpractice.apta.org/. Accessed August 26, 2018.

88. American Occupational Therapy Association, American Physical Therapy Association, American Speech-Language-Hearing Association. *Workload Approach: A Paradigm Shift for Positive Impact on Student Outcomes.* 2014. https://pediatricapta.org/special-interest-groups/SB/pdfs/APTA-ASHA-AOTA-Joint-Doc-Workload-Approach-.pdf. Accessed September 10, 2018.

89. APTA. Peer Review Resources. Alexandria, VA: American Physical Therapy Association. http://www.apta.org/PeerReview/. Accessed September 10, 2018.

90. van Brussel M, van der Net J, Hulzebos E, Helders PJ, Takken T. The Utrecht approach to exercise in chronic childhood conditions: the decade in review. *Pediatr Phys Ther.* 2011;23(1):2-14. doi:10.1097/PEP.0b013e318208cb22.

91. Verschuren O, Ada L, Maltais DB, Gorter JW, Scianni A, Ketelaar M. Muscle strengthening in children and adolescents with spastic cerebral palsy: considerations for future resistance training protocols. *Phys Ther.* 2011;91(7):1130-1139. doi:10.2522/ptj.20100356.

92. Demchak MA, Greenfield RG. A transition portfolio for Jeff, a student with multiple disabilities. *Teach Excep Child.* 2000;32(6):44-49. doi:10.1177/004005990003200606.

93. Modell SJ, Valdez LA. Beyond bowling transition planning for students with disabilities. *Teach Except Child.* 2002;34(6):46-52. doi:10.1177/004005990203400607.

94. Squatrito Millar D, Renzaglia A. Factors affecting guardianship practices for young adults with disabilities. *Except Child.* 2002;68(4):465-484. doi:10.1177/001440290206800404.

95. Erson T. *Courageous Pacers.* Therapro. 1993. http://www.therapro.com/Browse-Category/Classroom-Fitness/The-Courageous-Pacers-Program.html. Accessed October 8, 2018.

RESOURCES

Active Living Research: https://activelivingresearch.org

American Physical Therapy Association: www.apta.org

APTA Academy of Pediatric Physical Therapy: www.pediatricapta.org

National Organization on Disability: www.nod.org

National Youth Leadership Network: www.nyln.org

Partnership for Prevention, Community Prevention: Obesity, Activity, and Nutrition. http://prevent.org/Topics.aspx?eaID=5&topicID=45

Ratey JJ. *SPARK: The Revolutionary New Science of Exercise and the Brain.* Little, Brown, and Company, New York, NY; 2008. http://www.johnratey.com/

SPARK. Research-Based Physical Education Programs, Physical Education Curriculum & More. San Diego State University Research Foundation. https://sparkpe.org/

US Department of Education, Office of Special Education Programs, Office of Special Education and Rehabilitation Services: https://www2.ed.gov/about/offices/list/osers/osep/index.html?src=mr

US Department of Education, ESSA: https://www.ed.gov/essa?src=ft

US Department of Education, IDEA: https://sites.ed.gov/idea/?src=ft

Aquatic Therapy

Elizabeth Ennis, PT, EdD, PCS, ATP

Water has been used as a modality for health and wellness for centuries, from "taking to the waters" in ancient civilizations, to more contemporary uses of aquatic therapy, including as a therapeutic intervention in rehabilitation.[1] The properties of water have been noted to be useful when addressing concerns with body functions and structures such as range of motion, muscle tone, strength, and balance. Immersion in water also allows the patient to work on functional activities in a safe, comfortable, and challenging environment, which can transfer to improved functional activities on land.[2-10] In the early 1900s, reconstruction aides in the United States used water as part of the rehabilitation process to address spasticity, polio, and arthritis.[1] Aquatic therapy has continued to evolve and has been shown to be useful for individuals with a variety of diagnoses. The benefits of aquatics for children with functional difficulties are beginning to be documented in preliminary studies and case series.[5,8,11-19] In addition to improving functional activities of children, use of aquatics can enhance participation in society, as swimming pools and various forms of water play are common environments and activities for children.

PROPERTIES OF WATER

Several properties of water need to be considered when determining the appropriateness of aquatics and the components of a therapy program. These include buoyancy, hydrostatic pressure, viscosity, and temperature. While each of these can be used to enhance a therapy program and improve the child's functional skills, care should be taken to understand the impact of each property related to limitations the child may have, to maintain the child's safety, and to use the property most effectively.

Connolly BH, Montgomery PC, eds. *Therapeutic Exercise for Children With Developmental Disabilities, Fourth Edition* (pp 451-468).
© 2020 Taylor & Francis Group.

Buoyancy

Buoyancy is the power of an object to float when immersed in a liquid, thanks to Archimedes principle that water will exert an upward force equal to that of the amount of water displaced.[20] Buoyancy provides relief from gravity, reducing the impact on joints, and decreasing the risk of falls. This is effective for children who are overweight, as well as those with significant weakness or difficulty with motor control in a gravity-resisted environment. It allows children with limited movement to access any movement they are able to perform, engage in repetitive practice, and gain increased range of movement because of the decreased influence of gravity. However, buoyancy can be a bit unsettling for children who have difficulty with upright control, and can cause them to float into a position that is uncomfortable or even compromising. The therapist needs to make sure children are able to maintain an appropriate position, either through manual contacts or use of strategically placed flotation devices when in the water.

Hydrostatic Pressure

Hydrostatic pressure provides a consistent force across the surface of anything submerged in the water at an equal depth, and increases with the depth of submersion.[20] Whereas pressure increases with depth, the pressure in a standard therapy pool is fairly consistent. This pressure can positively affect edema, as well as increase proprioceptive awareness in children with altered sensation, as in children with sensory-processing difficulties. The challenge with hydrostatic pressure is that it can overpower some systems, such as in children with significantly weak respiratory muscles; therefore, depth of immersion should be considered when determining activities for children with compromised pulmonary systems or significant weakness. For example, a child with weakness in inhalation might be limited to immersion only to the level of the lower rib cage, allowing some strength training of the diaphragm, but not allowing an external force on the rib cage that would restrict expansion.

Viscosity

Viscosity is the "thickness" of the water that provides resistance ("drag") consistently to submerged objects.[20] This resistance makes the use of aquatics a bit deceptive in its intensity. Children in the water are consistently working against resistance, although the intensity can be altered through speed of movement, length of lever arm, and surface area being moved through the water. Moving more rapidly or with a larger surface area can increase the intensity of the work being performed. However, the lack of gravity and warmth of the water can make it appear less intense, and children often are surprised at how tired they are following a session in the pool.

Water Temperature

Water temperature also is important to consider, as this can affect children's core temperature, depending on their level of activity. Heat loss in water is significantly increased compared with air at a given temperature, and this needs to be taken into account when developing an activity program.[20] Warm water can be beneficial in addressing increased tone, muscle tightness, and anxiety. However, strenuous activity in warm water can increase core temperature significantly, and, in some instances, increase fatigue, which can be detrimental. Children with diagnoses such as muscular dystrophies that respond negatively to fatigue need to have carefully developed aquatic programs to minimize the potential for significant heating and fatigue. Conversely, minimal activity in cooler temperatures can be uncomfortable and cause a drop in core temperature. If a cooler pool is being used, the therapist should consider using wetsuits or similar garments in children who will not be constantly active. Wetsuits provide some temperature stability and comfort. Generally, a pool temperature between 91°F and 93°F is recommended if children are not participating in vigorous activities.[1,21]

Factors Related to Therapeutic Use

Purposes for Aquatic Therapy

Aquatics is used as a therapeutic modality to address a wide variety of conditions and concerns. Given the properties of water discussed previously, aquatic therapy can be used for relaxation, strengthening, postural control/balance, ambulation, cardiovascular strengthening and endurance, coordination, and proprioception, with the goal of transferring skills learned in the water to similar skills on land.[11-13,16,22,23] Aquatic therapy protocols are individualized to the child's current goals and the available facilities and equipment. The therapist often provides handling and cuing, similar to what is done on land, and many of the same outcome measures are used to measure progress.

Considerations (Safety, Fear, Sensory Processing)

Therapists considering using aquatics with a child need to consider multiple factors to determine whether aquatics is an appropriate modality. Safety issues should be a primary concern, especially related to the child's medical condition. For example, a child with a history of seizures may still be considered for aquatic therapy, depending on the type and frequency of seizures, any known triggers, and the availability of additional support personnel in the pool area. Issues related to fear should not be considered contraindications, as fear often relates to difficulty with sensory processing, which can be addressed with gradual introduction to the water. Using aquatics as a modality to address sensory processing issues related to hypo- or hyperresponsiveness of the proprioceptive system often can improve daily activities, such as showering or bathing, and increase the child's participation in community activities (eg, swimming and water play).

Coding Issues

When seeking third-party reimbursement, the aquatic current procedural terminology code may be used. However, not all third-party payers reimburse for the aquatic current procedural terminology code. Many therapists prefer to code for the issues they are treating, and use therapeutic activities, therapeutic exercise, neuromuscular reeducation, or gait to code for the activities that best represent the emphasis of intervention during aquatic therapy sessions.

Participation Restrictions

Therapists should consider the use of aquatics to address participation restrictions in children with mild motor delays and or developmental disabilities (DD). Children with significant DD often are isolated from typical community activities with peers because of lack of access, as well as lack of time because of attending multiple medical appointments. Working with children to ensure familiarity with water and providing families with activities that can be beneficial will allow children to engage in pool activities with peers in the community, decreasing their isolation and improving their participation. The 5 cases used throughout this text will be discussed based on the appropriateness of aquatic therapy as a treatment modality and what should be considered in each case. Examples of aquatic activities can be viewed in Video 16-1.

Case Study #1: Jason

> *Medical Diagnosis:* Cerebral palsy, right hemiparesis
> *Gross Motor Function Classification System:* Level I
> *Age:* 24 months

History

Jason was a preterm infant, and at his 6-month neonatal intensive care unit follow-up, asymmetries in use of the 2 sides of his body were noted, and he was referred to early intervention (EI). He receives occupational therapy and developmental intervention through EI, with speech and physical therapy obtained through private insurance. Jason is not currently taking any medications and has not needed surgical intervention to this point. He presents with right hemiparesis, but walked at age 15 months.

Participation Restrictions

Jason has difficulty keeping up with his twin sibling and other children during play, especially outside. Because he falls frequently, he is not exposed to a wide variety of environments and age-appropriate social situations unless closely supervised.

Significant Examination Findings

> Decreased muscle bulk on the right.
> Altered gait pattern.
> Increased activity with tactile stimulation (unclear if this is overstimulation or arousal with stimulation); possible tactile defensiveness.
> Orients primarily to the left.
> Poor coordination of the right side.
> Slow righting and protective reactions.
> Generalized weakness on the right side.
> Anterior pelvic tilt with right retraction.
> Observable rib cage asymmetry.
> Neglect of the right side.

Therapeutic Goals

General goals are for Jason to demonstrate improved age-appropriate mobility and play with peers, a reduction in falls, and improved coordination and bilateral use of extremities. Specific activity/functional goals for Jason in his aquatic therapy program are for him to be able to accomplish the following:

1. Stand in waist-deep water with symmetrical lower extremity weight bearing.
2. Walk backward 10 steps down a ramp.
3. Maintain bilateral grip on kick board and flutter kick for minimum of 5 seconds.
4. Place face in water and blow bubbles for 3 seconds.

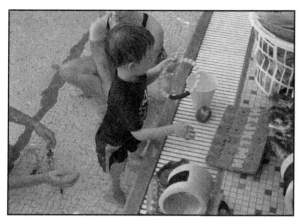

Figure 16-1. Tactile cues at the child's hips cue hip extension and increase stance time on the right with elongation of the trunk.

Aquatic Program for Jason

Jason has issues with coordination, neglect, and perceptual-motor awareness, and is at an age at which children become fussy when tasks become difficult. The pool provides a "fun" place to address his therapy goals, even if the tasks are a challenge for him, which should increase his motivation and cooperation during aquatic sessions.

Hydrostatic pressure can decrease tactile hypersensitivity while providing proprioceptive input to increase awareness of his right side. Introduction to water should be gradual because of his sensitivity. Chest-deep immersion with a swim vest or chest belt will allow free use of all 4 extremities and provide maximum proprioceptive input.

Standing activities can be performed in shallow water to encourage hip extensor activity and decreased retraction of his right pelvis during stance. Walking can be performed with tactile cues at his hips to cue hip extension and to increase stance time on right with elongation of the trunk (Figure 16-1).

If there is a ramp, the amount of support from the water can be varied, tibial translation during stance can be encouraged going up the ramp, and backward walking can be used to encourage hip extension.

Performing prone activities on a float mat can increase hip extension as well as core stability due to the unstable surface. Over time, the child can transition up to tall kneeling, with or without cuing (Figure 16-2).

Flutter kicks with a kick board or prone on elbows on a mat for play also can encourage extension movements. Sitting activities on the mat, such as dumping and filling a bucket, can encourage core activation and bilateral upper extremity use, as well as work on balance and protective reactions in sitting (Figure 16-3).

"Monkey crawling" along the pool wall will encourage bilateral reciprocal use of extremities in midrange position, and facilitate motor planning and out-of-synergy movements (ie, increased upper extremity extension while working on lower extremity flexion).

Handling to address core/rib asymmetries can be performed while Jason is seated on a dynamic surface during play (eg, float mat in tailor or heel-sit positions) with rotation to either side, and 2-handed bucket activities to increase use of the right arm, especially out of typical flexor patterns (ie, using shoulder flexion with elbow extension). Bubble and blowing activities with the chest in the water allow resisted respiration and breath support.

Figure 16-2. Performing tall kneeling activities on a float mat can increase hip extension, as well as core stability due to the unstable surface.

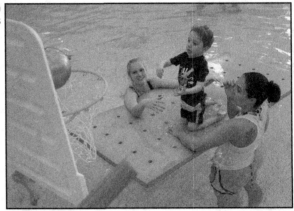

Figure 16-3. Sitting activities on the mat can encourage core activation and bilateral upper extremity use, as well as work on balance and protective reactions in sitting.

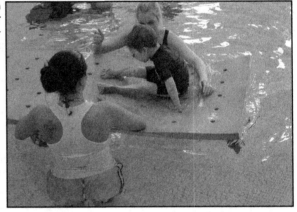

Water allows movement without fear of falling. Ideally, extremity floats would not be used for this child in shallow water or on float mats to make sure core muscles are active. Jason should remain in a depth where the water is chest deep except for float mat/kick board work. Once he is more comfortable in the water, swimming activities and deeper water activities can be incorporated into his aquatic therapy sessions.

Weekly sessions for 2 to 3 months with land practice interspersed should allow Jason to gain strength, improve coordination, and decrease neglect of his right side. While short-term goals can address improvement in skills related to the pool, long-term goals should address function, such as improved balance, improved gait pattern, increased speed of protective reactions, and improved mobility in everyday activities. His home program should focus on the parents' ability to perform activities with him in the water during family recreational times that continually address his therapeutic goals.

CASE STUDY #2: JILL

▸ *Medical Diagnosis:* Cerebral palsy, spastic quadriparesis, microcephaly, intellectual deficits, seizure disorder
▸ *Gross Motor Function Classification System:* Level V
▸ *Age:* 7 years

History

Jill was a full-term infant. Following neonatal seizures, she was admitted to the neonatal intensive care unit and was ventilated for several days. She initially had feeding difficulties, but was bottle-feeding well on discharge. At her 4-month follow-up visit, she was noted to have decreased head growth, with normal eye and ear exams.

Participation Restrictions

Jill has significant limitations in active movements and few independent functions. Her play and social opportunities are very limited because of her severe motor and cognitive impairments.

Significant Examination Findings

- Has seizures, but triggers are unknown.
- Uses wheelchair and prone stander; is nonambulatory with poor prognosis for ambulation.
- Has poor sitting balance.
- Has limited mobility in her ribs and shoulder girdle, poor head control, poor voluntary movement in all extremities, and generalized weakness.
- Has limited active movement of arms to 60 degrees of abduction.
- Demonstrates hyperactive reflexes throughout, and presents with increased tone in all extremities. Movement through space results in autonomic distress, but it is unclear if this is due to fear of movement, lack of awareness of where she is in space, or other perceptual concerns.
- Respiration is difficult because of her immobile rib cage, which makes her susceptible to upper respiratory infections.

Therapeutic Goals

General intervention goals are to promote all active movements possible in a reduced-gravity environment, improve tolerance to movement through increased proprioceptive activities and slow rhythmic movements in water, increase range of motion, and produce relaxation in muscles. Specific activity/functional goals for Jill in her aquatic therapy program are for her to be able to accomplish the following:

1. Maintain lower extremity extension in supported standing when wearing ankle weights.
2. Demonstrate tolerance of the water environment by smiling and making excited vocalizations.
3. Make voluntary limb movements in supine when instructed to "go swimming!"
4. Maintain bilateral grasp on kick board for 3 seconds while supported in sitting.
5. Maintain upright head control when tilted 20 degrees in supported sitting on float mat.

Aquatic Program for Jill

Activities for Jill will consist primarily of non–weight-bearing tasks, allowing the warmth of the water to decrease the stiffness in her muscles, and the reduced impact of gravity to encourage any available movements. Her therapist could use a neck collar to keep Jill's head above water and stable, decreasing the risk of swallowing water. Any session should allow free float time for initiation of active movement, directed by the therapist to encourage purposeful activities.

Figure 16-4. Slow, rhythmic movements can be used to relax trunk muscles, activate limb motions, and promote relaxation.

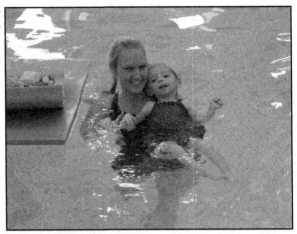

Figure 16-5. Tasks performed prone on a float mat can be used to generate controlled extension.

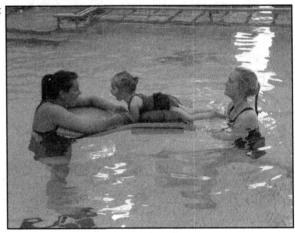

Slow, rhythmic movements can be used to relax trunk muscles, activate limb motions, and promote relaxation. Starting with Jill in supine, the therapist can support her under her upper trunk and shoulders, using slow lateral movements to the left and right (Figure 16-4).

The resistance of the water on one side can activate muscles while the other side relaxes. Jill can later be shifted to being supported at her hip and shoulder with similar movements, then to supporting her lower legs with a flotation device under her head to keep her head above water during the lateral movements.

After activities to promote relaxation and any active movement, tasks performed prone on a kick board or with her trunk on a float mat can be used to generate controlled extension (Figure 16-5).

Because Jill has seizures, it is important to know any triggers, and also to have support personnel on the deck if Jill were to have a seizure. If her seizures are related to any external stimuli, the therapist needs to take care to reduce stimulation such as flashing lights or excessive visual input.

Jill can work on upright positioning and weight bearing, beginning in chest-deep water and progressing to waist deep, which requires more trunk activity. Ankle weights can increase foot contact with the bottom of the pool, and encourage lower extremity extension, allowing the therapist to focus on Jill's hips and trunk (Figure 16-6).

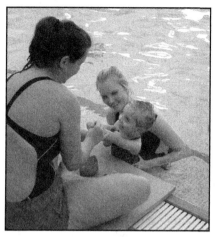

Figure 16-6. Work in an upright position with weight bearing, beginning in chest-deep water and progressing to waist-deep, requires more trunk activity.

CASE STUDY #3: TAYLOR

> *Medical Diagnosis:* Myelomeningocele, repaired L1-2
> *Age:* 4 years

History

Taylor is a 4-year-old boy with L1-2 myelomeningocele and a ventricular-peritoneal shunt. He had a suspected Arnold-Chiari malformation that was treated by surgical release of the posterior fossa. He receives occupational therapy once each week and physical therapy twice each week in his preschool program. The school district is considering placement for Taylor in a regular kindergarten classroom next year.

Participation Restrictions

Taylor cannot keep up with peers when pushing his manual wheelchair. Both when floor sitting and in his manual wheelchair, he cannot access some environments for exploration, play, and social interactions.

Significant Examination Findings

> Lower extremities are small in proportion to upper extremities and trunk.
> Head is slightly larger (95th percentile) in proportion to his body because of hydrocephalus.
> Visual-perceptual problems, which have made cognitive testing difficult. His performance suggests his intellectual skills are in the low normal range. He has good attention skills and usually is cooperative and motivated in the classroom.
> Uses an anterior walker and a reciprocating gait orthosis. He self-propels a manual wheelchair. External support is necessary for standing. He is beginning to use long leg braces and crutches.
> Balance reactions are slow in sitting and standing. He has good protective reactions in sitting, but not in standing.
> Loss of motor function in his lower extremities; poor active trunk extension.
> Good head control in all positions and normal upper extremity coordination.

> Generalized weakness is noted in upper extremities and trunk, especially in abdominal muscles.
> Able to transition in and out of sitting and into all fours independently; attempts to pull to kneeling.
> Uses reciprocating gait orthosis or long leg braces for standing activities.
> Range of motion is within functional limits; slightly tight hip flexors and hip adductors.
> Tends to hold his breath when using his upper extremities for weight-bearing or strenuous tasks; he has inadequate abdominal strength to support sustained exhalation.
> Overall endurance for physical activity is decreased compared with peers.

Therapeutic Goals

General goals for Taylor are to improve strength and endurance for propelling his manual wheelchair to keep up with classmates; and to improve balance, strength, and endurance for walking with long leg braces and forearm crutches. Specific activity/functional goals for Taylor in his aquatic therapy program are for him to be able to accomplish the following:

1. Maintain sitting balance on kick board while being tilted 10 degrees in any direction (ie, laterally, forward/backward).
2. Use lower extremity muscles to "walk" in parallel bars in pool.
3. Use a bubble wand and blow bubbles for one minute while chest is submerged in water.
4. Use a bilateral grasp on a kick board to "swish" it back and forth in water (while sitting on pool steps) for 10 seconds.

Aquatic Program for Taylor

The pool is an excellent environment for Taylor to work on overall endurance, strengthening of trunk muscles, and core stability. Children with spina bifida at mid to high lumbar levels often use excessive trunk movements because of a lack of lower extremity activation. Increased strength and core stability will be key for Taylor to be successful in using long leg braces and crutches for ambulation.

Taylor's aquatic session can begin in deep water with a pool noodle under his arms. This will allow him to activate his trunk and legs as much as he is able, with his therapist encouraging him to move through the water. Other activities to work on Taylor's trunk include seated activities on a kick board with the therapist shifting the board laterally and in an anterior-posterior direction; and sitting on a float mat using a bucket for dump and fill activities (Figures 16-7 and 16-8).

Taylor can work on trunk activation while sitting on the pool steps in the water—push-pull with the kick board will strengthen his arms and engage his trunk muscles for stability. Weights can be placed around his ankles for standing activities in the parallel bars in the pool. Weight-shifting activities can be coupled with input for appropriate trunk movements. Taylor can work on ambulating in the water, with weights around his ankles and blocking at his knees. The therapist can use manual cues for weight-shift and lower extremity advancement (Figure 16-9).

Taylor should work on respiration, such as breathing during forceful activities. When his trunk is submerged, inhalation is resisted by the hydrostatic pressure of the water, and can be manually cued with quick stretch techniques or other manual cues.

Weekly sessions for a few months can provide strengthening that can be carried over to land activities, especially standing and ambulation activities with braces and crutches in which Taylor wants to participate. Increasing his comfort in the water will allow him to engage in water-play activities with peers.

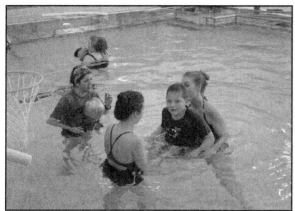

Figure 16-7. Support of the child in a seated position allows him to activate his trunk and legs as much as he is able, with his therapist encouraging him to move through the water.

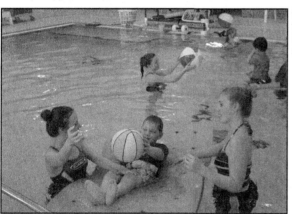

Figure 16-8. Other activities to work on Taylor's trunk include seated activities on a float mat board, with the therapist shifting the board laterally and in an anterior-posterior direction.

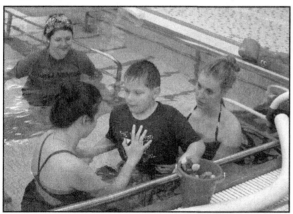

Figure 16-9. The child can work on ambulating in the water, with weights around the ankles and blocking at the knees.

Case Study #4: Ashley

> *Medical Diagnosis:* Down syndrome
> *Age:* 15 months

History

Ashley is a 15-month-old girl with Down syndrome. She had esophageal atresia, and primary repair was not possible. A gastrostomy was present for her first 6 months. She had a ventricular-septal defect that was surgically repaired at age 8 months. Cardiac issues in children with Down syndrome tend to delay development further because of decreased tolerance to activity. Ashley has a history of chronic otitis media with mild conductive hearing loss. Pressure-equalizing tubes were inserted at age 12 months. Ashley did not begin EI services until she was age 10 months. Ashley and her mother attend a parent/caregiver-infant EI program twice weekly with consultative physical therapy, occupational therapy, and speech therapy services available at each session. The family has declined home-based services.

Participation Restrictions

Ashley avoids other children when in a group setting. She is unable to keep up with her peers in play and demonstrates hypersensitivity to many environmental stimuli. Her limited play and environmental opportunities negatively affect her motor-skill development and social and cognitive experiences.

Significant Examination Findings

> Needs encouragement and stimulation to attend to motor and cognitive tasks.
> Pulls to stand but is not yet attempting to cruise at furniture. She will walk with maximal assistance with 2 hands held. She has slow and usually ineffective protective and equilibrium reactions in sitting, all fours, and standing.
> Hypermobility is noted in all upper and lower extremity proximal and distal joints.
> Demonstrates a variety of movement patterns but movements are very slow; postural reactions are delayed.
> Multiple repetitions of cognitive and motor tasks for skill achievement and retention are needed.
> Good head control in all positions. She rolls independently, transitions in and out of sitting and in and out of a hands-and-knees position. She pulls to kneeling and pulls to stand at furniture.
> Tends to use straight-plane movements without using trunk rotation. She does not appear hypersensitive to tactile input. She generally is apprehensive about movement activities. She grasps objects but cannot release them with control. She cannot pick up pellet-sized objects.
> Decreased respiratory-phonatory functioning. She is a mouth breather and occasionally drools.

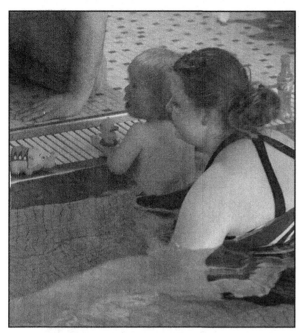

Figure 16-10. Ashley could work on sit to stand from the therapist's leg to the ledge.

Therapeutic Goals

General intervention goals are to increase Ashley's tolerance to sensory experiences, particularly proprioceptive and vestibular, and to improve her balance for improved floor mobility and ambulation. Specific activity/functional goals for Ashley in her aquatic therapy program are for her to be able to accomplish the following:

1. Cruise laterally 3 steps in either direction while standing in water holding onto the pool ledge with the therapist supporting her at the waist.
2. "Slap" water with her hands for 5 to 10 seconds while sitting on the pool steps.
3. Tolerate being tilted laterally 10 degrees in either direction while seated on a kick board.
4. Place her face in water for 1 second, 3 of 5 attempts.

Aquatic Program for Ashley

Ashley had pressure-equalizing tubes inserted 3 months ago; therefore, getting water in her ears is not a concern. However, protective earplugs can be used. Given the need to encourage voluntary movement, the therapist should determine what activities Ashley enjoys and use similar activities to motivate her in the pool.

Having Ashley floating with support and slowly changing positions should be performed initially to help her become accustomed to the water. Eventually, multiplanar position changes should be used, as she does not perform many activities with rotation or diagonal movements. Standing in the water at a ledge would allow the therapist to encourage cruising to move toward objects of interest. Ashley could work on sit to stand from the therapist's leg to the ledge (Figure 16-10).

Strength and core stability can be addressed with Ashley working in prone/quadruped on a float mat (Figure 16-11), with manual cues to reach with one hand while maintaining the hands-and-knees position, or moving forward on her belly on an unstable surface.

Figure 16-11. Strength and core stability can be addressed with Ashley working in prone/quadruped on a float mat.

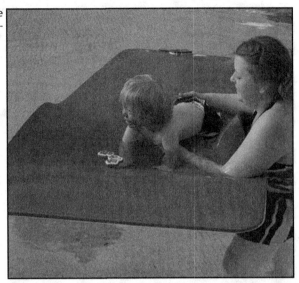

Figure 16-12. A float mat can be used for sitting activities, with Ashley reaching for objects while on the unstable surface to develop protective reactions and core stability.

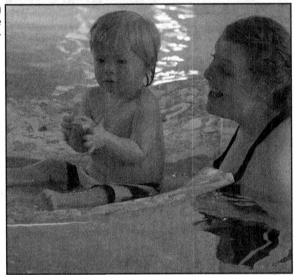

The float mat could be used for sitting activities, with Ashley reaching for objects while on the unstable surface to develop protective reactions and core stability (Figure 16-12). Similar activities could be performed sitting on a kick board with the therapist motivating movement as needed and providing manual cuing. Breathing activities in chest-deep water, with the therapist encouraging blowing activities, can help to develop respiratory muscles.

Pool sessions for Ashley can be 30 minutes once weekly to start, increasing to 45 minutes as tolerated, and her parents should be encouraged to be in the pool with the therapist. Since the family is familiar with the consultative model of services, the therapist should encourage the family to take Ashley to a pool as a family activity and perform some of the activities they are taught, along with just having a fun family outing.

CASE STUDY #5: JOHN

> *Medical Diagnosis:* Developmental coordination disorder/attention-deficit hyperactivity disorder

> *Age:* 5 years

History

John is a 5-year-old boy, born prematurely, who has been very active physically but is easily frustrated. He is noted to be "clumsy" and is unable to perform gross and fine motor tasks as well as his peers. Following evaluations by a developmental pediatrician and neuropsychologist, he received dual diagnoses of developmental coordination disorder and attention-deficit hyperactivity disorder. He has been placed on Ritalin (methylphenidate). John is in a half-day kindergarten program, but does not qualify for special education services. He is receiving occupational and physical therapy (each 2 times per month) through a private agency.

Participation Restrictions

John avoids movement-based activities with peers, both at school during recess and at the neighborhood playground. He does not attempt new activities and has poor endurance to keep up with his peers or family during age-appropriate gross motor activities, such as bike riding.

Significant Examination Findings

> Walks independently, but occasionally walks on his toes. He can walk with a heel-toe gait when reminded. He tends to walk too quickly with poor balance, often bumping into environmental objects or other people. He cannot walk a 4-inch (10-cm) balance beam without falling off and can maintain his balance on one foot for only 1 to 2 seconds.

> Has difficulty varying the speed of movement and coordinating upper and lower extremities, such as required when performing jumping jacks. He has motor planning problems and has difficulty learning new motor tasks. He requires more practice than his peers to master each motor skill. Skills do not generalize easily.

> Upper extremity strength is decreased for his age. Endurance for age-appropriate activities, such as soccer, is decreased compared with his peers.

> Ambulates independently; he can run, although he does so in a poorly coordinated pattern. He cannot skip but gallops instead. He has difficulty with ball skills (eg, catching, throwing, dribbling) and eye-hand coordination. He uses a modified lateral pinch for coloring and printing.

> Occasionally demonstrates signs of tactile defensiveness.

> Tends to walk with stiff legs and a decreased arm swing. He often leans forward as he walks.

Therapeutic Goals

General goals are for John to improve his overall strength and endurance for physical activity, and to improve motor planning abilities to enable participation in age-appropriate gross motor activities. Specific activity/functional goals for John in his aquatic therapy program are for him to be able to accomplish the following:

Figure 16-13. Eye-hand coordination can be addressed through toss-and-catch ball play while standing in mid-chest depth water or sitting on a float mat.

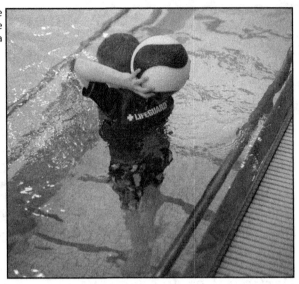

1. Throw and catch a beach ball without falling while sitting on a float mat, 3 of 5 attempts.
2. Swim through a hula hoop without touching the sides.
3. Swim (any stroke) or jog one length of pool without stopping.
4. Turn a forward somersault in the water.
5. Jump off a ledge of the pool and perform a "cannonball" (ie, tucking arms and legs).

Aquatic Program for John

The pool is a wonderful place to work with John for several reasons: (1) the resistance of the water can slow down an inappropriate increased rate of activity, (2) the pressure of the water can improve body awareness and decrease hypersensitivity, and (3) multistep activities can be developed without the fear of falling or bumping into objects or people.

Eye-hand coordination can be addressed through toss-and-catch ball play while standing in mid–chest-deep water or sitting on a float mat. Starting with larger beach balls and progressing to smaller balls encourages success while providing a fun target (eg, therapist, basketball hoop, parent), which can add motivation to the activity (Figure 16-13).

Walking or running in chest-deep water and jumping off a ledge with verbal and manual cuing provides experience with bilateral activities enhanced by the pressure of the water, which gives John intrinsic feedback about his movements.

Promising "free swimming" time is useful with children like John as a motivation to complete an activity. Saying "If we do this, then you can have 2 minutes to do what you want" can help with compliance to the program (Figure 16-14).

Free swim then can be turned into a multistep obstacle course to encourage following multistep commands and sequential motor planning. Hula hoops, diving toys, buckets of water, and other objects can be used to develop the activities in the obstacle course.

At first, success is completion of the tasks. Once a multistep course can be completed, improved time of completion can be used to measure progress.

The aquatic program can be initiated once weekly for 45 to 60 minutes, and a community program should be developed as soon as possible, allowing John to engage with peers in a typical social environment. When in the community pool, John may feel as skilled as his peers, and will be able to participate in age-appropriate water play with his friends.

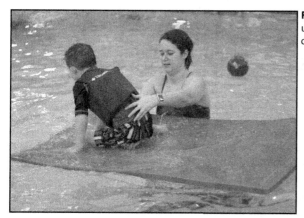

Figure 16-14. Promising "free swimming" time is useful with children like John as a motivation to complete an activity.

Summary

Aquatic therapy is an excellent adjunct to traditional physical therapy interventions. Therapy activities in water have unique characteristics because of the buoyancy of water and the opportunity for increased musculoskeletal relaxation and mobility. Aquatic therapy activities can be adapted to meet the needs of a wide variety of children with varying diagnoses and impairments. One of the most positive features of aquatic therapy is its potential to provide children with DD the opportunity to participate in an age-appropriate social environment and water play. Eliminating participation restrictions is a primary focus in physical therapy, and aquatic therapy often can accomplish this goal.

References

1. Cole AJ, Becker BE. *Comprehensive Aquatic Therapy*. 3rd ed. Pullman, WA: Washington State University Press; 2010.
2. Villalta EM, Peiris CL. Early aquatic physical therapy improves function and does not increase risk of wound-related adverse events for adults after orthopedic surgery: a systematic review and meta-analysis. *Arch Phys Med Rehabil*. 2013;94(1):138-148. doi:10.1016/j.apmr.2012.07.020.
3. Resende SM, Rassi CM, Viana FP. Effects of hydrotherapy in balance and prevention of falls among elderly women. *Rev Bras Fisioter*. 2008;12(1):57-63. doi:10.1590/S1413-35552008000100011.
4. Prins J, Cutner D. Aquatic therapy in the rehabilitation of athletic injuries. *Clin Sports Med*. 1999;18(2):447-461. doi:10.1016/S0278-5919(05)70158-7.
5. McManus BM, Kotelchuck M. The effect of aquatic therapy on functional mobility of infants and toddlers in early intervention. *Pediatr Phys Ther*. 2007;19(4):275-282. doi:10.1097/PEP.0b013e3181575190.
6. Marinho-Buzelli AR, Bonnyman AM, Verrier MC. The effects of aquatic therapy on mobility of individuals with neurological diseases: a systematic review. *Clin Rehabil*. 2015;29(8):741-751. doi:10.1177/0269215514556297.
7. Lima TB, Dias JM, Mazuquin BF, et al. The effectiveness of aquatic physical therapy in the treatment of fibromyalgia: a systematic review with meta-analysis. *Clin Rehabil*. 2013;27(10):892-908. doi:10.1177/0269215513484772.
8. Fragala-Pinkham MA, Dumas HM, Barlow CA, Pasternak A. An aquatic physical therapy program at a pediatric rehabilitation hospital: a case series. *Pediatr Phys Ther*. 2009;21(1):68-78. doi:10.1097/PEP.0b013e318196eb37.
9. Ennis E. The effects of a physical therapy-directed aquatic program on children with autism spectrum disorders. *J Aquat Phys Ther*. 2011;19(1):4-10.
10. Becker BE. Aquatic therapy: scientific foundations and clinical rehabilitation applications. *PM R*. 2009;1(9):859-872. doi:10.1016/j.pmrj.2009.05.017.
11. Kelly M, Darrah J. Aquatic exercise for children with cerebral palsy. *Dev Med Child Neurol*. 2005;47(12):838-842. doi:10.1017/S0012162205001775.
12. Fragala-Pinkham MA, Smith HJ, Lombard KA, Barlow C, O'Neil ME. Aquatic aerobic exercise for children with cerebral palsy: a pilot intervention study. *Physiother Theory Pract*. 2014;30(2):69-78. doi:10.3109/09593985.2013.825825.
13. Retarekar R, Fragala-Pinkham MA, Townsend EL. Effects of aquatic aerobic exercise for a child with cerebral palsy: single-subject design. *Pediatr Phys Ther*. 2009;21(4):336-344. doi:10.1097/PEP.0b013e3181bebo39.

14. Lai CJ, Liu WY, Yang TF, Chen CL, Wu CY, Chan RC. Pediatric aquatic therapy on motor function and enjoyment in children diagnosed with cerebral palsy of various motor severities. *J Child Neurol*. 2015;30(2):200-208. doi:10.1177/0883073814535491.

15. Dimitrijevic L, Aleksandrovic M, Madic D, Okicic T, Radovanovic D, Daly D. The effect of aquatic intervention on the gross motor function and aquatic skills in children with cerebral palsy. *J Hum Kinet*. 2012;32(1):167-174. doi:10.2478/v10078-012-0033-5.

16. Oriel KN, Kanupka JW, DeLong KS, Noel K. The impact of aquatic exercise on sleep behaviors in children with autism spectrum disorder: a pilot study. *Focus Autism Other Dev Disabil*. 2016;31(4):254-261. doi:10.1177/1088357614559212.

17. Lee J, Porretta DL. Enhancing the motor skills of children with autism spectrum disorders: A pool-based approach. *J Phys Educ Recreat Dance*. 2013;84(1):41-45. doi:10.1080/07303084.2013.746154.

18. Lawson LM, Mazurowski M, Petersen S. Sensory processing patterns and swim skill acquisition of children with autism spectrum disorder. *Am J Recreat Ther*. 2017;16(2):29-40. doi:10.5055/ajrt.2017.0131.

19. Fabrizi SE. Splashing our way to playfulness! An aquatic playgroup for young children with autism, a repeated measures design. *J Occup Ther Schools Early Intervent*. 2015;8(4):292-306. doi:10.1080/19411243.2015.1116963.

20. Norm A, Hanson B. *Aquatic Exercise Therapy*. Philadelphia, PA: WB Saunders; 1996.

21. Becker BE. Biophysiologic aspects of hydrotherapy. In: Cole AJ, Becker BE, eds. *Comprehensive Aquatic Therapy*. 3rd ed. Pullman, WA: Washington State University Publishing; 2010:23-53.

22. Peterson T. Pediatric aquatic therapy. In: Cole AJ, Becker BE, eds. *Comprehensive Aquatic Therapy*. 3rd ed. Pullman, WA: Washington State University Publishing; 2010:323-361.

23. Karklina B, Declerck M, Daly DJ. Quantification of aquatic interventions in children with disabilities: a systematic literature review. *Int J Aquatic Res Educ*. 2013;7(4):344-379. doi:10.25035/ijare.07.04.07.

The Children
Physical Therapy Management

17

Patricia C. Montgomery, PT, PhD, FAPTA
Barbara H. Connolly, PT, DPT, EdD, C/NDT, FAPTA

A major focus of this text has been to move away from conceptualizing issues relevant to physical therapists as being based on the medical diagnoses of children with developmental disabilities (DD). Instead, the authors of the various chapters have emphasized using the World Health Organization's *International Classification of Functioning, Disability and Health* (ICF).[1] Physical therapists typically do not address underlying pathology, such as occurs with genetic syndromes, destruction of brain tissue associated with anoxia, or cardiac defects. Emphasis in physical therapy is on the sequelae of pathology and the relationship to participation restrictions and activity limitations.

The purpose of this chapter is to summarize the primary participation restrictions and activity limitations for each of the children in the 5 case studies. We also hypothesize about the primary impairments that are contributing to functional limitations. Although for teaching purposes, examination, evaluation, and intervention strategies related to specific problem areas have been presented in separate chapters, physical therapists must address the "big picture" and attempt to identify the primary issues related to intervention for children who demonstrate a variety of multiple interacting variables.

We also have taken the position that physical therapists are engaging more in prediction and management of physical therapy needs for children with DD. In that regard, we have hypothesized about future considerations for case management, intervention, and periodic episodes of care.

CASE STUDY #1: JASON

> *Medical Diagnosis:* Cerebral palsy, right hemiparesis
> *Gross Motor Function Classification System:* Level I
> *Age:* 24 months

Connolly BH, Montgomery PC, eds. *Therapeutic Exercise for Children With Developmental Disabilities, Fourth Edition* (pp 469-489).
© 2020 Taylor & Francis Group.

Primary Participation Restrictions

› Unable to keep up with peers in gross motor play situations, especially outdoors, limiting social interactions
› Unable to eat the same foods as sibling or same-age peers at snack and mealtime, limiting oral-motor stimulation and nutrition
› Has difficulty manipulating objects and toys requiring bilateral upper extremity control, limiting play opportunities and cognitive learning
› Limited play environments because he falls frequently, thereby decreasing opportunities for environmental exploration

Primary Activity/Functional Limitations

› Unable to use his right arm and hand effectively for self-care tasks or manipulation of toys
› Does not protect himself adequately with loss of balance
› Falls frequently, especially when attempting to move quickly or run
› Demonstrates difficulty eating textured food, often losing food out of his mouth or choking
› Does not communicate well using speech, relying more on gestures

Primary Impairments

› Poor sensory awareness on the right side of the body/mild disregard
› Motor control deficits on right side of body
› Sensory and motor deficits in oral-motor musculature
› Immature balance reactions and postural control
› Generalized weakness of right extremities
› Limited flexibility of muscles on right side of the body
› Poor respiratory control

Participation/Activity Goals

Self-Care and Domestic Life

Jason will be able to accomplish the following:
› Use both hands to take off his socks.
› Eat soft meats without losing food out of his mouth.
› Maintain symmetrical lip closure on a cup rim without losing liquid.
› Remove food from spoon without losing food out of mouth.
› Sit on a bench and assist with removing a T-shirt.

Mental Functions

Jason will be able to accomplish the following:
› Communicate using words in addition to gestures.

Neuromotor Development and Sensory Processing

Jason will be able to accomplish the following:
› Use both hands to catch and throw a 12-inch (30-cm) diameter ball, 2 of 3 trials.

- Reach forward for a 12-inch (30-cm) diameter ball with both elbows extended, 3 of 3 attempts.
- Grasp a hat with both hands and reach overhead with both arms to place it on his head.
- Begin to "scribble" and "color" with the right hand using large color markers.
- Run 10 to 20 feet (3 to 6 m) and keep up with his peers.
- Be able to play "leap frog" bearing weight on both upper extremities for several seconds.
- Spontaneously position toys at midline or slightly to the right side of the body during play, 2 of 5 trials.
- Demonstrate awareness of temperature differences in environmental objects with both hands.

Balance

Jason will be able to accomplish the following:
- Climb on and off furniture using reciprocal movements in his upper and lower extremities.
- Ambulate on a community playground, mounting and dismounting from at least 4 pieces of equipment without falling.
- Walk up and down 3 to 5 steps, holding on to a railing, using a reciprocal pattern.
- Walk in his playroom at home picking up and carrying an item requiring 2 hands for support, then placing the item on a shelf at shoulder height.
- Fall fewer than 3 times a day.
- Use his arms to catch himself when he falls, 3 of 5 losses of balance.
- When standing, not fall over when bumped or pushed by another child, 2 of 3 occasions.
- Demonstrate ability when walking outdoors to change direction quickly without falling, 2 of 3 attempts.

Posture

Jason will be able to accomplish the following:
- Independently bench-sit with symmetrical weight bearing.

Ventilation and Respiration

Jason will be able to accomplish the following:
- Sustain the volume of vocal sounds for simple songs and noises.
- Take 3 to 4 sips of liquid from an open cup before pausing to breathe with no gasping or choking.

Interventions

- Improve sensory awareness on the right side of his body, as well as in oral-motor structures.
- Improve balance reactions and postural control, especially in standing.
- Improve coordination and speed during gross motor tasks, such as running.
- Improve coordination during bilateral fine motor tasks.
- Increase strength of right trunk and extremities.
- Increase range of motion (ROM) of his right extremities and trunk.
- Improve coordination of respiration with eating, drinking, sound/speech production tasks, and during gross motor skills.
- Increase symmetry during sitting, standing, and fine motor activities.

Additional Considerations/Prognosis

Although age-appropriate gross motor skills, such as balancing on one foot or walking a balance beam, may never be accomplished at the same level as his peers, Jason's physical therapy prognosis for functional gross motor skills (eg, stepping up and down curbs, ramps, stairs) is excellent. Studies of potential for ambulation indicate that almost all children with spastic hemiparesis become independent ambulators.[2] When Jason's current level of motor performance is examined in relation to the Gross Motor Function Classification System (GMFCS),[3-5] he is classified at Level I, or the highest level of independent mobility in children with cerebral palsy (CP).

In predicting and managing Jason's physical therapy needs, the physical therapist will want to emphasize intervention directed to the upper extremity. Lack of upper extremity dexterity and hand function presents the greatest potential for difficulties with fine motor skills and activities of daily living (ADL) tasks as Jason matures. A direct therapeutic focus on the involved upper extremity in some children with hemiplegia may result in frustration and withdrawal from the activity.[6] An alternative strategy would be to adapt activities and toys in such a way that the 2 hands must be used to successfully complete the activity. One innovative method for increasing motivation and sustaining involvement in practicing bimanual tasks was demonstrated in a program that incorporated "magic" hand tricks during a 2-week summer camp (6 hours per day) for children with hemiplegia.[7] This program resulted in significant improvement in upper extremity function. The challenge for the physical therapist is to collaborate with the family, school staff, and others involved with Jason to determine appropriate activities and toys during various episodes of care that will promote bilateral upper extremity use and improved functional skills.

Several studies of children with hemiplegia suggest that constraint-induced movement therapy (CIMT) may be of benefit in improving function of the involved upper extremity (see Chapter 13), and this treatment strategy should be explored with Jason and his family. Neuroplasticity is present throughout the life span and functional magnetic resonance imaging (fMRI) can been used to measure cortical plasticity. Manning et al[8] used resting state fMRI to evaluate central nervous system changes in 11 children following CIMT and 4 untreated children with hemiplegia. Sensorimotor resting-state network reorganization in children after receiving CIMT correlated with positive changes on tests of motor function.

Bodimeade and colleagues[9] documented that children and adolescents with hemiplegia, when compared with typically developing (TD) control individuals, demonstrated difficulties in executive functions, including attention, cognitive flexibility, goal setting, and information processing. Although Jason's cognitive abilities are difficult to predict at age 2 years, he appears to have age-appropriate play skills and does not have negative comorbidities, such as a seizure disorder. Jason likely will be able to attend the neighborhood elementary and high schools with his peer group. He may not demonstrate intellectual difficulties as he matures, but if learning difficulties should become evident, he would qualify for special education services.

Jason's motor needs may be addressed sufficiently through school and community-based programs. Private physical therapy services, however, may be indicated on an episodic basis to monitor his motor-skill progress. He also should be monitored for the need of a lower extremity orthosis as he ages. There is evidence that lower extremity orthotics, particularly hinged ankle-foot orthotics, improve some gait parameters and decrease energy expenditure in children with hemiparetic CP.[10] However, the authors of one study of children with CP suggested complementary training may need to augment the immobilizing effects of braces on calf muscles.[11]

Antispasticity intervention often is considered for children with CP. One study of lower-limb muscles in 17 children with spastic diplegia evaluated the effect of 3 consecutive botulinum toxin-A (BoNT-A) injections.[12] Gait quality was assessed using 2-dimensional video gait assessment. Improvements in gait quality were statistically significant, but did not reach the smallest real difference value of 4 points. The authors suggested that repeated lower-extremity BoNT-A injections to improve quality of gait in children with CP should be reconsidered. Schasfoort et al[13] compared

2 groups of children (GMFCS Levels I to III) age 4 to 12 years (mean 7.3; SD 2.3) receiving 12 weeks of comprehensive rehabilitation. One group (N=41) received BoNT-A prior to intervention and the second group (N=24) did not receive BoNT-A. After the primary intervention and at 24 weeks' follow-up, there was no difference between groups in improving impairments, gait kinematics, or goal attainment. These authors also suggested that BoNT-A should be critically examined for children at GMFCS Levels I to III between ages 4 to 12 years.

Studies comparing the use of BoNT-A in the upper extremities of children with CP receiving therapy with children receiving therapy without BoNT-A have resulted in different conclusions. One study found receiving occupational and physical therapy without BoNT-A was preferred, as the BoNT-A injections caused weakness and did not lead to better outcomes than therapy alone.[14] A separate study found more children in the BoNT-A-plus-occupational therapy group improved when compared with children in the therapy-only group.[15]

In 2015, García Salazar and colleagues[16] completed a systematic review of intrinsic factors and functional changes in spastic muscle after application of BoNT-A in children with CP. Of 2182 papers reviewed, only 17 met the inclusion criteria. The conclusion was that application of BoNT-A failed to demonstrate changes in passive stiffness of spastic muscle and that evidence related to functional level is controversial. Pediatric therapists should continue to monitor the empirical evidence surrounding BoNT-A injections as well as the positive or negative responses to injections in children they may treat.

Jason and his family should be encouraged to explore community resources as his motor skill level increases and his interest in sports or fitness-related activities becomes evident.

As an adolescent and adult, Jason should be able to manage his care in relation to his hemiparesis. Periodic consultation with a physical therapist may be helpful to solve any difficulties he may encounter at home or work or to address home program or fitness needs.

Case Study #2: Jill

- > *Medical Diagnosis:* Cerebral palsy, spastic quadriparesis, microcephaly, intellectual deficits, seizure disorder
- > *Gross Motor Function Classification System:* Level V
- > *Age:* 7 years

Primary Participation Restrictions

- > Unable to sustain visual contact with peers, limiting social interactions
- > Unable to communicate effectively for social interaction and independence
- > Unable to move independently to interact with peers
- > Unable to maintain head control and stable visual field for classroom learning
- > Unable to eat same food as peers and interact during snack time, limiting social interaction and nutrition

Primary Activity/Functional Limitations

- > Nonambulatory
- > Unable to maintain balance in any position
- > Limited floor mobility
- > Poor voluntary grasp and release for fine motor skills
- > Problems eating and drinking

> Problems with visual tracking and focusing
> Limited communication skills
> Inability to perform self-care skills

Primary Impairments

> Lack of motor control
> Limited intellectual skills
> Limited ROM of trunk and extremities
> Generalized weakness
> Sensory hypersensitivity
> Seizure disorder
> Limited respiratory function
> Poor ocular control

Participation/Activity Goals

Self-Care and Domestic Life

Jill will be able to accomplish the following:

> When positioned in her adapted wheelchair, maintain lip and jaw closure during feeding and appropriately close lips and jaw on the rim of a drinking glass.
> Tolerate having a toothbrush brought into her mouth for oral hygiene, without increased cheek/lip retraction.
> Maintain elbow extension while she pushes her arm through a coat sleeve.

Mental Functions

Jill will be able to accomplish the following:

> Produce a vowel sound for 2 to 3 seconds to communicate that she wants an adult's attention.
> Reach above 60 degrees, 3 of 5 attempts in supported sitting, to touch a communication (ie, picture) board.

Range of Motion

Jill will be able to accomplish the following:

> Maintain ROM to be comfortable in her wheelchair and stander and while positioned prone on the floor.

Neuromotor Development and Sensory Processing

Jill will be able to accomplish the following:

> Tolerate being lifted from her wheelchair and carried during movement transitions without signs of distress.
> Right and maintain her head in vertical when being lifted or carried as part of her daily care at home and school.
> Roll from prone to supine, 1 of 5 attempts.
> Lift her head in prone-on-elbows position and maintain the position for 5 seconds to visually locate a toy placed in front of her.
> Grasp an object placed in her hand, 5 of 10 attempts in supported sitting.
> Release an object that is stabilized by an adult, 1 of 5 attempts in supported sitting.
> Use one upper extremity to bat at a joystick in preparation for a trial with a power wheelchair.

Balance

Jill will be able to accomplish the following:

> Maintain assisted standing balance for 3 to 5 seconds during standing pivot transfers.
> Stand and transfer, with the assist of one adult supporting her around the upper chest area, from her wheelchair to a classroom chair of equal height, requiring her to take 2 steps.

Muscle Performance

Jill will be able to accomplish the following:

> Participate in 20 minutes of aerobic exercise with her peers when assisted by an adult while positioned either in a partial-body weight-bearing device, a gait trainer, or a mobile stander.

Education Life

Jill will be able to accomplish the following:

> Hold head erect for 5 minutes when positioned in her vertical stander to watch a classroom activity or video.

Interventions

> Increase attention to visual and auditory stimuli.
> Increase strength in lower extremities.
> Improve motor control.
> Improve ability to tolerate sensory input.
> Maintain or improve ROM.
> Improve ability to bear weight in standing.
> Improve coordination of respiration with oral and pharyngeal activity during eating, drinking, and sound/speech production.
> Achieve a sustained whole-hand grasp and voluntary release.
> Improve ocular control with emphasis on downward gaze.

Additional Considerations/Prognosis

Jill's cognitive and communication skills are adversely affected by the presence of microcephaly and a seizure disorder. Epilepsy is estimated to occur in approximately one-third of children with CP and is more common in children with hemiplegia or quadriplegia than in children with diplegia.[17] Seizure disorders may be related to cortical involvement and the severity of brain damage in children with hemiplegia and quadriplegia compared with brain damage that is more periventricular (ie, children with diplegia). Reid et al[18] used population data of individuals with CP to assess frequency of intellectual disability and strength of associations with impairments. Intellectual disability was present in 45% of the cohort and was associated with nonambulation (47% vs 8%), quadriparesis (42% vs 5%), and epilepsy (52% vs 12%).

Jill's prognosis for independent motor function is poor. She has multiple severe impairments that interfere with her ability to develop gross motor and functional skills.

Jill likely will require moderate to maximal assist for ADLs as she matures. She is classified at Level V of the GMFCS,[3-5] representing children with CP with the most limited independent function and mobility. Although it will be difficult, and extensive modifications may be needed, a trial with power mobility is indicated to determine whether any level of independence in mobility can be achieved.

Emphasis in physical therapy management will be on minimizing the development of secondary impairments and maximizing Jill's ability to assist with her care, thereby minimizing the level of assistance required of her caregivers and increasing her independence. Additional resources should be directed at developing a functional communication system for Jill so she will be able to express her needs to her caregivers to the greatest extent possible.

An ongoing maintenance program (administered by caregivers as part of Jill's daily routine) to maintain ROM would be an important component of intervention for Jill. Although a systematic review of multiple databases for stretch interventions with children with neuromuscular disabilities age 0 to 19 years provided only low-grade evidence for positive outcomes,[19] specific protocols may be beneficial. Gibson et al[20] demonstrated positive effects of using standing frames in contracture management of nonmobile children with CP. Empirical evidence suggests that a protocol of standing 1 hour daily in a standing frame 5 days per week during her school program might be beneficial to maintain lower extremity ROM.

Weight-bearing protocols also are important for many children with CP. Alvarez Zaragoza and colleagues[21] demonstrated a relationship between low bone mineral density (BMD) and motor impairment (ie, quadriplegic CP, GMFCS Level V), methods of feeding, anthropometric indicators, and malnutrition. Higher probability of low BMD was found in tube-feeding patients and those who were malnourished (in relation to weight/age and body mass indices). Jill's feeding difficulties may contribute to poorer nutrition and be a contributing factor to low BMD, placing her at a risk for fractures. Fractures have been documented as occurring at any time during the life span of an individual with CP.[22] Fractures may occur because of a variety of reasons with the combination of osteoporosis, long lever arms, and contractures being cited as increasing the risk of nontraumatic fractures. Brunner and Döderlein[23] identified a total of 54 nontraumatic fractures in 37 individuals with CP over a 20-year period. The fractures were found to have occurred between ages 12 and 16 years, with the most common site being the supracondylar region of the distal femur. These researchers identified hip dislocations or contractures of major joints as being predisposing factors to the fractures. Furthermore, they found that 41% of the fractures occurred within 9 months of surgery and that the majority of fractures occurred during physical therapy intervention.

If Jill's limited ROM and stiffness in her trunk and extremities increase, antispasticity interventions may be considered. As discussed with Jason, intervention in this area would have to be considered carefully. The least invasive procedures (ie, serial casting or BoNT-A injections) should be considered before surgical types of intervention. Because Jill can assist with standing pivot transfers and has some head control, it would be important to preserve these functions. In that regard, insertion of a baclofen pump would be preferable to a selective dorsal rhizotomy (SDR). If there are negative functional sequelae (due to loss of stiffness and ability to bear weight or maintain head control), the dosage can be adjusted or the pump removed. SDR, however, would be a permanent, nonreversible procedure.

Morton et al[24] studied intrathecal baclofen infusion in nonambulant children with CP (GMFCS Levels IV and V). Intrathecal baclofen over the first 18 months improved quality of life in terms of comfort and ease of care; however, there was less effect on function, participation in society, or overall cost of new equipment. A retrospective review of 44 children undergoing SDR at British Columbia Children's Hospital demonstrated that SDR yielded reduction in spasticity after 10 years.[25] Early improvements in motor function were present but attenuated in children in GMFCS Levels II and III and were not sustained in children in GMFCS Levels IV and V.

As she ages, Jill's scoliosis may increase, and she is at risk for hip subluxation or dislocation. Huser and colleagues[26] stated that hip displacement occurs in more than one-third of children with CP, with a higher prevalence in nonambulatory children.

Hip subluxation and/or dislocation can result in pain and difficulty with sitting and perineal care. Zhang et al[27] reviewed radiological outcome of reconstructive hip surgery (ie, varus derotational proximal femoral osteotomy with or without additional pelvic osteotomy) in children with CP GMFCS Levels IV and V. Overall, hip reconstruction tended to fail earlier in children at GMFCS Level V than in children at GMFCS Level IV. In a prospective study of 37 children (GMFCS Levels III to V) with hip subluxation, the positive effect of soft-tissue releases (ie, bilateral tenotomies of adductors and iliopsoas) was reviewed.[28] The only independent preoperative risk factor for poor outcome was migration percentage greater than 50% prior to the surgery. Unfortunately, high-quality evidence on prevention of hip displacement for children with CP is lacking.[29] Because Jill is at a high risk for hip displacement because of her lack of mobility, there should be a specific protocol for monitoring her hip status.

Episodic physical therapy care may be indicated to periodically review Jill's status and her equipment, update her home program, and train her caregivers. As Jill ages, her family should be in contact with community-based services that can provide information on possible vocational training, group home living arrangements, and financial assistance to meet Jill's long-term needs.

CASE STUDY #3: TAYLOR

> *Medical Diagnosis:* Myelomeningocele, repaired L1-2
> *Age:* 4 years

Primary Participation Restrictions

> Unable to keep up with peers when walking with assistive device or propelling wheelchair
> Unable to make transitions to and from wheelchair to play with classmates
> Unable to access areas of playground to join peers
> Unable to communicate effectively for social interactions
> Unable to perform at same skill level with fine motor tasks, such as tracing, as peers

Primary Activity/Functional Limitations

> Requires external support to stand and ambulate
> Has difficulty maintaining balance in sitting and on hands and knees when reaching outside his base of support
> Requires assistance for lower body dressing
> Demonstrates limited independent transitions during floor mobility
> Requires assistance for wheelchair and toilet transfers
> Communication often limited to 3- to 4-word sentences

Primary Impairments

> Loss of cutaneous and proprioceptive sensation below L1-2
> Loss of motor function below L1-2
> Problems with visual processing, especially figure-ground discrimination
> Inadequate balance reactions
> Generalized muscle weakness
> Limited endurance for motor activities
> Limited ROM in hip musculature
> Poor respiratory function

Participation/Activity Goals

Self-Care and Domestic Life

Taylor will be able to accomplish the following:

› Put on and remove sweat pants with minimal assistance while sitting on the floor leaning against furniture or a wall.
› Correctly put on shoes and socks, eliminating potential pressure areas every time.
› Perform 5 to 10 sitting push-ups each hour to decrease potential pressure areas on sacrum or heads of femur.

Mental Functions

Taylor will be able to accomplish the following:

› Be able to walk with his walker, wheel his wheelchair, and make movement transitions while producing coordinated sounds such as in singing, yelling, or counting for up to 30 seconds.

Neuromotor Development and Sensory Processing

Taylor will be able to accomplish the following:

› Use his walker and follow a visual pattern (trail) on the floor without becoming unsteady or losing his balance.
› From standing, actively fall forward on a 3-inch (7.6-cm) thick mat and catch himself with his arms without hitting his head on the mat.

Balance

Taylor will be able to accomplish the following:

› Maintain standing balance in his new orthotics for 15 seconds with his eyes closed (with crutches).
› Maintain standing balance in his new orthotics for 1 minute while moving his head up, down, right, and left (with crutches).

Muscle Performance

Taylor will be able to accomplish the following:

› Independently lift his body weight with his arms during transfers.
› Actively participate in movement games and activities for 30 minutes daily without needing a rest.
› Propel his wheelchair from the classroom to the cafeteria at the same speed as his peers.
› Self-propel his wheelchair for 10 to 15 minutes during community outings with 3 brief rest breaks.

Education Life

Taylor will be able to accomplish the following:

› Transfer in and out of his wheelchair to a classroom chair with standby assist.

Ventilation and Respiration

Taylor will be able to accomplish the following:

› Drink 3 to 4 sips of liquid from a cup before stopping to breathe.
› Produce sentences of 3 to 4 words on 1 exhalation without running out of breath support.

Interventions

> Improve visual perceptual skills, especially figure-ground discrimination.

> Improve balance reactions in all positions.

> Increase strength of upper extremity and trunk muscles.

> Decrease frequency of skin breakdown.

> Increase independence in transfers.

> Decrease sensitivity to head bending in standing.

> Increase endurance for ambulation and propelling wheelchair.

> Improve protective reactions in standing.

> Increase speed of ambulation.

> Improve coordination of respiration with oral and pharyngeal activities during speech and feeding activities.

> Increase ROM in lower extremities for proper alignment in orthotics.

> Improve independence in self-care skills.

Additional Considerations/Prognosis

Taylor has an L1-2 or high-lumbar myelomeningocele, which is associated with a guarded prognosis for independent ambulation (with orthoses and assistive devices). Williams et al[30] examined age-related walking in children with spina bifida (SB). In the sample of children they followed, there were 10 children with high lumbar-level lesions. Five of these children walked at an average age of 5 years, 2 months, but 3 ceased walking at an average age of 6 years, 11 months. Therefore, by age 7 years, only 2 of the 10 children were ambulating. Roach and colleagues[31] completed a retrospective review of 84 adults with SB. The average age was 31 years (range, 20 to 64 years). Thirty-one percent of the individuals had thoracic lesions and all were wheelchair dependent. Of the 12% at L1-L3, all but 1 used a wheelchair. Thirty-three percent had lesions at L4-L5, and of these 78% used a wheelchair at least part time. The remaining 24% of individuals with lesions at S1 or lower all walked. Yasmeh et al[32] suggested that decreased walking activity in children with mid- to high-lumbar myelomeningocele puts them at risk for obesity, muscle weakening, and disuse osteoporosis. Many long-term follow-up studies with children with myelomeningocele were initiated before the advent of fetal surgery. Long-term outcomes may be improving because of more recent advances in surgical interventions for children with SB. In one study, 54 patients undergoing fetal surgery before 26 weeks' gestation were followed for a median of 10 years.[33] Of the 42 children participating in follow-up, 33 (79%) were community ambulators, 3 (7%) were household ambulators, and 6 (14%) were wheelchair dependent. Preschool ambulation was predictive of long-term ambulation.

The increased energy expenditure required to ambulate often is excessive when combined with energy requirements to perform other ADL and academic tasks.[34] Additional variables that can adversely affect achieving an expected level of ambulation in children with SB have been documented to include balance disturbances, occurrence of spasticity in knee and hip movement, an increased number of shunt revisions, and lack of motivation.[35] Physical therapists should provide education to children with SB and their families regarding warning signs of tethering of the spinal cord,[36] which is a complication that occurs as a result of pathological fixation of the spinal cord, resulting in traction on neural tissue. Ischemia and progressive neurologic deterioration will occur unless there is a surgical intervention. Symptoms can include increased scoliosis, gait changes, increased spasticity in the lower extremities, back and leg pain, decreased muscle strength, lower extremity contractures, urinary bladder changes, and changes in motor or sensory level in extremities.

Another health risk for children with SB is latex allergy. Latex allergy is a reaction to certain proteins found in natural rubber latex, which, in some individuals, may cause skin irritation, hives, or a potential anaphylactic reaction that may be life threatening. Because symptoms increase with increased frequency of exposure, patients with SB are at high-risk because of repeated exposures during procedures at home (eg, catheterization) and in the hospital (eg, multiple surgeries).[37] Latex allergy, in addition to dental caries, difficulty in mouth opening, and difficulty sitting in a dental chair, has been reported as a common problem in dentistry.[38] Therefore, avoidance of latex should be enforced whenever possible. In one study, children with SB who had surgery under latex-free conditions demonstrated significantly decreased latex sensitization and allergy when compared with a previous non–latex-free operated-on group of children.[37]

Individuals with SB are at risk for learning disabilities due to malformations of the central nervous system (neural tube defect). Preschool-aged children with SB demonstrate difficulty with early numeracy skills[39], and school-aged children demonstrate difficulty with math that persists into adulthood. Children with SB also have difficulty with verbal working memory, visual-spatial memory, and fine motor skills. Roach et al,[31] in their retrospective review of 84 adults with SB, found 42% had normal intelligence quotients (IQs), 44% attended regular education classes, and 8% had college degrees.

Taylor's perceptual-motor difficulties and academic performance will need to be monitored throughout his school years and intervention strategies and goals individualized to enhance his motor, intellectual, and social skills. Taylor likely will need some level of special education services throughout his academic career.

As Taylor matures, he may wish to explore a combination of mobility devices, including a sports wheelchair and power mobility. It would be beneficial to obtain a wheelchair that moves him from sitting to supported standing to increase the time he spends weight bearing and to maintain lower-extremity ROM. As an adult, he may develop the ability to live independently, but will need many architectural adaptations to accommodate his functional limitations and his primary use of a wheelchair for mobility. He also may need some level of support services in an independent-living situation. Bellin et al[40] in a study of 50 adults (age 18 to 25 years) with myelo-meningocele found that men were more likely to report employment. However, women had greater success in transitioning into independent-living situations. Overall, low rates of employment and independent living, however, suggest limited success in development of self-management skills. Lindsay and colleagues[41] reviewed the challenges of youth with SB in transitioning to postsecondary education and employment. These authors suggested that health care providers should help children with SB prepare for school-to-work transitions by fostering independence, mastery of life skills, and ability to self-manage their SB-related symptoms. As Taylor becomes a young adult, resources and information on finances, housing, transportation, and employment support will be crucial to maximize his quality of life.

Taylor's physical therapist (private and or school based) should work with him to improve his transfer skills, mobility, self-care skills, and fitness level as he matures. Physical therapy would not be provided continuously, but would be "episodic" as new needs or issues arise.

CASE STUDY #4: ASHLEY

> *Medical Diagnosis:* Down syndrome
> *Age:* 15 months

Primary Participation Restrictions

> Avoids movement-based activities, limiting sensory input and experiences
> Avoids interacting with peers, limiting social interactions

- Unable to keep up with peers during play at the weekly early intervention (EI) sessions or at the community "mothers' day out" program
- Unable to manipulate toys effectively for play and cognitive learning
- Unable to eat some foods and does not participate in snack time with peers

Primary Activity/Functional Limitations

- Avoids movement
- Does not attempt to cruise at furniture
- Falls over easily in all positions
- Does not assist in self-cares
- Loses liquid and food from her mouth during feeding
- Cannot pick up small objects

Primary Impairments

- Hypermobile joints
- Low muscle tone
- Mild conductive hearing loss
- Intellectual deficits
- Poor balance reactions and postural control
- Generalized weakness
- Poor endurance
- Poor oral sensory awareness
- Poor motor control

Participation/Activity Goals

Self-Care and Domestic Life

Ashley will be able to accomplish the following:

- Use her lower lip to stabilize under a cup rim when a cup is presented for drinking with minimal loss of fluid.
- Lose only a minimal amount of food out of her mouth during snack time.
- Pick up Cheerios independently during snack time.
- While sitting on the floor, take off her shoes (laces undone) independently.

Mental Functions

Ashley will be able to accomplish the following:

- Smile or produce sounds during movement activities such as swinging in a swing, rocking in a chair, or propelling a small riding toy.

Neuromotor Development and Sensory Processing

Ashley will be able to accomplish the following:

- Move from standing to sitting to an all fours position, with minimal assist with no indications of apprehension.

> Move around the EI playroom (any method) to obtain a toy without prompting or assist from an adult.
> Release objects into containers independently during play.

Balance

Ashley will be able to accomplish the following:
> Begin to cruise at a support surface, 3 to 4 steps in either direction, to obtain a toy.
> Be able to reach laterally for a toy while sitting without loss of balance.
> Catch herself 50% of the time without loss of balance in all fours.

Gait

Ashley will be able to accomplish the following:
> Take steps to "walk" 5 feet (1.5 m) between her parents in play.
> Push a push toy in standing for 10 to 15 feet (3 to 4.5 m) with standby assistance for safety.

Interventions

> Increase stability in all positions.
> Increase strength and endurance for motor activities.
> Decrease apprehension regarding movement activities.
> Improve balance reactions and postural control in all positions.
> Improve oral-motor skills for feeding and sound/speech production tasks.
> Develop voluntary controlled release and pinch.
> Demonstrate goal-directed play.
> Assist with self-cares.

Additional Considerations/Prognosis

Children with Down syndrome (DS) have a good prognosis for developing motor skills, and the average age for achieving independent ambulation is around 2 years.[42] Treadmill training has been found to be beneficial for children with DS (see Chapter 12). Looper and Ulrich[43] studied the effect of treadmill training and use of supramalleolar orthoses (SMOs) on motor skills development in infants with DS. Seventeen infants with DS were randomly assigned to either (1) an experimental group of children who wore SMOs 8 hours per day, 5 days per week and received treadmill training or (2) a control group of children who received treadmill training but no SMOs until training ceased. Treadmill training started when the child could pull to stand and ended when the child could take 3 independent steps. At 1 month postintervention, the control group had higher Gross Motor Function Measure scores with standing, walking, running, and jumping subscale scores. The conclusion was that orthoses may have a detrimental effect on overall gross motor skills development, and SMOs should not be prescribed for children with DS until they are walking.

Physical therapists should be aware of the possibility of atlantoaxial instability in individuals with DS. Various reports suggest atlantoaxial instability is present in 6.8% to 27% of the population with DS.[44] Although neurologic examination to detect early symptoms of spinal cord compression has been suggested as an alternative to X-ray examinations, radiographs are recommended at age 2 years and periodically administered in childhood and adolescence. Children with asymptomatic instability typically do not require surgery, but should not engage in contact sports, gymnastics, diving, or other activities that might result in injury to the cervical spine. An X-ray examination is obligatory for special education athletes to determine the sport(s) in which the athlete safely may participate. After the EI and preschool period, Ashley may not require motor-based services other than consultative physical therapy through her school district and adaptive physical education. Ashley's physical therapist should encourage the family to participate in school- and community-based motor programs that will address fitness and lifelong leisure skills for Ashley.

Cognitive deficits are a component of DS. Although longitudinal studies are limited, memory impairments are reported to be one of the cognitive impairments that are present throughout the life span.[45] Children with DS show gradually declining IQ scores during childhood, as cognitive gains do not keep up with their chronological age. In early childhood mild cognitive delays are noted.[46] By school age, cognitive delays become more pronounced. Nonverbal skills remain closer to mental age, but verbal deficits emerge and persist. Expressive language is delayed when compared with comprehension.

The presence of praxis issues in children with DS has been studied for many years.[47-50] In 2005, Fidler et al[50] studied 18 toddlers with DS (mean age 33.8 months), 16 DD toddlers matched for cognitive age, and 19 TD toddlers (mean age 18 months) to assess praxis abilities. These researchers found that the toddlers with DS were significantly worse overall in praxis compared with the matched DD group, as well as with the TD group. A strong relationship was noted between praxis and adaptive functioning in the children with DS. Additionally, motivation was an issue noted in the DS group. The researchers suggested that the young child with DS may need targeted interventions that focus both on praxis skills and motivational orientation. During the childhood years, the most marked deficits in children with DS are in attention and executive functions.

Because of the cognitive deficits associated with DS, Ashley will be eligible for special education services throughout her school years. Individualized Education Program goals during her academic career and eventual vocational goals and training will need to be matched to Ashley's individual profile of motor abilities.

It is anticipated that, as an adult, Ashley will be able to function in a group-home situation unless she remains at home with her parents. She also should be able to attend vocational training and work in a supervised setting within the community or through a work program for adults with DD. Unfortunately, recent studies have documented that many individuals with DS begin to develop dementia as they reach middle age (see Chapter 18). Virtually all individuals with DS develop neuropathology similar to Alzheimer disease after age 40 years.[51] Physical therapists and occupational therapists should be aware of early signs of dementia in individuals with DS and be prepared to intervene as necessary to retain as much adaptive functioning as possible.

CASE STUDY #5: JOHN

> *Medical Diagnosis:* Developmental coordination disorder/attention-deficit hyperactivity disorder
> *Age:* 5 years

Primary Participation Restrictions

> Unable to keep up with peers on the playground
> Self-limits interactions with peers during motor activities
> Unable to communicate effectively with adults or peers
> Unable to maintain attention and social interactions with classmates in learning/academic activities

Primary Activity/Functional Limitations

> Avoids physical activity
> Has difficulty performing age-appropriate fine and gross motor skills
> Demonstrates general "clumsiness" during daily activities, falling or bumping into objects
> Intelligibility in speech is variable
> Limits variety of drinks and food he will accept
> Has decreased attention span for motor tasks
> Poor handwriting and printing skills are evident in an academic environment

Primary Impairments

> Attention deficit
> Expressive language delay
> Poor motor control and motor planning
> Weakness in upper extremities
> Limited endurance
> Difficulties with sensory processing, especially tactile discrimination and kinesthesia

Participation/Activity Goals

Self-Care and Domestic Life

John will be able to accomplish the following:

> Use utensils during mealtime to stab food (fork) and butter bread (knife).
> Independently button and unbutton large buttons on a shirt.
> Independently zip and unzip the zipper on his jacket after being assisted to engage the zipper.

Mental Functions

John will be able to accomplish the following:

> Produce the consonants "t" and "d" when they appear at the end of a word in sentences of 3 to 4 words in length.
> Speak intelligibly enough to be understood by peers in a play situation.

Neuromotor Development and Sensory Processing

John will be able to accomplish the following:

> Use both hands to throw and catch a 10-inch (25-cm) diameter ball.
> Play safely and appropriately on equipment in a local fast food restaurant playground with other children present.

Balance

John will be able to accomplish the following:

> Walk independently, changing speeds and directions as needed on even and uneven terrain without falling.

Gait

John will be able to accomplish the following:

> Walk in a crowded environment, such as the mall, without bumping into objects or people.

Muscle Performance

John will be able to accomplish the following:

> Participate in physical activity with peers for 15 to 20 minutes without undue fatigue.
> Ride his bike (with training wheels) for 5 miles (8 km) during family bike trips.

Interventions

> Improve motor planning skills.
> Increase upper body strength.
> Increase endurance for gross motor activities.
> Improve balance reactions and postural control.
> Increase frequency of practice of self-selected motor activities.
> Improve speech/sound production skills.
> Complete self-cares independently.
> Participate with peers in age-appropriate gross motor activities.

Additional Considerations/Prognosis

John's medical diagnosis includes developmental coordination disorder (DCD) and attention-deficit hyperactivity disorder (ADHD). Barnhart et al[52] reviewed the general parameters of DCD, which is considered a chronic, usually permanent condition in children that is characterized by motor impairment significant enough to interfere with ADLs. To be diagnosed with DCD, children must not have abnormal muscle tone or movements or sensory loss. In addition, children should have an IQ greater than 70 and not meet criteria for a diagnosis of pervasive developmental disorder. Apraxia and dyspraxia often have been equated with DCD. Ayres[53] was one of the first therapists to address children with motor-planning problems, and she defined "developmental dyspraxia" as a motor-planning disorder, which was a "disorder of sensory integration interfering with the ability to plan and execute skilled or nonhabitual tasks."[53(p8)] Ayres discussed the lack of homogeneity of observations among children with dyspraxia. She also recommended criteria for using the diagnosis of development dyspraxia, which included a meaningful constellation of low scores on tests of praxis, normal IQ, and normal conventional neurological examination. Miyahara and Möbs[54] suggested that apraxia and dyspraxia primarily refer to problems in motor sequencing and selection, which not all children with DCD exhibit. They proposed various criteria to distinguish among these conditions.

ADHD is a chronic condition associated with inattention, hyperactivity, and impulsivity. In one longitudinal study of 476 children diagnosed with ADHD who were retrospectively evaluated in adulthood, 60% demonstrated symptom persistence and 41% met both symptom and impairment criteria.[55]

McLeod et al[56] performed resting-state fMRI on 7 children with DCD, 21 with ADHD, 18 with DCD and ADHD, and 23 TD controls. Resting-state connectivity of the primary motor cortex was compared among groups. Children with DCD and/or ADHD exhibited similar reductions in functional connectivity between the primary motor cortex and several brain areas, as well as different age-related patterns of connectivity as compared with the TD control children. These findings suggest disruptions in motor circuitry in children with DCD and/or ADHD, which may contribute to problems with motor functioning and attention. Gabbard and Bobbio[57] proposed an "internal modeling deficit" hypothesis in children with DCD that is characterized by significant limitations in the ability to accurately generate and use internal models of motor planning and control.

One intervention study with children with DCD demonstrated that similar gains can be made with group-based training and individual-based intervention.[58] One of the major goals for children with DCD is to improve their "sequencing" skills, and there are many opportunities for sequencing in groups (eg, "Tommy goes first, you go second"; "We need to get the mat and ramp before the scooter board"). Physical fitness has been shown to be poorer in children with low motor competence,[59] and one study demonstrated that a 13-week intervention to improve aerobic fitness, strength, and self-perception had a positive impact on adolescent physical self-perception in children with low motor competence, particularly in male participants.[60] Wii Fit interventions also have been shown to produce positive outcomes in children with DCD or balance problems.[61,62] Smits-Engelsman et al[63] in a meta-analysis of motor interventions for children with DCD stated that intervention was shown to produce benefits for motor performance as compared with no intervention. A comparison of types of intervention showed strong effects for task-oriented interventions by occupational and physical therapists.

John's prognosis for independent motor function is good. He may not develop motor skills adequate for athletic competition, but should have motor skills sufficient to enable him to participate in social recreational activities with peers (eg, bowling, swimming). Children with John's motor problems generally improve with maturation and practice of specific skills.

John developing competence in an area of interest to improve his self-image is important. Noncompetitive sports, such as karate, may be selected initially and would improve John's motor control while providing an outlet for his high energy level. Physical therapy services would be primarily consultative for John and his family. Emphasis would be on providing suggestions for home-based activities and community programs that would meet his individual needs as his motor abilities improve and interest in motor-related activities increases.

Summary

Although the child with DD may need physical therapy on an episodic basis throughout the life span, the goal is *not* lifelong physical therapy. Rather, the goal of the physical therapist is to enable independence and self-management in the child and family. The physical therapist should strive to consider the "whole" child and emphasize appropriate goals related to the child's participation in societal roles.

When performing examination and evaluation of children, identifying participation restrictions and activity limitations and hypothesizing about related underlying impairments are the essential elements in establishing a framework for determining goals and intervention strategies. A variety of treatment techniques often can be used to meet the same therapeutic objective or several objectives simultaneously. Although repetition is important in treatment, using a variety of activities contributes to making intervention enjoyable and motivating for children and therapists. Creativity, therefore, is the art of pediatric therapy.

References

1. World Health Organization. *International Classification of Functioning, Disability and Health (ICF)*. Geneva, Switzerland: World Health Organization; 2001.
2. Wu YW, Day SM, Strauss DJ, Shavelle RM. Prognosis for ambulation in cerebral palsy: a population-based study. *Pediatrics*. 2005;224(5):1264-1271. doi:10.1542/peds.2004-0114.
3. Palisano RJ, Rosenbaum PL, Walter SD, Russell D, Wood E, Galuppi B. Development and reliability of a system to classify gross motor function in children with cerebral palsy. *Dev Med Child Neurol*. 1997;39(4):214-223. doi:10.1111/dmcn.1997.39.issue-4.
4. Palisano RJ, Hanna SE, Rosenbaum PL, et al. Validation of a model of gross motor function for children with cerebral palsy. *Phys Ther*. 2000;80(10):974-985. doi:10.1093/ptj/80.10.974.

5. Rosenbaum PL, Walter SD, Hanna SE, et al. Prognosis for gross motor function in cerebral palsy: creation of motor development curves. *JAMA*. 2002;288(11):1357-1363. doi:10.1097/01.OGX.0000055751.17527.56.

6. Peterson P, Peterson CE. Bilateral hand skills in children with mild hemiplegia. *Phys Occup Ther Pediatr*. 1984;41(1):77-87. doi:10.1080/J006v04n01_08.

7. Green D, Schertz M, Gordon AM, et al. A multi-site study of functional outcomes following a themed approach to hand-arm bimanual intensive therapy for children with hemiplegia. *Dev Med Child Neurol*. 2013;55(6):527-533. doi:10.1111/dmcn.12113.

8. Manning KY, Menon RS, Gorter JW, et al. Neuroplastic sensorimotor resting state network reorganization in children with hemiplegic cerebral palsy treated with constraint-induced movement therapy. *J Child Neurol*. 2016;31(2):220-226. doi:10.1177/0883073815588995.

9. Bodimeade HL, Whitingham K, Lloyd O, Boyd RN. Executive function in children and adolescents with unilateral cerebral palsy. *Dev Med Child Neurol*. 2013;55(10):926-933. doi:10.1111/dmcn.12195.

10. Aboutorabi A, Arazpour M, Ahmadi Bani M, Saeedi H, Head JS. Efficacy of ankle foot orthoses types on walking in children with cerebral palsy: a systematic review. *Ann Phys Rehabil Med*. 2017;60(6):393-402. doi:10.1016/j.rehab.2017.05.004.

11. Hösl M, Böhm H, Arampatzis A, Döderlein L. Effects of ankle-foot braces on medial gastrocnemius morphometrics and gait in children with cerebral palsy. *J Child Orthop*. 2015;9(3):209-219. doi:10.1007/s11832-015-0664-x.

12. Read FA, Boyd RN, Barber LA. Longitudinal assessment of gait quality in children with unilateral cerebral palsy following repeated lower limb intramuscular Botulinum toxin-A injections. *Res Dev Disabil*. 2017;68(9):35-41. doi:10.1016/j.ridd.2017.07.002.

13. Schasfoort F, Pangalila R, Sneekes E, et al. Intramuscular botulinum toxin prior to comprehensive rehabilitation has no added value for improving impairments, gait kinematics and goal attainment in walking children with spastic cerebral palsy. *J Rehabil Med*. 2018;50(8):732-742. doi:10.2340/16501977-2369.

14. Rameckers EA, Speth LA, Duysens J, Vles JS, Smits-Engelsman BC. Botulinum toxin-A in children with congenital spastic hemiplegia does not improve upper extremity motor-related function over rehabilitation alone: a randomized controlled trial. *Neurorehabil Neural Repair*. 2009;23 (3):218-225. doi:10.1177/1545968308326629.

15. Lidman G, Nachemson A, Peny-Dahlstrand M, Himmelmann K. Botulinum toxin A injections and occupational therapy in children with unilateral spastic cerebral palsy: a randomized controlled trial. *Dev Med Child Neurol*. 2015;57(8):754-761. doi:10.1111/dmcn.12739.

16. García Salazar LF, dos Santos GL, Pavão SL, Rocha NA, de Russo TL. Intrinsic properties and functional changes in spastic muscle after application of BTX-A in children with cerebral palsy: systematic review. *Dev Neurorehabil*. 2015;18(1):1-14. doi:10.3109/17518423.2014.948640.

17. Singhi P, Jagirdar S. Khandelwal N, Malhi P. Epilepsy in children with cerebral palsy. *J Child Neurol*. 2003;18(3):174-179. doi:10.1177/08830738030180030601.

18. Reid SM, Meehan EM, Arnup ST, Reddihough DS. Intellectual disability in cerebral palsy: a population-based retrospective study. *Dev Med Child Neurol*. 2018;60(7):607-694. doi:10.1111/dmcn.13773.

19. Craig J, Hilderman C, Wilson G, Misovic R. Effectiveness of stretch interventions for children with neuromuscular disabilities: evidence-based recommendations. *Pediatr Phys Ther*. 2016;28(3):262-275. doi:10.1097/PEP.0000000000000269.

20. Gibson SK, Sprod JA, Maher CA. The use of standing frames for contracture management of non-mobile children with cerebral palsy. *Int J Rehabil Res*. 2009;32(4):316-323. doi:10.1097/MRR.0b013e32831e4501.

21. Alvarez Zaragoza C, Vasquez Garibay EM, García Contreras AA, et al. Bone mineral density and nutritional status in children with quadriplegic cerebral palsy. *Arch Osteoporos*. 2018;13(1):17. doi:10.1007/s11657-018-0434-8.

22. Rapp CE Jr, Torres MM. The adult with cerebral palsy. *Arch Fam Med*. 2000;9(5):466-472. doi:10.1001/archfami.9.5.466.

23. Brunner R, Döderlein L. Pathological fractures in patients with cerebral palsy. *J Pediatri Orthop B*. 1996;5(4):232-238. doi:10.1097/01202412-199605040-00003.

24. Morton RE, Gray N, Vloeberghs M. Controlled study of the effects of continuous intrathecal baclofen infusion in non-ambulant children with cerebral palsy. *Dev Med Child Neurol*. 2011;53(8):736-741. doi:10.1111/j.1469-8749.2011.04009.x.

25. Ailon T, Beauchamp R, Miller S, et al. Long-term outcome after selective dorsal rhizotomy in children with spastic cerebral palsy. *Child Nerv Syst*. 2015;31(3):415-423. doi:10.1007/s00381-015-2614-9.

26. Huser A, Mo M, Hosseinzadeh P. Hip surveillance in children with cerebral palsy. *Orthop Clin North Am*. 2018;49(2):181-190. doi:10.1016/j.ocl.2017.11.006.

27. Zhang S, Wilson NC, Mackey AH, Stott NS. Radiological outcome of reconstructive hip surgery in children with gross motor function classification system IV and V cerebral palsy. *J Pediatr Orthop B*. 2014;23(5):430-434. doi:10.1097/BPB.0000000000000075.

28. Terjesen T. To what extent can soft-tissue releases improve hip displacement in cerebral palsy? *Acta Orthop*. 2017;88(6):695-700. doi:10.1080/17453674.2017.1365471.

29. Miller SD, Juricic M, Hesketh K, et al. Prevention of hip displacement in children with cerebral palsy: a systematic review. *Dev Med Child Neurol*. 2017;59(11):1130-1138. doi:10.1111/dmcn.13480.

30. Williams EN, Broughton NS, Menelaus MB. Age-related walking in children with spina bifida. *Dev Med Child Neurol.* 1999;41(7):446-449. doi:10.1017/S0012162299000985.

31. Roach JW, Short BF, Saltzman HM. Adult consequences of spina bifida: a cohort study. *Clin Orthop Relat Res.* 2011;469(5):1246-1252. doi:10.1007/s11999-010-1594-z.

32. Yasmeh P, Mueske NM, Yasmeh S, Ryan DD, Wren TAL. Walking activity during daily living in children with myelomeningocele. *Disabil Rehabil.* 2017;39(14):1422-1427. doi:10.1080/09638288.2016.1198429.

33. Danzer E, Thomas NH, Thomas A, et al. Long-term neurofunctional outcome, executive (EF) functioning, and behavioral adaptive skills (BAS) following fetal myelomeningocele surgery. *Am J Obstet Gynecol.* 2016;214(2):269.e1-269.e8. doi:10.1016/j.ajog.2015.09.094. Epub 2015 Oct 9.

34. Franks CA, Palisano RJ, Darbee JC. The effect of walking with an assistive device and using a wheelchair on school performance in students with myelomeningocele. *Phys Ther.* 1991;71:(8):570-577; discussion 577-579. doi:10.1097/01241398-199205000-00057.

35. Bartonek A, Saraste H. Factors influencing ambulation in myelomeningocele: a cross-sectional study. *Dev Med Child Neurol.* 2001;43(6):253-260. doi:10.1111/j.1469-8749.2001.tb00199.x.

36. Iqbal N, Qadeer M, Sharif SY. Variation in outcome in tethered cord syndrome. *Asian Spine J.* 2016;10(4):711-718. doi:10.4184/asj.2016.10.4.711.

37. Blumchen K, Bayer P, Buck D, et al. Effects of latex avoidance on latex sensitization, atopy and allergic diseases in patients with spina bifida. *Allergy.* 2010;65(12):1585-1593. doi:10.1111/j.1398-9995.2010.02447.x.

38. Garg A, Utreja A, Singh SP, Angurana SK. Neural tube defects and their significance in clinical dentistry: a mini review. *J Investig Clin Dent.* 2013;4(1):3-8. doi:10.1111/j.2041-1626.2012.00141.x.

39. Raghubar KP, Barnes MA, Dennis M, Cirino PT, Taylor H, Landry S. Neurocognitive predictors of mathematical processing in school-aged children with spina bifida and their typically developing peers: attention, working memory, and fine motor skills. *Neuropsychology.* 2015;29(6):861-873. doi:10.1037/neu0000196.

40. Bellin MH, Dicianno BE, Levey E, et al. Interrelationships of sex, level of lesion, and transition outcomes among young adults with myelomeningocele. *Dev Med Child Neurol.* 2011;53(7):647-652. doi:10.1111/j.1469-8749.2011.03938.x.

41. Lindsay S, McPherson AC, Maxwell J. Perspectives of school-work transitions among youth with spina bifida and health care providers. *Disabil Rehabil.* 2017;39(7):641-652. doi:10.3109/09638288.2016.1153161.

42. Shea AM. Chapter 23. Motor attainments in Down syndrome. In: Lister E, ed. *Proceedings of the II STEP Conference; Contemporary Management of Motor Control Problems.* Alexandria, VA: Foundation for Physical Therapy; 1991:225-236.

43. Looper J, Ulrich DA. Effect of treadmill training and supramalleolar orthosis use on motor skills development in infants with Down syndrome: a randomized clinical trial. *Phys Ther.* 2010;90(3):382-390. doi:10.2522/ptj.20090021.

44. Mysliwiec A, Posłuszny A, Saulicz E, et al. Atlanto-axial instability in people with Down's syndrome and its impact on the ability to perform sports activities—a review. *J Hum Kinet.* 2015;48(11):17-24. doi:10.1515/hukin-2015-0087.

45. Godfrey M, Lee NR. Memory profiles in Down syndrome across development: a review of memory abilities through the lifespan. *J Neurodev Disord.* 2018;10(1):5. doi:10.1186/s11689-017-9220-y.

46. Greco J, Pulsifer M, Seligsohn K, Skotko B, Schwartz A. Down syndrome: cognitive and behavioral functioning across the lifespan. *Am J Med Genet C Semin Med Genet.* 2015;169(2):135-149. doi:10.1002/ajmg.c.31439.

47. Bruni M, Cameron D, Dua S, Noy S. Reported sensory processing of children with Down syndrome. *Phys Occup Ther Pediatr.* 2010;30(4):280-293. doi:10.3109/01942638.2010.486962.

48. Connolly BH, Michael BT. Performance of retarded children with and without Down syndrome on the Bruininks Oseretsky Test of Motor Proficiency. *Phys Ther.* 1986;66(3):344-348. doi:10.1093/ptj/66.3.344.

49. Latash ML. Learning motor synergies by persons with Down syndrome. *J Intellect Disabil Res.* 2007;51(12):962-971. doi: 101111/j.1365-2788.2007.01008.x.

50. Fidler DJ, Hepburn SL, Mankin G, Rogers SJ. Praxis skills in young children with Down syndrome, other developmental disabilities, and typically developing children. *Am J Occup Ther.* 2005;59(2):129-138. doi:10.5014/ajot.59.2.129.

51. Rafii MS. Improving memory and cognition in individuals with Down syndrome. *CNS Drugs.* 2016;30(7):567-573. doi:10.1007/s40263-016-0353-4.

52. Barnhart RC, Davenport MJ, Epps SB, Nordquist VM. Developmental coordination disorder. *Phys Ther.* 2003;83(8):722-731. doi:10.1093/ptj/83.8.722.

53. Ayres AJ. *Developmental Dyspraxia and Adult-Onset Apraxia.* Torrance, CA: Sensory Integration International; 1985:58.

54. Miyahara M, Möbs I. Developmental dyspraxia and developmental coordination disorder. *Neuropsychol Rev.* 1995;5(4):245-268. doi:10.1007/BF02214648.

55. Sibley MH, Swanson JM, Arnold LE, et al. Defining ADHD symptom persistence in adulthood: optimizing sensitivity and specificity. *J Child Psychol Psychiatry.* 2017;58(6):655-662. doi:10.1111/jcpp.12620.

56. McLeod KR, Langevin LM, Goodyear BG, Dewey D. Functional connectivity of neural motor networks is disrupted in children with developmental coordination disorder and attention-deficit/hyperactivity disorder. *Neuroimage Clin.* 2014;4(C):566-575. doi:10.1016/j.nicl.2014.03.010.

57. Gabbard C, Bobbio T. The inability to mentally represent action may be associated with performance deficits in children with developmental coordination disorder. *Int J Neurosci.* 2011;121(3):113-120. doi:10.3109/0020745 4.2010.535936.

58. Hung WW, Pang MY. Effects of group-based versus individual-based exercise training on motor performance in children with developmental coordination disorder: a randomized controlled study. *J Rehabil Med.* 2010;42(2):122-128. doi:10.2340/16501977-0496.

59. Haga M. Physical fitness in children with high motor competence is different from that in children with low motor competence. *Phys Ther.* 2009;89(10):1089-1097. doi:10.2522/ptj.20090052.

60. McIntyre F, Chivers P, Larkin D, Rose E, Hands B. Exercise can improve physical self perceptions in adolescents with low motor competence. *Hum Mov Sci.* 2015;42(8):333-343. doi:10.1016/j.humov.2014.12.003.

61. Ferguson GD, Jelsma D, Jelsma J, Smits-Engelsman BC. The efficacy of two task-oriented interventions for children with developmental coordination disorder: neuromotor task training and Nintendo Wii Fit training. *Res Dev Disabil.* 2013;34(9):24449-2461. doi:10.1016/j.ridd.2013.05.007.

62. Jelsma D, Geuze RH, Mombarg R, Smits-Engelsman BC. The impact of Wii Fit intervention on dynamic balance control in children with probable developmental coordination disorder and balance problems. *Hum Mov Sci.* 2014;33(2):404-418. doi:10.1016/j.humov.2013.12.007.

63. Smits-Engelsman BC, Blank R, van der Kaay AC, et al. Efficacy of interventions to improve motor performance in children with developmental coordination disorder: a combined systematic review and meta-analysis. *Dev Med Child Neurol.* 2013;55(3):229-337. doi:10.1111/dmcn.12008.

Issues in Aging in Individuals With Lifelong Disabilities

Barbara H. Connolly, PT, DPT, EdD, C/NDT, FAPTA

As individuals with lifelong disabilities (LLDs) are living longer, interest in their physical health and wellness management has grown in those professionals providing adult health care. Between 2000 and 2010 the population of nondisabled individuals 65 years and older increased at a faster rate (15.1%) than the total US population (9.7%) according to the 2010 US Bureau of the Census report.[1] The actual number of people 65 years and older had grown from 34.9 million in 2000 to 40.3 million in 2010.[1] With biomedical advances and health care improvements, the number of adults with LLDs also seems to be increasing. Statistics on individuals with LLDs most commonly are available for individuals with cerebral palsy (CP), Down syndrome (DS), spina bifida (SB), and intellectual disabilities (ID). In the United States, 18% (12.6 million) of children younger than 18 years were reported to have a chronic physical, developmental, behavioral, or emotional condition.[2] The United Cerebral Palsy Association estimated there are 764,000 children and adults in the United States with CP[3], and a 1998 estimate of the number of adults with CP was about 400,000.[4] Ninety-five percent of children with diplegia CP and 75% of children with quadriplegia CP survive until age 30 years,[5] whereas the overall survival rate of all children with CP to age 20 years is 90%.[6] Thus, the survival rate to adulthood may depend on the clinical status of the individual with CP.[7]

DS is a physical and cognitive developmental disorder with an incidence in the United States estimated to be 1 per 700 to 800 newborns.[8] DS is the most common cognitive disorder at birth and the prevalence is roughly 250,000.[8] Life expectancy of individuals with DS in the United States is currently about 60 years.[8]

Individuals with developmental disabilities (DDs) are being served in the community and are frequently living to be older than 60 years.[9,10] Based on the 1994 to 1995 National Health Interview Survey, the number of individuals (all ages) with ID or DD was reported to be 3.9 million with a prevalence rate of 1.49%.[11] As the younger individuals age, soon there may be between 670,200 and 4,021,300 individuals with ID older than 65 years living in the United States.[12]

Connolly BH, Montgomery PC, eds. *Therapeutic Exercise for Children With Developmental Disabilities, Fourth Edition* (pp 491-516).
© 2020 Taylor & Francis Group.

According to the 2015 Centers for Disease Control and Prevention analysis of the National Birth Defects Prevention Network data for 1999 to 2011, the frequency of live born infants with SB is 3.10 per 10,000 births.[13] The overall medical management and lifestyles of these children have changed, which has had an impact on life expectancy. Statistics suggest 90% of children with SB survive until age 30 years and then may live for decades longer.[14]

In pediatric rehabilitation, the tenet that children cannot be addressed as if they were small adults has been widely embraced. However, the difficulty in transition of services for the child with DD to services for the adult with DD has not been fully explored or perhaps appreciated by occupational or physical therapists with pediatric experience. Additionally, therapists in adult practice settings may be presented with unique problems in the adult with DD that they are not prepared to address. Although individual needs of people with DD vary greatly, knowledge of the effects of aging on this group of individuals can facilitate more effective health care by occupational therapists and physical therapists. Based on the need for therapists in pediatrics and in adult rehabilitation to gain more knowledge in the area of aging in individuals with LLDs, the American Physical Therapy Association House of Delegates passed RC 34-05 in 2005.[15] The goals set by RC 34-05 included development of educational materials and a plan to ensure that all physical therapists are adequately trained in providing care to individuals with LLDs across the life span.

DEFINING THE POPULATION

Definition of Developmental Disabilities and Intellectual Disability

DD is defined in Public Law 106-402—the Developmental Disabilities Assistance and Bill of Rights Act of 2000:

A developmental disability is a severe chronic disability of an individual which[16]:

1. is attributable to a mental or physical impairment or a combination of mental and physical impairments;
2. is manifested before the individual attains age 22;
3. is likely to continue indefinitely;
4. results in substantial functional limitations in 3 or more of the following areas of major life activity: self-care, receptive and expressive language, learning, mobility, self-direction, capacity for independent living, economic self-sufficiency; and
5. reflects the individual's need for a combination and sequence of special, interdisciplinary, or generic services, or other forms of assistance that are of lifelong or extended duration and are individually planned and coordinated.

ID is a disability characterized by significant limitations both in intellectual functioning and in adaptive behavior. Adaptive behavior is a collection of conceptual, social, and practical skills that are learned and performed in everyday life. The disability originates before the age of 18 years.[17]

Biological-Cognitive Signs of Aging

Although DD and ID have been carefully defined through legislation and practice, the definition of *aged* as applied to these populations is not as clear. Aging typically has been defined using a normative-statistical approach (chronological age), whereas others have used a biological approach related to signs and symptoms of aging. For example, in individuals with LLDs such as DS, aging may begin as early as 35 years.[18] Almost all adults with DS who are older than 40 years

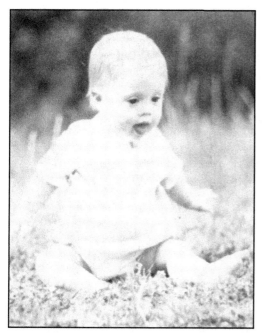

Figure 18-1. WM at age 1 year.

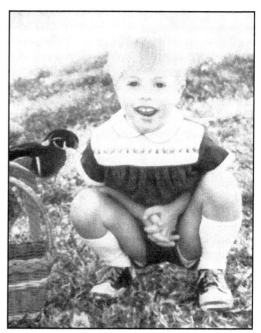

Figure 18-2. WM at age 3 years.

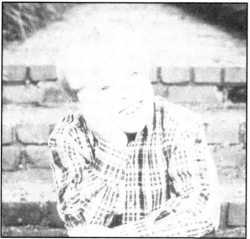

Figure 18-3. WM at age 7 years.

have been found to display neuropathology consistent with Alzheimer disease (AD), although not all will have clinical signs of AD.[19] Burt et al found that adults with DS showed evidence of loss of previously attained adaptive skills more frequently than individuals with ID, but without DS.[20] For adults with DS older than 55 years, the incidence of AD has been estimated at 55%.[20,21] Few studies have examined the presence of AD in geriatric populations of adults without DS, but with ID. However, 2 studies based on postmortem examinations seem to indicate that individuals with ID may be at risk for AD at ages roughly comparable to those of adults without ID.[22,23] Janicki and MacEachron[24] also documented that individuals with ID and neuromotor disorders may experience effects of aging on mobility and activities of daily living (ADLs) earlier than individuals without ID. However, most researchers have selected the mid-50s as a definition of aged in adults with DD based on observations of changing functional status in normative age-related activities (Figures 18-1 through 18-7).[25]

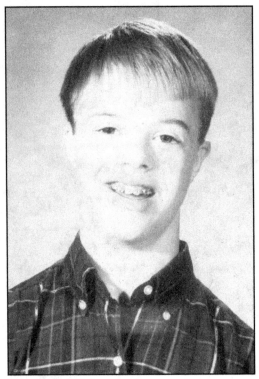

Figure 18-4. WM at age 9 years.

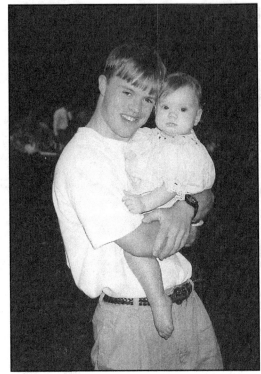

Figure 18-5. WM at age 18 years.

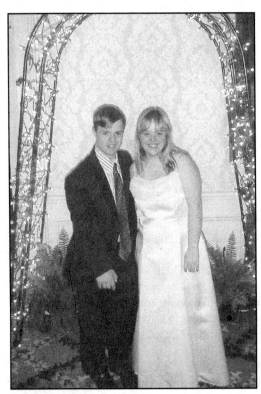

Figure 18-6. WM at age 21 years.

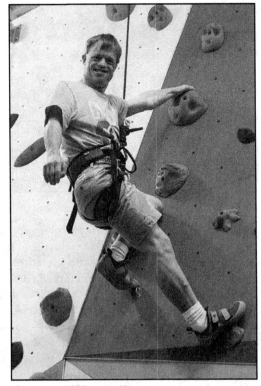

Figure 18-7. WM at age 43 years.

Prevalence

The number of adults with DD/ID is projected to nearly double from 642,860 in 2000 to 1.2 million by 2030.[26] For individuals with CP, a 2006 survey of CP registries across the world revealed a prevalence rate of approximately 2 cases of CP per 1000 live births.[27] However, data from the United States reveals a higher prevalence, with 3 or 4 cases of CP per 1000 school-aged children.[28] As noted previously, 1 per 700 to 800 infants with DS are born in the United States[8] and the frequency of live-born infants with SB is 3.10 per 10,000 births.[13]

The exact number of individuals with disabilities is important to social services agencies, state developmental disabilities planning councils, and state units on aging because, for the first time in history, adults with LLDs are beginning to outlive their parents and are in need of broad-based services. These services include medical, physical, emotional, and financial support.

Mortality

Life expectancy for all individuals with DD/ID has increased, but is less than for the general population.[1,29] Data from US state intellectual and developmental service system administrative data sets and from deidentified state Medicaid claims have been used to determine age of death in people with DD/ID. The average age at death for people in the state service systems was 50.4 to 58.7 years and 61.2 to 63.0 years in the Medicaid data. The crude adult mortality rate was 15.2 per thousand. Thus, the age at death remains lower and the mortality rates higher for people with DD/ID compared with individuals without DD/ID.[29]

The life expectancy for individuals with DS has increased from 9 years in 1929[30] to 12 years in 1949,[30] to 35 years in 1982,[30] to 55 years or older currently.[31] In individuals with CP, 2 periods of the life span have to be considered when discussing mortality. The first period is through infancy and childhood into adulthood, with the second period being survival in adulthood. Mortality in individuals with CP is concentrated in infancy; however, survival in adults with CP is lower than in the general population.[32]

In the 1980s, Jacobson et al[33] found the greatest life expectancy in individuals with LLDs to be in women, people who are ambulatory and/or have mild levels of cognitive impairments, and those who have remained in community settings. Early mortality has been linked in several studies to the loss of the ability to ambulate.[34,35] In 1999, Shavelle and Strauss,[36] in a study of 1812 individuals who had left institutions to move into the community, found that the community death rate was 88% higher than expected for comparable persons living in institutions. They also found that relative mortality in the community seemed to be greatest among the highest functioning persons. Causes of death included diseases of circulation, cancer, pneumonia, aspiration pneumonia, choking, trauma, and cardiac arrest (in some cases due to infection).

As individuals with DD/ID age, they experience age-related disorders similar to individuals without such disabilities.[37] However, in addition to these disorders, secondary medical problems that may contribute to mortality have been described, including obesity, heart disease, deterioration of functional ambulation, chronic skin problems, hygiene-related problems, and early aging[38,39] (Figure 18-8).

EFFECTS OF AGING ON THE SENSES

Even minor functional changes related to aging in areas such as vision, hearing, and vestibular functioning may cause major problems for individuals who have LLDs. An understanding of how some of the general needs of these individuals can be served by medical and community systems is essential for physical therapists and occupational therapists who serve this population.

Figure 18-8. Obesity in an individual with developmental disabilities.

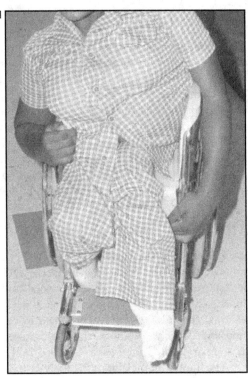

Vision

Age-related eye diseases and conditions include macular degeneration, cataracts, diabetic eye disease, glaucoma, low vision, and blepharitis.[40] However, other changes in the eye related to aging include loss in the photoreceptors and decreased function of the ganglion cells within the retina[41]; poor integrity of the visual fields, dark adaptation, and loss of color spectrum by the fourth decade[42,43]; and decreased pupillary responses.[44] With aging, convergence is compromised, ptosis is seen, and a symmetric restriction in upward gaze is experienced.[42] Additionally, loss of vision with aging may occur because of glaucoma, macular degeneration, or diabetic retinopathy.

Implications for Individuals With Developmental Disabilities

Although limited information is available about the prevalence of visual problems in individuals with DD, it is likely that a greater number of people with DD have uncorrected or unidentified visual problems than in the general population. Hand, in a study of older people with lifelong ID, found that 32% had visual problems.[45] Additionally, Good et al[46] reported that the incidence of cortical visual impairment is increasing in children with neurological deficits. These authors speculated that better medical care has lowered the mortality rate of children with severe neurological problems and thus these children survive for longer periods of time. Although the residual vision of the child with cortical visual impairment often improves over time, the child may be left with diminished visual acuity.

The prevalence of visual impairment in adults with DS who are age 65 to 74 years is 70%. This prevalence is much greater than the 6.5% of adults of the same age who are not intellectually challenged and 17.4% of adults of the same age who are intellectually challenged, but who do not have DS.[47] Types of visual problems include cataracts, blepharitis, keratoconus, and excessive myopia.[48]

Another factor that may contribute to a high number of individuals with DD/ID having undiagnosed visual problems is the examiner's difficulty in gathering subjective information from the individual. The extent of visual loss may not be identifiable if the individual cannot respond to a standard eye chart consisting of letters, numbers, or words. In general, physiological changes in tandem with environmental and preexisting disease factors in individuals with LLDs may cause greater impairments in vision than would be anticipated in the general population. Signs that might indicate a change in vision include rubbing the eyes, squinting, shutting or covering one eye, or tilting the head. Changes in daily functions, such as stumbling during gait, hesitancy on steps or curbs, holding reading materials closer than usual, or sitting close to the television, also might suggest visual changes. Considerations that need to be made for individuals with DD/ID may include early cataract removal before declining function impairs the individual's ability to cooperate with postoperative care, soft lighting, reduced glare in the environment, use of color, use of high contrast, or referral to a low-vision rehabilitation specialist. Reinforcement with tactile or verbal cues also may be necessary to improve visual responses.

Hearing

Prevalence studies indicate that 26.3% of nondisabled individuals older than 70 years exhibit some degree of hearing loss, with the most common cause of sensorineural hearing loss being presbycusis.[49] Presbycusis can be related to a number of factors, including cellular aging in the peripheral, auditory, and central nervous system pathways, acoustic trauma, cardiovascular disease, and cumulative effects of ototoxic medications.[50] Problems noted with presbycusis include a slowly progressive bilateral hearing loss, difficulty with word recognition, and a decline in perceptual processing of the temporal characteristics of speech.

Implications for Individuals With Developmental Disabilities

Conductive hearing losses can occur because of external ear disease and acute or chronic diseases of the middle ear. Otitis media (ie, inflammation of the middle ear) is one of the most common causes of conductive hearing loss. Otitis media usually is treated with medication but can result in permanent ear damage and hearing loss.[51] Individuals with DD may be more likely to develop this type of hearing loss than the general population because of the occurrence of repeated otitis media that is undetected and untreated. Conductive and sensorineural hearing losses have been reported to occur in up to 70% of people with DS.[52] The conductive hearing loss noted in early adulthood may have resulted from frequent childhood middle ear infections.[53] In general, sensorineural hearing loss is associated with the general aging population. However, the sensorineural hearing loss in individuals with DS can begin to develop during the second decade of life.

A hearing loss in many adults with DD/ID can be "hidden" because of their limited communication abilities and sheltered lifestyles. Therefore, many aging adults with DD/ID may have an undetected hearing loss that interferes with an already limited communication ability and contributes to social isolation and depression. Clinical signs that might indicate a hearing loss include turning up the television or radio very loud, speaking loudly, responding to questions inappropriately, appearing to be stubborn, or becoming confused in noisy environments.

Considering the possibility of a greater incidence of hearing losses in adults with DD/ID, health care providers should insist on audiological testing for all these individuals. Auditory testing every 2 years is recommended for people with DS.[52] The testing should be conducted by an audiologist with special training in evaluating individuals with DD/ID. Hearing aids can be helpful in increasing responsiveness to sound, but only if tolerated by the wearer. For those who cannot tolerate hearing aids, functional hearing can be improved through minimizing background noise, facing the person being spoken to, and speaking slowly with good articulation. If the hearing loss is identified early, communication through use of sign language or augmentative communication might be used as alternative strategies.

Taste and Smell

Evidence suggests that some nondisabled older individuals experience less pleasure during meals because of impaired ability to taste and smell, which results from higher thresholds for these senses.[54] Increases in the thresholds of taste and smell may make food seem tasteless and less appealing. For individuals with DD, this may cause changes in their oral-motor skills, eating habits, and nutritional intake. Additionally, Turk et al[55] found that in adult women with CP (34% with concurrent ID), there was a high prevalence of poor dental health and gastroesophageal reflux. A decreased appetite also may result as a side effect from some medications. With any of these problems, a lack of interest in food may occur and the nutritional health of the individual may be affected.

Implications for Individuals With Developmental Disabilities

Being under ideal body weight can be a problem for people with DD.[56,57] In particular, male individuals with lower levels of cognitive functioning, multiple disabilities, and feeding difficulties typically are underweight.[57] The lack of interest in eating because of changes in taste and smell in these individuals may lead to further debilitation, susceptibility to opportunistic infections, and even death. Nutritional supplements may be necessary for maintaining ideal body weight and meeting daily nutritional requirements. Additionally, emphasis should be placed on the visual appearance of food, as well as on texture, to increase the meal's appeal. Separating food rather than mixing food on a plate and varying textures of food might increase interest in eating. Use of condiments, other than salt, also may be used to increase overall flavor.

Dental problems may cause problems with eating in individuals with DD. The greatest dental problem faced by the adult with DD is periodontal disease. The incidence of severe, destructive periodontal disease in individuals with DS is higher than in non-DS individuals.[58] The immunologic deficiencies in persons with DS may be related to this increased prevalence and severity of periodontal disease.[59]

Somatosensory

Although the degree of change may vary in nondisabled individuals, touch and the related senses of proprioception and kinesthesia appear to decrease with age. Age-related changes that contribute to problems with touch and position sense have been noted in the peripheral nervous system both anatomically as well as physiologically.[60,61] Morphologic changes in the nerve cells, nerve roots, peripheral nerves, and specialized nerve terminals have been linked with the aging process. With aging, Meissner corpuscles decrease in concentration,[62] Pacinian corpuscles decrease in density,[63] and afferent nerve fibers decrease in number.[64] Degeneration of the dorsal columns occurs as one ages. This degeneration is thought to be due to the loss of centrally directed axons of the dorsal root ganglion cells.[65] Additionally, action potentials may take longer than usual to reach the central nervous system in the aging adult. This delay is due to a gradual shortening of the internodal length that contributes to an increased conduction velocity.

Quantitative studies have shown that a progressive impairment of sensory detection occurs with aging. An example of this gradual decline is the perception of touch/pressure, which approaches a 4-fold reduction in men older than 40 years.[66] Schmidt et al[63] found an age-related decline in response to "flutter" and "tap," which they related to changes in the peripheral sensory units rather than conduction along the afferent nerves.

Proprioception has been reported as being similar in young and older individuals without disabilities.[67] However, passive movement thresholds have been reported to be twice as high for the hip, knee, and ankle in people older than 50 years compared with individuals younger than 40 years.[68] No change in upper extremity perception was noted. Skinner et al,[69] in a study of knee joint position sense, found that the abilities to reproduce passive knee position and to detect motion deteriorated with age.

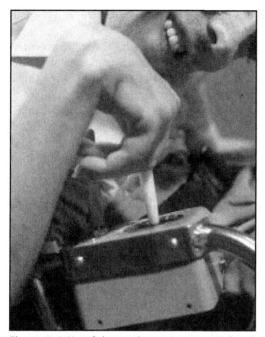

Figure 18-9. Use of abnormal posturing to access hand-held controls.

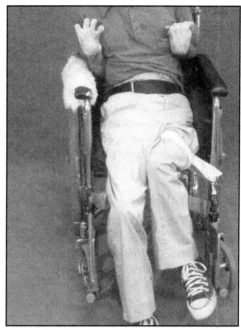

Figure 18-10. An individual propelling his wheelchair using his feet.

Implications for Individuals With Developmental Disabilities

Loss of somatosensory function in aging adults with DD may be devastating. For the individual who depends on tactile input to guide movement, the decrease in tactile function may lead to decreases in movement and possibly result in immobility. For example, the individual may no longer be able to access communication boards or to independently propel a wheelchair without sustaining injuries to the upper extremities (Figure 18-9).

With the loss of proprioceptive abilities, particularly in the lower extremities, functional patterns of movement may be lost. For example, many adults with neuromotor disorders propel their wheelchairs with their feet (Figure 18-10).

If joint sense is decreased or lost in the hips, knees, or ankles, the coordination needed for efficiently moving from one place to another in the wheelchair may be compromised. If the individual is ambulatory, a loss of proprioceptive abilities with age may necessitate use of a different type of ambulation assistance, such as a walker rather than crutches or canes. Assistance from another person during ambulation may be necessary for some individuals who are no longer "safe" during independent ambulation because of loss of proprioceptive function.

EFFECTS OF AGING ON THE
NEUROMUSCULOSKELETAL SYSTEM

Flexibility

Changes in collagen are a biological cause for decreases in flexibility as one ages. With age, collagen fibers become irregular in shape owing to cross-linking. This pattern results in a decreased linear-pull relationship in the collagen tissue and leads to decreased mobility in the body's tissues.[70] Poor nutrition also may lead to collagen changes, and this problem may be seen in the population with DD. In particular, deficiency of Vitamin C appears to interfere with normal tissue integrity and may affect muscle functioning and elasticity of collagen.

Muscles, skin, and tendons become less flexible and mobile as one ages. The spine becomes less flexible because of collagen changes in the annulus and to decreased water content in the nucleus pulposus. Furthermore, osteoporotic changes in the vertebral bones may lead to fractures of the vertebrae, increased collagen scarring, and decreased flexibility of the spine.

Hypokinesis or decreased activity can be a functional cause of loss of flexibility. Older individuals who remain sitting or immobile for long periods of time may develop tightness in those muscles that are shortened in that particular position and that may form collagenous adhesions. In particular, decreased passive and active range of motion (ROM), particularly in the flexor musculature, may be seen in elders who sit for extended periods of time during the day.

Implications for Individuals With Developmental Disabilities

Loss of flexibility in the aging adult with DD may be even more dramatic than for the typical aging adult. The New York State Developmental Disabilities Planning Council identified loss of flexibility as one of the possible causes of decreased function and mobility in adults with CP.[71] Loss of flexibility was identified as a secondary condition that occurred as a result of the primary neuromotor pathology. Secondary conditions in older persons with neuromotor problems such as CP may be seen because of multiple body systems that were affected during the developmental years. If the individual has been inactive or if there was limited weight bearing, adequate bone density and mass may not have developed. Therefore, that individual is likely to experience an accelerated loss of bone density and mass with age. A link between the use of some medications (such as Dilantin [phenytoin]) and osteoporosis has been documented.[72] This risk appears to be particularly high in individuals who use the medications for long periods of time and those who are nonambulatory or sedentary. Study of the mechanism by which the medications may be associated with metabolic bone disease has been focused on Vitamin D metabolism and bone turnover. Many physicians recommend that regular periods of sunlight be part of a daily schedule to offset the effects of anticonvulsants on bone loss in those individuals who are at greatest risk. Additionally, individuals with neuromotor problems may be at an increased risk for osteoporosis because of limitations in mobility, inadequate calcium intake in the diet, and decreased sun exposure leading to low circulating levels of Vitamin D. Multiple studies have found that individuals with DD have a high prevalence of low bone mineral density (BMD).[73-75] Individuals with low BMD were more likely to be older, non-weight bearing, Caucasian, and severely cognitively delayed. Other osteoporotic risk factors noted were low body weight, small body size, hypogonadism, endocrine disorders, sedentary lifestyle, and poor nutrition. All these factors commonly are found in individuals with DD.

A pathological cause of loss of flexibility in people of any age is arthritis. Osteoarthritis (OA), a commonly occurring disorder in the elderly, is characterized by deterioration of articular cartilage and formation of new bone in the subchrondral areas as well as at the margins of the joint. Age is one of the strongest risk factors for OA for all joints. The increase with age is thought to be due to a number of factors, including biologic changes, obesity, joint injury, joint deformities, and muscle weakness.[76]

Arthritic changes in the joints of aging adults with DD may be noted at earlier ages. Individuals with more severe cases of CP tend to develop OA at a higher rate than those with less severe cases.[77] The factors that contribute to the early development of OA appear to be compromised ambulation, reduced muscular activity, restriction in ROM, and diminished BMD.[78] OA has been cited as a cause of pain as well as loss of flexibility in individuals with CP.[77,79] Cathels and Reddihough[77] found clinical evidence of arthritis in 27% of a group of 149 adolescents and young adults with CP. Individuals who walked were more affected than those who did not walk. Opheim et al studied 226 individuals with unilateral or bilateral spastic CP (ages 24 to 76 years) over a 7-year period. They found that 52% of the individuals reported deterioration in walking due to pain frequency and intensity at the end of the study compared with 39% at the beginning of the study.[80] Trauma to a joint predisposes it to OA, as has been noted in the high incidence of OA in the shoulders and elbows of baseball pitchers, ankles of ballet dancers, and knees of basketball players. Therefore, disturbances of the joint mechanics or repeated abnormal stresses to a joint in those individuals who are ambulatory may predispose them to early-onset OA. Pain and weakness usually are associated with OA, but in individuals with DD who cannot communicate easily, these symptoms may be missed or misinterpreted.

Arthritic changes in different joints may lead to loss of functional abilities in individuals with DD.[80] For example, the ability to transfer oneself from a wheelchair to the bed or tub may become extremely difficult if soreness in the shoulders, elbows, and wrists is experienced. Many individuals who were ambulatory may opt to use a wheelchair if pain is experienced in the spine, hips, knees, or ankles during walking activities. Additionally, more adaptive equipment may be necessary in the home for the person to be as independent as possible with ADLs.

Strength

Muscle strength, as defined by the ability to produce force or torque, declines with age in typically developing men and women.[81] A common change noted in aging muscle is reduction of mass and loss of strength, both related to the activity level of the individual.[82] Additionally, decreased strength may be due to smaller numbers of muscle fibers and muscle motor units, as well as a decrease in size of the muscle fibers. Functioning motoneurons appear to decline with aging and thus problems may be noted in coordination and speed of muscle contraction.

Additionally, decreases in muscle strength as a person ages may be related to decreased time spent in vigorous work or athletic activities. For example, Keller and Engelhardt found that a decline in muscle strength was noted between people younger than 40 years to those older than 40 years between 16.6% to 40.9% for knee flexion and extension.[81] Muscles that appear most likely to show a decrease in muscle strength during periods of inactivity are the active antigravity muscles, such as the quadriceps, hip extensors, ankle dorsiflexors, latissimus dorsi, and triceps.

Implications for Individuals With Developmental Disabilities

Individuals with physical disabilities have been noted to experience additional problems in the musculoskeletal system as they age.[7,79,80,83] The musculoskeletal problems may be related to deformities, including subluxations and dislocations of the hip; abnormalities of the foot such as flat feet, varus, valgus, or equinus; patella alta; cervical stenosis; spondylolysis; scoliosis; pelvic obliquity; and contractures[79,80,83] (Figure 18-11).

These musculoskeletal problems may cause secondary conditions, such as decreased strength, due to the inability of the individual to move in a variety of patterns. Additionally, CP may cause a cycle of deconditioning of the individual followed by a further decrease in physical activity, which then leads to a functional decline.

Pain, soreness, weakness of muscles, energy decline, and the tendency to be more susceptible to injury all increase in people with long-standing disabilities, not just in those with CP. Loss of muscle strength in individuals who have had difficulty with movement all their lives may be even greater than that expected solely due to the aging process. Janicki and Jacobson,[84] in a study of more than 10,000 individuals who were intellectually challenged, found a decline in motoric skills began at about age 50 years, even for those who were mild to moderately challenged. Among those who were more severely and profoundly challenged, motoric skills remained relatively stable until they reached their late 70s. However, this delayed decline was related most probably to more limited motoric abilities even at younger ages when compared with the individuals with mild to moderate intellectual impairments. Muscle weakness has been documented in studies of young people with spastic diplegia, particularly regarding the impact on ambulation and stair climbing.[82,85-87] However, it appears that other groups of people with neuromotor problems also experience increasing problems with movement as they age. This loss of movement may be related to pain

Figure 18-11. Pronation of the foot in an individual with a developmental disability.

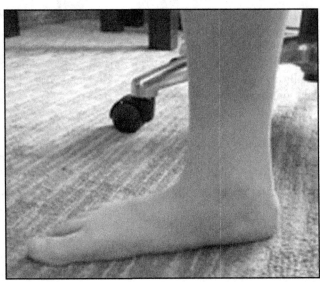

or degenerative joint disease, either of which could lead to decreased use of or less force exerted by certain muscles during movement.

Strength training is a popular form of exercise for individuals with and without disabilities. However, questions have been raised over time about the appropriateness of such programs with individuals with spasticity. Andersson et al[88] found that a progressive strength training program for individuals with spastic diplegia (age 25 to 47 years) provided significant improvement in isometric strength (hip extensors $P = .006$, hip abductors $P = .01$) and in isokinetic concentric work at 30 degrees per second (knee extensors $P = .02$). The results of the intervention also yielded significant improvements in the Gross Motor Function Measure dimensions D (standing) and E (walking, running, and jumping) as well as in the Timed Up and Go test. No increase in spasticity as measured by the modified Ashworth Scale was noted in individuals who underwent strength training. Similar positive findings were reported by Ross et al in a systematic review of the effect of strength training on the mobility of adults with CP.[89]

Therefore, as with most nondisabled adults, moderate regular exercise is essential for maintaining mobility in adults with DD. Loss of even a small amount of strength may lead to loss of functional abilities in this population because of the very sensitive balance between muscle groups that has been developed over time for some functional activities. Weakness can result in loss of functional abilities, such as walking, climbing stairs, transferring, or getting up from a chair. Additionally, increased occurrences of complications such as pressure sores, contractures, and pneumonia may result from immobility in some adults who have lifelong limitations in movement. Bed rest or chair rest should be avoided if at all possible, and gross motor activities should be included as a part of the day's activities.

Posture and Positioning

Posture is derived from the relationship of body parts, one to another, as well as to the maturation and interaction of the musculoskeletal, neuromuscular, and cardiopulmonary systems. Additionally, psychological well-being may have an impact on the "posture" of an individual.

Upright posture, either in sitting or in standing, reflects the most noticeable changes as one ages. Sitting postural changes in many older adults include the head held forward, the shoulders rounded, and the upper back kyphotic. In sitting or standing, a flatter lumbar lordosis may be seen in the low back. In standing, flexion at the hips and knees may be more noticeable. These changes in the spine and in the lower extremities most frequently are caused by changes in intervertebral discs as well as to decreased mobility or hypokinesis.

Intervertebral Discs

Age-related changes in the intervertebral discs begin during the third decade of life in the "normal" population.[90,91] Water content in the nucleus pulposus ranges from 70% to 90%, with diminishing amounts with age. By the sixth to seventh decades, the water content is decreased by 30%.[92] With age, the annulus, which is composed of collagen, becomes less elastic. Together, the decreased water in the nucleus and the increased fibers of the annulus result in the disc becoming flatter and less resilient. These changes lead to diminishing height and flexibility of the spine in aging individuals.

Age-related changes also take place in the ligaments of the spine with degeneration of tensile ability with age. Tkaczuk[93] determined that tensile characteristics of the anterior and posterior ligaments of the lumbar spine decreased with age. Additionally, Nachemson and Evans[94] determined that the "resting" tension of the ligamentum flavum also decreased. The loss of this resting tension could lead to further spinal instability in the aging individual.

Hypokinesis

Prolonged periods of time in one position also can lead to postural changes in aging individuals. Older people tend to remain in one position (usually sitting) for longer periods of time, and thus the body's flexor musculature tend to shorten. Resulting limitations in extensor musculature then may occur. In particular, the older individual may present with increased hip and knee flexion, increased kyphosis of the upper trunk, and decreased lumbar lordosis. Additionally, a relationship has been established between osteoporosis and inactivity. In humans, weight-bearing produces stress on the bone, and collagen acts as the crystal, which transforms the stimulus into an osteoblastic effect. New bone tissue then is laid down along the stress lines. Thus, lack of muscular stress, as well as lack of weight bearing on the bone, will contribute to osteoporosis.[95] Numerous studies have shown an increased risk of osteoporosis (and fractures) in individuals with ID and in adults with CP.[38,73,96,97]

Implications for Individuals With Developmental Disabilities

The spine may be a focal point of difficulty for persons with LLDs. A scoliosis that has been present since childhood may further progress as the individual ages (Figure 18-12). In particular, older people with CP who have been immobile or relatively inactive may not have developed adequate bone density and mass at a younger age and are likely to experience an accelerated loss of bone density and mass as they age. Individuals with severe scoliosis also may have increasing problems with mobility, skin integrity, and hygiene care, resulting in greater dependency on caregivers. Spondylolysis, which is commonly seen in ambulatory adults with diplegia, may progress to spondylolisthesis if not detected early.[98] Cervical stenosis and cervical degenerative changes are seen in adults with CP, especially in those with dystonia or athetosis.[98] Symptoms of progression of cervical degeneration include new spasticity, new weakness, paresthesias, and urinary incontinence, all of which can lead to a loss of function.

In individuals who have taken medications for seizure disorders, a decrement in BMD density may be noted.[72] Seizures are present in approximately 30% of individuals with CP, and the type of medication taken for control of their seizures may place them at risk.[99] This increased risk for osteoporosis may cause a predisposition for fracture rates at earlier ages than in the general population. For example, compression fractures of the spine may be noted with increased frequently in those individuals with seizure and neuromotor disorders, and the resultant pain from the fractures may further contribute to hypokinesis.

Figure 18-12. Severe scoliosis in an adult with DD.

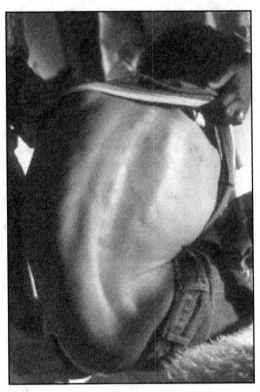

Clinical suggestions for older individuals with DD are similar to those given to other aging individuals. Increased activity in positions other than supine or sitting are suggested along with increased weight-bearing positions. Caution, however, must be taken regarding the amount of stress that is placed on joints that have been misaligned for many decades. In many cases, therapists and others assisting aging individuals with DD must realize that they are working with structures that have never been "normal." Therefore, some procedures used with geriatric clients without DD or with children with DD may not be appropriate. For example, placing an individual with a severe scoliosis in a side-lying position should be attempted only with close supervision, because fractures of the rib cage may occur because of long-term osteoporosis. Stretching of contractures that have been long term also should be performed with much caution because of the risk of fracture if undue pressure is placed around the joint.

Fractures

Fractures have been documented as occurring at any time during the life span of an individual with CP.[7,100] Fractures may occur for a variety of reasons with the combination of osteoporosis, long lever arms, and contractures being cited as increasing the risk of nontraumatic fractures. Brunner and Döderlein[100] identified a total of 54 nontraumatic fractures in 37 individuals with CP over a 20-year period. The fractures were found to have occurred between ages 12 and 16 years, with the most common site being the supracondylar region of the distal femur. These researchers identified hip dislocations or contractures of major joints as being predisposing factors to the fractures. Furthermore, they found that 41% of the fractures occurred within 9 months of a surgery and that the majority of the fractures occurred during physical therapy intervention. The fractures not associated with a surgery occurred during ADLs. Brunner and Döderlein[100] also described stress fractures occurring at the patella, associated with a crouched gait and overactivation of the quadriceps. These findings further illustrate the importance of maintaining good bone health in individuals with CP through exercise, strengthening, and prevention of injuries.

Gait and Balance

Three major factors contribute to adequate balance during stance and gait. The first factor is the appropriate processing of input from the visual, vestibular, and somatosensory (primarily proprioceptive) systems that allows a person to acquire information about his or her body in space. A second factor is central processing or the ability of the body to determine, in advance, the correct sequence of responses. Lastly, the body must be able to carry out the appropriate response via the effector system (strength, ROM, flexibility, and endurance).

Changes in stance and gait with aging may be affected by changes in any of these 3 factors. Changes noted with aging include mild rigidity, slowed postural reaction times, decreased stride length, increased stride width, decreased gait speed, decreased vertical displacement, decreased excursion of legs during the swing phase, decreased rotation of the trunk, reduced ankle joint power, and decreased velocity of limb motions.[101] Additionally, decreased back extension and neck ROM may interfere with upright posture and balance. Processing of sensory input may be diminished in aging adults and may result in loss of balance. Inadequate processing of proprioceptive input may interfere with the processing of information regarding motion of the body with respect to the support surface and to motion of the body segments. Additionally, older adults may have increased response times due to poor central processing of sensory information.[102,103] This delay in response has been speculated as contributing to instability during stance and ambulation in older people who fall. For example, a loss of balance was noted in older participants during a study in which they were asked to quickly perform unilateral knee flexion during standing.[99] Additionally, gait speed has been shown to decrease with older age during fast-speed walking as compared with usual-speed walking.[101]

Different strategies for responding to unexpected postural perturbations have been noted in older adults in comparison with healthy young adults. A higher incidence of proximal to distal sequencing has been noted in older adults than in young adults.[103] This change in the sequencing pattern has been speculated as being an indicator of altered postural control and central processing in the older adult.

Implications for Individuals With Developmental Disabilities

As people with DD become older, they become more like those in their nondisabled peer group in relationship to gait and balance problems. For example, Hresko et al found progressive hip instability after skeletal maturity in individuals with DS, which led to a decrease in ambulation skills.[104] Foot pronation also was noted to lead to an increased incidence of pedal arthritis in adults with DS, but at an earlier age than would be expected in a nondisabled peer group.[105]

Years of toe walking and cavus foot deformities in some individuals can lead to pain in the metatarsal heads and difficulty during walking (Figure 18-13). However, in individuals with CP, ambulation and balance appear to decline at an earlier age than in the general population for a variety of reasons, such as degenerative hip disease, abnormalities of the ankle-foot system, and spinal abnormalities.[80] Andersson and Mattsson cited decreased walking ability over time in a group of 221 individuals with CP due to knee and balance problems, increased spasticity, and lack of physical training.[106] Other studies documented that individuals with CP (with and without cognitive impairments) experienced declines in ambulation abilities from adolescence to adulthood.[80,107-109] In a study of 406 adults with CP (age 18 years and older), 75% walked at the time of the survey, but nearly 50% reported declines in walking abilities, often before their mid-30s.[108] In another study of 72 adults with CP between ages 19 to 65, 72% were able to walk, but of these 24% had stopped walking before age 40 years.[109]

The risk of falling may occur at an earlier age in non-CP individuals as well. Center and colleagues[73] found that falls were the second most likely cause of injury in a group of individuals with ID who were institutionalized. These researchers found that individuals with ID were 3.5 times more likely to have a fracture than the general population. Additionally, the fracture rate

Figure 18-13. Long-standing deformity of the foot.

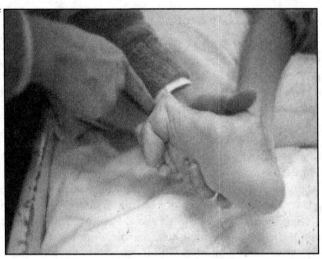

was higher among those who could ambulate independently and among those who needed assistive devices to ambulate. A further complication is the deconditioning that may occur after a hip fracture or dislocation that necessitates a reduction in the daily amount of gross motor activity. Some individuals who were ambulatory prior to a hip fracture may never again attain the coordination or endurance needed for independent ambulation. Compression fractures of the spine also may contribute to pain and loss of upright mobility. For older individuals who have lost functional ambulation, consideration should be given for use of a wheelchair or other adaptive equipment.

Although independent ambulation may not be possible for the older individual with DD, daily amounts of moderate regular exercise are essential to maintain mobility. Appropriate exercise can improve strength, flexibility, and balance, and therefore reduce the chance of future falls and injuries. The importance of physical activity has to be stressed with individuals with LLDs beginning in childhood. Low levels of physical activity in these individuals might increase the risk for related chronic diseases and with poor health-related physical fitness. All individuals with LLDs at any age should be encouraged to participate, to the extent they are able, in aerobic, anaerobic, and muscle strengthening activities.[110]

CARDIOPULMONARY/CARDIOVASCULAR CHANGES DURING THE AGING PROCESS

Anatomic and Physiologic Changes

Most researchers agree that changes in cardiac and pulmonary function occur as one ages, regardless of lifestyle. The lung matures by age 20 to 25 years, and after that age a progressive decrease in chest wall and bronchiolar compliance occurs because of structural changes in the bones, cartilage, and elastic structures.[111] With aging there are structural changes in the thoracic cage (such as reduced height of the thoracic vertebrae and calcification of the rib cage), causing a reduction in chest wall compliance. As has been discussed previously, cross-linking of collagen fibers and a decrease in resiliency of elastic and cartilaginous tissue occur. The elastic fibers in the lungs also are compromised, resulting in increased lung compliance and decreased elastic recoil.[111] These anatomical changes contribute to a resultant overall decrease in total lung compliance by age 60 years.[111,112]

Aging also is associated with increased air trapping and an increase in airspace size due to loss of supporting tissue.[111] A decreased efficiency of gas exchange occurs as one ages due to loss of tissue from the alveolar walls and septra as well as an increase in the size and number of alveolar fenestra.[112] Additionally, respiratory muscle strength decreases with age, occurring more so in men than in women.[111]

The total lung compliance changes that are noted with age have an important impact on the pulmonary function of an individual. Vital capacity declines whereas functional residual capacity and residual volume increase.[111]

With aging, there are significant structural changes in the heart and vasculature, such as vascular stiffening and increased left ventricular wall thickness. Fibrosis that occurs with aging can lead to diastolic dysfunction, increased afterload, and heart failure.[113,114] There is also a progressive increase in the prevalence of cardiovascular disease (eg, coronary artery disease, hypertension, and diabetes).[114]

Pathological Changes

One of the most common diseases in people older than 65 years in the United States is coronary disease, with an incidence of approximately 14% in those age 65 to 74 years and 25% in those 75 years and older.[115] Hypertension occurs more frequently in the aging population, with more than 55% of individuals older than 65 years presenting with hypertension.[115] As previously noted, Kapell et al[47] found that people with intellectual deficits have a greater incidence of nonischemic heart disease when compared with their age- and gender-matched peers in the general population. Strauss et al[116] documented excess mortality among adults with CP from ischemic heart disease. However, they stated that the excess mortality may be due to a failure to detect subtle clues of ischemic heart disease in this population.

Implications for Individuals With Developmental Disabilities

Detailed studies on the prevalence of heart and pulmonary disease among people with DD are not available. However, the age-associated problems of high cholesterol, hypertension, and heart disease are noted to occur in elders with LLDs. Additionally, secondary conditions involving the musculoskeletal and cardiopulmonary systems that affect fitness have been reported.[4,117]

In some individuals with LLDs, the risk for some of the age-associated problems may actually be less than for the general population because of restrictions in lifestyle, such as the inability to smoke, drink alcohol, or overeat. Exercise programs are as important in improving cardiovascular fitness in individuals with LDDs as in the general population.[118] The Surgeon General report on physical activity and health states that for people with lifelong disabling conditions, regular physical activity can improve stamina, muscular strength, and quality of life.[118] Evidence exists that supervised exercise programs for adults with LLDs can result in improved cardiovascular fitness.[119-127] In adults with DS, aerobic exercise programs improved mobility and physical capacity,[119,120,122] resistance exercise programs increased muscle strength and performance,[121,123] and combined aerobic and resistance exercise programs improved submaximal and peak exercise capacity.[123] For people with CP, strengthening programs have been associated with improvements in ambulation as well as in fitness levels.[89,126,127] In individuals with severe physical disabilities, the physical, occupational, or recreational therapist should be consulted during the development of the exercise program. For older individuals, the role of the physical or occupational therapists also might include consultation with fitness center staff about facility accessibility.

Individuals with DD have additional problems, however, with respiratory diseases. Respiratory disease, historically, has been a major cause of death in individuals with DD. The increased mortality in the DD population due to respiratory infections is attributed to the presence of CP, epilepsy, and reduced efficiency in coughing, feeding, and breathing.[128,129]

TABLE 18-1. AGE-ADJUSTED PERCENTAGE DISTRIBUTION OF BODY MASS INDEX AMONG ADULTS AGE 18 YEARS AND OLDER: UNITED STATES 2016

AGE (YEARS)	HEALTHY WEIGHT	OVERWEIGHT	OBESE
All ages	34.0%	34.6%	29.5%
18 to 44	38.3%	31.8%	27.6%
45 to 64	27.5%	36.9%	34.7%
65 to 74	26.8%	40.5%	31.5%
75 and older	37.4%	38.3%	21.2%

Adapted from the Centers for Disease Control and Prevention. National Center for Health Statistics. National Health Interview Survey, 2016. https://www.cdc.gov/nchs/nhis/SHS/tables.htm.

TABLE 18-2. PERCENTAGE OF OBESITY BY AGE AND DISABILITY STATUS

CHILDREN AGES 2 TO 17 YEARS WITH DISABILITIES BMI at or above 95th percentile	CHILDREN AGES 2 TO 17 YEARS WITHOUT DISABILITIES BMI at or above 95th percentile	ADULTS WITH DISABILITIES BMI of 30 or higher	ADULTS WITHOUT DISABILITIES BMI of 30 or higher
22%	16%	36%	23%

Abbreviation: BMI, body mass index.

Adapted from the Centers for Disease Control and Prevention. National Center for Health Statistics. 2003-2008 National Health and Nutrition Examination Survey Data. Hyattsville, MD: Centers for Disease Control and Prevention and 2008 Behavioral Risk Factor Surveillance system. https://www.cdc.gov/brfss/annual_data/annual_2016.html.

AGING AND OBESITY

Obesity is becoming a major health problem for all age groups throughout the industrialized world. In the 2016 National Health Interview Survey,[115] 30% of adults age 18 years and older were classified as overweight and 27% were identified as obese (Table 18-1).

Researchers have identified obesity as a major problem with individuals with DD/ID, with their prevalence data either similar to or higher than their non-DD/ID counterparts[57,130,131] (Table 18-2). Studies have also shown that when comparing ID and non-ID individuals, that women, older individuals, and those with less severe disabilities and certain genetic disorders (ie, DS) were more likely to be obese[130-135] (Table 18-3). The lack of healthy eating habits and regular physical activity are thought to be contributory factors in the DD/ID population similar to the factors in the general population.

TABLE 18-3. PERCENTAGE OF ADULTS— OVERWEIGHT, OBESITY, OR EXTREME OBESITY BY DIAGNOSIS

DIAGNOSIS	OVERWEIGHT (BMI ≥ 25)	OBESITY (BMI ≥ 30)	EXTREME OBESITY (BMI ≥ 40)
Down syndrome	87.9%	70.7%	19.0%
Intellectual impairments	84.8%	60.6%	12.1%
General population	64.5%	30.5%	4.7%

Abbreviation: BMI, body mass index.

Adapted from Rimmer JH, Wang E. Obesity prevalence among a group of Chicago residents with disabilities. *Arch Phys Med Rehabil.* 2005;86(7):1461-1464.

COGNITIVE CHANGES IN INDIVIDUALS WITH DOWN SYNDROME

As previously noted, almost all adults with DS older than age 40 years display neuropathology consistent with AD, although not all will have clinical signs of AD.[19] The prevalence rates for AD among adults with DS increase with age, with reported rates of 10% at age 30 to 39 years, up to 55% at age 50 to 59 years, and almost 75% at age 60 to 65 years.[19,52] Wisniewski et al[136] identified loss of vocabulary, recent memory loss, impaired short-term visual retention, difficulty in object identification, and loss of interest in surroundings as early cognitive changes. Dalton and Crapper[137] described memory loss in people with DS age 39 to 58 years over a 3-year period. Four of the 11 participants deteriorated over the 3 years to the point that they could no longer learn a simple discrimination task. Fenner and colleagues[138] found that the greatest decline in function was in a 45- to 49-year-old age group.

Physical therapists and occupational therapists should be aware of early signs of dementia in individuals with DS and be prepared to intervene as necessary to retain as much adaptive functioning as possible. Higher functioning people with DS will present with the same signs of AD as noted in the general population.[139] These signs include memory loss, temporal disorientation, and decreased verbal output. Early signs of dementia in lower-functioning individuals with DS might include apathy, inattention, decreased social interaction, irritability, aggression, daytime sleepiness, gait deterioration, and seizures.

As noted in the letter from a parent of an adult with DS, not all adults with DS may experience the physical and cognitive declines as they age. In fact, many adults with DS are able to function well in the community, have employment for many years, and enjoy an active social life (Table 18-4).

SUMMARY

Physical therapists and occupational therapists should be effective health advocates and health care providers throughout the life span of individuals with DD. Although people with DD share similar changes and risks of aging as others their age, the sequelae of lifelong physical and cognitive impairments present special challenges to many therapists. At some point, individuals with DD may need rehabilitation rather than habilitation to regain abilities after injury or illness. An understanding of the effects of aging on the general population, plus identification of special

TABLE 18-4. FROM A PARENT'S PERSPECTIVE

EARLY YEARS

WM was born full term and diagnosed at birth. He had a slight heart murmur in infancy, which was resolved at age 6 months. He was "floppy" but had no other medical issues. Over time, he has been prone to have ear blockages from wax buildup (even now at age 43 years).

From the time of WM's diagnosis with Down syndrome, I wanted to know what I could do to make him better, and the first thing I discovered was that it was possible to actually affect his physical growth and development. We started early intervention when he was 5 weeks old. For a long time, his physical and overall development followed the usual curve for infants and small children. The tricks we learned to coax him from one developmental level to another actually worked. By the time he was almost 2 and his youngest sister was born, he had reached my goal of him walking independently. His older sister worked tirelessly with him every day after school, placing Cheerios on the piano bench and coaxing him to toddle toward them until he was walking independently and soon running everywhere.

WM attended a private school for children with special needs until he was 16 years old, and then attended a local high school until he was 21 years. The information I learned in those Early Intervention Classes about what he should be doing next also made me a good observer of when it was time to move him from one program to another, and we were really fortunate to find the very best teachers and programs at every stage of the game. All of his early education encouraged healthy habits, including physical activity, and they made it fun for the students.

Having a nearly same-age sibling made staying on track seem like the right thing to do for him and the whole family. When his sister learned to pump the swing or ride a tricycle or swim, so did he. I was recently stunned to learn that many of his peers had never learned to ride a 2-wheeler because he had been riding one since he was about 8 years old. We are not a particularly athletic family, but we just did what other families did with their kids: threw a softball, kicked soccer balls, and went swimming. When his school entered him in Special Olympics activities, we were there to cheer him on. Initially he competed in track and field and swimming and gymnastics. Later on, he did weight lifting, and competed on the state level in both weight lifting and swimming. I believe those 2 sports set the pattern for his adult life.

ADULT HABITS AND PATTERNS

WM is naturally slim as is his father. He doesn't watch his diet particularly, although as he has matured he has discovered that some foods agree with him more than others, and he is extremely disciplined about avoiding those foods. He eats a hefty breakfast on work mornings of sausage, cheese, and egg biscuits, which he prepares in the microwave. He eats a variety of foods for lunch at work, and a meat and vegetable dinner with family at night. Because he is so well muscled, he has no trouble keeping his weight down; in fact, his dietary changes have resulted in weight loss that we are watching carefully.

WM got a job as a grocery bagger when he was 23 years old and holds the same job today. He will soon celebrate his 20-year anniversary there. He works 7 hours a day, 4 days a week. He loves his job and has become very proficient at it through the years,

continued

TABLE 18-4. FROM A PARENT'S PERSPECTIVE (CONTINUED)

discovering how to pack neatly and to the customers' preferences … lightly for the "little old ladies" who can't carry heavy bags, and packing a lot in for other customers to minimize bag usage. This job also includes gathering carts from the parking lot, and that has presented the only challenge to his fitness. He has a tendency to try to push too many carts at once, and since he's still a pretty small guy (height barely 5 feet and weight 115 pounds), he has had a few back sprains through the years involving a rib that occasionally slips out of place.

CURRENT PHYSICAL AND MENTAL HEALTH

Those minor injuries are basically the only visits to the doctor outside his annual physical, and occasional bacterial skin infections. His eye and hearing screenings are normal. As I said when I was asked to write this letter about WM's health, there's very little of interest. He is showing some signs of aging at 43. He has a little gray in his beard, and he likes his down time after work. He enjoys an active social life with his girlfriend, made possible by the personal assistants provided by the state. He continues to receive weekly speech therapy to increase intelligibility and encourage appropriate responses and conversational skills. This serves as a form of mental health therapy as well since he opens up to his beloved therapist about many concerns that he doesn't discuss with others. He attends an enrichment class at the local university and is an enthusiastic member of the college community. He's active in several Bible and religious groups and has a strong faith. He is active on Facebook and adept at posting photos and using all the features of his smartphone. He is a happy man as evidenced by his posts and enthusiastic attitude with occasional, perfectly normal ups and downs common to young adults. He often expresses gratitude for having a life that is good (Figure 18-14).

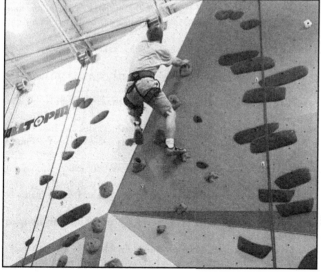

Figure 18-14. WM participating in the community.

implications for people with DD, is mandatory for health care professionals, including physical therapists and occupational therapists. Knowledge of issues related to aging will assist therapists in providing appropriate interventions not only for the population of aging nondisabled individuals, but also for those with LLDs.

References

1. United States Census Bureau. The Older Population: 2010. http://www.census.gov/prod/cen2010/briefs/c2010br-09.pdf. Accessed May 1, 2018.

2. Newacheck PW, Strickland B, Shonkoff JP, et al. An epidemiologic profile of children with special health care needs. *Pediatrics*. 1998;102(1 pt 1):117-123. doi:10.1542/peds.102.1.117.

3. United Cerebral Palsy Association. UCP Fact Sheet. http://ucp.org/wp-content/uploads/2013/02/cp-fact-sheet.pdf. Accessed May 1, 2018.

4. Murphy KP, Molnar GE, Lankasky K. Medical and functional status of adults with cerebral palsy. *Dev Med Child Neurol*. 1995;37(12):1075-1084. doi:10.1111/j.1469-8749.1995.tb11968.x.

5. Crichton JU, Mackinnon M, White CP. The life-expectancy of persons with cerebral palsy. *Dev Med Child Neurol*. 1995;37(7):567-576. doi:10.1111/j.1469-8749.1995.tb12045.x.

6. Evans PM, Evans SJ, Alberman E. Cerebral palsy: why we must plan for survival. *Arch Dis Child*. 1990;65(12):1239-1333. doi:10.1136/adc.65.12.1329.

7. Rapp CE Jr, Torres MM. The adult with cerebral palsy. *Arch Fam Med*. 2000;9(5):466-472. doi:10.1001/archfami.9.5.466.

8. Roberts M, Skotko BG. Down syndrome. In: Domino FJ, ed. *The 5-Minute Clinical Consult Standard 2017*. 25th ed. Philadelphia, PA: Wolters Kluwer Health; 2016:310-311.

9. Eyman RK, Grossman HJ, Chaney RH, Call TL. Survival of profoundly disabled people with severe mental retardation. *Am J Dis Child*. 1993;147(5):329-336. doi:10.1001/archpedi.1993.02160270091029.

10. Martin BA. Primary care of adults with mental retardation living in the community. *Am Fam Physician*.1997;56(2):485-494.

11. Larson SA, Lakin KC, Anderson L, Kwak LN, Lee JH, Anderson D. Prevalence of mental retardation and developmental disabilities: estimates from the 1994/1995 National Health Interview Survey Disability Supplements. *Am J Ment Retard*. 2001;106(3):231-252. doi:10.1352/0895-8017(2001)106<0231:POMRAD>2.0.CO;2.

12. Silverman W, Zigman WB, Kim H, McHale S, Wisniewski HM. Aging and dementia among adults with mental retardation and Down syndrome. *Top Geriatr Rehabil*. 1998;13(3):49-69. doi:10.1097/00013614-199803000-00007.

13. Martin JA, Hamilton BE, Osterman MJ, Curtin SC, Mathews TJ. Births: final data for 2012. *Natl Vital Stat Rep*. 2013;62(9):1-68.

14. Bergman JS. Protecting the mobility of the aging person with cerebral palsy or spina bifida. https://www.sbawp.org/the-stages-of-life/aging-with-spina-bifida. Accessed May 1, 2018.

15. American Physical Therapy Association. RC 34-05.

16. Developmental Disabilities Assistance and Bill of Rights Act of 2000, Public Law 106-402 U.S. Congress, Senate, 106th Congress, 2000.

17. Schalock RL, Borthwick-Duffy SA, Bradley VJ, et al. *Intellectual Disability: Definition, Classification, and Systems of Support*. 11th ed. Washington, DC: American Association on Intellectual and Developmental Disabilities; 2010.

18. Barnhart RC, Connolly B. Aging and Down syndrome: implications for physical therapy. *Phys Ther*. 2007;87(10):1399-1406. doi:10.2522/ptj.20060334.

19. Shamas-Ud-Din S. Genetics of Down's syndrome and Alzheimer's disease. *Br J Psychiatry*. 2002;181(2):167-168; author reply 168. doi:10.1192/bjp.181.2.167.

20. Burt DB, Loveland KA, Lewis KR. Depression and the onset of dementia in adults with mental retardation. *Am J Ment Retard*. 1992;96(5):502-511.

21. Rabe A, Wisniewski KE, Schupf N, et al. Relationship of Down's syndrome to Alzheimer's disease. In: Deutsch SI, Weizman A, Weizman R, eds. *Application of Basic Neuroscience to Child Psychiatry*. New York, NY: Plenum; 1990.

22. Barcikowska M, Silverman W, Zigman W, et al. Alzheimer-type neuropathology and clinical symptoms of dementia in mentally retarded people without Down syndrome. *Am J Ment Retard*. 1989;93(5):551-557.

23. Popovitch ER, Wisniewski HM, Barcikowska M, et al. Alzheimer neuropathology in non-Down's mentally retarded adults. *Acta Neuropathol*. 1990;80(4):362-367. doi:10.1007/BF00307688.

24. Janicki MP, MacEachron AE. Residential, health and social service needs of elderly developmentally disabled persons. *Gerontologist*. 1984;24(2):128-137. doi:10.1093/geront/24.2.128.

25. Janicki MP, Otis JP, Puccio PS, et al. Service needs among older developmentally disabled persons. In: Janicki MP, Wisniewski HM, eds. *Aging and Developmental Disabilities, Issues and Approaches*. Baltimore, MD: Paul H. Brookes; 1985.

26. Heller T. People with intellectual and developmental disabilities growing old: an overview. *Impact*. 2010;23(1):2-4.

27. Paneth N, Hong T, Korzeniewski S. The descriptive epidemiology of cerebral palsy. *Clin Perinatol*. 2006;33(2):251-267. doi:10.1016/j.clp.2006.03.011.

28. Yeargin-Allsopp M, Van Naarden Braun K, Doernberg NS, Benedict RE, Kirby RS, Durkin MS. Prevalence of cerebral palsy in 8-year-old children in three areas of the United States in 2002: a multisite collaboration. *Pediatrics*. 2008;121(3):547-554. doi:10.1542/peds.2007-1270.

29. Lauer E, McCallion P. Mortality of people with intellectual and developmental disabilities from select US state disability service systems and medical claims data. *J Appl Res Intellect Disabil.* 2015;28(5):394-405. doi:10.1111/jar.12191.

30. Bittles AH, Glasson EJ. Clinical, social, and ethical implications of changing life expectancy in Down syndrome. *Dev Med Child Neurol.* 2004;46(4):282-286. doi:10.1111/j.1469-8749.2004.tb00483.x.

31. Glasson EJ, Sullivan SG, Hussain R, Petterson BA, Montgomery PD, Bittles AH. The changing survival profile of people with Down's syndrome: implications for genetic counselling. *Clin Genet.* 2002;62(5):390-393. doi:10.1034/j.1399-0004.2002.620506.x.

32. Peterson H, Lenski M, Hidecker MJC, Min L, Paneth N. Cerebral palsy and aging. *Dev Med Child Neurol.* 2009;51(4):16-23. doi:10.1111/j.1469-8749.2009.03428.x.

33. Jacobson JW, Sutton MS, Janicki MP. Demography and characteristics of aging and aged mentally retarded persons. In: Janicki MP, Wisniewski HM, eds. *Aging and Developmental Disabilities: Issues and Approaches.* Baltimore, MD: Paul H. Brookes; 1985.

34. Hutton JL, Pharoah POD. Life expectancy in cerebral palsy. *Arch Dis Child.* 2006;91(3):254-258. doi:10.1136/adc.2005.075002.

35. Strauss D, Ojdana K, Shavelle R, Rosenbloom L. Decline in function and life expectancy of old persons with cerebral palsy. *NeuroRehabilitation.* 2004;19(1):69-78.

36. Shavelle R, Strauss D. Mortality of persons with developmental disabilities after transfer into community care: a 1996 update. *Am J Mental Retard.* 1999;104(2);143-147. doi:10.1352/0895-8017(1999)104<0143:MOPWDD>2.0.CO;2.

37. Orlin MN, Cicirello NA, O'Donnell AE, Doty AK. The continuum of care for individuals with lifelong disabilities: role of the physical therapist. *Phys Ther.* 2014;94(7):1043-1053. doi:10.2522/ptj.20130168.

38. Henderson CM, Rosasco M, Robinson LM, et al. Functional impairment severity is associated with health status among older persons with intellectual disability and cerebral palsy. *J Intellect Disabil Res.* 2009;53(11):887-897. doi:10.1111/j.1365-2788.2009.01199.x.

39. Rimmer JH, Yamaki K. Obesity and intellectual disability. *Ment Retard Dev Disabil Res Rev.* 2006;12(1):22-27. doi:10.1002/mrdd.20091.

40. National Institutes of Health, National Eye Institute. Age-related eye diseases. http://nei.nih.gov/healthyeyes/aging_eye. Accessed May 3, 2018.

41. Fozard JL, Wolf E, Bell B, et al. Visual perception and communication. In: Birren JE, Schaie KW, eds. *Handbook of the Psychology of Aging,* New York, NY: Van Nostrand Reinhold; 1977.

42. Cohen MM, Lessell S. The neuro-ophthalmology of aging. In: Albert ML, ed. *Clinical Neurology of Aging.* New York, NY: Oxford University Press; 1984.

43. Kallman H, Vernon MS. The aging eye. A family physician discusses some inevitable changes and suggests methods for dealing with them. *Postgrad Med.* 1987;81(2):108-109, 123.

44. Lowenfield IR. Pupillary changes related to age. In: Thompson HS, ed. *Topics in Neuro-Ophthalmology.* Baltimore, MD: Williams & Wilkins; 1979.

45. Hand JE. Report of a national survey of older people with lifelong intellectual handicap in New Zealand. *J Intellect Disabil Res.* 1994;38(pt 3):275-287. doi:10.1111/j.1365-2788.1994.tb00395.x.

46. Good WV, Jan JE, deSa L, Barkovich AJ, Groenveld M, Hoyt CS. Cortical visual impairment in children. *Surv Ophthalmol.* 1994;38(4):351-364. doi:10.1016/0039-6257(94)90073-6.

47. Kapell D, Nightingale B, Rodriguez A, Lee JH, Zigman WB, Schupf N. Prevalence of chronic medical conditions in adults with mental retardation: comparison with the general population. *Ment Retard.* 1998;36(4):269-279. doi:10.1352/0047-6765(1998)036<0269:POCMCI>2.0.CO;2.

48. Krinsky-McHale SJ, Silverman W, Gordon J, Devenny DA, Oley N, Abramov I. Vision deficits in adults with Down syndrome. *J Appl Res Intellect Disabil.* 2014;27(3):247-263. doi:10.1111/jar.12062.

49. Dillon CF, Gu Q, Hoffman HJ, Ko CW. Vision, hearing, balance, and sensory impairment in Americans aged 70 years and over: United States, 1999-2006. *NCHS Data Brief.* 2010;(31):1-8.

50. Vernon M, Griffin DH, Yoken C. Hearing loss. *J Fam Pract.* 1981;12(6):1153-1158.

51. Northern JL, Downs MP. *Hearing in Children.* 6th ed. San Diego, CA: Plural Publishing; 2014.

52. Smith DS. Health care management of adults with Down syndrome. *Am Fam Physician.* 2001;64(6):1031-1038.

53. Kreicher KL, Weir FW, Nguyen SA, Meyer TA. Characteristics and progression of hearing loss in children with Down syndrome. *J Pediatr.* 2018;193(2):27-33.e2. doi:10.1016/j.jpeds.2017.09.053.

54. Stevens JC, Cain WS. Smelling via the mouth: effect of aging. *Percept Psychophys.* 1986;40(3):142-146. doi:10.3758/BF03203009.

55. Turk MA, Scandale J, Rosenbaum PF, Weber RJ. The health of women with cerebral palsy. *Phys Med Rehabil Clin N Am.* 2001;12(1):153-168. doi:10.1016/S1047-9651(18)30088-3.

56. Hove O. Weight survey on adult persons with mental retardation living in the community. *Res Dev Disabil.* 2004;25(1):9-17. doi:10.1016/j.ridd.2003.04.004.

57. Emerson E. Underweight, obesity and exercise among adults with intellectual disabilities in supported accommodation in Northern England. *J Intellect Disabil Res.* 2005;49(pt 2):134-143. doi:10.1111/j.1365-2788.2004.00617.x.

58. Armitage GC. Development of a classification system for periodontal diseases and conditions. *Ann Periodontol.* 1999;4(1):1-6. doi:10.1902/annals.1999.4.1.1.

59. Ferreira R, Michel RC, Greghi SL, et al. Prevention and periodontal treatment in Down syndrome patients: a systematic review. *PLoS One.* 2016;11(6):e0158339. doi:10.1371/journal.pone.0158339.

60. Sabin TD, Venna N. Peripheral nerve disorders in the elderly. In: Albert ML, ed. *Clinical Neurology of Aging.* New York, NY: Oxford University Press; 1984.

61. LaFratta CW, Canestrari R. A comparison of sensory and motor nerve conduction velocities as related to age. *Arch Phys Med Rehabil.* 1966;47(5):286-290.

62. Bolton CF, Winkelmann RK, Dyck PJ. A quantitative study of Meissner's corpuscles in man. *Neurology.* 1966;16(1):1-9.

63. Schmidt RF, Wahren LK, Hagbarth KE. Multiunit neural responses to strong finger pulp vibration. I. Relationship to age. *Acta Physiol Scand.* 1990;140(1):1-10. doi:10.1111/j.1748-1716.1990.tb08969.x.

64. Corbin KB, Gardner ED. Decrease in number of myelinated fibers in human spinal roots with age. *Anat Rec.* 1937;68(1):63-74. doi:10.1002/ar.1090680105.

65. Mufson EJ, Stein DG. Degeneration in the spinal cord of old rats. *Exp Neurol.* 1980;70(1):179-186. doi:10.1016/0014-4886(80)90016-3.

66. Dyck PJ, Schultz PW, O'Brien PC. Quantitation of touch-pressure sensation. *Arch Neurol.* 1972;26(5):465-473. doi:10.1001/archneur.1972.00490110099010.

67. Kokmen E, Bossemeyer RW Jr, Barney J, Williams WJ. Neurological manifestations of aging. *J Geronotol.* 1977;32(4):411-419. doi:10.1093/geronj/32.4.411.

68. Laidlaw RW, Hamilton MA. A study of thresholds in perception of passive movement among normal control subjects. *Bull Neurol Inst.* 1937;6:268-340.

69. Skinner HB, Barrack RL, Cook SD. Age-related decline in proprioception. *Clin Orthop Rel Res.* 1984;184(4):208-211. doi:10.1097/00003086-198404000-00035.

70. Bailey AJ. Molecular mechanisms of ageing in connective tissues. *Mech Ageing Dev.* 2001;122(7):735-755. doi:10.1016/S0047-6374(01)00225-1.

71. Turk MA, Geremski CA, Rosenbaum PF. *Secondary Conditions of Adults With Cerebral Palsy: Final Report.* Syracuse, NY: State University of New York, Health Science Center at Syracuse, Department of Physical Medicine and Rehabilitation; 1997.

72. Lee RH, Lyles KW, Colón-Emeric C. A review of the effect of anticonvulsant medications on bone mineral density and fracture risk. *Am J Geriatr Pharmacother.* 2010;8(1):34-46. doi:10.1016/j.amjopharm.2010.02.003.

73. Center J, Beange H, McElduff A. People with mental retardation have an increased prevalence of osteoporosis: a population study. *Am J Ment Retard.* 1998;103(1):19-28. doi:10.1352/0895-8017(1998)103<0019:PWMRHA>2.0.CO;2.

74. Hess M, Campagna EJ, Jensen KM. Low bone mineral density risk factors and testing patterns in institutionalized adults with intellectual and developmental disabilities. *J Appl Res Intellect Disabil.* 2018;31(suppl 1):157-164. doi:10.1111/jar.12341.

75. Lin LP, Hsu SW, Yao CH, et al. Risk for osteopenia and osteoporosis in institution-dwelling individuals with intellectual and/or developmental disabilities. *Res Dev Disabil.* 2015;36C:108-113. doi:10.1016/j.ridd.2014.09.022.

76. Zhang Y, Jordan JM. Epidemiology of osteoarthritis. *Clin Geriatr Med.* 2010;26(3):355-369. doi:10.1016/j.cger.2010.03.001.

77. Cathels BA, Reddihough DS. The health care of young adults with cerebral palsy. *Med J Aust.* 1993;159(7):444-446. doi:10.5694/j.1326-5377.1993.tb137961.x.

78. Carter DR, Tse B. The pathogenesis of osteoarthritis in cerebral palsy. *Dev Med Child Neurol.* 2009;51(suppl 4):79-83. doi:10.1111/j.1469-8749.2009.03435.x.

79. Tosi LL, Maher N, Moore DW, Goldstein M, Aisen ML. Adults with cerebral palsy: a workshop to define the challenges of treating and preventing secondary musculoskeletal and neuromuscular complications in this rapidly growing population. *Dev Med Child Neurol.* 2009;51(suppl 4):2-11. doi:10.1111/j.1469-8749.2009.03462.x.

80. Opheim A, Jahnsen R, Olsson E, Stanghelle JK. Walking function, pain, and fatigue in adults with cerebral palsy: a 7-year follow-up study. *Dev Med Child Neurol.* 2009;51(5):381-388. doi:10.1111/j.1469-8749.2008.03250.x.

81. Keller K, Engelhardt M. Strength and muscle mass loss with aging process. Age and strength loss. *Muscles Ligaments Tendons J.* 2013;3(4):346-350. doi:10.11138/mltj/2013.3.4.346.

82. Damiano DL, Abel ME. Functional outcomes of strength training in spastic CP. *Arch Phys Med Rehabil.* 1998;79(2):119-125. doi:10.1016/S0003-9993(98)90287-8.

83. Horstmann HM, Hosalkar H, Keenan MA. Orthopaedic issues in the musculoskeletal care of adults with cerebral palsy. *Dev Med Child Neurol.* 2009;51(suppl 4):99-105. doi:10.1111/j.1469-8749.2009.03417.x.

84. Janicki MP, Jacobson JW. Generational trends in sensory, physical, and behavioral abilities among older mentally retarded persons. *Am J Ment Defic.* 1986;90(5):490-500.

85. Wiley ME, Damiano DL. Lower-extremity strength profiles in spastic cerebral palsy. *Dev Med Child Neurol.* 1998;40(2):100-107. doi:10.1111/j.1469-8749.1998.tb15369.x.

86. Dodd KJ, Taylor NF, Damiano DL. A systematic review of the effectiveness of strength-training programmes for people with CP. *Arch Phys Med Rehabil.* 2002;83(8):1157-1164. doi:10.1053/apmr.2002.34286.

87. Dodd KJ, Taylor NF, Graham HK. A randomized clinical trial of strength training in young people with cerebral palsy. *Dev Med Child Neurol.* 2003;45(10):652-657. doi:10.1111/j.1469-8749.2003.tb00866.x.

88. Andersson C, Grooten W, Hellsten M, Kaping K , Mattsson E. Adults with cerebral palsy: walking ability after progressive strength training. *Dev Med Child Neuro.* 2003;45(5):220-228.

89. Ross SM, MacDonald M, Bigouette JP. Effects of strength training on mobility in adults with cerebral palsy: a systematic review. *Disabil Health J.* 2016;9(3):375-384. doi:10.1016/j.dhjo.2016.04.005.

90. Naylor A, Happey F, MacRae T. Changes in the human intervertebral disc with age: a biophysical study. *J Am Geriatr Soc.* 1955;3(12):964-973. doi:10.1111/j.1532-5415.1955.tb01009.x.

91. White AA, Panjabi MM. *Clinical Biomechanics of the Spine.* Philadelphia, PA: JB Lippincott; 1978.

92. Borenstein DG, Burton JR. Lumbar spine disease in the elderly. *J Am Geriatr Soc.* 1993;41(2):167-175. doi:10.1111/j.1532-5415.1993.tb02053.x.

93. Tkaczuk H. Tensile properties of human lumbar longitudinal ligaments. *Acta Orthop Scand Suppl.* 1968;(suppl 115):1-69. doi:10.3109/ort.1968.39.suppl-115.01.

94. Nachemson AL, Evans JH. Biomechanical study of human lumbar ligamentum flavum. *J Anat.* 1969;105(pt 1):188-189.

95. Lewis CB. Musculoskeletal changes with age: clinical implications. In Lewis CB, ed. *Aging: The Health Care Challenge.* 3rd ed. Philadelphia, PA: FA Davis Co; 1996.

96. Matute-Llorente Á, González-Agüero A, Gómez-Cabello A, Vicente-Rodríguez G, Casajús JA. Decreased levels of physical activity in adolescents with Down syndrome are related with low bone mineral density: a cross-sectional study. *BMC Endocr Disord.* 2013;13(1):22. doi:10.1186/1472-6823-13-22.

97. Srikanth R, Cassidy G, Joiner C, Teeluckdharry S. Osteoporosis in people with intellectual disabilities: a review and brief study of risk factors for osteoporosis in a community sample of people with intellectual disabilities. *J Intellect Disabil Res.* 2011;55(1):53-62. doi:10.1111/j.1365-2788.2010.01346.x.

98. Murphy KP. Cerebral palsy lifetime care—four musculoskeletal conditions. *Dev Med Child Neuro.* 2009;51(suppl 4):30-37. doi:10.1111/j.1469-8749.2009.03431.x.

99. Aksu F. Nature and prognosis of seizures in patients with cerebral palsy. *Dev Med Child Neuro.* 1990;32(8):661-668. doi:10.1111/j.1469-8749.1990.tb08426.x.

100. Brunner R, Döderlein L. Pathological fractures in patients with cerebral palsy. *J Pediatri Orthop B.* 1996;5(4):232-238. doi:10.1097/01202412-199605040-00003.

101. Ko SU, Hausdorff JM, Ferrucci L. Age-associated differences in the gait pattern changes of older adults during fast-speed and fatigue conditions: results from the Baltimore longitudinal study of ageing. *Age Ageing.* 2010;39(6):688-694. doi:10.1093/ageing/afq113.

102. Woollacott MH. Changes in posture and voluntary control in the elderly: Research findings and rehabilitation. *Top Geriatr Rehabil.* 1990;5(1):1-11.

103. Woollacott MH, Shumway-Cook A, Nashner LM. Aging and posture control: changes in sensory organs and muscular coordination. *Int J Aging Hum Dev.* 1986;23(2):97-114. doi:10.2190/VXN3-N3RT-54JB-X16X.

104. Hresko MT, McCarthy JC, Goldberg MJ. Hip disease in adults with Down syndrome. *J Bone Joint Surg Br.* 1993;75(4):604-607. doi:10.1302/0301-620X.75B4.8331117.

105. Roizen NJ, Patterson D. Down's syndrome. *Lancet.* 2003;361(9365):1281-1289. doi:10.1016/S0140-6736(03)12987-X.

106. Andersson C, Mattsson E. Adults with cerebral palsy: a survey describing problems, needs, and resources, with special emphasis on locomotion. *Dev Med Child Neurol.* 2001;43(1):76-82. doi:10.1017/S0012162201.

107. Sandström K, Alinder J, Oberg B. Descriptions of functioning and health and relations to a gross motor classification in adults with cerebral palsy. *Disabil Rehabil.* 2004;26(17):1023-1031. doi:10.1080/09638280410001703503.

108. Jahnsen R, Villien L, Egeland T, Stanghelle JK, Holm I. Locomotion skills in adults with cerebral palsy. *Clin Rehabil.* 2004;18(3):309-316. doi:10.1191/0269215504cr735oa.

109. Bottos M, Feliciangeli A, Sciuto L, Gericke C, Vianello A. Functional status of adults with cerebral palsy and implications for treatment of children. *Dev Med Child Neurol.* 2001;43(8):516-528. doi:10.1111/j.1469-8749.2001.tb00755.x.

110. Maltais DB, Wiart L, Fowler E, Verschuren O, Damiano DL. Health-related physical fitness for children with cerebral palsy. *J Child Neurol.* 2014;29(8):1091-1100. doi:10.1177/0883073814533152.

111. Sharma G, Goodwin JS. Effect of aging on respiratory system physiology and immunology. *Clin Interv Aging.* 2006;1(3):253-260. doi:10.2147/ciia.2006.1.3.253.

112. Pump KK. Fenestrae in the alveolar membrane of the human lung. *Chest.* 1974;65(4):431-436. doi:10.1378/chest.65.4.431.

113. Lakatta EG. Cardiovascular regulatory mechanisms in advanced age. *Physiol Rev.* 1993;73(2):413-467. doi:10.1152/physrev.1993.73.2.413.

114. Strait JC, Lakatta EG. Aging-associated cardiovascular changes and their relationship to heart failure. *Heart Fail Clin.* 2012;8(1):143-164. doi:10.1016/j.hfc.2011.08.011.

115. Centers for Disease Control and Prevention. National Center for Health Statistics. National Health Interview Survey, 2016. https://www.cdc.gov/nchs/nhis/SHS/tables.htm. Accessed May 15, 2018.

116. Strauss D, Cable W, Shavelle R. Causes of excess mortality in cerebral palsy. *Dev Med Child Neurol.* 1999;41(9):580-585. doi:10.1111/j.1469-8749.1999.tb00660.x.

117. Traci MA, Seekins T, Szalda-Petree A, Ravesloot C. Assessing secondary conditions among adults with developmental disabilities: a preliminary study. *Ment Retard.* 2002;40(2):119-131. doi:10.1352/0047-6765(2002)040<0119:ASC AAW>2.0.CO;2.

118. US Department of Health and Human Services. Office of Disease Prevention and Health Promotion. Healthy people 2020. http://www.healthypeople.gov/.

119. Beasley CR. Effects of a jogging program on cardiovascular fitness and performance in mentally retarded adults. *Am J Ment Defic.* 1982;86(6):609-613.

120. Dodd KJ, Shields N. A systematic review of the outcomes of cardiovascular exercise programs for people with Down syndrome. *Arch Phys Med Rehabil.* 2005;86(10):2051-2058. doi:10.1016/j.apmr.2005.06.003.

121. Shields N, Taylor NF, Dodd KJ. Effects of a community-based progressive resistance training program on muscle performance and physical function in adults with Down syndrome: a randomized controlled trial. *Arch Phys Med Rehabil.* 2008;89(7):1215-1220. doi:10.1016/j.apmr.2007.11.056.

122. Andriolo RB, EI Dib RP, Ramos L, Atallah AN, da Silva EM. Aerobic exercise training programmes for improving physical and psychosocial health in adults with Down syndrome. *Cochrane Database Syst Rev.* 2010;(5):CD005176. doi:10.1002/14651858.CD005176.pub4.

123. Mendonca GV, Pereira FD, Fernhall B. Effects of combined aerobic and resistance exercise training in adults with and without Down syndrome. *Arch Phys Med Rehabil.* 2011;92(1):37-45. doi:10.1016/j.apmr.2010.09.015.

124. Li C, Chen S, Meng How Y, Zhang AL. Benefits of physical exercise intervention on fitness of individuals with Down syndrome: a systematic review of randomized-controlled trials. *Int J Rehabil Res.* 2013;36(3):187-195. doi:10.1097/MRR.0b013e3283634e9c.

125. Silva A, Campos C, Sá A, et al. Wii-based exercise program to improve physical fitness, motor proficiency and functional mobility in adults with Down syndrome. *Int J Rehabil Res.* 2017;61(8):755-765. doi:10.1111/jir.12384.

126. Rimmer JH. Physical fitness levels of persons with cerebral palsy. *Dev Med Child Neurol.* 2001;43(3):208-212. doi:10.1017/S0012162201000391.

127. Andersson C, Grooten W, Hellsten M, Kaping K, Mattsson E. Adults with cerebral palsy: walking after progressive strength training. *Dev Med Child Neurol.* 2003;45(3):220-228. doi:10.1111/j.1469-8749.2003.tb00335.x.

128. Haak P, Lenski M, Hidecker MJ, Min L, Paneth N. Cerebral palsy and aging. *Dev Med Child Neurol.* 2009;51(suppl 4):16-23. doi:10.1111/j.1469-8749.2009.03428.x.

129. Holmes L Jr, Joshi A, Lorenz Z, Miller F, Dabney K. Pediatric cerebral palsy life expectancy: has survival improved over time? *Pediat Therapeut.* 2013;3(1):146. doi:10.4172/2161-0665.1000146.

130. Centers for Disease Control and Prevention. National Center for Health Statistics. 2003-2008 National Health and Nutrition Examination Survey Data. Hyattsville, MD; U.S.

131. Centers for Disease Control and Prevention. 2008 Behavioral Risk Factor Surveillance system. https://www.cdc.gov/brfss/annual_data/annual_2016.html. Accessed May 16, 2018.

132. Yamaki K. Body weight status among adults with intellectual disability in the community. *Ment Retard.* 2005;43(1):1-10. doi:10.1352/0047-6765(2005)43<1:BWSAAW>2.0.CO;2.

133. Rubin SS, Rimmer JH, Chicoine BA, Braddock DL, McGuire DE. Overweight prevalence in persons with Down syndrome. *Mental Retard.* 1998;36(3):175-181. doi:10.1352/0047-6765(1998)036<0175:OPIPWD>2.0.CO;2.

134. Rimmer JH, Yamaki K. Obesity and intellectual disability. *Ment Retard Dev Disabil Res Rev.* 2006;12(1):22-27. doi:10.1002/mrdd.20091.

135. Rimmer JH, Wang E. Obesity prevalence among a group of Chicago residents with disabilities. *Arch Phys Med Rehabil.* 2005;86(7):1461-1464. doi:10.1016/j.apmr.2004.10.038.

136. Wisniewski KE, Wisniewski HM, Wen GY. Occurrence of neuropathological changes and dementia of Alzheimer's disease in Down's syndrome. *Ann Neurol.* 1985;17(3):278-282. doi:10.1002/ana.410170310.

137. Dalton AJ, Crapper DR. Down's syndrome and aging of the brain. In: Mittler P, ed. *Research to Practice in Mental Retardation: Biomedical Aspects.* Vol. III. Baltimore, MD: University Park Press; 1977.

138. Fenner ME, Hewitt KE, Torpy DM. Down's syndrome: intellectual and behavioural functioning during adulthood. *J Ment Defic Res.* 1987;31(3):241-249. doi:10.1111/j.1365-2788.1987.tb01367.x.

139. Alzheimer's Association. Down syndrome and Alzheimer's disease. https://www.alz.org/dementia/down-syndrome-alzeimers-symptoms.asp. Accessed May 16, 2018.

Financial Disclosures

Dr. Rona Alexander receives royalties from Clinician's View and the Hammill Institute on Disabilities.

Dr. Joanell A. Bohmert has no financial or proprietary interest in the materials presented herein.

Dr. David D. Chapman has no financial or proprietary interest in the materials presented herein.

Dr. Barbara H. Connolly has no financial or proprietary interest in the materials presented herein.

Dr. Susan K. Effgen has no financial or proprietary interest in the materials presented herein.

Dr. Elizabeth Ennis has no financial or proprietary interest in the materials presented herein.

Dr. Roberta Gatlin has instructional CEU courses on the topic of therapeutic interventions in the NICU with Educational Resources Inc and an online course with MedBridge.

Dr. Dora J. Gosselin has no financial or proprietary interest in the materials presented herein.

Dr. Maria Jones has no financial or proprietary interest in the materials presented herein.

Dr. Lisa K. Kenyon has no financial or proprietary interest in the materials presented herein.

Dr. Helen L. Masin has no financial or proprietary interest in the materials presented herein.

Dr. Anita Witt Mitchell has no financial or proprietary interest in the materials presented herein.

Dr. Patricia C. Montgomery has several online courses on the topic of therapeutic interventions with MedBridge.

Dr. Anne H. Zachry has no financial or proprietary interest in the materials presented herein.

Index

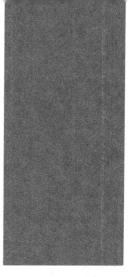

Printed in the United States
by Baker & Taylor Publisher Services